AUTISM

The Movement Sensing Perspective

FRONTIERS IN NEUROSCIENCE

Series Editor
Sidney A. Simon, PhD

Published Titles

Apoptosis in Neurobiology
Yusuf A. Hannun, MD, Professor of Biomedical Research and Chairman, Department of Biochemistry and Molecular Biology, Medical University of South Carolina, Charleston, South Carolina
Rose-Mary Boustany, MD, tenured Associate Professor of Pediatrics and Neurobiology, Duke University Medical Center, Durham, North Carolina

Neural Prostheses for Restoration of Sensory and Motor Function
John K. Chapin, PhD, Professor of Physiology and Pharmacology, State University of New York Health Science Center, Brooklyn, New York
Karen A. Moxon, PhD, Assistant Professor, School of Biomedical Engineering, Science, and Health Systems, Drexel University, Philadelphia, Pennsylvania

Computational Neuroscience: Realistic Modeling for Experimentalists
Eric DeSchutter, MD, PhD, Professor, Department of Medicine, University of Antwerp, Antwerp, Belgium

Methods in Pain Research
Lawrence Kruger, PhD, Professor of Neurobiology (Emeritus), UCLA School of Medicine and Brain Research Institute, Los Angeles, California

Motor Neurobiology of the Spinal Cord
Timothy C. Cope, PhD, Professor of Physiology, Wright State University, Dayton, Ohio

Nicotinic Receptors in the Nervous System
Edward D. Levin, PhD, Associate Professor, Department of Psychiatry and Pharmacology and Molecular Cancer Biology and Department of Psychiatry and Behavioral Sciences, Duke University School of Medicine, Durham, North Carolina

Methods in Genomic Neuroscience
Helmin R. Chin, PhD, Genetics Research Branch, NIMH, NIH, Bethesda, Maryland
Steven O. Moldin, PhD, University of Southern California, Washington, D.C.

Methods in Chemosensory Research
Sidney A. Simon, PhD, Professor of Neurobiology, Biomedical Engineering, and Anesthesiology, Duke University, Durham, North Carolina
Miguel A.L. Nicolelis, MD, PhD, Professor of Neurobiology and Biomedical Engineering, Duke University, Durham, North Carolina

The Somatosensory System: Deciphering the Brain's Own Body Image
Randall J. Nelson, PhD, Professor of Anatomy and Neurobiology, University of Tennessee Health Sciences Center, Memphis, Tennessee

The Superior Colliculus: New Approaches for Studying Sensorimotor Integration
William C. Hall, PhD, Department of Neuroscience, Duke University, Durham, North Carolina
Adonis Moschovakis, PhD, Department of Basic Sciences, University of Crete, Heraklion, Greece

New Concepts in Cerebral Ischemia
Rick C.S. Lin, PhD, Professor of Anatomy, University of Mississippi Medical Center, Jackson, Mississippi

DNA Arrays: Technologies and Experimental Strategies
Elena Grigorenko, PhD, Technology Development Group, Millennium Pharmaceuticals, Cambridge, Massachusetts

Methods for Alcohol-Related Neuroscience Research
Yuan Liu, PhD, National Institute of Neurological Disorders and Stroke, National Institutes of Health, Bethesda, Maryland
David M. Lovinger, PhD, Laboratory of Integrative Neuroscience, NIAAA, Nashville, Tennessee

Primate Audition: Behavior and Neurobiology
Asif A. Ghazanfar, PhD, Princeton University, Princeton, New Jersey

Methods in Drug Abuse Research: Cellular and Circuit Level Analyses
Barry D. Waterhouse, PhD, MCP-Hahnemann University, Philadelphia, Pennsylvania

Functional and Neural Mechanisms of Interval Timing
Warren H. Meck, PhD, Professor of Psychology, Duke University, Durham, North Carolina

Biomedical Imaging in Experimental Neuroscience
Nick Van Bruggen, PhD, Department of Neuroscience Genentech, Inc.
Timothy P.L. Roberts, PhD, Associate Professor, University of Toronto, Canada

The Primate Visual System
John H. Kaas, Department of Psychology, Vanderbilt University, Nashville, Tennessee
Christine Collins, Department of Psychology, Vanderbilt University, Nashville, Tennessee

Neurosteroid Effects in the Central Nervous System
Sheryl S. Smith, PhD, Department of Physiology, SUNY Health Science Center, Brooklyn, New York

Modern Neurosurgery: Clinical Translation of Neuroscience Advances
Dennis A. Turner, Department of Surgery, Division of Neurosurgery, Duke University Medical Center, Durham, North Carolina

Sleep: Circuits and Functions
Pierre-Hervé Luppi, Université Claude Bernard, Lyon, France

Methods in Insect Sensory Neuroscience
Thomas A. Christensen, Arizona Research Laboratories, Division of Neurobiology, University of Arizona, Tuscon, Arizona

Motor Cortex in Voluntary Movements
Alexa Riehle, INCM-CNRS, Marseille, France
Eilon Vaadia, The Hebrew University, Jerusalem, Israel

Neural Plasticity in Adult Somatic Sensory-Motor Systems
Ford F. Ebner, Vanderbilt University, Nashville, Tennessee

Advances in Vagal Afferent Neurobiology
Bradley J. Undem, Johns Hopkins Asthma Center, Baltimore, Maryland
Daniel Weinreich, University of Maryland, Baltimore, Maryland

The Dynamic Synapse: Molecular Methods in Ionotropic Receptor Biology
Josef T. Kittler, University College, London, England
Stephen J. Moss, University College, London, England

Animal Models of Cognitive Impairment
Edward D. Levin, Duke University Medical Center, Durham, North Carolina
Jerry J. Buccafusco, Medical College of Georgia, Augusta, Georgia

The Role of the Nucleus of the Solitary Tract in Gustatory Processing
Robert M. Bradley, University of Michigan, Ann Arbor, Michigan

Brain Aging: Models, Methods, and Mechanisms
David R. Riddle, Wake Forest University, Winston-Salem, North Carolina

Neural Plasticity and Memory: From Genes to Brain Imaging
Frederico Bermudez-Rattoni, National University of Mexico, Mexico City, Mexico

Serotonin Receptors in Neurobiology
Amitabha Chattopadhyay, Center for Cellular and Molecular Biology, Hyderabad, India

TRP Ion Channel Function in Sensory Transduction and Cellular Signaling Cascades
Wolfgang B. Liedtke, MD, PhD, Duke University Medical Center, Durham, North Carolina
Stefan Heller, PhD, Stanford University School of Medicine, Stanford, California

Methods for Neural Ensemble Recordings, Second Edition
Miguel A.L. Nicolelis, MD, PhD, Professor of Neurobiology and Biomedical Engineering, Duke University Medical Center, Durham, North Carolina

Biology of the NMDA Receptor
Antonius M. VanDongen, Duke University Medical Center, Durham, North Carolina

Methods of Behavioral Analysis in Neuroscience
Jerry J. Buccafusco, PhD, Alzheimer's Research Center, Professor of Pharmacology and Toxicology, Professor of Psychiatry and Health Behavior, Medical College of Georgia, Augusta, Georgia

In Vivo Optical Imaging of Brain Function, Second Edition
Ron Frostig, PhD, Professor, Department of Neurobiology, University of California, Irvine, California

Fat Detection: Taste, Texture, and Post Ingestive Effects
Jean-Pierre Montmayeur, PhD, Centre National de la Recherche Scientifique, Dijon, France
Johannes le Coutre, PhD, Nestlé Research Center, Lausanne, Switzerland

The Neurobiology of Olfaction
Anna Menini, PhD, Neurobiology Sector International School for Advanced Studies, (S.I.S.S.A.), Trieste, Italy

Neuroproteomics
Oscar Alzate, PhD, Department of Cell and Developmental Biology, University of North Carolina, Chapel Hill, North Carolina

Translational Pain Research: From Mouse to Man
Lawrence Kruger, PhD, Department of Neurobiology, UCLA School of Medicine, Los Angeles, California
Alan R. Light, PhD, Department of Anesthesiology, University of Utah, Salt Lake City, Utah

Advances in the Neuroscience of Addiction
Cynthia M. Kuhn, Duke University Medical Center, Durham, North Carolina
George F. Koob, The Scripps Research Institute, La Jolla, California

Neurobiology of Huntington's Disease: Applications to Drug Discovery
Donald C. Lo, Duke University Medical Center, Durham, North Carolina
Robert E. Hughes, Buck Institute for Age Research, Novato, California

Neurobiology of Sensation and Reward
Jay A. Gottfried, Northwestern University, Chicago, Illinois

The Neural Bases of Multisensory Processes
Micah M. Murray, CIBM, Lausanne, Switzerland
Mark T. Wallace, Vanderbilt Brain Institute, Nashville, Tennessee

Neurobiology of Depression
Francisco López-Muñoz, University of Alcalá, Madrid, Spain
Cecilio Álamo, University of Alcalá, Madrid, Spain

Astrocytes: Wiring the Brain
Eliana Scemes, Albert Einstein College of Medicine, Bronx, New York
David C. Spray, Albert Einstein College of Medicine, Bronx, New York

Dopamine–Glutamate Interactions in the Basal Ganglia
Susan Jones, University of Cambridge, United Kingdom

Alzheimer's Disease: Targets for New Clinical Diagnostic and Therapeutic Strategies
Renee D. Wegrzyn, Booz Allen Hamilton, Arlington, Virginia
Alan S. Rudolph, Duke Center for Neuroengineering, Potomac, Maryland

The Neurobiological Basis of Suicide
Yogesh Dwivedi, University of Illinois at Chicago

Transcranial Brain Stimulation
Carlo Miniussi, University of Brescia, Italy
Walter Paulus, Georg-August University Medical Center, Göttingen, Germany
Paolo M. Rossini, Institute of Neurology, Catholic University of Rome, Italy

Spike Timing: Mechanisms and Function
Patricia M. Di Lorenzo, Binghamton University, Binghamton, New York
Jonathan D. Victor, Weill Cornell Medical College, New York City, New York

Neurobiology of Body Fluid Homeostasis: Transduction and Integration
Laurival Antonio De Luca Jr., São Paulo State University–UNESP, Araraquara, Brazil
Jose Vanderlei Menani, São Paulo State University–UNESP, Araraquara, Brazil
Alan Kim Johnson, The University of Iowa, Iowa City, Iowa

Neurobiology of Chemical Communication
Carla Mucignat-Caretta, University of Padova, Padova, Italy

Itch: Mechanisms and Treatment
E. Carstens, University of California, Davis, California
Tasuku Akiyama, University of California, Davis, California

Translational Research in Traumatic Brain Injury
Daniel Laskowitz, Duke University, Durham, North Carolina
Gerald Grant, Duke University, Durham, North Carolina

Statistical Techniques for Neuroscientists
Young K. Truong, University of North Carolina, Chapel Hill, North Carolina
Mechelle M. Lewis, Pennsylvania State University, Hershey, Pennsylvania

Neurobiology of TRP Channels
Tamara Luti Rosenbaum Emir, Instituto de Fisiología Celular, Universidad Nacional Autónoma de México (UNAM)

Autism: The Movement Sensing Perspective
Elizabeth B. Torres, Psychology Department, Rutgers, The State University of New Jersey
Caroline Whyatt, Psychology Department, Rutgers, The State University of New Jersey

AUTISM

The Movement Sensing Perspective

Edited by

Elizabeth B. Torres

Caroline Whyatt

CRC Press
Taylor & Francis Group
Boca Raton London New York

CRC Press is an imprint of the
Taylor & Francis Group, an **informa** business

CRC Press
Taylor & Francis Group
6000 Broken Sound Parkway NW, Suite 300
Boca Raton, FL 33487-2742

First issued in paperback 2020

ISBN-13: 978-1-4822-5163-0 (hbk)
ISBN-13: 978-0-367-65766-6 (pbk)

Library of Congress Cataloging-in-Publication Data

Names: Torres, Elizabeth B., editor. | Whyatt, Caroline, editor.
Title: Autism : the movement sensing perspective / [edited by] Elizabeth B. Torres and Caroline Whyatt.
Description: Boca Raton : Taylor & Francis, 2018. | Includes bibliographical references.
Identifiers: LCCN 2017015110 | ISBN 9781482251630 (hardback : alk. paper)
Subjects: | MESH: Autistic Disorder | Autism Spectrum Disorder | Psychomotor Performance
Classification: LCC RC553.A88 | NLM WS 350.8.P4 | DDC 616.85/882--dc23
LC record available at https://lccn.loc.gov/2017015110

Visit the Taylor & Francis Web site at
http://www.taylorandfrancis.com

and the CRC Press Web site at
http://www.crcpress.com

Contents

Preface xiii
Foreword xv
Contributors xvii

SECTION I The Big Question: Why Study Movement?

Chapter 1 Why Study Movement Variability in Autism? 3
Maria Brincker and Elizabeth B. Torres

Chapter 2 The Autism Phenotype: Physiology versus Psychology? 23
Caroline Whyatt

Chapter 3 Can Cognitive Theories Help to Understand Motor Dysfunction in Autism Spectrum Disorder? 43
Nicci Grace, Beth P. Johnson, Peter G. Enticott, and Nicole J. Rinehart

Concluding Remarks to Section I: Top-Down versus Bottom-Up Approaches to Connect Cognition and Somatic Motor Sensations 57

SECTION II Basic Research: Movement as a Social Model

Chapter 4 Dissecting a Social Encounter from Three Different Perspectives 63
Elizabeth B. Torres

Chapter 5 More Than Meets the Eye: Redefining the Role of Sensory-Motor Control on Social Skills in Autism Spectrum Disorders 73
Caroline Whyatt

Chapter 6 Action Evaluation and Discrimination as Indexes of Imitation Fidelity in Autism 89
Justin H. G. Williams

Chapter 7 ADOS: The Physiology Approach to Assess Social Skills and Communication in Autism Spectrum Disorder 103
Caroline Whyatt and Elizabeth B. Torres

Chapter 8 On the Brainstem Origin of Autism: Disruption to Movements of the Primary Self 119
Jonathan Delafield-Butt and Colwyn Trevarthen

Chapter 9 The Gap between Intention and Action: Altered Connectivity and GABA-mediated Synchrony in Autism 139

John P. Hussman

SECTION III Let's Get the Math Right to Improve Diagnosis, Research, and Treatment Outcomes

Preface to Section III: First Things First–Let Us Get the Math Right 153

Chapter 10 Non-Gaussian Statistical Distributions Arising in Large-Scale Personalized Data Sets from Biophysical Rhythms of the Nervous Systems 155

Jorge V. José

Chapter 11 Excess Success for a Study on Visual Search and Autism: Motivation to Change How Scientists Analyze Data 165

Gregory Francis

Chapter 12 Contemporary Problems with Methods in Basic Brain Science Impede Progress in ASD Research and Treatments 177

Elizabeth B. Torres

Chapter 13 Inherent Noise Hidden in Nervous Systems' Rhythms Leads to New Strategies for Detection and Treatments for Core Motor Sensing Traits in ASD 197

Elizabeth B. Torres

Chapter 14 Micromovements: The s-Spikes as a Way to "Zoom In" the Motor Trajectories of Natural Goal-Directed Behaviors 217

Di Wu, Elizabeth B. Torres, and Jorge V. José

SECTION IV The Therapeutic Model: Movement as a Percept to Awaken the Mind

Preface to Section IV 227

Chapter 15 Rhythm and Movement for Autism Spectrum Disorder: A Neurodevelopmental Perspective 229

Blythe LaGasse, Michelle Welde Hardy, Jenna Anderson, and Paige Rabon

Chapter 16 Use of Video Technology to Support Persons Affected with Sensory-Movement Differences and Diversity 243

Sharon Hammer, Lisa Ladson, Max McKeough, Kate McGinnity, and Sam Rogers

Chapter 17 Argentinian Ambulatory Integral Model to Treat Autism Spectrum Disorders........253

Silvia Baetti

Chapter 18 Autism Sports and Educational Model for Inclusion (ASEMI)........271

Marcelo Biasatti and Maximiliano Lombardo

Chapter 19 Reframing Autism Spectrum Disorder for Teachers: An Interdisciplinary Task........281

Corinne G. Catalano

Concluding Remarks to Section IV........289

SECTION V Autism, the Untold Story from the Perspectives of Parents and Self-advocates

Preface Section V........293

Chapter 20 Seeing Movement: Implications of the Movement Sensing Perspective for Parents........295

Pat Amos

Chapter 21 Shiloh: The Outstanding Outlier........327

Summer Pierce

Chapter 22 Ada Mae: Our Magical Fairy........333

Jonathan Grashow and Kathryn Grashow

Chapter 23 It's a Girl's Life........339

Jadyn Waiser, Michelle Stern Waiser, and Anita Breslin

Chapter 24 Treat the Whole, Not the Parts........347

Chapter 25 Anthony's Story: Finding Normal........353

Cynthia Baeza

Chapter 26 Autism: A Bullying Perspective........357

Sejal Mistry and Caroline Whyatt

Chapter 27 Turning the Tables: Autism Shows the Social Deficit of Our Society 367
Elizabeth B. Torres

Conclusions 379

Index 381

Preface

Neuroscience—a diverse field of study—provides a unique insight into the most complex system of all: the human. Reflecting technological advances, modern neuroscience draws on the foundations of engineering, mathematics, and statistics to provide a rich and nuanced field of inquiry aimed at transforming some of the current psychological and psychiatric approaches to study the mind. The work outlined in this book is arguably at one of the forefronts of this new era of psychology and neuroscience. Combining principles from clinical psychology or psychiatry with the study of motor control and perception, this work aims to open new dialogue and push at the boundaries of our understanding of autism.

Initially conceived in the 1950s as a mental illness in the *Diagnostic and Statistical Manual of Mental Disorders* of the American Psychiatric Association, by the 1980s autism had evolved into a phenotype with a more specific psychological profile. Clinical psychology provided an early definition focusing on the role of deficits in social interactions and communication; primary axes of symptomatology that have since been discussed within the broader context of repetition and ritualistic behaviors. In so doing, the field of clinical psychology initiated the path to systematically diagnose this developmental disorder and deliver treatment. The new movement helped create an infrastructure for education and training that, without a doubt, advanced the clinical practices and influenced policy making for special education and inclusion.

Notwithstanding the many advances in the clinical and educational arenas, basic research on autism has made more modest progress over the years, partly due to a paucity of studies involving objective assessments of the physiological underpinnings of nervous systems' development. A new era of autism basic research has been marked by an integrative neuroscientific approach that combines elements of foundational levels of electrophysiology with higher-level concepts from the psychological sciences. One of the threads weaving the fabric of this new symbiotic collaborative effort has been computational neuroscience. Indeed, new methods and technological advances in areas of movement neuroscience have begun to promote the notion that autism and its coping neurodevelopment can be longitudinally quantified.

This book is the culmination of a journey that started with ample resistance from the research community to the very notion that movements and their sensation could provide a new quantitative lens to gain insight into many of the problems that self-advocates and parents had described so vividly since autism was defined in the 1950s. It also marks the beginning of a new interdisciplinary era of collaborative work across disciplines as diverse as philosophy, theoretical physics, applied mathematics, psychology, and the neurosciences at large.

The book is divided into five sections that aims to provide an overview of an integrative approach driven by psychology and neuroscience. Section I provides some motivational thoughts on how to connect movement and its sensations with the emergence of cognition, using a combination of high-level psychological and foundational physiological techniques. Section II delves into the social definition of autism, integrating information across many layers of inquiry, from genes to behavior, and using a complex systems approach aimed at discovering scale-invariant emergent properties of the developing nervous systems. Section III focuses on mathematical principles and statistical techniques that can help redefine many concepts in basic behavioral physiology and psychological approaches to the study of behavior, highlighting caveats in our current assumptions for data analyses, inference, and interpretation. Section IV includes some examples of less conventional therapeutic interventions tailored to enhance social exchange, while Section V brings in the perspective of parents and their journey through the diagnoses and therapies for autism.

The book closes with a positive note, thanking the fields of clinical psychology and psychiatry for their pioneering efforts that have enabled today's critical inflection point in a new computational neuroscience–driven research era. Indeed, it is these foundational concepts that have facilitated the launch of today's accelerated rate of change of discovery that will lead to new personalized target treatments and new methods to longitudinally track their effectiveness and their risks.

We dedicate this collective effort to those touched by this condition and embrace them as an integral part of our broad human spectrum.

Elizabeth B. Torres
Caroline Whyatt
Rutgers University
New Brunswick, New Jersey

Foreword

As a scientist and clinician who has spent decades trying to better understand and help people with autism, I read Elizabeth Torres and Caroline Whyatt's book, *Autism: The Movement Sensing Perspective*, with great interest. In fact, over the past several years, I've made a special point of following the work of Elizabeth Torres and her collaborators. It was clear from their earliest papers that they were describing a unique perspective on autism that has the potential to fundamentally change the way we understand, assess, and treat this complex disorder.

In this book, Torres and Whyatt and their co-authors make a strong case that movement offers an essential dynamic window into neurodevelopment and autism. It has long been recognized that impairments in motor abilities and sensory processing are part of the autism syndrome. In his original descriptions of eleven children with autism, Kanner's observations included "a failure to assume an anticipatory posture," "limitation in the variety of spontaneous activity," and clumsiness in "gait and gross motor performance." More recently, researchers have discovered that delays and differences in motor development are among the earliest symptoms of autism evident in infancy. However, such characteristics have been relegated to the category of associated features. The model described in this book turns this conceptualization upside down, positing that differences in motor and sensory abilities are primary and social interaction deficits are the secondary consequences of underlying differences in moving and sensing. This leads to different ways of thinking about how best to treat autism, as well as novel ways of measuring response to treatment.

A key concept introduced is that individual variability in movement is a form of kinesthetic sensory feedback flowing, in closed loop, from the peripheral to the central nervous system. As such, movement sensation helps the person to prospectively guide social interaction dynamics. From the vantage point of the researcher and the clinician, the objective quantification of motion offers a new form of feedback to guide interventions with unprecedented precision. Indeed, the new model provides a rich lens through which we can understand neurodevelopment, both typical and atypical. Torres and Whyatt demonstrate how this concept can help us understand autism and its cardinal symptoms and lead to innovative approaches to assessment. Specifically, they suggest that the recording of dynamic, continuous micro-movements will uncover different types of fluctuations in amplitude and timing that will have direct clinical relevance for understanding complex behaviors, such as social interaction. In a sense, this approach can be likened to using a microscope to uncover patterns and meaning that are evident in behavior that simply can't be seen with the naked eye. The authors also suggest that different statistical approaches are needed to capture the nonlinear patterns inherent in such data. Rapid advances in the field of computational neuroscience will provide powerful tools for analyzing and interpreting such data.

Drawing parallels to how clinicians originally characterized Parkinson's disease using subjective observation, the authors describe how our current diagnostic and assessment methods for autism, which rely on clinical observation, fall short. The quantification of dynamic motor features of Parkinson's disease provided a more detailed, objective way of assessing the progression of this condition and its response to treatment. Furthermore, such quantitative approaches yielded important new insights about Parkinson's disease that simply were not possible through subjective clinical observation. Can a similar path of discovery help us better understand and quantify autism?

This book is revolutionary in its approach to autism. Inherently interdisciplinary in its focus, Torres and Whyatt's book will delight and expand the perspectives of clinicians, physiologists, neuroscientists, and computer scientists who care about understanding and improving the lives of persons with autism.

Geraldine Dawson, PhD
Professor of Psychiatry and Behavioral Sciences
Director, Duke Center for Autism and Brain Development Duke University
Past President, International Society for Autism Research

Contributors

Pat Amos
Ardmore, Pennsylvania

Jenna Anderson
Therapy Foundations, LLC
Phoenix, AZ

Silvia Baetti
Child Psychiatry and Neurology
Hospital Italiano de Buenos Aires
Buenos Aires, Argentina

Cynthia Baeza
Piscataway, New Jersey

Marcelo Biasatti
Child Psychiatry and Neurology
Hospital Italiano de Buenos Aires
Buenos Aires, Argentina

Anita Breslin
Private Practice
East Brunswick, New Jersey

Maria Brincker
Philosophy Department
University of Massachusetts
Boston, Massachusetts

Corinne G. Catalano
Center for Autism and Early Childhood Mental Health
College of Education and Human Services
Montclair State University
Montclair, New Jersey

Jonathan Delafield-Butt
Faculty of Humanities and Social Sciences
University of Stratchclyde
Glasgow, United Kingdom

Peter G. Enticott
Deakin Child Study Centre
School of Psychology
Deakin University
Melbourne, Victoria, Australia

Gregory Francis
Department of Psychological Sciences
Purdue University
West Lafayette, Indiana
and
Brain Mind Institute
École Polytechnique Fédérale de Lausanne
Lausanne, Switzerland

Nicci Grace
Monash Institute of Cognitive and Clinical Neurosciences
Monash University
Melbourne, Victoria, Australia

Jonathan Grashow
Pittsburgh, Pennsylvania

Kathryn Grashow
Pittsburgh, Pennsylvania

Sharon Hammer
Verona, Wisconsin

Michelle Welde Hardy
Pediatric Neurology Therapeutics
San Diego, CA

John P. Hussman
Hussman Institute for Autism
Baltimore, Maryland

Beth P. Johnson
Monash Institute of Cognitive and Clinical Neurosciences
Monash University
Melbourne, Victoria, Australia

Jorge V. José
Physics Department
Indiana University
Bloomington, Indiana
and
Stark Neuroscience Institute
and
Department of Cellular and Integrative Physiology
Indiana University School of Medicine
Indianapolis, Indiana

Lisa M. Ladson
Educational and Behavioral Consultant
Imagine a Child's Capacity
Madison, WI

Blythe LaGasse
Music Therapy Faculty University Colorado State
Fort Collins, Colorado

Maximiliano Lombardo
Child Psychiatry and Neurology
Hospital Italiano de Buenos Aires
Buenos Aires, Argentina

Kate McGinnity
Cambridge, Wisconsin

Max McKeough
Portage, Wisconsin

Sejal Mistry
School of Arts and Sciences
Rutgers University
New Brunswick, New Jersey

Paige Rabon
Music Therapist
Highlands Ranch, CO

Nicole J. Rinehart
Deakin Child Study Centre
School of Psychology
Deakin University
Melbourne, Victoria, Australia

Sam Rogers
Verona, Wisconsin

Elizabeth B. Torres
Psychology Department
Rutgers University
New Brunswick, New Jersey

Colwyn Trevarthen
Child Psychology
The University of Edinburgh
Edinburgh, United Kingdom

Jadyn Waiser
Branchburg, New Jersey

Michelle Stern Waiser
Branchburg, New Jersey

Caroline Whyatt
Psychology Department
Rutgers University
New Brunswick, New Jersey

Justin H. G. Williams
The Institute of Medical Sciences
The University of Aberdeen
Aberdeen, United Kingdom

Di Wu
Physics Department
Indiana University
Bloomington, Indiana

Section I

The Big Question

Why Study Movement?

1 Why Study Movement Variability in Autism?

Maria Brincker and Elizabeth B. Torres

CONTENTS

Introduction ... 3
Movements as Richly Layered Reafference ... 4
Reafference Principle ... 5
Movements as Output Revealing Many Layered Influences ... 6
Movements as Input Revealing What Must Be Coped With ... 7
Continuous Reentrant Historicity, Integration, and (Voluntary) Control ... 7
Voluntary Control and Stability: How Being Still on Command Is Itself an Accomplishment... 8
New Data and New Analyses Are Needed ... 10
Using Movement Variability to Move Autism Research Forward ... 12
Methodological and Conceptual Barriers ... 12
Institutional Barriers: Clinical Assessments and Conflicts of Interest ... 13
Warning Against Motor Reductionism and Neat Cognitive Modularity ... 17
Conclusion and Take-home Message ... 18
References ... 19

Movement variability has emerged as a critical research component in the field of neural motor control. This chapter explains why movement variability can be seen as such a rich resource for studying neural development and autism spectrum disorder. This cannot be done without a unifying framework for understanding the relationship between neural control, movement, and movement sensing. Thus, in the process of explaining why we should study movements, several analytical and empirical aspects of motor-sensed variability from self-generated actions are recast, as are their putative role in the development of motor-sensory-sensed maps of external stimuli present in social settings. This chapter offers a new lens for the research and treatment of neurodevelopmental disorders on a spectrum. This chapter thus proposes a general re-conceptualization of movement sensation and control. Through this a new framework for research and treatment of neurodevelopmental disorders in general we study ASD in particular.

INTRODUCTION

Autism has been defined as a disorder of social cognition, interaction, and communication where ritualistic, repetitive behaviors are commonly observed. But how should we understand the behavioral and cognitive differences that have been the main focus of so much autism research? Can high-level cognitive processes and behaviors be identified as the core issues people with autism face, or do these characteristics perhaps often rather reflect individual attempts to cope with underlying physiological issues? Much research presented in this volume will point to the latter possibility, that is, that people on the autism spectrum cope with issues at much lower physiological levels pertaining not only to central nervous system (CNS) function, but also to the peripheral nervous (PNS) and autonomic nervous (ANS) systems (Torres et al. 2013a). The following are questions that we pursue in this chapter: What might be

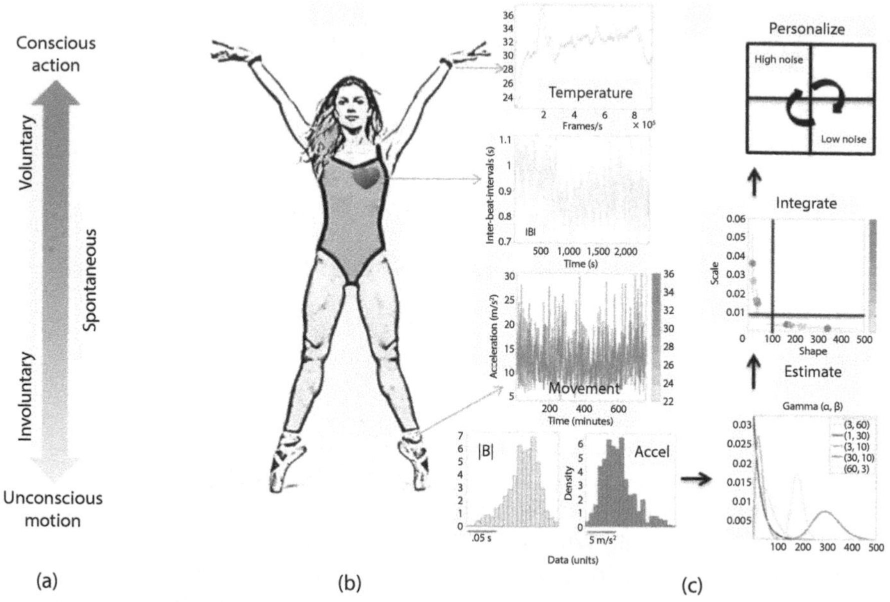

FIGURE 1.1 Characterization of multilayered sensory-motor systems. (a) Taxonomy of layers of motor control. (b) Different waveforms registered with wearable sensors across different layers of the nervous systems give rise to different types of minute fluctuations in amplitude and timing (micromovements). (c) Analytics for personalized medicine integrate multisensory micromotions and characterize noise-to-signal transitions across multiple levels in a and b.

fruitful ways of gaining objective measures of the large-scale systemic and heterogeneous effects of early atypical neurodevelopment? How should we track their evolution over time? How should we identify critical changes along the continuum of human development and aging?

We suggest that the study of movement variability—very broadly conceived as including all minute fluctuations in bodily rhythms and their rates of change over time (coined micromovements [Figure 1.1a and b] [Torres et al. 2013a])—offers a uniquely valuable and entirely objectively quantifiable lens to better assess, understand, and track not only autism but also cognitive development and degeneration in general. This chapter presents the rationale first behind this focus on micromovements and second behind the choice of specific kinds of data collection and statistical metrics as tools of analysis (Figure 1.1c).

In brief, the proposal is that the micromovements obtained using various timescales applied to different physiological data types (some examples are shown in Figure 1.1) contain information about layered influences and temporal adaptations, transformations, and integrations across anatomically semi-independent subsystems that cross talk and interact. Further, the notion of sensorimotor reafference is used to highlight the fact that these layered micromotions are sensed, and that this sensory feedback plays a crucial role in the generation and control of self-generated movements in the first place. In other words, the measurements of various motoric and rhythmic variations provide an access point not only to the "motor systems," but also to much broader central and peripheral sensorimotor and regulatory systems. Lastly, we posit that this new lens can also be used to capture influences from systems of multiple entry points or collaborative control and regulation, such as those that emerge during dyadic social interactions (further explained in Chapter 7).

MOVEMENTS AS RICHLY LAYERED REAFFERENCE

We now turn to the first core aspect of bodily movement that we want to highlight in this chapter, namely, that movement contains complex reafferent system information. This reafferent complexity serves to ground and justify our core methodological proposal that the microstructures of movement variability and their shifting statistical signatures can be measured and therefore represent a rich opportunity for objective assessment of neural and autoregulatory functioning.

Reafference Principle

The concept of reafference stems from the work of Von Holst and Mittelstaedt in the 1950s as they tried to capture the circularity of movement and sensation. They wrote, "Voluntary movements show themselves to be dependent on the returning stream of afference which they themselves cause." The core idea is that a movement-dependent sensory signal, that is, the "reafference," is ever present in the organism that moves at will as it interacts with its surroundings, and thus that the overall afferent is layered and due to both self- and externally generated causes. The self-recognition and eventual anticipatory prediction of the system's own self-initiated movements has gained influence in the context of the contemporary notion of "smart (probabilistically predictive) sensing" used today in portable media such as cell phones, tablets, appliances, and cars. Yet the concept is rooted back in the pioneering works of these physiologists: Von Holst and Mittelstaedt (1950), Von Holst (1954), and Grusser (1995). We see their principle of sensorimotor reafference as a tremendously important insight that is still overlooked in many areas of neuroscience and clinical practice today. Most crucially, reafference has been ignored in nearly all areas dealing with autism spectrum disorders (ASDs).

Von Holst and Mittelstaedt were interested in how we can sense the external world, given this predicament of sensing through self-generated movement. Like earlier theorists, such as Dewey (1896) in philosophy, Uexküll (1928) in theoretical biology, and later Gibson (1960, 1979) in psychology, they challenged the notion of the "stimulus" as something that simply appears passively as an "input" for the organism. Rather, the isolation of the stimulus is in a sense already an accomplishment of the active sensorimotor organism. The predicament of the organism seems to be that it needs a certain predictive knowledge of self and world in order to perceive these in the first place. In other words, the organism is always in a sort of hermeneutically circular situation where its sensorimotor history serves as the anchor for both perception and action in the present.

Interestingly, it is only fairly recently that the field of predictive coding and Bayesian statistics has brought these insights and Von Holst's reafference principle to mainstream perception research (Friston et al. 2012). However, the reafference principle has been enormously influential in the area of motor control, and many theories about "internal models," "efference copies," "corollary discharge," and "error minimization" have been developed (Wolpert and Miall 1996; Wolpert and Kawato 1998; Wolpert et al. 1998; Haruno et al. 2001) trying to map how this principle of reafference might be more precisely implemented physiologically and/or computationally. Questions have been raised pertaining to the actual nature of the efferent command, how this efferent signal is linked to the expected afferent input, how this expectation is compared and used to interpret the actual afference input, and which of these "signals" are used as "posteriors" to update which parts of systems of "priors" and so forth (Kording and Wolpert 2004, 2006). We shall not here try to settle these still live theoretical and empirical debates over how best to understand specific reafference processes, nor try to model how various aspects of these feedback mechanisms are embodied at different levels of the nervous system.

However, we do want to draw attention to the problematic simplicity by which these questions of implementation are typically posed—not only by many contemporary motor control theorists but also by Von Holst himself. Models, for example, mostly assume that we are dealing with one efferent signal at the time, being compared with a reafferent such that a simple subtraction can generate an error signal that might directly translate to an "ex-afferent" signal pertaining to the perception of the external world. But in actuality, our movements are temporally continuous and highly layered also within single motor channels. In this sense, sensory feedback might be used to adjust movement across many anatomically distinct loops and hierarchical levels. When reading the literature on motor control, one could be misled into believing that all movement is goal directed and under high-level intentional control (Shadmehr and Wise 2005). However, such types of movements actually represent a rather small fraction of our overall bodily movements. Thus, the question is how we also understand the regulation and reafference of more spontaneous and non-goal-directed actions (Torres 2011), and further how this sort of reafference might work in concert with—and perhaps inform—our cortical priors for goal-directed and intentional action control.

As mentioned, it is a core aspect of Von Holst and Mittelstaedt's original principle that raw sensory input is not simply a passive reflection of the external world, but always sensed throughout one's own active movements. One way to think of this central insight is that our perception of the external world in a sense always involves an active "subtraction of self." To get to what Von Holst and Mittelstaedt called the ex-afference, that is, the perception of the world beyond the expected effects of one's own self-produced movement, various subtractions seem to take place. However, the question is, how does the organism know what part of the overall afference is the reafference, that is, the expected product of its own movement? A big complication here is the fact that we are actually physically embodied living creatures—that we are not simply dealing with abstract motor commands executed to digital perfection. Rather, our bodies represent an intricate orchestration of multitudes of subsystems at mind-boggling plentiful levels of description. The question is, how do we know what to subtract from what? To produce controlled movements, it seems that we need to empirically update our predictions not only about the physical and social world but also about our own bodies. And by bodies, we do not here simply mean our sensorimotor machinery, but our bodies as autonomically regulated and physically and socially impacted. Accordingly, we need a model of reafference that accounts for our continuous exploration of multiple simultaneously changing aspects of self, others, and the world.*

To elucidate this need for a more complex model, it might be helpful to take a closer look at this extreme complexity of our embodiment, and thus of what might be seen as forms of reafference to begin with. To do this, in the following two sections, for the purposes of analysis, we will look in turn at movements as outputs and inputs, respectively. Note that this division is purely methodological, not a claim that these can be isolated in practice. To the contrary, the reafference principle reminds us that movements and bodily rhythms are always simultaneously produced and sensed.

Movements as Output Revealing Many Layered Influences

Our bodily movements and rhythms are products of many complex and heterogeneous influences stemming from within the CNS and PNS and spanning phylogeny and ontogeny. Further, movements also carry effects of a whole host of other physiological and external physical and social influences. One can thus see the continuous stream of bodily motions and rhythms not only as a product of some current conscious mental state or regional brain activity but also as an expression of the state of the entire contextually embedded organism.

This layered nature of the peripheral movement is extremely important to keep in mind as we analyze the complex data measured and collected, for example, by wearable sensors on bodily parts during a particular set of contextually situated activities. If one, to the contrary, thought of the cortical motor system more or less as a digital command center, functioning in relative isolation and independently from other bodily processes and influences, and as producing each output independently of previously sensed movement, then one might think that what movement sensors would measure would be revealing of only this modular cortical motor function. However, such abstract assumptions ignore not only the reentrant and complex integrative nature of the cortical motor output, but also the entire subcortical, peripheral, and physical embodiment of the movement system, which all contribute to the patterns of variability found at the level of the actual embodied movement. To make this point

* Note that Von Holst and Mittelstaedt avoided some of these complexities through their focus on eye movements rather than body movements. They took the main afferent in vision to simply be the retinal modulation and showed a minimal regard for bodily proprioceptive channels involving a far higher number of degrees of freedom than the eye.

about dynamic complexity and heterogeneity palpable, it is informative to look beyond cognitive neuroscience to the fields of evolutionary, developmental, and functional anatomy.

In the following, we return to the question of control, but here just notice that the movement "output" measured at the periphery is subject to both physical forces and biological regulatory influences far beyond our volitional and narrowly cortical control.

Movements as Input Revealing What Must Be Coped With

By objectively measuring and characterizing the current variabilities and patterns of movement change, one can see this as a readout not only of the movements (actively) self-produced by a given embodied system, but also of what the nervous system of this person has to cope with. In other words, the continuous and distributed brain–body feedback circularities are layered into overlapping movement sequences (discussed in Chapter 7), and also serve as kinesthetic inputs. Whether these movements are consciously tracked or transpire largely beneath awareness, they feed back into the system. When considering the fact that our movements are sensed and serve as input, the quality and characteristics of this sensory input become important, that is, does it read as a useful or noisy, random, or confusing signal? What would it mean for a typically developing system to receive a given type of kinesthetic input rather than another? What tools would be needed to extract systematized information from the variations at hand? Consensus is growing that the PNS and CNS must contain various priors, that is, expectations about the barrage of sensory changes that happens at the body's many receptors. These priors can then help us sort out the many layers of influences contained in the sensory input.

Following the hypothesis of Von Holst and Mittelstaedt, there might be some sort of internal signal—perhaps an efference copy—that allows a system to sort its overall afferent input into reafference and ex-afference, respectively. However, as we have underscored earlier, the actual efference, in the sense of the actual peripheral movement, is a rather complex and layered affair. In other words, the efference copy or, more broadly, embodied expectation had better be layered and complex as well, to be able to tease apart and decompose the signals of the returning afferent barrage. The simplistic picture of one isolated afference quantity minus one isolated efference quantity is simply not going to cut it even if we limit our consideration to one sensory modality or even one receptor channel in isolation.

Also note that in a broad sense of priors, many such expectations are precisely distributed and embedded in the functional anatomy of both peripheral and central systems. One can thus see not only cortical sensory feedback expectations, but also baseline firing rates, average conduction times given myelination, and so forth, as involving priors. The idea here is that the baseline firing rate gives rise to expectations that are communicable at least in the sense that the broader expectations of the sensorimotor system have been adapted to these. With this notion of anatomically distributed priors, we now start to see how the expectations pertaining to higher-level events and volitional action not only carry traces of the overall embodiment but also rely on the predictable behavior of this broader physiological system. This is an important part of our interpretation of the reafference hypothesis, as it would suggest that we should think of deliberate action control and high-level perception as always interacting with and dependent on much broader peripheral—and often cultural and social—systems. This means similarly that one might interpret some priors about the physical and social environment as not explicitly represented, but as more distributed and implicitly adapted to. These are all issues that need more empirical elucidation. However, they alert us to the possibility of "corrupted" or unreliable priors at all these levels.

Continuous Reentrant Historicity, Integration, and (Voluntary) Control

Now we have looked at the complexity of the measurable movements at the periphery, and how this both reflects the many causal influences and can be seen as a complex sensory input that the organism needs to try to understand, anticipate the consequences of, and control. So far, we have mostly focused on the sensory "understanding" part. However, this understanding is intimately linked to processes of action control necessarily requiring estimation, prediction, and confirmation about the current and impending actions and their sensory consequences. How we tease apart what is conducive of positive reward for the system from what to avoid in future encounters will require evaluation schemas that "remember," store, and retrieve information in some (prospective) statistical sense.

Given sensorimotor circularity, separating active willed movement variability from supportive spontaneous variability may actually be possible when considering long histories of sensory consequences continuously sampled in unbroken reafferent sensorimotor loops. It is a core aspect of our proposal that this temporal feedback circularity is not just adding random noise, as others have pointed out (Faisal et al. 2008), but also serves a key feature of adaptive and integrative sensorimotor and regulatory control. As we have expressed in an earlier paper, "not all variability is created equal" (Brincker and Torres 2013), and clearly self-sensing movement variability influences noise that comes from other parts of its own body and over time might become a meaningful signal in the overall reafferent economy. Mechanisms that help the nervous systems recognize internal phase transition from spontaneous random noise to systematic, well-structured noise (i.e., signal) will aid in the detection and distinction of deliberateness versus spontaneity (Kalampratsidou and Torres 2016) present both in one's own movements and in those of other social interaction partners. This is a testable hypothesis under the new proposed lens of micromovements' kinesthetic sensing.

In sum, we hypothesize the existence of a proper sensory-motor variability environment as a necessary ingredient to scaffold the emergence of a predictive, anticipatory code realizable from the inherent statistical properties of actively generated movements. Such movements generated under schemas that successfully compensate for transduction and transmission delays within the nervous systems will go on to form a foundation for the sort of anticipatory coding required for adaptive and fruitful behavior and social exchange. The question is how the actual embodied and embedded historical organism succeeds in this feat of knowing, predicting ahead, and controlling its own movements and isolating and interpreting relevant sensory signals while temporarily discarding or downplaying irrelevant ones within a given context. It is clear that this intricate resolution within the individual's nervous systems could fail to develop properly or break down in multiple ways, and one should not be surprised to find atypical sensorimotor variations in babies born with complications (Torres et al. 2016b) (Figure 1.2a–c) conducive in some cases to neurodevelopmental disorders, such as ASD, compared with neurotypical controls (Figure 1.2d and e). Disorders of sensory-motor systems are also quantifiable in neurodegenerative cases, such as Parkinson's disease, and in deafferentation (Torres et al. 2014). In the latter case, stochastic signatures overlapping with those of ASD individuals have been quantified at the motor output (Torres et al. 2016a). Further, individual reafference sets the stage for social exchange with others—and can be reciprocally shaped by such exchanges (De Jaegher and Di Paolo 2007). Many of the estimation, transformation, and prediction processes that take place within the person (Figure 1.1) are thus bound to extend to the social dyad (see Chapter 7 for an expansion on this proposition).

Voluntary Control and Stability: How Being Still on Command Is Itself an Accomplishment

With this notion of reafference in hand, not only singling out the stimulus but also holding the body still becomes an accomplishment. To paraphrase the American polymath of the nineteenth century Charles Sanders Peirce, given the historicity of the world, what needs explaining is not instances of change but rather instances of apparent stability (Peirce 1891). In other words, in terms of biological and cognitive development, how do we succeed in developing stable structures and relations, and what are the active processes of maintenance that go into the creation of these stabilities? Take the simple command of remaining still while participating in a regular cognitive neuroscience experiment.

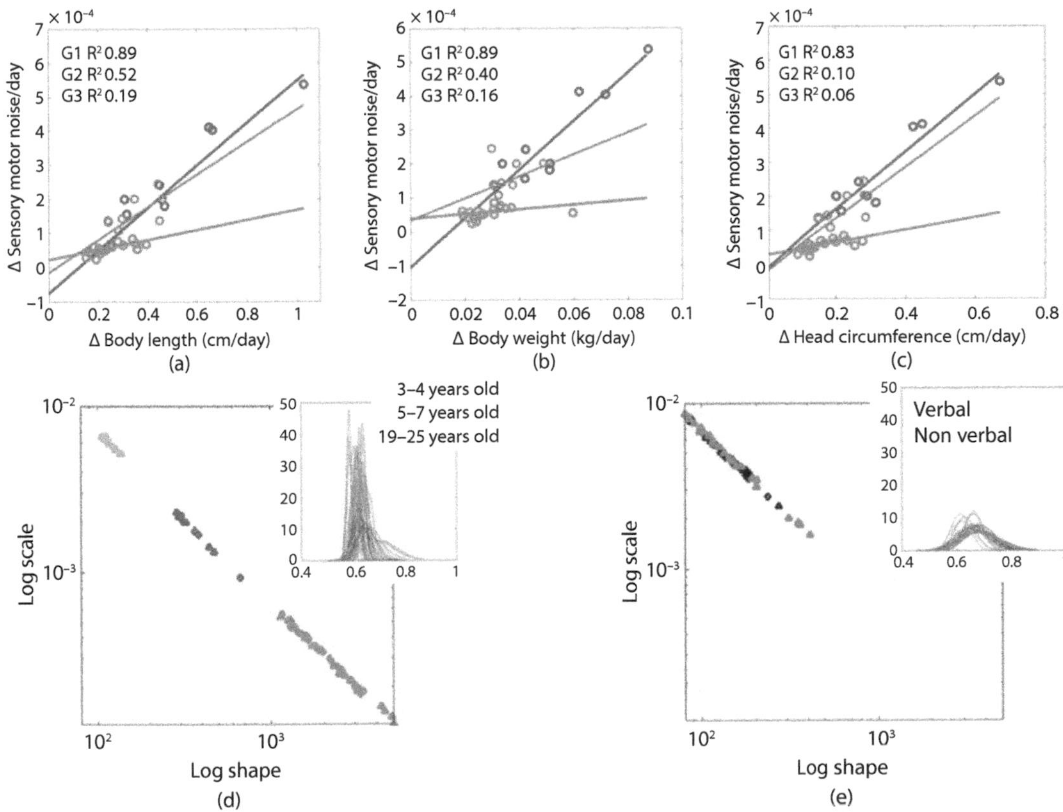

FIGURE 1.2 Stagnation in neuromotor development in the newborn and beyond. (a–c) Index of risk for neurodevelopmental derailment characterized by lack of noise-to-signal transitions in acceleration-dependent micromovements measured as a function of the rate of physical growth (weight, body length, and head circumference) longitudinally tracked in newborn babies for 6 months. G1, G2 and G3 are classified according to patterns of growth and readiness to walk (see Torres et al. 2016). (d) Maturation in noise-to-signal transition in typical development (cross-sectional data from 3 to 25 years old) showing the decrease in noise and the shift from skewed to symmetric shapes of probability distribution functions from velocity-dependent micromovements. (e) Stagnation in noise-to-signal transitions in ASDs (cross-sectional data from 3 to 25 years old) lacking the decrease in noise and the absence of shifts to symmetric Probability Density Functions (PDFs). Available at: http://journal.frontiersin.org/article/10.3389/fped.2016.00121/full and http://journal.frontiersin.org/article/10.3389/fnint.2013.00032/full.

Most existing techniques and analytical methods to study cortical surface activity require such stillness to minimize motion artifacts. Yet the field rarely admits to (1) the artificial nature of such an imposed condition and (2) the level of volition that is required in order to maintain such stillness even for a few minutes.

Recent work involving 1048 participants has revealed that excess noise accumulation in involuntary micromotions of the head (while the person is in a resting state) is present in individuals with ASD and attention deficit hyperactivity disorder (ADHD) but absent from neurotypical controls (Figure 1.3a). Such excess noise signatures were consistently found regardless of differences in ages, Autism Diagnostic Observation Schedule (ADOS) severity scores, IQ levels, and levels of social difficulties (Torres and Denisova 2016). For our purposes here, note that any excess involuntary micromotions in these neurodevelopmental disorders are bound to interfere with the ability to remain still on command. This ability, taken for granted in neurotypicals, is indeed a great accomplishment of their nervous systems. We further hypothesize that the extent to which this ability is

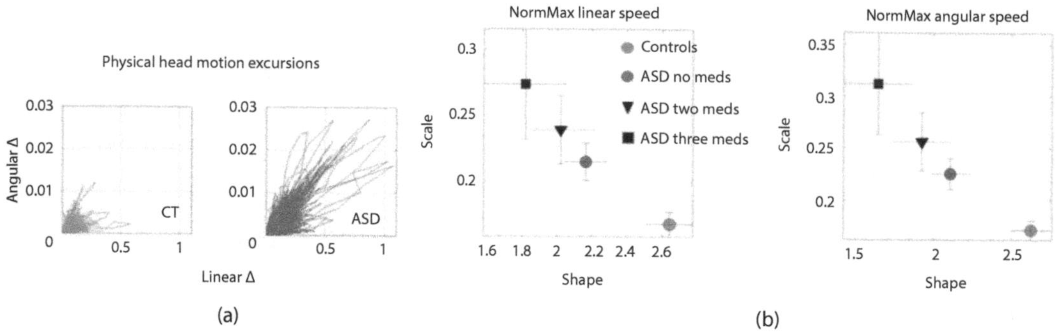

FIGURE 1.3 Excess noise accumulation from involuntary head micromotions in ASD is present with or without psychotropic medication intake (a), indicated by empirically estimated stochastic signatures in (b) using involuntary head micromotions in ASD. Data extracted from involuntary head micromotions of 1048 individuals (including ASD and controls) registered in the Autism Brain Imaging Data Exchange (ABIDE) publicly available to researchers.

compromised may be revealing of the level of severity concerning disconnects between the (intentional) desire to voluntarily control bodily motions and the actual realization of this will.

NEW DATA AND NEW ANALYSES ARE NEEDED

This idea of reafference and embodied heterogeneity and historicity is absent from most traditional cognitive theories of mind and action, and therefore also from common methodologies and practices of data collection and statistical analyses. Given this absence, it is perhaps not surprising that the very information sought is entirely missing from the core description of autism. One critical problem in this regard is that the methods employed in the current key disciplines defining and treating autism often predefine global-level behavioral categories and formulate discrete segments unambiguously captured by the naked eye (Figure 1.4a). In so doing, these definitions result in researchers missing, for example, intermediate, more ambiguous (spontaneous) segments of the actions (see also Chapter 7). Such segments occur much too fast or at frequencies that escape the naked eye. In this sense, conceptual categories are in part to blame for the failure to capture and analyze the rich variability of multiple influences across many layers and control levels of the ever-interacting CNS and PNS (Figure 1.1a). This use of high-level categorization of behavior seems analogous to if one were to use biased instrumentation with poor spatiotemporal resolution, and then, without any awareness of or attention to these limitations, conclude that the data collected represented all the relevant phenomena.

Further, another set of problems may arise when low-level variability is studied, but most researchers, in the areas of motor control, (1) acquire data under highly practiced tasks with an exclusive focus on goal-directed movements, (2) analyze the data under preimposed linear models, and (3) use parametric statistics under a priori assumptions of normality, further enforcing a notion of stationarity in data that is inherently stochastic with shifting dynamics (Figure 1.4b). Such impositions undermine our ability to empirically study the sensorimotor maturations and dynamic adaptations occurring in typical development. With the paucity of motor control data reflecting the highly nonlinear nature of neurodevelopment (Smith and Thelen 1993; Thelen and Smith 1994), along with its true stochastic and nonstationary features (Torres et al. 2016b), it has been extremely challenging to even begin to frame the problems that an atypically developing nervous system may face (Torres et al. 2013a, 2013b, 2016a), let alone propose a solution.

Assessing the dynamics, acquisitions, and temporal developments of statistical distributions characterizing physical sensorimotor parameters during typical neurodevelopment can add that missing layer of objective information that current psychological definitions of autism have failed to provide

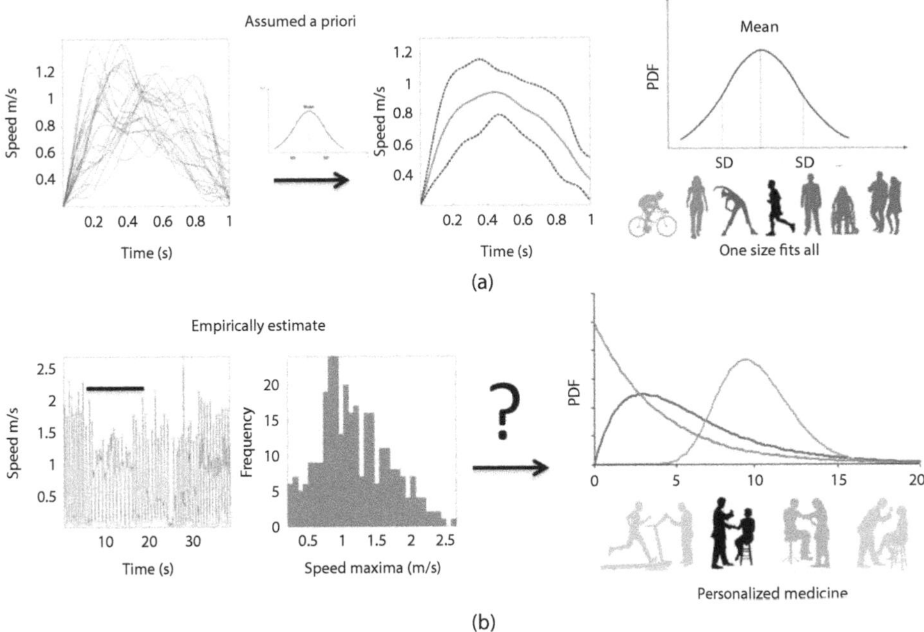

FIGURE 1.4 Moving beyond the one-size-fits-all model used to analyze the statistics of human behavior. (a) Assuming and enforcing normality in data that is inherently not normally distributed. Kinematic parameters (speed, meters per second; temporal profiles) taken across epochs (e.g., pointing trials) of a motor control experiment are averaged under the assumption of Gaussian mean and variance, thus smoothing out the minute fluctuations that provide information about the noise-to-signal ratios and their transitions from spontaneous random noise to systematic, well-structured noise (signal) with predictive power. The a priori imposed Gaussian assumption is applied to all population data discarding as well as individual features critical for the implementation of personalized medicine models. (b) The individualized approach does not assume a theoretical distribution but rather estimates it from the empirical data. A kinematics data time series has a segment highlighted with a bar representing the data in (a) continuously registered and used as it accumulates information about the person. The historicity of the data is then reflected in the changing shapes and dispersions of the nonstationary data. Each person spans a family of probability distributions, and it is the rates of change of noise-to-signal transitions that uniquely define the person's responses to context, goals, and treatments. The minute fluctuations in the data and their cumulative history are preserved in this individualized approach amenable for the personalized medicine model as applied to the fields of neurology and neuropsychiatry.

(Torres et al. 2013a, 2016a). Such a step seems essential if we want to understand how the growing and developing nervous systems adapt and gain familiarity and control in the face of constantly changing bodies and environments. Only after we characterize the multilayered influences of the nervous systems in typical neurodevelopment will we begin to identify and characterize atypical manifestations. This will enable us to pose new questions and gain new insights into atypical processes partaking in any social exchange between the individual with neurodevelopmental challenges and others in the social medium. Note how this approach differs from current "deficit models" in psychiatry—where atypical development is seen as a failure to develop high-level abilities without a systemic characterization of how this typical development dynamically comes about or of which systemic lower-level issues might make other behaviors and abilities adaptive for a given person.

Further, and very importantly for our present purposes, scientists who do look at physical bodily variabilities typically enforce a priori assumptions of normality and linearity in the data (Kuczmarski et al. 2002; Flegal and Cole 2013). We argue that this practice completely fails to acknowledge the evidence that probability distributions change over time and in response to new conditions.

Thus, while some parameters of well-practiced movements of Typically Developing (TD) adults often can be approximated by normal distributions, early and atypical development is precisely linked to skewed distributions of those same parameters and a prevalence of noisy and random movement variabilities. We now have multiple sources of evidence of neurodevelopmental stagnations where movement variabilities do not undergo the maturation and transitions quantified in typical development (Figure 1.2) (Torres et al. 2013a, 2016a, 2016b). We propose that such stagnant variabilities—otherwise interpreted as corrupted movement priors—can be approximately mapped and precisely tracked over time if one lets go of a priori imposed assumptions of normality, linearity, and stationarity. Movement variabilities thus present us with extremely valuable data types not only for understanding both typical and atypical developmental trajectories but also for tracking learning and the effectiveness of therapeutic interventions. They provide the counterintuitive notion that some noise is signal in the nervous systems.

USING MOVEMENT VARIABILITY TO MOVE AUTISM RESEARCH FORWARD

Movements, their microfluctuations, and their sensations provide a flow of feedback measurable in noninvasive ways. We argue that this continuous reentrant information simultaneously reflecting a layered peripheral output and input makes movement variations an incredibly rich lens through which to study neurodevelopment and, in particular, the systems' ability to adapt to new tasks and integrate and transform feedback across various sensorimotor and autonomic channels and subsystems. In other words, rather than simply assuming we have a nervous system in control, we seek to measure the system's ability to integrate across semiautonomous subsystems and recover stability and control given constant change and perturbation. The advent of rapidly advancing wearable sensing technologies now makes this project very feasible. These technologies enable noninvasive data collection and studies of peripheral micromotions, as well as micromotions of coupled bodily rhythms and various cognitive tasks. All these movement variabilities can be accessed completely objectively at high resolutions and relatively low cost while the person naturally interacts with the surrounding social medium.

In the context of autism research, the theoretical conception of "movement as reentrant smart (predictive) sensory feedback" and the use of its inherent variabilities as outcome measures thus seem like potent tools. However, there are some methodological, conceptual, and institutional barriers to progress that bear mentioning.

METHODOLOGICAL AND CONCEPTUAL BARRIERS

Movement issues in autism have been highlighted for decades (see, e.g., Damasio and Maurer 1978; Donnellan et al. 2012; Donnellan and Leary 2012; Torres and Donnellan 2015), but with little consequence. One reason could be that there has been a lack of proper methodology to address its continuous, dynamic, and stochastic flow in naturalistic social exchanges.

There is now broad mounting evidence of the presence of sensory-motor issues in autism (Jones and Prior 1985; Rogers et al. 1996; Rinehart et al. 2001; Williams et al. 2001; Noterdaeme et al. 2002; Teitelbaum et al. 2002, 2004; Minshew et al. 2004; Mostofsky et al. 2006; Jansiewicz et al. 2006; Gowen et al. 2008; Fournier et al. 2010a, 2010b; Brincker and Torres 2013; Torres et al. 2013a, 2016a; Mosconi and Sweeney 2015; Mosconi et al. 2015). Yet, in the field of autism sensorimotor issues are sadly still bluntly denied and excluded from consideration within core clinical and research constituencies.

It is worth highlighting the arguments against movement issues as being central to ASD. Many have, for example, pointed to (1) an absence of narrowly motor or gross-level isolated movement issues in many people with autism and also (2) the skillful and amazingly precise movements of certain musical prodigies on the spectrum (for such a diverse account, see Silberman 2015). Thus, at this level of description it looks like a strong double dissociation of ASD and movement issues. Yet a paucity of actual physical quantification and measurements with millisecond timescale precision has accompanied such claims, claims that have been primarily based on categorical interpretation of the observed phenomena. Accordingly, autism has been clinically defined in purely descriptive cognitive and behavioral terms, as if behaviors in general did not involve movement and their sensations. As argued above, this definition assumes that all relevant evidence should follow preexisting high-level categorizations, and ignores that the naked eye cannot possibly see how the PNS and the CNS exchange feedback from actively produced motions.

Institutional Barriers: Clinical Assessments and Conflicts of Interest

Given what we know about sensorimotor issues, we suggest that the current clinical definition and use in assessment not only seems inaccurate, but also seems epistemically and morally problematic. A look at the current ADOS assessment practices is instructive here. The ADOS-2 manual (Lord et al.), under the "Guidelines for Selecting a Module" section, proposes the following—to many, innocent sounding—caveat:

> Note that the ADOS-2 was developed for and standardized using populations of children and adults without significant sensory and motor impairments. Standardized use of any ADOS-2 module presumes that the individual can walk independently and is free of visual or hearing impairments that could potentially interfere with use of the materials or participation in specific tasks.

The above statement implicitly assumes that the person administering the test and selecting the module a priori knows whether the child has significant sensory-motor issues that could impede performance. Yet the naked eye of that person has limited capacity to make that determination with any degree of certainty, not to mention that they would have to know beforehand what they were looking for.

The crucial point is that we neither need to exclude sensorimotor issues nor assess these a priori or intuitively. Objective quantification and characterization of physiological disturbances tied to sensory-motor phenomena are now possible. We can also empirically assess and track such disturbances longitudinally, and thus objectively judge the sensory and somatic motor effects of various medications. Such assessment is equally possible in relation to behavioral therapies.

Additionally, one can use similar methods during cognitive-social performance evaluated by the *Diagnostic and Statistical Manual of Mental Disorders* (DSM) and ADOS criteria. Specifically, it is possible to use the new statistical platform for individualized behavioral analysis (SPIBA) and wearable sensors to assess dyadic social exchange with millisecond time precision (see Chapter 7).

The idea here is to expand the notion of reafference to the social domain, and accordingly continuously track and analyze coupled rhythms and their mutual output–feedback loops during social exchange. In particular, this can be done during the types of staged social exchanges that observational inventories such as the ADOS-2 carry out (see Chapter 7). These observational inventories have yet to go beyond the manual scores and their interpretation. Actually quantifying physiological signatures of nervous systems with neurodevelopmental issues as social exchanges unfold could reveal physiological signatures of entrained and disjointed exchange. Nervous systems persistently receiving corrupted sensory-motor feedback are likely bound to operate in rather disjointed ways that we have yet to characterize (Brincker and Torres 2013). For example, Figure 1.5 shows some of the signatures of involuntary head motions polluting the resting-state behavior of individuals with various forms of ADHD that occur with and without psychotropic medication intake. In terms of the social dyad, the effects of such corrupted feedback tend to be reflected in both agents, as the reciprocal interaction continuously unfolds in a given context (Whyatt et al. 2015).

Likewise, Figure 1.6a further stresses this point as it shows the interplay of the noise-to-signal ratio characterizing the signatures of involuntary head micromotions in individuals with ASD as a function of ordinal data from incremental IQ scores across ages. These signatures change in Figure 1.6b in controls as they age and develop, but remain stunted across 6–60 years of age in ASD. Color bars

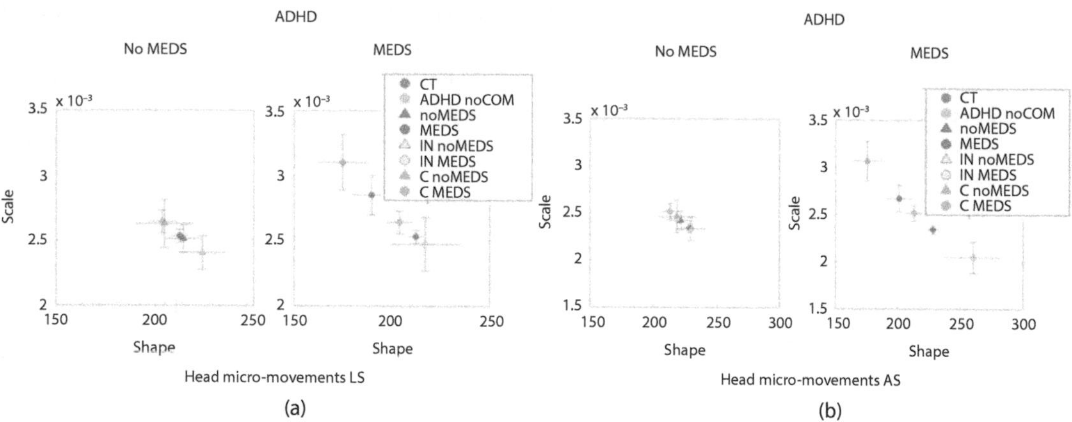

FIGURE 1.5 Stochastic signatures of involuntary head micromotions in ADHD estimated for the normalized peak fluctuations in linear and angular velocities: (a) linear speed and (b) angular speed. Medication effects in ADHD subtypes (inattentive [IN] and combined [C], denoting hyperactive plus inattentive) on the stochastic signatures of involuntary head micromotions for the normalized linear and angular peak velocities. Panels show the empirically estimated gamma shape and scale parameters for cases without and with medication corresponding to participants in the ADHD-200 database.

show differences in the incremental values of the IQ as well. Each dot in this graph represents the gamma moments of individuals above and below the median change in IQ scores for five age groups. There are 10 points in each class of subjects, 2 per age group denoting the median ranked group. Gradients of gray denote the controls' IQ changes per age, while blue shades denote those of the ASD. The size of the marker is the kurtosis of the probability distribution estimated from the micromovements extracted from involuntary head motions. The *z*-axis is the shape (skewness) of the distribution whereby the controls converge to symmetric, Gaussian-like shapes, while the ASD remain with very skewed shapes tending toward the exponential range of the gamma parameter plane (Torres and Denisova 2016).

Along these lines of involuntary motions polluting the nervous systems of the individuals with ASD, the pervasive use of psychotropic medication across neurodevelopmental conditions poses a question about the long-term effects that combinations and dosages of such substances may have on a young, rapidly growing and developing nervous system. We simply do not know the answer to this question, but recent work involving large cross-sectional data from individuals with ASD and ADHD (Torres and Denisova 2016) reveals excess noise and randomness in the involuntary head motions that systematically increases with the use of psychotropic medication in relation to individuals with such disorders who do not take medication. Table 1.1 lists some of the commonly reported medication in the ABIDE I database used in this recent study.

It should be underscored once more that the central tenet of this volume is to bridge current discrete criteria emphasizing cognitive and social issues with continuous criteria characterizing the biorhythms of natural behaviors flowing during social exchange. The explicit goal is to reach a much more precise and individualized understanding of the entire spectrum of experiences that self-advocates and practitioners have expressed so forcefully against too narrow deficit models (Donnellan et al. 2012; Donnellan and Leary 2012; Robledo et al. 2012). Thus, we stress that what we propose is a methodological and diagnostic use of the micromovements as a new lens to understand the complex heterogeneous characteristics people experience on the autism spectrum both at an individual level and at the level of dyadic (and multiparty) social exchange. Accordingly, the idea is by no means to exclude the many autonomic, sensory, cognitive, behavioral, and social challenges. Quite the contrary, the idea is to attempt to characterize these low- and

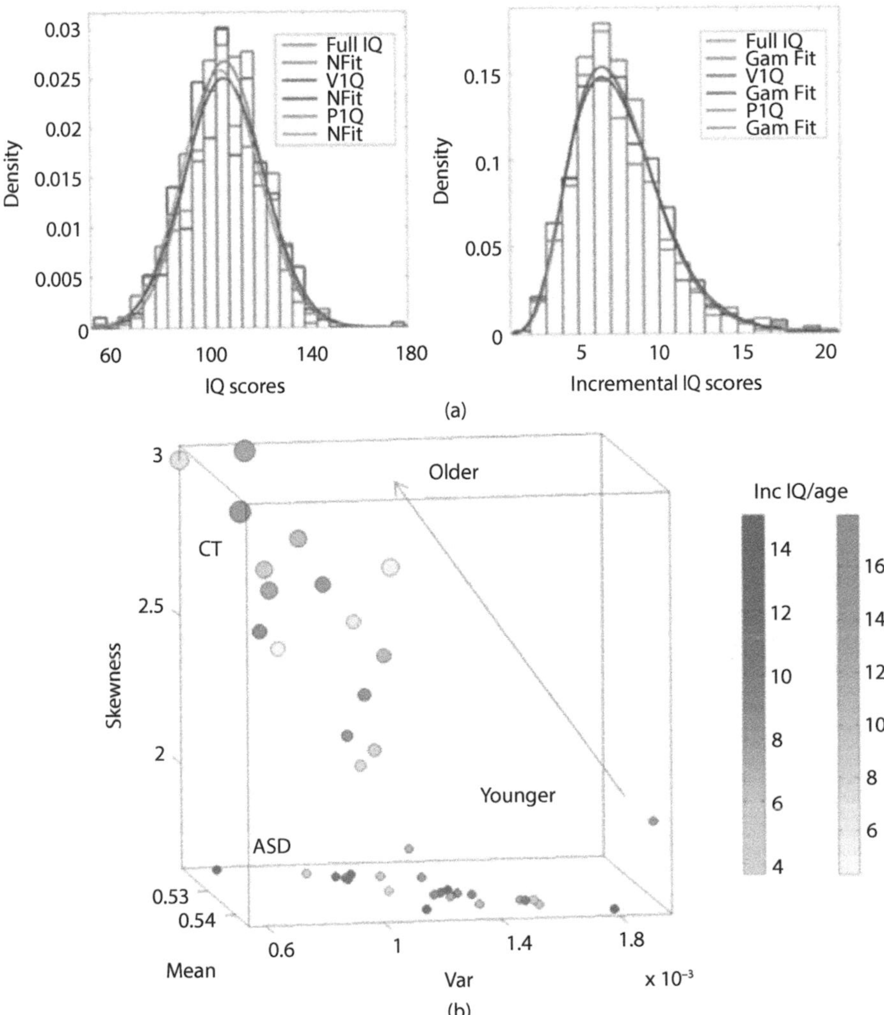

FIGURE 1.6 Stochastic signatures of head micromovements differ with incremental changes in IQ with age. (a) Probability distribution functions fit to the frequency histograms of full IQ, verbal IQ, and performance IQ scores for the case of absolute scores (Gaussian fit) and incremental scores (gamma fit) corrected by age for both control typical (CT) and ASD participants. (b) Incremental scores for different age groups in CT and ASD obtained for age groups ranging from 6 to 60 years old. Color corresponds to the rate of change of incremental full IQ with age. Values of 3 (excess skewness index) correspond to symmetric distributions, while values below 3 are skewed distributions with a heavy right tail. The youngest CTs are 6 years old, on the bottom of the graph of the empirically estimated summary statistics. Note that the CT moments evolve with age. The mean values increase, tending to slower rates of involuntary head micromotions in the linear displacement domain. The variance decreases as the CTs age and the distributions become more symmetric, with higher kurtosis as well. In the ASD group from 6 to 60 years old, their distributions remain heavily skewed at the level of the TD of 6 years old.

high-level ambiguous descriptions from a more systemic *physiological perspective*—with basis in the evidence that physical data can be collected noninvasively, under unrestrained conditions, and continuously while employing contemporary wearable sensors.

New analytics designed for the personalized use of wearable sensors now enable the objective characterization of such signals and their use in near real time, making biofeedback available in

TABLE 1.1
Subset of Psychotropic Medications Taken by Participants with ASD in Figure 1.3b Shown by Medication Class, and Their Reported Motor and Bodily Related Side Effects

Class (Psychotropic Medication)	Medication Names	Motor and Bodily Related Side Effects
Antidepressants	Fluoxetine, sertraline hydrochloride, trazodone, escitalopram, citalopram, bupropion, mirtazapine, duloxetine hydrochloride, venlafaxine, paroxetine	Tremors; paraesthesia; dizziness, drowsiness
Stimulants	Amphetamine and dextroamphetamine, lisdexamfetamine, methylphenidate extended release, dexmethylphenidate, dextroamphetamine sulfate	Dizziness, drowsiness; twitching; convulsions
Anticonvulsants	Oxcarbazepine, valproic acid, lamotrigine	Tremors; drowsiness
Atypical antipsychotics	Risperidone, ziprasidone hydrochloride, asenapine, quetiapine, aripiprazole	Tremors, twitching; restlessness
Benzodiazepine anticonvulsant	Lorazepam	Drowsiness; muscle trembling
Alpha-agonists	Guanfacine, clonidine	Restlessness; shakiness; dizziness
Atypical ADHD medication Noreprinephrine Reuptake Inhibitor (NRI)	Atomoxetine	Tremors; dizziness, drowsiness
Nonbenzodiazepine sedative-hypnotic	Eszopiclone	Clumsiness; difficulty with coordination
Nonbenzodiazepine anxiolytic	Buspirone	Nervousness

parametric form during activities of daily living, therapeutic interventions, and basic research (Torres et al. 2013a, 2013c; Whyatt et al. 2015). Under these conditions, such variability is now conceptualized as reentrant sensory flow that can become predictive (or not). It is in this potential for prospective (predictive) control and the self-discovery of cause-and-effect relations from actively self-generated motions that we will rest our hopes for habilitation and improvement of social exchange across the spectrum of neurodevelopmental disorders. Indeed, as it has been already demonstrated, in nonverbal children with ASD, the reentrant flow can begin to transition from random and noisy to predictive and systematic within a matter of minutes of using bio-sensory-motor feedback to evoke self-exploration and self-discovery of goals conducive of agency in the person's motions (Torres et al. 2013c; Torres 2016).

This methodology aiming to elicit and build self-emerging control is thus in a sense the inverse of the currently widely used methods of prompting and reinforcing predefined action types by external rewards, as done in the behaviorists' tradition of animal conditioning. Indeed, allowing self-exploration and autonomous detection of goals and voluntary control rewards the child internally simply by enabling active identification of action generation with sensory-motor consequences during motor learning. Such schemas exploiting self-discovery of self-generated movements and their sensory consequences lead to the nontransient dampening of sensory-motor noise (Torres et al. 2013c) and retained gains even 4–5 weeks later, in the absence of practice.

WARNING AGAINST MOTOR REDUCTIONISM AND NEAT COGNITIVE MODULARITY

Note that the proposal is not that autism uniquely or reductively should be characterized as a problem of micromovements. The central tenet of our work is to characterize current cognitive and behavioral symptom descriptions with objective means in noninvasive ways. The ubiquitous presence of micromotions of different timescales and frequencies in all aspects of behavior enables the development and use of a statistical platform to measure these minute fluctuations in the nervous systems' output. This methodology can be also applied in naturalistic social exchanges, by measuring the forms of social–output–feedback loops simultaneously co-occurring within the person and between the agents in the social dyad. Using the changing signatures of micromovements in such multilayered contexts further allows advancing our understanding of such complex and heterogeneous phenomena as ASD above and beyond verbal descriptions and interpretations of the continuous flow of actions, largely missed by the naked eye.

Theoretically, our proposal to think of movements and their inherent variability as important forms of feedback to estimate sensory and somatic motor consequences is rooted in a nonmodular and more contextual and organismic view of human cognition. We are acutely aware that many researchers work under different, more modular and brain–body dualistic paradigms that treat the brain as a bodiless organ and describe the emergent mental states in complete disconnect from physical states of the nervous systems. In fact, one can see the classifications used in the DSM-5 as, to a large extent, simply assuming what the philosopher Susan Hurley has labeled the "classical sandwich of cognition," that is, the idea that there are neat divisions between sensory and motor systems and that central cognitive processes rely on a relatively modular neurological machinery that is independent not only of sensorimotor processes but also of peripheral and autonomic systems more broadly (Hurley 2001). Similarly, Daniel Rogers has documented in great detail how twentieth-century psychiatry is ripe with examples of theoretically based arguments either denying or isolating motor and neurological issues from our understanding of psychiatric cases and psychological function more broadly (Rogers 1992).

However, we see little current empirical evidence in support of blindly assuming such abstract models or of letting our assessment and classification of neurodevelopment depend on them. Given evidence pertaining to contextual influences and feedback in development, evolution, physiology, neurology, and so many areas of molecular and cognitive neuroscience, it seems that one would have to empirically prove any clean modularity of, for example, the motor system from the sensory systems, or of cognitive or cortical processes from subcortical, peripheral, and autonomic systems. In short, it seems that the burden of proof might be on the researcher that assumes isolation rather than the one that starts with an assumption of possible integration and cross talk between the many regulatory subsystems. To repeat the insight from Peirce, in a historical system it is stability rather than change that primarily calls for an explanation (Peirce 1891). We thus do not deny or attempt to ignore that there are anatomically differentiated subsystems that function with relative autonomy. Rather, what we hope to do is to explain why and how this feat of relative autonomy, isolation, and stability gradually self-emerges and is ultimately accomplished in typical neurodevelopment. In other words, how do we succeed in isolating and using meaningful signals in the cacophony of variabilities and noise that we are embodied and embedded in? We aim at discovering the specific ways in which such processes might be disrupted in various clinical cases, and thereby be better positioned to aid and support such processes when the organism faces developmental challenges. To summarize, we are not claiming that people with autism cannot move—we are hypothesizing that individually heterogeneous difficulties with various forms of regulatory and adaptive control will be reflected in the microstructure of movement variability continuously registered as the person naturally interacts with physical objects or, for example, the social medium of a clinician.

However, as discussed, highly modular and narrow theoretical conceptions of movement prevail in the current clinical definition of autism, and symptoms are typically based on predefined cognitive categories associated with studies of a "bodiless brain" (Baron-Cohen et al. 1985; Happe et al. 2001; Chakrabarti and Baron-Cohen 2006; Happe and Frith 2006; Ramachandran and Oberman 2006; Sucksmith et al. 2013). Reducing the level of inquiry to discrete descriptions and subjective interpretations of observable phenomena makes the problem unnecessarily intractable. But more importantly, ignoring the continuity and physical bases of behavior misses the opportunity to therapeutically close the feedback loops within the person's nervous systems and also between the person's nervous systems and those of the participating interlocutor in the social dyad.

Further, in terms of moving the research forward, existing approaches leave little room for blind reproducibility of results and limit constructive diversified discussion of possible methods to pose new questions and advance our basic understanding of this complex problem. Additionally, current cognitive theoretical constructs are not conducive to empirical questions that enable bridging the layer of inventories that these theories promote (Baron-Cohen and Wheelwright 2004; Baron-Cohen et al. 2005; Wheelwright et al. 2006) with the layers of genetic research that could advance target treatments.

We thus see pervasive human, financial, therapeutic, and scientific consequences of the current too narrow cognitivist definitions, and hope that our new approach can contribute to a broadening of the conceptual landscape, and thus the empirical science of autism. The new proposed approach can hopefully also contribute to the expansion and diversification of available therapies in the United States by virtue of providing a concrete framework for outcome measures to enable insurance coverage (see Chapter 27). Note that this is independent of whether the intervention in question is medical or behavioral. In terms of empathic understanding, we hope that looking at the dynamics of micro-movements will help transform the perception of this condition, and thereby, to some extent, reframe actual interactions. One aspect here that is often assumed in both clinical and educational settings is that the affected person is in full control of his or her behavior, but we suggest that such control is precisely an accomplishment that can be aided by special accommodations and therapeutic and medical expertise in various fields. Further, many symptomatic behaviors, such as "stimming," averted gaze, and ritualistic routines, might be understood as coping mechanisms supporting stability and control of perception and action. Thus, rather than being taken as focal intended and communicative behaviors in the interaction, these might better be seen as personal accommodations, much like posture adjustments and autonomic responses such as blinking. Overall, one could hope that some of the bullying the children suffer today (Zablotsky et al. 2014) might be dampened in the face of new, more scientific definitions of the condition and the potential of public knowledge of the core physiological symptoms.

CONCLUSION AND TAKE-HOME MESSAGE

In short, much like one might look at marine sediment and ice cores in order to infer and assess climate conditions of the past and further use this understanding to analyze the present, we suggest that biophysical rhythms output by the nervous systems contain a rich interlayered basis for assessing neurodevelopment. Further—and in contrast to the ice core analogy—because of the dynamic and stochastic nature of the motions embedded in the nervous systems' rhythms and property of self-sensing their own self-produced movements, these motions (in the broadest sense of the word) can also provide an important handle for intervention and developmental support. Movement, in this sense, gives a dynamic window into neurodevelopment and the many influences of early interventions that are at present blindly performed. We need to know, for instance, the effects that combinations of different drug classes (psychotropic or otherwise) may have on a developing nervous system. They were not tested in the first place with neurodevelopment in mind. We do not know what effects behavioral modifying techniques may have on the children's nervous systems, beyond tantrums, self-injurious behaviors, and anxiety attacks reported by self-advocates, parents, and therapists. We do not know how to objectively and automatically track the balance between benefit and risk of any intervention today. Even without directly revealing the causes of autism, movement variability does provide a new powerful physiological lens into all these issues. As such, motion and its sensations are bound to become our great ally in beginning to unravel the dynamic evolving complexities of ASDs, in terms of both development and when subject to treatments. It would be foolish not to take advantage of such a powerful new access point. In Chapter 2, we look at autism through this new physiological lens to go beyond purely psychological constructs. Through this lens, we learn much more about autism than meets the eye.

REFERENCES

Baron-Cohen, S., A. M. Leslie, and U. Frith. 1985. Does the autistic child have a "theory of mind"? *Cognition* 21 (1):37–46. doi: 0010-0277(85)90022-8 [pii].

Baron-Cohen, S., and S. Wheelwright. 2004. The empathy quotient: An investigation of adults with Asperger syndrome or high functioning autism, and normal sex differences. *J Autism Dev Disord* 34 (2):163–75.

Baron-Cohen, S., S. Wheelwright, J. Robinson, and M. Woodbury-Smith. 2005. The Adult Asperger Assessment (AAA): A diagnostic method. *J Autism Dev Disord* 35 (6):807–19. doi: 10.1007/s10803–005–0026–5.

Brincker, M., and E. B. Torres. 2013. Noise from the periphery in autism. *Front Integr Neurosci* 7:34. doi: 10.3389/fnint.2013.00034.

Chakrabarti, B., and S. Baron-Cohen. 2006. Empathizing: Neurocognitive developmental mechanisms and individual differences. *Prog Brain Res* 156:403–17. doi:10.1016/S0079–6123(06)56022–4.

Damasio, A. R., and R. G. Maurer. 1978. A neurological model for childhood autism. *Arch Neurol* 35 (12):777–86.

De Jaegher, H., and E. Di Paolo. 2007. Participatory sense-making: An enactive approach to social cognition. *Phenomenol Cogn Sci* 6 (4):485–507.

Dewey, J. 1896. The reflex arc concept in psychology. *Psychol Rev* 3:357–60.

Donnellan, A. M., D. A. Hill, and M. R. Leary. 2012. Rethinking autism: Implications of sensory and movement differences for understanding and support. *Front Integr Neurosci* 6:124. doi: 10.3389/fnint.2012.00124.

Donnellan, A. M., and M. R. Leary. 2012. *Autism: Sensory-Movement Differences and Diversity.* 1st ed. Cambridge, WI: Cambridge Book Review Press.

Faisal, A. A., L. P. Selen, and D. M. Wolpert. 2008. Noise in the nervous system. *Nat Rev Neurosci* 9 (4): 292–303. doi:10.1038/nrn2258.

Flegal, K. M., and T. J. Cole. 2013. Construction of LMS parameters for the Centers for Disease Control and Prevention 2000 growth charts. *Natl Health Stat Report* (63):1–3.

Fournier, K. A., C. J. Hass, S. K. Naik, N. Lodha, and J. H. Cauraugh. 2010a. Motor coordination in autism spectrum disorders: A synthesis and meta-analysis. *J Autism Dev Disord* 40 (10):1227–40. doi: 10.1007/s10803–010–0981–3.

Fournier, K. A., C. I. Kimberg, K. J. Radonovich, M. D. Tillman, J. W. Chow, M. H. Lewis, J. W. Bodfish, and C. J. Hass. 2010b. Decreased static and dynamic postural control in children with autism spectrum disorders. *Gait Posture* 32 (1):6–9. doi: 10.1016/j.gaitpost.2010.02.007.

Friston, K., C. Thornton, and A. Clark. 2012. Free-energy minimization and the dark-room problem. *Front Psychol* 3:130. doi: 10.3389/fpsyg.2012.00130.

Gibson, J. J. 1960. The concept of the stimulus in psychology. *Am Psychol* 15:694–703.

Gibson, J. J. 1979. *The Ecological Approach to Visual Perception.* Boston: Houghton Mifflin.

Gowen, E., J. Stanley, and R. C. Miall. 2008. Movement interference in autism-spectrum disorder. *Neuropsychologia* 46 (4):1060–8. doi: 10.1016/j.neuropsychologia.2007.11.004.

Grusser, O. J. 1995. On the history of the ideas of efference copy and reafference. *Clio Med* 33:35–55.

Happe, F., J. Briskman, and U. Frith. 2001. Exploring the cognitive phenotype of autism: Weak "central coherence" in parents and siblings of children with autism. I. Experimental tests. *J Child Psychol Psychiatry* 42 (3):299–307.

Happe, F., and U. Frith. 2006. The weak coherence account: Detail-focused cognitive style in autism spectrum disorders. *J Autism Dev Disord* 36 (1):5–25. doi: 10.1007/s10803–005–0039–0.

Haruno, M., D. M. Wolpert, and M. Kawato. 2001. Mosaic model for sensorimotor learning and control. *Neural Comput* 13 (10):2201–20. doi: 10.1162/089976601750541778.

Hurley, S. L. 2001. Perception and action: Alternative views. *Synthese* 129:3–40.

Jansiewicz, E. M., M. C. Goldberg, C. J. Newschaffer, M. B. Denckla, R. Landa, and S. H. Mostofsky. 2006. Motor signs distinguish children with high functioning autism and Asperger's syndrome from controls. *J Autism Dev Disord* 36 (5):613–21. doi: 10.1007/s10803-006-0109-y.

Jones, V., and M. Prior. 1985. Motor imitation abilities and neurological signs in autistic children. *J Autism Dev Disord* 15 (1):37–46.

Kalampratsidou, V., and E. B. Torres. 2016. Outcome measures of deliberate and spontaneous motions. Presented at the Third International Symposium on Movement and Computing MOCO'16, Thessaloniki, Greece, July 5–6.

Kording, K. P., and D. M. Wolpert. 2004. Bayesian integration in sensorimotor learning. *Nature* 427 (6971): 244–7. doi: 10.1038/nature02169

Kording, K. P., and D. M. Wolpert. 2006. Probabilistic mechanisms in sensorimotor control. *Novartis Found Symp* 270:191–8; discussion 198–202, 232–7.

Kuczmarski, R. J., C. L. Ogden, S. S. Guo, L. M. Grummer-Strawn, K. M. Flegal, Z. Mei, R. Wei, L. R. Curtin, A. F. Roche, and C. L. Johnson. 2002. 2000 CDC growth charts for the United States: Methods and development. *Vital Health Stat* 11 (246):1–190.

Lord, C., M. Rutter, P. C. DiLavore, S. Risi, and Western Psychological Services. *Autism Diagnostic Observation Schedule ADOS Manual*. Torrance, CA: Western Psychological Services.

Minshew, N. J., K. Sung, B. L. Jones, and J. M. Furman. 2004. Underdevelopment of the postural control system in autism. *Neurology* 63 (11):2056–61. doi: 63/11/2056 [pii].

Mosconi, M. W., S. Mohanty, R. K. Greene, E. H. Cook, D. E. Vaillancourt, and J. A. Sweeney. 2015. Feedforward and feedback motor control abnormalities implicate cerebellar dysfunctions in autism spectrum disorder. *J Neurosci* 35 (5):2015–25. doi: 10.1523/JNEUROSCI.2731-14.2015.

Mosconi, M. W., and J. A. Sweeney. 2015. Sensorimotor dysfunctions as primary features of autism spectrum disorders. *Sci China Life Sci* 58 (10):1016–23. doi: 10.1007/s11427-015-4894-4.

Mostofsky, S. H., P. Dubey, V. K. Jerath, E. M. Jansiewicz, M. C. Goldberg, and M. B. Denckla. 2006. Developmental dyspraxia is not limited to imitation in children with autism spectrum disorders. *J Int Neuropsychol Soc* 12 (3):314–26.

Noterdaeme, M., K. Mildenberger, F. Minow, and H. Amorosa. 2002. Evaluation of neuromotor deficits in children with autism and children with a specific speech and language disorder. *Eur Child Adolesc Psychiatry* 11 (5):219–25. doi: 10.1007/s00787-002-0285-z.

Peirce, C. S. 1981. The Architecture of Theories. *The Monist. Reprinted in Philosophical Writings of Peirce,* ed. Buchler, J. New York: Dover, 1955.

Ramachandran, V. S., and L. M. Oberman. 2006. Broken mirrors: A theory of autism. *Sci Am* 295 (5):62–9.

Rinehart, N. J., J. L. Bradshaw, A. V. Brereton, and B. J. Tonge. 2001. Movement preparation in high-functioning autism and Asperger disorder: A serial choice reaction time task involving motor reprogramming. *J Autism Dev Disord* 31 (1):79–88.

Robledo, J., A. M. Donnellan, and K. Strandt-Conroy. 2012. An exploration of sensory and movement differences from the perspective of individuals with autism. *Front Integr Neurosci* 6:107. doi: 10.3389/fnint.2012.00107.

Rogers, D. M. 1992. *Motor Disorder in Psychiatry: Towards a Neurological Psychiatry*. Chichester: J. Wiley & Sons.

Rogers, S. J., L. Bennetto, R. McEvoy, and B. F. Pennington. 1996. Imitation and pantomime in high-functioning adolescents with autism spectrum disorders. *Child Dev* 67 (5):2060–73.

Shadmehr, R., and S. P. Wise. 2005. *The Computational Neurobiology of Reaching and Pointing: A Foundation for Motor Learning, Computational Neuroscience*. Cambridge, MA: MIT Press.

Silberman, S. 2015. *Neurotribes: The Legacy of Autism and the Future of Neurodiversity*. New York: Avery, an imprint of Penguin Random House.

Smith, L. B., and E. Thelen. 1993. *A Dynamic Systems Approach to Development: Applications*. MIT Press/Bradford Books Series in Cognitive Psychology. Cambridge, MA: MIT Press.

Sucksmith, E., C. Allison, S. Baron-Cohen, B. Chakrabarti, and R. A. Hoekstra. 2013. Empathy and emotion recognition in people with autism, first-degree relatives, and controls. *Neuropsychologia* 51 (1):98–105. doi: 10.1016/j.neuropsychologia.2012.11.013.

Teitelbaum, O., T. Benton, P. K. Shah, A. Prince, J. L. Kelly, and P. Teitelbaum. 2004. Eshkol-Wachman movement notation in diagnosis: The early detection of Asperger's syndrome. *Proc Natl Acad Sci USA* 101 (32): 11909–14. doi: 10.1073/pnas.0403919101.

Teitelbaum, P., O. B. Teitelbaum, J. Fryman, and R. Maurer. 2002. Infantile reflexes gone astray in autism. *J Dev Learn Disord* 6:15.

Thelen, E., and L. B. Smith. 1994. A dynamic systems approach to the development of cognition and action. In: *MIT Press/Bradford Books Series in Cognitive Psychology*. Cambridge, MA: MIT Press.

Torres, E. B. 2011. Two classes of movements in motor control. *Exp Brain Res* 215 (3–4):269–83. doi: 10.1007/s00221-011-2892-8.

Torres, E. B. 2016. Rethinking the study of volition for clinical use. In *Progress in Motor Control: Theories and Translations*, ed. J. Lazcko and M. Latash. New York: Springer, pp 229–254.

Torres, E. B., M. Brincker, R. W. Isenhower, P. Yanovich, K. A. Stigler, J. I. Nurnberger, D. N. Metaxas, and J. V. Jose. 2013a. Autism: The micro-movement perspective. *Front Integr Neurosci* 7:32. doi: 10.3389/fnint.2013.00032.

Torres, E. B., J. Cole, and H. Poizner. 2014. Motor output variability, deafferentation, and putative deficits in kinesthetic reafference in Parkinson's disease. *Front Hum Neurosci* 8:823. doi: 10.3389/fnhum.2014.00823.

Torres, E. B., and K. Denisova. 2016. Motor noise is rich signal in autism research and pharmacological treatments. *Sci Rep* 6:37422. doi: 10.1038/srep37422.

Torres, E. B., and A. M. Donnellan. 2015. Autism: the movement perspective. *Front. Integr. Neurosci.* 9:12. doi: 10.3389/fnint.2015.00012.

Torres, E. B., R. W. Isenhower, J. Nguyen, C. Whyatt, J. I. Nurnberger, J. V. Jose, S. M. Silverstein, T. V. Papathomas, J. Sage, and J. Cole. 2016a. Toward precision psychiatry: Statistical platform for the personalized characterization of natural behaviors. *Front Neurol* 7:8. doi: 10.3389/fneur.2016.00008.

Torres, E. B., R. W. Isenhower, P. Yanovich, G. Rehrig, K. Stigler, J. Nurnberger, and J. V. Jose. 2013b. Strategies to develop putative biomarkers to characterize the female phenotype with autism spectrum disorders. *J Neurophysiol* 110 (7):1646–62. doi: 10.1152/jn.00059.2013.

Torres, E. B., B. Smith, S. Mistry, M. Brincker, and C. Whyatt. 2016b. Neonatal diagnostics: Toward dynamic growth charts of neuromotor control. *Front Pediatr* 4 (121):1–15. doi: 10.3389/fped.2016.00121.

Torres, E. B., P. Yanovich, and D. N. Metaxas. 2013c. Give spontaneity and self-discovery a chance in ASD: Spontaneous peripheral limb variability as a proxy to evoke centrally driven intentional acts. *Front Integr Neurosci* 7:46.

Uexküll, J. von. 1928. *Theoretische biologie*. Berlin: J. Springer.

Von Holst, E. 1954. Relations between the central nervous system and the peripheral organs. *Br J Anim Behav* 2 (3):89–94.

Von Holst, E., and H. Mittelstaedt. 1950. The principle of reafference: Interactions between the central nervous system and the peripheral organs. In *Perceptual Processing: Stimulus Equivalence and Pattern Recognition*, ed. P. C. Dodwell, 41–72. New York: Appleton-Century-Crofts.

Wheelwright, S., S. Baron-Cohen, N. Goldenfeld, J. Delaney, D. Fine, R. Smith, L. Weil, and A. Wakabayashi. 2006. Predicting autism spectrum quotient (AQ) from the systemizing quotient-revised (SQ-R) and empathy quotient (EQ). *Brain Res* 1079 (1):47–56. doi: 10.1016/j.brainres.2006.01.012.

Whyatt, C., A. Mars, E. DiCicco-Bloom, and E. B. Torres. 2015. Objective characterization of sensory-motor physiology underlying dyadic interactions during the Autism Diagnostic Observation Schedule-2: Implications for research and clinical diagnosis. Presented at the Annual Meeting of the Society for Neuroscience, Chicago, October 17–21.

Williams, J. H., A. Whiten, T. Suddendorf, and D. I. Perrett. 2001. Imitation, mirror neurons and autism. *Neurosci Biobehav Rev* 25 (4):287–95. doi: S0149-7634(01)00014-8 [pii].

Wolpert, D. M., and M. Kawato. 1998. Multiple paired forward and inverse models for motor control. *Neural Netw* 11 (7–8):1317–29. doi: S0893-6080(98)00066-5 [pii].

Wolpert, D. M., and R. C. Miall. 1996. Forward models for physiological motor control. *Neural Netw* 9 (8): 1265–79. doi: S0893608096000354 [pii].

Wolpert, D. M., R. C. Miall, and M. Kawato. 1998. Internal models in the cerebellum. *Trends Cogn Sci* 2 (9): 338–47.

Zablotsky, B., C. P. Bradshaw, C. M. Anderson, and P. Law. 2014. Risk factors for bullying among children with autism spectrum disorders. *Autism* 18 (4):419–27. doi: 10.1177/1362361313477920.

2 The Autism Phenotype
Physiology versus Psychology?

Caroline Whyatt

CONTENTS

Introduction....23
The ASD Phenotype: Role of Associated Secondary Symptoms....24
Autism Spectrum Disorder: Psychological versus Physiological....25
Behavior: A Physiological Stance....26
Development of Behavior....26
ASD: A By-Product of Underdeveloped Nervous Systems? The Developmental Trajectory....28
Associated Sensory Symptoms....28
Associated Motor Symptoms....29
Parallels With Physiologically Grounded Disorders: Parkinson's Disease—A Model for ASD?....32
ASD and PD: The Missing Link?....34
ASD: Does the Evidence Suggest It Is Time for a New Model?....34
References....35

In Chapter 1, the role of movement, and movement sensing, was eloquently illustrated, positing the need for a reconceptualization of autism spectrum disorders (ASDs). In particular, the limited perspective of ASD as a psychiatric disorder, viewed and conceptualized through an isolated cognitivist lens, was discussed in light of academic evidence to the contrary. Throughout this chapter, evidence is presented illustrating the pervasive nature of sensory processing and motor control to higher-level outcomes, such as social and cognitive skills. Viewed from a developmental perspective, questions will be posed regarding the isolated and artificial segregation of higher-level symptomatology to characterize ASD, and the repeated resistance to the inclusion of such secondary or "associated" sensory and movement skills. This chapter thus aims to further discuss and elucidate the impact and limitation of this arguably restricted view, and further asks, is it time for a new model of ASD?

INTRODUCTION

Introduced in the fifth edition of the *Diagnostic and Statistical Manual of Mental Disorders* (DSM-5) (APA 2013), *autism spectrum disorder* (ASD) is an umbrella term encompassing autism, Asperger's syndrome (AS), and pervasive developmental disorder—not otherwise specified (PDD-NOS). Clinically defined and characterized by "classical" behavioral symptomatology (impaired social and communicative ability, and restricted and repetitive behaviors) (APA 2013), ASD is broadly conceptualized as a social-cognitive disorder—a characterization that persists across both the clinical and academic fields.

Within the clinical domain, ASD is defined and examined through a "triad" of behavioral impairments—socialization, communication, and imagination—all of which reflect this overarching conceptualization (Wing and Gould 1979). These core behavioral difficulties are assessed using clinical diagnostic tools, such as the Autism Diagnostic Observation Schedule 2 (ADOS-2)

(Lord et al. 2012) and Autism Diagnostic Interview–Revised (ADI-R) (Lord et al. 1994). A focus on key behavioral impairment within this framework facilitates the diagnosis procedure, which in turn enables the timely provision of developmental and educational services. As such, the impact of this arguably restricted conceptualization of ASD is unknown, and may be limited within the clinical arena (Donnellan 1984).

Within the academic domain, these classical, overt behavioral difficulties have been extensively researched, leading to a long-standing focus on three predominant theories of ASD, all of which have a strong social-cognitive thread: theory of mind (Baron-Cohen et al. 1985), weak central coherence theory (Frith 1989), and executive functioning theory (Ozonoff et al. 1991; Ozonoff and McEvoy 1994). Yet, the integrity of this clinically reinforced perception of ASD, and the corresponding cognitive theoretical constructs, has been repeatedly questioned within the academic community—from the testing metrics used to the discriminant ability of such models to isolate ASD from other developmental conditions (see De Jaegher 2013; Whyatt and Craig 2013a). Indeed, these functionalized and fragmented social-cognitivist theories, despite being popularized within the clinical and academic arenas, fail to account for the diverse, heterogeneous spectrum phenotype of ASD (see also Whyatt and Craig 2013a; De Jaegher 2013). Given the recent amalgamation of neurodevelopmental disorders into the umbrella of ASD, questions are raised over the persistent clinical and academic conceptualization of a social-cognitive disorder entrenched within the psychological, psychiatric that endorses a symptom-based approach.

THE ASD PHENOTYPE: ROLE OF ASSOCIATED SECONDARY SYMPTOMS

First presented in the seminal works of Leo Kanner (1943) and Hans Asperger (1944), autism and AS were long considered distinct developmental disorders in terms of both epidemiology and nosology. In particular, both were quantified and classified by levels of language and intellectual ability. Critically, however, Asperger noted a range of lower-level motor peculiarities:

> Gross motor movements are clumsy and ill-coordinated. Posture and gait appear odd [90% of the 34 cases mentioned above] are poor at games involving motor skills. (Asperger, translated in Wing 1981, p. 116)

Further quantified and discussed by British psychiatrist Lorna Wing (1981), these motor difficulties were proposed to be a critical component isolating the two disorders:

> The one area in which … comparison does not seem to apply is in motor development. Typically, autistic children tend to be good at climbing and balancing when young. Those with Asperger's syndrome, on the other hand, are notably ill-coordinated in posture, gait and gestures. (Wing 1981, p. 123)

Despite this distinction, Wing argued for the consideration of AS and autism as part of a larger group of conditions characterized by a range of communal symptoms—introducing the "triad of impairments" (Wing and Gould 1979; Wing 1981). This rather controversial view of a "spectrum of autism" (Nordin and Gillberg 1996; Wing 1997) led to a flurry of research examining the true extent of communal symptoms. This research served to illustrate the broader phenotype of autism (e.g., Dawson et al. 2002), with similarities across a range of axes, including lower-level motor characteristics. Specifically, through the use of modern standardized behavioral tools of movement assessment and pioneering technologies, a growing range of evidence has illustrated the ubiquitous nature of motor peculiarities. Early results cited abnormal gait, postural control, bradykinesia, hyperagility, and dystonia as some of the most prevalent movement abnormalities within both autism and AS, supporting Wing's spectrum of autism (Damasio and Maurer 1978; Vilensky et al. 1981; Kohen-Raz et al. 1992; Hallett et al. 1993).

It was in the publication of the DSM-4 (APA 1994) that autism and AS were first viewed on a spectrum or continuum of a single disorder, a reconceptualization that was completed with the publication of the DSM-5 (APA 2013). Yet, despite this amalgamation, the building evidence for the presence of sensory-motor difficulties across the entire spectrum of ASD remains largely abandoned, even within recent diagnostic criteria.* Rather, the triad of impairments remains characteristic of the spectrum's phenotype. Sensory-motor difficulties remain a secondary or associated symptom contained within the ambiguous category of symptomatology "restricted and repetitive behaviors"—rather than as a fourth axis of impairment (Wing and Gould 1979; Ming et al. 2007). This omission may reflect an ongoing tension between our conceptualization of ASD as a psychological or physiological construct.

AUTISM SPECTRUM DISORDER: PSYCHOLOGICAL VERSUS PHYSIOLOGICAL

ASD—and its predecessors—has been traditionally considered a psychological or psychiatric condition, reflected in a social-cognitive conceptualization and theoretical foundation. Diagnosed through behavioral observation—reflecting the working model of the DSM-5—ASD continues to be viewed as a mental disorder characterized by behavioral disturbance. However, from a computational perspective these behavioral outcomes may be indicative of underlying etiology. Unlike mental health disorders, such as dementia or depression, there is a dearth of clinical, medical, and academic knowledge of, and importantly consensus on, the underlying physical etiology of ASD—perhaps, in part, reflective of this psychological position. By subsuming sensory-motor difficulties under "restricted and repetitive behaviors," the diagnostic and clinical domains retain a psychological stance—with such behaviors tied to existing social-cognitive theoretical frameworks, particularly weak central coherence and executive functioning theories (Frith 1989; Ozonoff et al. 1991; Ozonoff and McEvoy 1994). However, in light of the recent quantification of persistent lower-level sensory-motor difficulties, should ASD be characterized as a psychological construct?

The 10th revision of the International Classification of Diseases (ICD-10) (WHO 1994), the core medical listing of "disease and related health problems," provides a comprehensive encyclopedia of both psychological and physiological conditions. ASD can be found in Section F80-F89 under "Disorders of Psychological Development" of the "Mental and Behavioral Disorders: Diagnostic Criteria."† This section block is prefaced with the following statement:

> The disorders included in this block have in common: (a) onset invariably during infancy or childhood; (b) impairment or delay in development of functions that are strongly related to *biological maturation of the central nervous system*; … affected include language, visuo-spatial skills, and motor coordination.

The DSM, published by the American Psychiatric Association (current version—APA 2013), operationalizes the working symptomatology of mental disorders listed in the ICD-10 and is the leading manual of mental disorders adopted across the United States and further afield.‡ Despite reference to potential physiological etiology and sensory and motor difficulties within the ICD-10, these features are omitted from the operationalization of ASD within the DSM—including the most recent version, DSM-5 (APA 2013)—in accordance with a psychological perspective.

Why does ASD remain viewed and characterized as a psychological construct founded upon, and diagnosed via, core social-cognitive deficits? This preserved characterization and conceptualization is perhaps unsurprising due to a number of factors. First, the clinical domain and the DSM hold strength within this arena, directly influencing and guiding diagnostic criteria, and thus conceptualization (see Chapter 27). Second, the existence of ASD on a continuum of ranging severity and

* Indeed, although serving an alternative purpose, namely, illustrating the continuity or spectrum of ASD, this research solidified evidence for the presence of significant sensory-motor difficulties, and led to the emergence of a new field of related inquiry.

† For full diagnostic information for ASD according to the ICD-10, see http://apps.who.int/classifications/icd10/browse/2016/en#/F80-F89.

‡ For full diagnostic information for ASD according to the DSM-5, see https://www.autismspeaks.org/what-autism/diagnosis/dsm-5-diagnostic-criteria.

symptomatology serves to magnify the difficulty of deconstructing complex behaviors into underlying physiological expressions. Specifically, the range of social-cognitive behaviors that are characteristic of the ASD phenotype are complex, and have yet to be comprehensively deconstructed to consider underlying neurophysiology. These core constructs, which remain firmly ensconced within the behavioral and psychological realm, are further hampered by the early disconnect between psychology and modern neuroscience. Indeed, as a field, psychology as defined by Descartes (1984) traditionally viewed the mind and brain as distinct—resulting in the disembodied perspective alluded to in Chapter 1. Despite this, however, behavioral outcomes from physical movement to complex higher-level social-cognitive processing can be fundamentally viewed as the physical reaction to, and active engagement with, our external environment.

BEHAVIOR: A PHYSIOLOGICAL STANCE

Behavior in its purest form can be conceptualized as a mediated* response, often physical, to incoming sensory stimuli. These afferent sensory stimuli are bound and synthesized, generating an internal percept to guide an appropriate response. Behavioral responses can be reflexive and automatic, or can be goal directed and voluntarily mediated by internal need, intention, and rewards (Haggard 2008). Higher-cortical control centers, such as the prefrontal cortex, differentiate such voluntary, top-down coordinated control from early or reflexive behaviors—leading to a focus on higher-level cognitive processes in the understanding of human behavior. This is reflected in the examination and understanding of ASD from a social-cognitive stance. However, even during cortically mediated voluntary actions sensory stimuli (and their consequences) remain the guiding factor in the planning, and thus organization, of simple and complex behavior. In particular, during development, the infant builds an internal representation or schematic based on these early exploratory behaviors. The consequences of behaviors, and the resulting sensory stimuli, are "sampled," building a stochastic, predictive platform from which an individual can predict the consequences of an action, and the identification of perceptual invariants to guide action (Fajen 2005)—allowing a level of prospective control. An inability to build this emergent internal representation will lead an individual to live in the "here and now," reflected in immature levels of prospective control impeding action and resulting in notable behavioral difficulties. Therefore, disruption in behavioral output should be viewed and considered within the context of sensory processing ability and fundamental motor control—both of which may impede behavioral outcomes.

Development of Behavior

A direct extension of the human nervous system, the sensory organs provide our line of communication with the external environment. The foundations for this level of sensory perception and control are laid during early neurulation within the embryo (Volpe 2008), with the initial development of the central and peripheral nervous systems. Subsequent neuronal cell proliferation, migration, and organization provide the foundations for neural control, a process that begins prenatally but continues postnatally. Indeed, postnatal neural plasticity leads to the strengthening and pruning of neural pathways in response to incoming stimuli—guiding neurodevelopment and subsequent behavioral outcomes.

The visual system illustrates this postnatal neurodevelopment and its role in the development of behavior. Born with undifferentiated retinal cells (photoreceptors) and a reliance on the use of subcortical structures for processes, including spatiotopical coding, infant vision is initially blurry and hazy (for review, see Braddick and Atkinson 2011). Postnatal visual development, due to anatomical differentiation and maturation of the nervous systems, leads to increased visual acuity, color vision, and depth perception (Held et al. 1980; Atkinson 2002), resulting in a newfound interest in objects and faces within the environment. This environmental inquisition drives subsequent active, volitional

* Mediation that differentiates this conceptualization from a pure stimuli-response paradigm.

exploratory behaviors, which provide the foundational building blocks for social and cognitive development. Indeed, infants born with impaired vision are known to display a limited range of infant exploratory and complex play behaviors (Tröster and Brambring 1994), resulting in delayed motor, cognitive, and social development (McAlpine and Moore 1995; Bouchard and Tetreault 2000; Levtzion-Korach et al. 2000; Brambring 2006).

A more overt example of nervous system and behavioral development is observed in motor outcomes during infancy. Born as altricial organisms, the human infant must develop postnatal motor patterns for the establishment of meaningful, volitional behaviors. Arnold Gesell, a pioneer in infant development tracking, observed invariant sequences and stages of infant development (Gesell and Amatruda 1945, 1947). These stages were used to create a motor and behavioral developmental trajectory that focused on morphological maturation (Gesell and Amatruda 1945). Similarly, McGraw (1940) argued that infant development is a direct result of underlying neural growth. Through neural maturation—proliferation, pruning, and migration—the infant develops new patterns of behavior, moving away from "primitive reflexes" (McGraw 1940; Hadders-Algra 2000) toward higher levels of goal-directed autonomy and intentionality. Theories of physiological maturation are reflected in common clinical tools, such as motor milestone charts (Wijnhoven et al. 2004) and standardized tests of motor control,* which were developed on the premise that an infant will logically progress through a pattern of motor coordination as, and when, the developing system adapts. Such frameworks thus seek to identify and profile neurodevelopment through the sequence of motor output or growth patterns.

In contrast to this linear predefined hierarchical maturational stance, the dynamical systems (DS) approach (Thelen and Smith 1994) considered development an emergent and self-organizing consequence of recursive interactions with the environment. Motor or behavioral development was considered a nonlinear, evolving dynamic dependent on the assimilation of afferent sensory feedback—explicitly coupling sensory and motor development in an iterative loop. This afferent sensory feedback can take many forms, including visual and auditory; yet, it can also be "kinesthetic sensation" (Thelen and Smith 1994, p. 193) or "kinesthetic reafference" (Holst and Mittelstaedt 1950)—the direct sensing of movement from the peripheral nervous system through the dorsal root ganglia and spinocerebellar tract—a concept introduced in Chapter 1. Thus, with concomitantly occurring multimodal afferent feedback, along with kinesthetic reafference from self-produced active movements, sensory-motor behaviors can become tightly coupled (e.g., Holst and Mittelstaedt 1950; Gibson and Walk 1960; Held 1965; Gibson 1988; Bushnell and Boudreau 1993). Recent evidence suggests that disruption of this form of afferent feedback results in impaired levels of corporeal self-awareness and sensory-motor acquisition, and impedes movement (Cole and Paillard 1995; Fourneret et al. 2002; Stenneken et al. 2006; Balslev et al. 2007; Torres et al. 2014). Indeed, early passive behavior has been linked to an underdevelopment of the visual cortex (e.g., Singer 1985) and poor levels of later motor coordination (Held 1965). Through this process, and by virtue of neural plasticity, a topographic somatosensory map is achieved—providing the infant foundations for allo- and egocentric transformations to guide spatial awareness across coordinate systems (e.g., Cartesian external coordinates transformed into internal torques and dynamics)—vital in the development of internal models of motor control (e.g., Uno et al. 1989; Wolpert et al. 1998; Kawato 1999). Importantly, optimal early exploratory behaviors contain high levels of variability allowing the "sampling" of multiple behavioral permutations (see Chapter 1 for additional information, as well as Thelen and Smith 1994). This active, variable sampling allows the infant to generate predictions—associating motor output and sensory feedback—a cornerstone of subsequent internal models of motor control (e.g., Uno et al. 1989; Wolpert et al. 1998). Therefore, a lack of early exploratory behaviors may impede subsequent levels of coordination and control (Whyatt and Craig 2013a). In addition, it has been proposed that this environmental sampling is retained at a microlevel across movements throughout

* For example, Peabody Developmental Motor Scales (Folio and Fewell 2000) and Movement Assessment Battery for Children (Henderson et al. 2007).

the life span—leading to minute variation or "micromovements" in the motor signature, as introduced in Chapter 1, and detailed further in Chapters 8, 13 and 14 (see also Torres et al. 2013, 2016). The stochastic probabilistic cumulative signature of these micromovements then provides a blueprint of underlying predictability of the system—aiding in the identification of levels of neurodevelopment and diversity (Torres et al. 2016).

From a computational motor perspective, physical behaviors are thus a response to an internal percept selected based on internal state and cortical control (e.g., needs [Haggard 2008]). Internal models of motor control formulated during early infancy—and continually refined—use error-based contingencies or optimal outcomes to guide coordinated behavioral actions in response (e.g., Wolpert and Kawato 1998; Wolpert et al. 1998; Uno et al. 1989). This breakdown encapsulates the overarching simplified process of behavior, from simple motor actions through to complex social responses or cognitive behaviors. As nervous system refinement and development provide the foundations of sensory and motor progression, both of which guide behavioral outcomes, these components provide valuable insight into underlying physiological functioning. Given the presence of sensory and motor associated symptoms, the role of the nervous systems in ASD is questioned, in line with inferences made by the ICD-10 (WHO 1994).

ASD: A BY-PRODUCT OF UNDERDEVELOPED NERVOUS SYSTEMS? THE DEVELOPMENTAL TRAJECTORY

In spite of the continued classification of ASD as a psychological construct, a myriad of sensory and motor difficulties implicate underlying physiological difficulties. Building on advances in technology, namely, noninvasive motion capture and brain imaging techniques, such as fMRI, EEG, and PET,* associated phenotypic behaviors of ASD are being further clarified—culminating in new evidence of the etiology and neurobiology of ASD.

Associated Sensory Symptoms

Statistics indicate that approximately 90% of children and adults with an ASD experience pronounced sensory difficulties (Leekam et al. 2007). These include hyper- and hyposensitivity to sensory stimulation, resulting in seeking (e.g. stimming) and aversion behaviors, and difficulty with multisensory integration (Wallace and Stevenson 2014). In addition to providing support to lower-level symptoms, these irregularities with sensory processing may result in overt behavioral difficulties—such as those used to characterize ASD (Wallace and Stevenson 2014). Intuitively, if the sensory system is over- or underwhelmed by external—or internal—sensory stimuli, how can one focus attention and cognitive resources to additional tasks? While often attributed to attention or cognitive processing within the psychological field, pivoting around the weak central coherence theory (Plaisted 2001; Plaisted et al. 2003; Pellicano et al. 2005; Happé and Frith 2006), these fundamental difficulties can be tied to an underlying etiology within the central nervous system. Indeed, behavioral paradigms have illustrated significant variation in the multisensory binding window of individuals with ASD—leading to perceived difficulty in the coherent coupling of independent sensory input (Foss-Feig et al. 2010; Kwakye et al. 2011). Specifically, evidence suggests that individuals with ASD have a prolonged window of multisensory binding, leading to disjointed internal sensory percepts. A reduction in gamma band neural oscillations has been further implicated as the physiological underpinnings of this impaired temporal synchronization and organization between primary sensory processing areas (40 Hz range) (e.g., Tallon-Baudry and Bertrand 1999; Brock et al. 2002). Moreover, despite inherent variability in brain imaging results, ASD has been considered a by-product of irregular neural connectivity—with higher levels of local and a reduction in long-range neural connections

* Functional magnetic resonance imaging, electroencephalogram, and positron emission tomography.

(Courchesne and Pierce 2005). Such variation in levels of connectivity has been repeatedly proposed as the foundational etiology behind classical sensory processing outcomes—often attributed to the cognitive weak central coherence theory (e.g., Minshew et al. 1997). Therefore, ASD has been and continues to be conceptualized, in part, as an information processing condition. However, more recent reports are questioning this interpretation, illustrating the potential role of uncontrolled head movement or "noise" and the resulting overreliance on post hoc "scrubbing" techniques in the interpretation of these fMRI findings (Power et al. 2012; Tyszka et al. 2014; Torres and Denisova 2016). In particular, this evidence implies that an overreliance on scrubbing techniques may artificially lead to conclusions of irregular connectivity. Yet in addition to calling into question the theoretical framework of connectivity at the heart of ASD, such results infer excessive levels of minute head movements associated with a diagnosis—even with preventative measures regularly employed during imaging protocol. Indeed, recent mouse models of ASD imply irregularities in the transduction of sensory information through the peripheral nervous system, leading to sensory processing difficulties and classical ASD behavioral symptomatology (Orefice et al. 2016). In line with new research, there are growing questions regarding the route and purpose of this excessive motor or peripheral noise of the peripheral nervous system (Brincker and Torres 2013)—questions that are discussed further below.

Associated Motor Symptoms

In addition to evidence for neurological underpinnings of sensory processing difficulties associated with ASD, studies have inferred a similar etiology for motor difficulties (see Fournier et al. 2010 for a partial review of motor evidence). Retrospective analysis of home videos illustrates the prevalence of motor difficulties during infancy, with infants who are later diagnosed with ASD displaying impaired acquisition of motor milestones—a potential noninvasive marker (Teitelbaum et al. 1998; Zwaigenbaum et al. 2005; Sutera et al. 2007). With reference to neuronal maturation, this restriction of motor development implies disruption at the level of nervous system development. Motor difficulties range from gross, global behaviors, such as gait and postural control (Vilensky et al. 1981; Minshew et al. 2004; Vernazza-Martin et al. 2005; Rinehart et al. 2006) through to goal-directed voluntary actions, such as fine motor control/visuomotor integration (Provost et al. 2007; Green et al. 2009; Whyatt and Craig 2012). In particular, pronounced difficulties in the timing, initiation, planning, and on-line control of actions have been illustrated (Hughes et al. 1994; Hughes 1996; Mari et al. 2003; Rinehart et al. 2006; Glazebrook et al. 2006, 2008, 2009; Whyatt and Craig 2013a, 2013b). The universal nature of such motor symptoms may imply a wide underlying etiology—with potential loci at subcortical levels, including the cerebellum and basal ganglia or, as this book points toward, the peripheral nervous system.

Phylogenetically old, both the cerebellum and basal ganglia play critical roles in the subcortical control of motor coordination and sensory integration. With a number of iterative loops to regions of the cerebral cortex, including the parietal and primary motor cortices (Bostan et al. 2013), the cerebellum has long been considered a core element of the motor control system. Drawing on internal models of kinematics and dynamics, the cerebellum facilitates the timing and coordination of actions through predictive muscle activation for precise control over multisegmented and complex actions—reducing movement error (e.g., Braitenberg 1967; Ivry et al. 1988; Sasaki and Gemba 1993; Heck 1993, 1995; Braitenberg et al. 1997; Bastian et al. 2000; Doya 2000). The climbing fibers of the inferior olive provide the cerebellum with key afferent information from the periphery for event detection—as coded by an error signal. Specifically, the excitatory action of the climbing fibers from the inferior olive—when concurrently stimulated with parallel fibers—results in a prolonged, yet selective, suppression of future activity of the associated Purkinje cells, which normally display high activation during voluntary behaviors (e.g., Albus 1971; Ito et al. 1982). Activated by a perceived error in performance, such as variation in movement gains or sensory feedback (Gilbert and Thach 1977; Kitazawa et al. 1998), the climbing fibers act as a teaching signal. Thus, subsequent stimulation of the same parallel fibers results in suppressed spike Purkinje cell activity—a modulated response shaped by the error coding of the climbing fibers—facilitating motor learning and modification of behaviors (Albus 1971; Ito et al. 1982; Itō 1984). Utilizing this information, corrective adjustments are made to ongoing actions, and importantly, reliable predictive computational internal models for action are refined (e.g., Wolpert and Kawato 1998; Wolpert et al. 1998; Kawato 1999)—models subsequently utilized to control further tasks.

There is a prevalence of studies implying specific difficulties in motor planning, motor timing, and "smooth" multisegmented actions associated with ASD (Asperger 1944; Hughes et al. 1994; Hughes 1996; Mari et al. 2003; Glazebrook et al. 2006, 2008; Nazarali et al. 2009). Such results have been viewed as evidence for a specific difficulty with motor program selection, reprogramming, and degradation—inferring an underlying difficulty with loci within the cerebellum. By understanding the role of the cerebellum within motor control, reduced levels of activation at two levels may be implied in pronounced motor peculiarities associated with ASD. First, observed behavioral difficulties may be rooted in an inability to control and modulate output activity of the Purkinje cells. Indeed, refinement of the Purkinje cell activity is vital, with excessive variability in activity linked to ataxia—a common phenomenon associated with a diagnosis of ASD (Åhsgren et al. 2005)—clinically characterized by a lack of motor coordination and voluntary control (ICD-10 [WHO 1994]). Indeed, recent studies illustrate a significant reduction in the number of Purkinje cells in individuals with ASD (Arin et al. 1991; Bailey et al. 1998; Bauman and Kemper 2005). Second, error coding modulated by the climbing fibers of the inferior olive (coding afferent feedback), which shape motor output and may provide the foundations of internal models, may be disrupted. Such difficulties would lead to a foundational impairment in sensory-motor acquisition and integration due to difficulty generating stable patterns for motor prediction (see Chapters 8, 11, and 14). Indeed, structural irregularities within the inferior olive have been noted in ASD (see Chapter 9 and Bailey et al. 1998; Bauman and Kemper 2005).

Coded through the peripheral nervous system, this error signal is dependent on sampling of the environment to formulate traditional computational internal models and statistical properties from which to generate error. Specifically, it is proposed that the a priori assumptions at the core of current internal models of computational motor control (Uno et al. 1989; Wolpert and Kawato 1998; Wolpert et al. 1998; Kawato 1999) must be derived through such environmental sampling. This sampling and "calibration" may occur through early active exploratory rhythmical behaviors during infancy that are known to decrease with the emergence of coordinated goal-directed behaviors (Thelen and Smith 1994). As mentioned, the active nature of these exploratory behaviors facilitates multimodal sensory convergence and binding to reduce perceptual uncertainty. Importantly, these exploratory behaviors allow the infant to actively sample the degrees of freedom or permutations available for the completion of a behavior (Thelen and Smith 1994)—allowing for assimilation into the behavioral understanding—building a platform for prediction. This calibration process facilitates the refinement of sensory afferent information (Fajen 2005), the identification of action affordances (Gibson 1966, 2014; Gibson 1969, 1988), and the generation of stable movement patterns or 'attractors" (Thelen and Smith 1994). Further, a new body of work has proposed that the stochastic signature or accumulation of variability at the microlevel within behaviors provides a blueprint of the predictability, and thus stability, of the internal system at all ages (Torres et al. 2016). Utilizing this framework, and the associated metrics for analysis, it is argued that one can examine the stability and predictability of the underlying system (see Chapter 1 and Torres 2011; Torres et al. 2014, 2016). Therefore, subsequent movement or motor control difficulties, viewed and interpreted from a computational perspective, may reflect a physiological impairment at the level of neural error coding, or peripheral transduction and transmission—with an inability to generate a stable motor "schema" for action prediction and performance. Recent evidence for irregularities in the coding and transduction of peripheral sensory information (Orefice et al. 2016) may indeed imply a role for the peripheral nervous system in incoherent and disjointed patterns of motor control. Further, as mentioned, research indicates that a lack of such peripheral feedback (i.e., kinesthetic reafference) may lead to a reduction in corporeal self-awareness and a disruption in the motor signature (Torres et al. 2014). Indeed, research comparing the stochastic signature of micromovements further implies reduced levels of kinesthetic reafference in individuals with ASD, with a profile similar to that of a deafferented participant (i.e., a participant with neuropathy—with a lack of afferent information from the neck down) (Torres et al. 2016). Such results of higher levels of noise and lower levels of statistical predictability illustrated in the actions of individuals with ASD therefore further support the proposal of a reduction in kinesthetic sensing. Overt repetitive behaviors, or stimming, may be a by-product of this microlevel variability in sensing—an attempt to find order in the chaos (Whyatt and Craig 2013a)—by actively repeatedly sampling the environment. Moreover, an inability to refine the internal model at this level, or to generate a predictive platform, may result in an overreliance on on-line control. This inability to generate stable or "automatic" patterns is perhaps alluded to, and neatly summarized, in the below quote from Asperger on his earliest case studies:

> He was never able to swing with the rhythm of the group. His movements never unfolded *naturally and spontaneously* ... from the proper co-ordination of the motor system as a whole. Instead, it seemed as if he could only manage to move those muscular parts to which he directed a conscious effort of will ... nothing was spontaneous or natural, everything was intellectual. (Asperger, in Frith 1991, p. 57, emphasis added)

Related difficulties with action initiation and timing, a characteristic feature of ASD, have been further attributed to, and interpreted within, the computational motor programming framework. Traditionally, the initiation of internally generated actions has been linked to the basal ganglia (Doya 2000)—the subcortical reward center. Similar to the cerebellum, the basal ganglia—and input from the striatum—generate error coding to modulate these behavioral outcomes. Specifically, through the modulation of dopamine secretion, the basal ganglia encode for both current and future rewarding behaviors (Doya 2000), facilitating action selection based on reinforced learning (e.g., Graybiel 1995; Balleine et al. 2007). Physiological variation in the size of basal ganglia has been demonstrated in individuals with ASD (Sears et al. 1999; Hollander et al. 2005; Langen et al. 2007). Furthermore, such neurological variation was alluded to in early pioneering work quantifying gross motor impairments across the autism spectrum (Damasio and Maurer 1978; Vilensky et al. 1981), drawing explicit parallels with individuals with Parkinson's disease (PD) at this stage. Despite this, explicit reference between these psychological and physiological conditions has since been sparse—yet repeatedly inferred in the independent interpretation of results (Mari et al. 2003; Vernazza-Martin et al. 2005; Rinehart et al. 2006; Hollander et al. 2009; Whyatt and Craig 2013a).

Given the mounting evidence at both a behavioral and a physiological level for an underlying etiology of ASD, questions are raised over the continued use of a psychologically driven framework. As noted, a social-economic model is prevalent and beneficial within the clinical arena, facilitating diagnosis and enabling the timely provision of services. However, this restricted interpretation and conceptualization is arguably limiting. By utilizing diagnostic tools and criteria drawn from a clinical and psychological perspective, the academic community is restricted in their scope and exploration of ASD. Moreover, with a reliance on subjective behavioral examination and relatively broad psychological interpretation, we fail to progress to a patient-oriented and personalized approach to both diagnosis and intervention. With recent developments ranging from the amalgamation of a range of neurodevelopmental disorders into an umbrella term of ASD, through to a new conceptualization of both the nosology and epidemiology since the seminal works of Kanner (1943) and Asperger (1944), a modified framework seems apt. In addition, viewed within the context of today's precision medicine platform and health agenda, a patient-oriented, physiological perspective to approach and define ASD seems timely. Yet, barriers remain with disconnect between academic disciplines. The distinction between the fields of psychology and the new burgeoning area of neuroscience—particularly computational neuroscience—although closing, is pertinent to this struggle. The move from behavioral observation using arguably subjective psychologically driven tools and metrics, to the use of robust objective empirical estimation for individualized patient-oriented models is a large one*—yet a model for this transition can be followed.

PARALLELS WITH PHYSIOLOGICALLY GROUNDED DISORDERS: PARKINSON'S DISEASE—A MODEL FOR ASD?

First described in the 1817 work "An Essay on the Shaking Palsy" by James Parkinson (2002), PD is a prevalent neurodegenerative disorder characterized by impaired motor control. Although universally considered a physiological, neurological condition, rooted in a lack of dopaminergic secreting neurons within the substantial nigra pars compacta of the basal ganglia, PD was once empirically characterized by subjective behavioral observation. It was with the systematic study of Parkinson's tremor by neurologist Charcot (1887, in Goetz 2011) that the systematic nature with which PD could be diagnosed and quantified was first illustrated. Considered one of the fathers of neurology, Charcot provided a robust patient-oriented framework to examine neurological features of PD, moving away from the large umbrella grouping of disorders by particularly evident, subjective observable behaviors (Goetz 2011). Such systematic empirical quantifications provided the foundations for new diagnostic tools that were designed and refined for the clinical field. Indeed, initial methods of behavioral observation—similar to those used heavily during the diagnosis of ASD—are still retained in modern clinical practice of PD, with preliminary quantification using the Unified Parkinson's Disease Rating Scale (UPD-RS) (Movement Disorder Society Task Force 2003) and the Hoehn and Yahr stages (Goetz et al. 2004). However, in contrast to the ASD approach, each of these tools was designed and created to build on scientific, empirical evidence of the trajectory and etiology of PD. Thus, despite utilizing observational methods, such tools for the characterization of PD are designed to encompass core components derived from objective, biologically grounded scientific metrics, such as unilateral versus bilateral symptomatology—a key distinctive marker of progressive PD.

Now firmly established as a "movement disorder," PD is associated with a complex symptomatology, including uncontrollable resting tremor, dyskinesias, dystonia, akinesia, and bradykinesia (Jankovic 2008). Similar to the programming deficit hypothesis proposed for observable motor peculiarities associated with ASD, distinguishing characteristics of PD, such as akinesia and bradykinesia, have long been considered the by-product of "an inability to select and/or maintain internal control over the algorithms" needed to generate actions (Robertson and Flowers 1990, p. 591). Indeed, given the evidence for diverse, universal sensory-motor difficulties associated with ASD, similarities between ASD and the field of PD have been detected. These include an early illustration of postural instability associated with ASD (Damasio and Maurer 1978; Vilensky et al. 1981), with explicit parallels with PD drawn at this stage. Further motor similarities have since been noted (Mari et al. 2003; Rinehart et al. 2006; Whyatt and Craig 2013a; Vernazza-Martin et al. 2005; Hollander et al. 2009; Torres et al. 2016). Research has extended this quantification to also include the micro-movement perspective, illustrating similarities in peripheral noise between individuals with ASD or PD and a deafferentated patient (Torres et al. 2016). Building on, and extending from, evidence for reduced corporeal sensation, and thus reduced proprioception, such results further imply a poor level of peripheral transduction and impaired levels of kinesthetic sensing associated with PD and ASD, which may contribute to the breakdown of reference frames for action. Moreover, similar to ASD, irregularities within the cerebellum have since been proposed in PD (Wu and Hallett 2013), and quantified in reduced levels of procedural learning (Joel et al. 2005) and specific functional impairments, including ataxia.

* An additional hurdle for the provision of personalized metrics, even with the use of high-end research-grade technology, is the provision of adequate statistical metrics. Chapters 11 and 13 provide the reader with an overview of these limitations, and present a novel, robust, statistical landscape to facilitate this endeavor.

These objective similarities associated with the motor profile of ASD and PD are further supported by a range of nonmotor symptoms that are associated with progressive PD, symptoms that bear a striking resemblance to "classical" social-cognitive elements of ASD, including pronounced difficulties with theory of mind, executive functioning tasks, and obsessive-compulsive behaviors (Saltzman et al. 2000; Mengelberg and Siegert 2003). Thus, despite being characterized by prevalent motor difficulties, PD is associated with symptomatology traditionally conceptualized as psychological or psychiatric in nature. Indeed, contrasted against the symptomatology of ASD, both can be conceptualized as inverted, yet similar models—one characterized by overt psychological behavioral outcomes, and the other characterized by overt physiological behavioral outcomes—yet both encompassing a range of characteristics spanning this spectrum (Figure 2.1). The dominance of motor symptoms in PD is in stark contrast to the characterization of ASD, in which cognitive and social symptoms are seen as core aspects, with sensory-motor difficulties often referred to as secondary by-products—a contrast that further illustrates the dichotomy between employing a psychological versus a physiological construct.

Specifically, viewing and interpreting PD from a physiological, neurological framework has facilitated the discovery and understanding of underlying etiology, led to a patient-oriented model for diagnosis and intervention, and provided the foundation for clinical screening tools, such as the UPD-RS and Hoehn and Yahr scale. As such, the field of PD has transformed, moving from the use of subjective behavioral observation and broad categorization using explicit symptoms (Goetz 2011), to an empirically driven framework utilizing objective methodologies to inform clinical practice. Through this framework the objective quantifications of the biomedical and academic arenas continue to drive the development and refinement of clinical tools and techniques. The transformation within the field of neurology, specifically PD, has been significant—with a range of cutting-edge therapies and interventions now available. Comparatively, ASD research is in its infancy—facing the need to expand in its scope and conceptualization. Will the growing evidence for ASD as a complex, yet physiologically grounded disorder, allow the field to learn from this evolving patient-oriented model of PD?

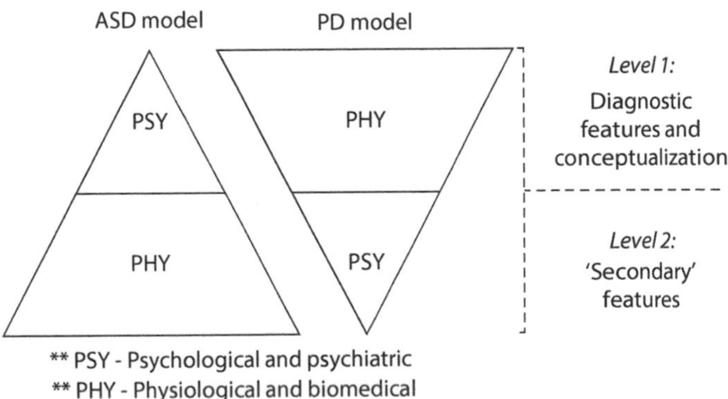

FIGURE 2.1 Inverted models of ASD and PD illustrating the prevalence of the neurological, physiological perspective in PD versus the psychological and psychiatric perspective of ASD. The psychological symptomatology characterizing ASD is arguably the tip of the iceberg, while similarly, the quantifiable objective physiological symptoms of PD are accompanied by similar psychological symptoms. Questions are thus raised over the utility of this model of ASD, with evidence for significant physiological sensory and motor symptomatology suggesting that a reconceptualization is required. Indeed, moving from this limited view to a patient-oriented physiological perspective of ASD may facilitate both our academic inquiry and the diversification of diagnostic and intervention techniques. Can we learn from the PD model?

ASD AND PD: THE MISSING LINK?

Despite significant parallels in the presence of motor and nonmotor elements of the phenotype between ASD and PD, there is currently no framework to explicitly tie these two seemingly disconnected disorders—helping to solidify ASD as a physiological construct. Interestingly, however, recent figures suggest that rates of PD diagnosis are significantly higher in adults with ASD than the population average (Starkstein et al. 2015). This implied link might infer a more substantial genotype connection between these neurodevelopmental and neurodegenerative disorders. Indeed, similar facets of epidemiology have been documented across both ASD and PD, including potentially higher incidence rates among males in both populations (Volkmar et al. 1993; Wooten et al. 2004). One area of potential cross talk currently being investigated by Torres and colleagues is the incidence of fragile X disorders (FXDs)—a spectrum of neurodevelopmental and neurodegenerative disorders, linked by a mutation or permutation of the FMR1 gene (Payton et al. 1989; De Boulle et al. 1993; Tsongalis and Silverman 1993). With a similar epidemiology—specifically a higher rate of incidence within males—FXDs may begin to provide a model between these neurodevelopmental and neurodegenerative ends of the spectrum.

The FMR1 gene, located on the X chromosome, is an area characterized by repetitions of the CGG trinucleotide. Under normal circumstances, the FMR1 gene has approximately 5–44 repeats; however, an increase in this repeat gives rise to varying levels of FXD expression. Specifically, 45–54 repeats, although associated with no measureable risk, have a probability of expansion in future generations (Reyniers et al. 1993); full mutation, more than 200 repeats, results in the expression of fragile X syndrome (FXS), and premutation with 55–200 repeats results in a range of fragile X–related disorders (including fragile X tremor ataxia syndrome [FXTAS] and fragile X premature ovarian insufficiency syndrome [FXPOI]). Approximately 30% of individuals with FXS receive a secondary diagnosis of ASD, while additional comorbidity occurs between individuals with ASD and permutation FMR1 gene carriers (Tassone et al. 2000a, 2000b; Aziz et al. 2003; Farzin et al. 2006; Clifford et al. 2007). Moreover, FXTAS, a permutation level of FXDs, caused by moderate expansion (55–199 repeats) (Hagerman and Hagerman 2004), is thought to be one of the most common single gene disorders leading to neurodegeneration in males. With core symptomatology including action tremor, neuropathy, cerebellar gait ataxia, parkinsonism, and executive dysfunction (Berry-Kravis et al. 2007; Bourgeois et al. 2007; Gonçalves et al. 2007; Leehey et al. 2007), FXTAS is often misdiagnosed as PD (Hall et al. 2014; Lozano et al. 2014; Niu et al. 2014).

With commonality in behavioral expression between FXDs and PD and comorbidity between FXDs and ASD, it is perhaps unsurprising that foundational similarities have been illustrated in underlying etiology. Physiological techniques have repeatedly illustrated significant variation in structural constructs, with neuronal disorganization implicated as a foundation of developmental conditions, including ASD and FXD (Volpe 2008). Further, evidence implies a similar molecular pathway between both neurodevelopmental disorders (for a review, see Coghlan et al. 2012), while brain imaging techniques have implied cerebellar irregularities in ASD, PD (as outlined above), and FXDs (Hagerman and Hagerman 2004; Hagerman et al. 2008; Leehey and Hagerman 2011). With this implied genetic or molecular comorbidity, and similarities at the phenotypic level, FXDs may provide a framework to connect both ASD and PD. With FXDs thought to be underdiagnosed, and the late detection of permutation carriers, the incidence and potential role of FMR1 gene repeats is arguably heightened. By examining genotype and phenotype similarities across these populations, Torres and colleagues intend to further explore these linkages. Drawing on previous models (Torres et al. 2016), and bespoke analytical metrics that retain a statistically valid approach, the team will provide a new layer of objective personalized phenotyping to bridge the gap between genetics and behavioral observation.

ASD: DOES THE EVIDENCE SUGGEST IT IS TIME FOR A NEW MODEL?

Throughout this chapter, evidence has been presented, both behavioral and biological, for a reconceptualization of ASD from a purely psychological construct to a physiologically grounded disorder.

This reconceptualization seems timely given recent redefinitions and classifications of this umbrella term—which encompasses a range of neurodevelopmental disorders. Indeed, this spectrum of neurodiversity now subsumed under the category ASD, when viewed within the spectrum of the general population, has led to a new ambiguity over arbitrary diagnostic thresholds, and illustrates the need to redefine our understanding of an ASD. By moving from the limited social-cognitivist model entrenched within the clinical domain to consider broad behavioral manifestations of ASD through objective measurement and in light of sensory and motor difficulties, we may map the foundations for a new model. During an era of precision medicine, and in light of the spectrum of both the ASD phenotype and genotype, this personalized, patient-oriented approach is apt—and may facilitate the refinement of both diagnostics and interventions. Drawing on the model of disorders such as PD, to which there are both implicit and explicit parallels, the avenues of exploration to identify and examine the etiology of ASD may be diversified while beginning an open dialogue between disciplines. As illustrated in the historical perspective of PD, our initial empirical behavioral observations, although critical, can be successfully augmented with additional techniques and approaches. By viewing the transformation of the field of PD to a patient-oriented, neurological approach that facilitates and informs the fields of clinical diagnostics and intervention, the model of ASD may look outdated. I suggest it is now time to begin considering ASD as a physiological construct so we may broaden and diversify the interventions available to individuals, move away from a psychological 'deficit model' that is harming and painful to the Autistic community, and begin to see the whole, not simply the parts.

REFERENCES

Åhsgren, I., I. Baldwin, C. Goetzinger-Falk, A. Erikson, O. Flodmark, and C. Gillberg. 2005. Ataxia, autism, and the cerebellum: A clinical study of 32 individuals with congenital ataxia. *Dev Med Child Neurol* 47 (3):193–8.

Albus, J. S. 1971. A theory of cerebellar function. *Math Biosci* 10 (1):25–61.

APA (American Psychiatric Association). 1994. *Diagnostic and Statistical Manual of Mental Disorders*, 4th ed. Washington, DC: APA.

APA (American Psychiatric Association). 2013. *Diagnostic and Statistical Manual of Mental Disorders*. 5th ed. Arlington, VA: APA.

Arin, D. M., M. L. Bauman, and T. L. Kemper. 1991. The distribution of Purkinje cell loss in the cerebellum in autism. *Neurology* 41 (Suppl 1):307.

Asperger, H. 1944. Die "Autistischen Psychopathen" im Kindesalter. *Eur Arch Psychiatry Clin Neurosci* 117 (1): 76–136.

Atkinson, J. 2002. *The Developing Visual Brain*. Oxford: Oxford University Press.

Aziz, M., E. Stathopulu, M. Callias, C. Taylor, J. Turk, B. Oostra, R. Willemsen, and M. Patton. 2003. Clinical features of boys with fragile X premutations and intermediate alleles. *Am J Medl Genet B* 121 (1):119–27.

Bailey, A., P. Luthert, A. Dean, B. Harding, I. Janota, M. Montgomery, M. Rutter, and P. Lantos. 1998. A clinicopathological study of autism. *Brain* 121 (5):889–905.

Balleine, B. W., M. R. Delgado, and O. Hikosaka. 2007. The role of the dorsal striatum in reward and decision-making. *J Neurosci* 27 (31):8161–5.

Balslev, D., J. Cole, and R. C. Miall. 2007. Proprioception contributes to the sense of agency during visual observation of hand movements: Evidence from temporal judgments of action. *J Cogn Neurosci* 19 (9):1535–41.

Baron-Cohen, S., A. M. Leslie, and U. Frith. 1985. Does the autistic child have a "theory of mind"? *Cognition* 21 (1):37–46.

Bastian, A. J., K. M. Zackowski, and W. T. Thach. 2000. Cerebellar ataxia: Torque deficiency or torque mismatch between joints? *J Neurophysiol* 83 (5):3019–30.

Bauman, M. L., and T. L. Kemper. 2005. Neuroanatomic observations of the brain in autism: A review and future directions. *Int J Dev Neurosci* 23 (2):183–7.

Berry-Kravis, E., C. G. Goetz, M. A. Leehey, R. J. Hagerman, L. Zhang, L. Li, D. Nguyen, D. A. Hall, N. Tartaglia, and J. Cogswell. 2007. Neuropathic features in fragile X premutation carriers. *Am J Med Genet A* 143 (1):19–26.

Bostan, A. C., R. P. Dum, and P. L. Strick. 2013. Cerebellar networks with the cerebral cortex and basal ganglia. *Trends in Cognitive Sciences* 17 (05):241–254. doi: 10.1016/j.tics.2013.03.003.

Bouchard, D., and S. Tetreault. 2000. The motor development of sighted children and children with moderate low vision aged 8–13. *J Vis Impair Blind* 94 (09):564–73.

Bourgeois, J. A., J. B. Cogswell, D. Hessl, L. Zhang, M. Y. Ono, F. Tassone, F. Farzin, J. A. Brunberg, J. Grigsby, and R. J. Hagerman. 2007. Cognitive, anxiety and mood disorders in the fragile X-associated tremor/ataxia syndrome. *Gen Hosp Psychiatry* 29 (4):349–56.

Braddick, O., and J. Atkinson. 2011. Development of human visual function. *Vis Res* 51 (13):1588–609.

Braitenberg, V. 1967. Is the cerebellar cortex a biological clock in the millisecond range? *Prog Brain Res* 25: 334–46.

Braitenberg, V., D. Heck, and F. Sultan. 1997. The detection and generation of sequences as a key to cerebellar function: Experiments and theory. *Behav Brain Sci* 20 (02):229–45.

Brambring, M. 2006. Divergent development of gross motor skills in children who are blind or sighted. *J Vis Impair Blind* 100 (10):620.

Brincker, M., and E. B. Torres. 2013. Noise from the periphery in autism. *Front Integr Neurosci* 7:34.

Brock, J., C. C. Brown, J. Boucher, and G. Rippon. 2002. The temporal binding deficit hypothesis of autism. *Dev Psychopathol* 14 (02):209–24.

Bushnell, E. W., and J. P. Boudreau. 1993. Motor development and the mind: The potential role of motor abilities as a determinant of aspects of perceptual development. *Child Dev* 64 (4):1005–21.

Clifford, S., C. Dissanayake, Q. M. Bui, R. Huggins, A. K. Taylor, and D. Z. Loesch. 2007. Autism spectrum phenotype in males and females with fragile X full mutation and premutation. *J Autism Dev Disord* 37 (4): 738–47.

Coghlan, S., J. Horder, B. Inkster, M. A. Mendez, D. G. Murphy, and D. J. Nutt. 2012. GABA system dysfunction in autism and related disorders: From synapse to symptoms. *Neurosci Biobehav Rev* 36 (9):2044–55.

Cole, J., and J. Paillard. 1995. Living without touch and peripheral information about body position and movement: Studies with deafferented subjects. In *The Body and Self*, ed. J. L. Bermudez, N. Eilan, and A. J. Marcel, pp. 245–66. Cambridge, MA: MIT Press.

Courchesne, E., and K. Pierce. 2005. Why the frontal cortex in autism might be talking only to itself: Local over-connectivity but long-distance disconnection. *Curr Opin Neurobiol* 15 (2):225–30.

Damasio, A. R., and R. G. Maurer. 1978. A neurological model for childhood autism. *Arch Neurol* 35 (12):777–86.

Dawson, G., S. Webb, G. D. Schellenberg, S. Dager, S. Friedman, E. Aylward, and T. Richards. 2002. Defining the broader phenotype of autism: Genetic, brain, and behavioral perspectives. *Dev Psychopathol* 14 (3): 581–611.

De Boulle, K., A. J. M. H. Verkerk, E. Reyniers, L. Vits, J. Hendrickx, B. Van Roy, F. Van Den Bos, and E. de Graaff. 1993. A point mutation in the FMR-1 gene associated with fragile X. *Nat Genet* 3 (1):31–5.

De Jaegher, H. 2013. Embodiment and sense-making in autism. Front Integr Neurosci 7:15.

Descartes, R. 1984. *The Philosophical Writings of Descartes*, trans. J. Cottingham, R. Stoothoff, and D. Murdoch. Vol. I. Cambridge: Cambridge University Press.

Donnellan, A. M. 1984. The criterion of the least dangerous assumption. *Behav Disord* 9:141–50.

Doya, K. 2000. Complementary roles of basal ganglia and cerebellum in learning and motor control. *Curr Opin Neurobiol* 10 (6):732–9.

Fajen, B. R. 2005. Perceiving possibilities for action: On the necessity of calibration and perceptual learning for the visual guidance of action. *Perception* 34 (6):717–40.

Farzin, F., H. Perry, D. Hessl, D. Loesch, J. Cohen, S. Bacalman, L. Gane, F. Tassone, P. Hagerman, and R. Hagerman. 2006. Autism spectrum disorders and attention-deficit/hyperactivity disorder in boys with the fragile X premutation. *J Dev Behav Pediatr* 27 (2):S137–44.

Folio, M. R., and R. R. Fewell. 2000. *Peabody Developmental Motor Scales: Examiner's Manual*. Austin, TX: Pro-ed.

Foss-Feig, J. H., L. D. Kwakye, C. J. Cascio, C. P. Burnette, H. Kadivar, W. L. Stone, and M. T. Wallace. 2010. An extended multisensory temporal binding window in autism spectrum disorders. *Exp Brain Res* 203 (2):381–9.

Fourneret, P., J. Paillard, Y. Lamarre, J. Cole, and M. Jeannerod. 2002. Lack of conscious recognition of one's own actions in a haptically deafferented patient. *Neuroreport* 13 (4):541–7.

Fournier, K. A., C. J. Hass, S. K. Naik, N. Lodha, and J. H. Cauraugh. 2010. Motor coordination in autism spectrum disorders: A synthesis and meta-analysis. *J Autism Dev Disord* 40 (10):1227–40.

Frith, U. 1989. *Autism: Explaining the Enigma*. Oxford: Basil Blackwell.

Gesell, A., and C. S. Amatruda. 1945. *The Embryology of Behavior: The Beginnings of the Human Mind.* Philadelphia: Lippincott.

Gesell, A., and C. S. Amatruda. 1947. *Developmental Diagnosis.* New York: Hoeber.

Gibson, E. J. 1988. Exploratory behavior in the development of perceiving, acting, and the acquiring of knowledge. *Annu Rev Psychol* 39 (1):1–42.

Gibson, E. J. 1969. *Principles of Perceptual Learning and Development.* New York: Appleton-Century-Crofts.

Gibson, E. J., and R. D. Walk. 1960. *The "Visual Cliff."* Vol. 1. San Francisco, CA: W. H. Freeman Company.

Gibson, J. J. 1966. *The Senses Considered as Perceptual Systems.* Boston, MA: Houghton Mifflin.

Gibson, J. J. 2014. *The Ecological Approach to Visual Perception: Classic Edition.* London: Psychology Press.

Gilbert, P. F. C., and W. T. Thach. 1977. Purkinje cell activity during motor learning. *Brain Res* 128 (2):309–28.

Glazebrook, C., D. Gonzalez, S. Hansen, and D. Elliott. 2009. The role of vision for online control of manual aiming movements in persons with autism spectrum disorders. *Autism* 13 (4):411–33.

Glazebrook, C. M., D. Elliott, and J. Lyons. 2006. A kinematic analysis of how young adults with and without autism plan and control goal-directed movements. *Motor Control* 10 (3):244–64.

Glazebrook, C. M., D. Elliott, and P. Szatmari. 2008. How do individuals with autism plan their movements? *J Autism Dev Disord* 38 (1):114–26.

Goetz, C. G. 2011. The history of Parkinson's disease: Early clinical descriptions and neurological therapies. *Cold Spring Harb Perspect Med* 1 (1):a008862.

Goetz, C. G., W. Poewe, O. Rascol, C. Sampaio, G. T. Stebbins, C. Counsell, N. Giladi, R. G. Holloway, C. G. Moore, and G. K. Wenning. 2004. Movement disorder society task force report on the Hoehn and Yahr staging scale: Status and recommendations. *Mov Disord* 19 (9):1020–8.

Gonçalves, M. R. R., L. P. Capelli, R. Nitrini, E. R. Barbosa, C. S. Porto, L. T. Lucato, and A. M. Vianna-Morgante. 2007. Atypical clinical course of FXTAS: Rapidly progressive dementia as the major symptom. *Neurology* 68 (21):1864–6.

Graybiel, A. M. 1995. Building action repertoires: Memory and learning functions of the basal ganglia. *Curr Opin Neurobiol* 5 (6):733–41.

Green, D., T. Charman, A. Pickles, S. Chandler, T. Loucas, E. Simonoff, and G. Baird. 2009. Impairment in movement skills of children with autistic spectrum disorders. *Dev Med Child Neurol* 51 (4):311–6.

Hadders-Algra, M. 2000. The neuronal group selection theory: A framework to explain variation in normal motor development. *Dev Med Child Neurol* 42 (8):566–72.

Hagerman, P. J., and R. J. Hagerman. 2004. Fragile X-associated tremor/ataxia syndrome (FXTAS). *Ment Retard Dev Disabil Res Rev* 10 (1):25–30.

Hagerman, R. J., D. A. Hall, S. Coffey, M. Leehey, J. Bourgeois, J. Gould, L. Zhang, A. Seritan, E. Berry-Kravis, and J. Olichney. 2008. Treatment of fragile X-associated tremor ataxia syndrome (FXTAS) and related neurological problems. *Clin Interv Aging* 3 (2):251.

Haggard, P. 2008. Human volition: Towards a neuroscience of will. *Nat Rev Neurosci* 9 (12):934–46.

Hall, D. A., R. C. Birch, M. Anheim, A. E. Jønch, E. Pintado, J. O'Keefe, J. N. Trollor, G. T. Stebbins, R. J. Hagerman, and S. Fahn. 2014. Emerging topics in FXTAS. *J Neurodev Disord* 6 (1):1.

Hallett, M., M. K. Lebiedowska, S. L. Thomas, S. J. Stanhope, M. B. Denckla, and J. Rumsey. 1993. Locomotion of autistic adults. *Arch Neurol* 50 (12):1304–8.

Happé, F., and U. Frith. 2006. The weak coherence account: Detail-focused cognitive style in autism spectrum disorders. *J Autism Dev Disord* 36 (1):5–25.

Heck, D. 1993. Rat cerebellar cortex in vitro responds specifically to moving stimuli. *Neurosci Lett* 157 (1): 95–8.

Heck, D. 1995. Sequential stimulation of guinea pig cerebellar cortex in vitro strongly affects Purkinje cells via parallel fibers. *Naturwissenschaften* 82 (4):201–3.

Held, R. 1965. Plasticity in sensory-motor systems. *Sci Am* 213 (5):84–94.

Held, R., E. Birch, and J. Gwiazda. 1980. Stereoacuity of human infants. *Proc Natl Acad Sci USA* 77 (9):5572–4.

Henderson, S. E., D. A. Sugden, and A. L. Barnett. 2007. *Movement Assessment Battery for Children-2: Movement ABC-2: Examiner's Manual.* São Paulo: Pearson.

Hollander, E., E. Anagnostou, W. Chaplin, K. Esposito, M. M. Haznedar, E. Licalzi, S. Wasserman, L. Soorya, and M. Buchsbaum. 2005. Striatal volume on magnetic resonance imaging and repetitive behaviors in autism. *Biol Psychiatry* 58 (3):226–32.

Hollander, E., A. T. Wang, A. Braun, and L. Marsh. 2009. Neurological considerations: Autism and Parkinson's disease. *Psychiatry Res* 170 (1):43–51.

Holst, E., and H. Mittelstaedt. 1950. Das reafferenzprinzip. *Naturwissenschaften* 37 (20):464–76.

Hughes, C. 1996. Brief report: Planning problems in autism at the level of motor control. *J Autism Dev Disord* 26 (1):99–107.

Hughes, C., J. Russell, and T. W. Robbins. 1994. Evidence for executive dysfunction in autism. *Neuropsychologia* 32 (4):477–92.

Itō, M. 1984. *The Cerebellum and Neural Control*. San Diego, CA: Raven Press.

Ito, M., M. Sakurai, and P. Tongroach. 1982. Climbing fibre induced depression of both mossy fibre responsiveness and glutamate sensitivity of cerebellar Purkinje cells. *J Physiol* 324:113.

Ivry, R. B., S. W. Keele, and H. C. Diener. 1988. Dissociation of the lateral and medial cerebellum in movement timing and movement execution. *Exp Brain Res* 73 (1):167–80.

Jankovic, J. 2008. Parkinson's disease: Clinical features and diagnosis. *J Neurol Neurosurg Psychiatry* 79 (4): 368–76.

Joel, D., O. Zohar, M. Afek, H. Hermesh, L. Lerner, R. Kuperman, R. Gross-Isseroff, A. Weizman, and R. Inzelberg. 2005. Impaired procedural learning in obsessive-compulsive disorder and Parkinson's disease, but not in major depressive disorder. *Behav Brain Res* 157 (2):253–63.

Kanner, L. 1943. Autistic disturbances of affective contact. *Nervous Child* 2:217–50.

Kawato, M. 1999. Internal models for motor control and trajectory planning. *Curr Opin Neurobiol* 9 (6): 718–27.

Kitazawa, S., T. Kimura, and P.-B. Yin. 1998. Cerebellar complex spikes encode both destinations and errors in arm movements. *Nature* 392 (6675):494–7.

Kohen-Raz, R., F. R. Volkman, and D. J. Cohen. 1992. Postural control in children with autism. *J Autism Dev Disord* 22 (3):419–32.

Kwakye, L. D., J. H. Foss-Feig, C. J. Cascio, W. L. Stone, and M. T. Wallace. 2011. Altered auditory and multisensory temporal processing in autism spectrum disorders. *Front Integr Neurosci* 4:129.

Langen, M., S. Durston, W. G. Staal, S. J. M. C. Palmen, and H. van Engeland. 2007. Caudate nucleus is enlarged in high-functioning medication-naive subjects with autism. *Biol Psychiatry* 62 (3):262–6.

Leehey, M. A., E. Berry-Kravis, S.-J. Min, D. A. Hall, C. D. Rice, L. Zhang, J. Grigsby, C. M. Greco, A. Reynolds, and R. Lara. 2007. Progression of tremor and ataxia in male carriers of the FMR1 premutation. *Mov Disord* 22 (2):203–6.

Leehey, M. A., and P. J. Hagerman. 2011. Fragile X-associated tremor/ataxia syndrome. *Handb Clin Neurol* 103: 373–386.

Leekam, S. R., C. Nieto, S. J. Libby, L. Wing, and J. Gould. 2007. Describing the sensory abnormalities of children and adults with autism. *J Autism Dev Disord* 37 (5):894–910.

Levtzion-Korach, O., A. Tennenbaum, R. Schnitzer, and A. Ornoy. 2000. Early motor development of blind children. *J Paediatr Child Health* 36 (3):226–9.

Lord, C., P. C. DiLavore, and K. Gotham. 2012. *Autism Diagnostic Observation Schedule*. Torrance, CA: Western Psychological Services.

Lord, C., M. Rutter, and A. Le Couteur. 1994. Autism diagnostic interview-revised: A revised version of a diagnostic interview for caregivers of individuals with possible pervasive developmental disorders. *J Autism Dev Disord* 24 (5):659–85.

Lozano, R., C. A. Rosero, and R. J. Hagerman. 2014. Fragile X spectrum disorders. *Intractable Rare Dis Res* 3 (4): 134–46.

Mari, M., U. Castiello, D. Marks, C. Marraffa, and M. Prior. 2003. The reach-to-grasp movement in children with autism spectrum disorder. *Philos Trans R Soc Lond B Biol Sci* 358 (1430):393–403.

McAlpine, L. M., and C. L. Moore. 1995. The development of social understanding in children with visual impairments. *J Vis Impair Blind* 89:349–58.

McGraw, M. B. 1940. Neuromuscular development of the human infant as exemplified in the achievement of erect locomotion. *J Pediatr* 17 (6):747–71.

Mengelberg, A., and R. Siegert. 2003. Is theory-of-mind impaired in Parkinson's disease? *Cogn Neuropsychiatry* 8 (3):191–209.

Ming, X., M. Brimacombe, and G. C. Wagner. 2007. Prevalence of motor impairment in autism spectrum disorders. *Brain Dev* 29 (9):565–70.

Minshew, N. J., G. Goldstein, and D. J. Siegel. 1997. Neuropsychologic functioning in autism: Profile of a complex information processing disorder. *J Int Neuropsychol Soc* 3 (04):303–16.

Minshew, N. J., K. Sung, B. L. Jones, and J. M. Furman. 2004. Underdevelopment of the postural control system in autism. *Neurology* 63 (11):2056–61.

Movement Disorder Society Task Force on Rating Scales for Parkinson's Disease. 2003. The Unified Parkinson's Disease Rating Scale (UPDRS): Status and recommendations. *Mov Disord* 18 (7):738.

Nazarali, N., C. M. Glazebrook, and D. Elliott. 2009. Movement planning and reprogramming in individuals with autism. *J Autism Dev Disord* 39 (10):1401–11.

Niu, Y.-Q., J.-C. Yang, D. A. Hall, M. A. Leehey, F. Tassone, J. M. Olichney, R. J. Hagerman, and L. Zhang. 2014. Parkinsonism in fragile X-associated tremor/ataxia syndrome (FXTAS): Revisited. *Parkinsonism Relat Disord* 20 (4):456–9.

Nordin, V., and C. Gillberg. 1996. Autism spectrum disorders in children with physical or mental disability or both. I. Clinical and epidemiological aspects. *Dev Med Child Neurol* 38 (4):297–313.

Orefice, L. L., A. L. Zimmerman, A. M. Chirila, S. J. Sleboda, J. P. Head, and D. D. Ginty. 2016. Peripheral mechanosensory neuron dysfunction underlies tactile and behavioral deficits in mouse models of ASDs. *Cell* 166 (2):299–313. doi: 10.1016/j.cell.2016.05.033.

Ozonoff, S., and R. E. McEvoy. 1994. A longitudinal study of executive function and theory of mind development in autism. *Dev Psychopathol* 6 (03):415–31.

Ozonoff, S., B. F. Pennington, and S. J. Rogers. 1991. Executive function deficits in high-functioning autistic individuals: Relationship to theory of mind. *J Child Psychol Psychiatry* 32 (7):1081–105.

Parkinson, J. 2002. An essay on the shaking palsy. *J Neuropsychiatry Clin Neurosci* 14 (2):223–36.

Payton, J. B., M. W. Steele, S. L. Wenger, and N. J. Minshew. 1989. The fragile X marker and autism in perspective. *J Am Acad Child Adolesc Psychiatry* 28 (3):417–21.

Pellicano, E., L. Gibson, M. Maybery, K. Durkin, and D. R. Badcock. 2005. Abnormal global processing along the dorsal visual pathway in autism: A possible mechanism for weak visuospatial coherence? *Neuropsychologia* 43 (7):1044–53.

Plaisted, K. C. 2001. Reduced generalization in autism: An alternative to weak central coherence. *Dev Autism* 2: 149–69.

Plaisted, K., L. Saksida, J. Alcántara, and E. Weisblatt. 2003. Towards an understanding of the mechanisms of weak central coherence effects: Experiments in visual configural learning and auditory perception. *Philos Trans R Soc Lond B Biol Sci* 358 (1430):375–86.

Power, J. D., K. A. Barnes, A. Z. Snyder, B. L. Schlaggar, and S. E. Petersen. 2012. Spurious but systematic correlations in functional connectivity MRI networks arise from subject motion. *Neuroimage* 59 (3): 2142–54.

Provost, B., B. R. Lopez, and S. Heimerl. 2007. A comparison of motor delays in young children: Autism spectrum disorder, developmental delay, and developmental concerns. *J Autism Dev Disord* 37 (2):321–8.

Reyniers, E., L. Vits, K. De Boulle, and B. Van Roy. 1993. The full mutation in the FMR-1 gene of male fragile X patients is absent in their sperm. *Nat Genet* 4 (2):143–6.

Rinehart, N. J., B. J. Tonge, R. Iansek, J. McGinley, A. V. Brereton, P. G. Enticott, and J. L. Bradshaw. 2006. Gait function in newly diagnosed children with autism: Cerebellar and basal ganglia related motor disorder. *Dev Med Child Neurol* 48 (10):819–24.

Robertson, C., and K. A. Flowers. 1990. Motor set in Parkinson's disease. *J Neurol Neurosurg Psychiatry* 53 (7): 583–92.

Saltzman, J., E. Strauss, M. Hunter, and S. Archibald. 2000. Theory of mind and executive functions in normal human aging and Parkinson's disease. *J Int Neuropsychol Soc* 6 (07):781–8.

Sasaki, K., and H. Gemba. 1993. Cerebro-cerebellar interactions: For fast and stable timing of voluntary movement. In *Role of the Cerebellum and Basal Ganglia in Voluntary Movement*, ed. N. Mano, I. Hamada, and M. DeLong, pp. 41–50. Amsterdam: Elsevier.

Sears, L. L., C. Vest, S. Mohamed, J. Bailey, B. J. Ranson, and J. Piven. 1999. An MRI study of the basal ganglia in autism. *Prog Neuropsychopharmacol Biol Psychiatry* 23 (4):613–24.

Singer, W. 1985. Activity-dependent self-organization of the mammalian visual cortex. In *Models of the Visual Cortex*, ed. D. Rose and V. Dobson, pp. 123–36. New York: Wiley.

Starkstein, S., S. Gellar, M. Parlier, L. Payne, and J. Piven. 2015. High rates of parkinsonism in adults with autism. *J Neurodev Disord* 7 (1):1.

Stenneken, P., W. Prinz, J. Cole, J. Paillard, and G. Aschersleben. 2006. The effect of sensory feedback on the timing of movements: Evidence from deafferented patients. *Brain Res* 1084 (1):123–31.

Sutera, S., J. Pandey, E. L. Esser, M. A. Rosenthal, L. B. Wilson, M. Barton, J. Green, S. Hodgson, D. L. Robins, and T. Dumont-Mathieu. 2007. Predictors of optimal outcome in toddlers diagnosed with autism spectrum disorders. *J Autism Dev Disord* 37 (1):98–107.

Tallon-Baudry, C., and O. Bertrand. 1999. Oscillatory gamma activity in humans and its role in object representation. *Trends Cogn Sci* 3 (4):151–62.

Tassone, F., R. J. Hagerman, W. D. Chamberlain, and P. J. Hagerman. 2000a. Transcription of the FMR1 gene in individuals with fragile X syndrome. *Am J Med Genet* 97 (3):195–203.

Tassone, F., R. J. Hagerman, D. Z. Loesch, A. Lachiewicz, A. K. Taylor, and P. J. Hagerman. 2000b. Fragile X males with unmethylated, full mutation trinucleotide repeat expansions have elevated levels of FMR1 messenger RNA. *Am J Med Genet* 94 (3):232–6.

Teitelbaum, P., O. Teitelbaum, J. Nye, J. Fryman, and R. G. Maurer. 1998. Movement analysis in infancy may be useful for early diagnosis of autism. *Proc Natl Acad Sci USA* 95 (23):13982–7.

Thelen, E., and L. B. Smith. 1994. A Dynamic Systems Approach to the Development of Cognition and Action. In: *MIT Press/Bradford Book Series in Cognitive Psychology*. Cambridge, MA: MIT Press, pp. 376.

Torres, E. B. 2011. Two classes of movements in motor control. *Exp Brain Res* 215 (3–4):269–83.

Torres, E. B., M. Brincker, R. W. Isenhower, P. Yanovich, K. A. Stigler, J. I. Nurnberger, D. N. Metaxas, and J. V. José. 2013. Autism: The micro-movement perspective. *Front Integr Neurosci* 7:32.

Torres, E. B., J. Cole, and H. Poizner. 2014. Motor output variability, deafferentation, and putative deficits in kinesthetic reafference in Parkinson's disease. *Front Hum Neurosci* 8:823.

Torres, E. B., and K. Denisova. 2016. Motor noise is rich signal in autism research and pharmacological treatments. *Sci Rep* 6:37422.

Torres, E. B., R. W. Isenhower, J. Nguyen, C. Whyatt, J. I. Nurnberger, J. V. Jose, S. M. Silverstein, T. V. Papathomas, J. Sage, and J. Cole. 2016. Toward precision psychiatry: Statistical platform for the personalized characterization of natural behaviors. *Front Neurol* 7:8.

Tröster, H., and M. Brambring. 1994. The play behavior and play materials of blind and sighted infants and preschoolers. *J Vis Impair Blind* 88:421–32.

Tsongalis, G. J., and L. M. Silverman. 1993. Molecular pathology of the fragile X syndrome. *Arch Pathol Lab Med* 117 (11):1121–5.

Tyszka, J. M., D. P. Kennedy, L. K. Paul, and R. Adolphs. 2014. Largely typical patterns of resting-state functional connectivity in high-functioning adults with autism. *Cereb Cortex* 24 (7):1894–905.

Uno, Y., M. Kawato, and R. Suzuki. 1989. Formation and control of optimal trajectory in human multijoint arm movement. *Biol Cybern* 61 (2):89–101.

Vernazza-Martin, S., N. Martin, A. Vernazza, A. Lepellec-Muller, M. Rufo, J. Massion, and C. Assaiante. 2005. Goal directed locomotion and balance control in autistic children. *J Autism Dev Disord* 35 (1): 91–102.

Vilensky, J. A., A. R. Damasio, and R. G. Maurer. 1981. Gait disturbances in patients with autistic behavior: A preliminary study. *Arch Neurol* 38 (10):646–9.

Volkmar, F. R., P. Szatmari, and S. S. Sparrow. 1993. Sex differences in pervasive developmental disorders. *J Autism Dev Disord* 23 (4):579–91.

Volpe, J. J. 2008. *Neurology of the Newborn*. Amsterdam: Elsevier Health Sciences.

Wallace, M. T., and R. A. Stevenson. 2014. The construct of the multisensory temporal binding window and its dysregulation in developmental disabilities. *Neuropsychologia* 64:105–23.

WHO (World Health Organization). 1994. *The ICD-10 Classification of Mental and Behavioural Disorders: Clinical Descriptions and Diagnostic Guidelines*. Geneva: WHO.

WHO (World Health Organization). 2016. Disorders of psychological development (F80–F89). *International Statistical Classification of Diseases and Related Health Problems 10th Revision (ICD-10).* http://apps.who.int/classifications/icd10/browse/2016/en#/F80-F89.

Whyatt, C., and C. Craig. 2013a. Sensory-motor problems in autism. *Front Integr Neurosci* 7:51.

Whyatt, C., and C. M. Craig. 2013b. Interceptive skills in children aged 9–11 years, diagnosed with autism spectrum disorder. *Res Autism Spectrum Disord* 7 (5):613–23.

Whyatt, C. P., and C. M. Craig. 2012. Motor skills in children aged 7–10 years, diagnosed with autism spectrum disorder. *J Autism Dev Disord* 42 (9):1799–809.

Wijnhoven, T. M. A., M. de Onis, A. W. Onyango, T. Wang, G.-E. A. Bjoerneboe, N. Bhandari, A. Lartey, and B. Al Rashidi. 2004. Assessment of gross motor development in the WHO Multicentre Growth Reference Study. *Food Nutr Bull* 25 (1 Suppl 1):S37–45.

Wing, L. 1981. Asperger's syndrome: A clinical account. *Psychol Med* 11 (01):115–29.

Wing, L. 1997. The autistic spectrum. *Lancet* 350 (9093):1761–6.

Wing, L., and J. Gould. 1979. Severe impairments of social interaction and associated abnormalities in children: Epidemiology and classification. *J Autism Dev Disord* 9 (1):11–29.

Wolpert, D. M., and M. Kawato. 1998. Multiple paired forward and inverse models for motor control. *Neural Netw* 11 (7):1317–29.

Wolpert, D. M., R. C. Miall, and M. Kawato. 1998. Internal models in the cerebellum. *Trends Cogn Sci* 2 (9): 338–47.

Wooten, G. F., L. J. Currie, V. E. Bovbjerg, J. K. Lee, and J. Patrie. 2004. Are men at greater risk for Parkinson's disease than women? *J Neurol Neurosurg Psychiatry* 75 (4):637–9.

Wu, T., and M. Hallett. 2013. The cerebellum in Parkinson's disease. *Brain* 136 (3):696–709.

Zwaigenbaum, L., S. Bryson, T. Rogers, W. Roberts, J. Brian, and P. Szatmari. 2005. Behavioral manifestations of autism in the first year of life. *Int J Dev Neurosci* 23 (2):143–52.

3 Can Cognitive Theories Help to Understand Motor Dysfunction in Autism Spectrum Disorder?

Nicci Grace, Beth P. Johnson, Peter G. Enticott, and Nicole J. Rinehart

CONTENTS

Motor Functioning in Autism Spectrum Disorder 43
Cognitive Theories in ASD 44
Movement Organization and Sequencing 45
How do Children with ASD Sequence their Movements? 45
Can Motor Sequencing Patterns in ASD Be Interpreted in the Context of Cognitive Theory? 46
Visuomotor Integration 47
Handwriting in ASD 49
Assessment of Handwriting Proficiency 49
Features of Poor Handwriting 49
Characterizing Handwriting Difficulties in ASD 50
Predictors of Handwriting Impairment in ASD 50
Can Handwriting Impairment Be Explained within Cognitive Theoretical Frameworks? 50
Conclusion 51
References 51

This chapter provides a literature review of various components necessary for adequate motor control. These range from the biomechanical aspects of motor sequencing to the complex interactions that take place during accurate eye–hand coordination. Both sources of motor acts are discussed within the context of tasks that require abstraction and have different degrees of cognitive loads. These include the various visuomotor components required for controlled handwriting, including important aspects of visuomotor integration that seem to develop differently in autism spectrum disorder (ASD). We discuss these findings in light of current cognitive theories of social and communication impairments in ASD to try and reconcile disparate notions on their possible links.

MOTOR FUNCTIONING IN AUTISM SPECTRUM DISORDER

Children with autism spectrum disorder (ASD) commonly experience a range of impairments in motor functioning, including poor coordination and/or fine motor skills (Fournier et al. 2010). The prevalence in rates of motor impairment has been reported to be as high as 82% in children with ASD (Green et al. 2009). Greater motor impairment is associated with greater disruptions in social functioning, including emotional and behavioral disturbance (Freitag et al. 2007; Hilton et al. 2007; Sipes et al. 2011; Papadopoulos et al. 2012b). For example, the ability to successfully interact with one's environment and peers (e.g., playing ball sports or climbing play equipment) may be significantly impeded by the presence of impaired motor skills (Pan et al. 2009).

The reasons for differences in the way individuals with ASD plan, execute, and regulate their movements are not yet widely understood, yet historically, empirical studies have interpreted these differences within the framework of a globally impaired motor system and/or an impaired ability for neural integration of sensory information (Sacrey et al. 2015). More recently, motor sequencing studies in ASD have increasingly suggested a strong interplay between the way in which individuals with ASD plan, execute, and regulate their movement, and their cognitive style (Cattaneo et al. 2007; Dowd et al. 2012). Indeed, this is akin to Leary and Hill's (1996) seminal work identifying the ways in which movement disturbance reported within the ASD literature could be related to the traditional social-communicative features of the disorder.

This chapter outlines the most prominent cognitive theories of ASD, which will later be explored in the context of movement organization and sequencing patterns typically reported within ASD populations. Specific attention is given to the way visuomotor integration relates to an individual's ability to plan, control, and execute his or her movements, using specific examples from studies of ocular motor control in ASD. Finally, these fields are brought together to examine how disruption of motor planning and visuomotor control gives rise to impairments in daily motor functioning. Here we use the example of handwriting, a highly automated motor task that is central to children's daily and academic lives.

COGNITIVE THEORIES IN ASD

Several cognitive theories have been proposed in an attempt to explain the characteristic symptoms of ASD (Hoy et al. 2004). The most prominent of these are executive dysfunction, theory of mind, and weak central coherence (Pellicano et al. 2006; Rajendran and Mitchell 2007). Initially, cognitive models were evaluated independently, with empirical support for one model negating the importance of another. It is now widely accepted that each provides important insight into the neuropsychological profile of ASD; however, there is continued debate regarding the nature of their relationships (Rinehart et al. 2000; Rajendran and Mitchell 2007; Brunsdon and Happé 2014; Kimhi 2014).

Executive dysfunction theory posits that impaired higher-order cognitive processes, such as mental flexibility, planning, and inhibitory control, may account for characteristic clinical features of ASD. For example, reduced inhibitory control and perseveration have been suggested to underlie the core features of the disorder, including restricted and repetitive motor behaviors. Importantly, executive dysfunction accounts of ASD are domain general and not inherently specific to ASD (Rajendran and Mitchell 2007). Indeed, executive dysfunction is common to several clinical populations, particularly those in which frontal lobe dysfunction is implicated, such as attention deficit hyperactivity disorder (ADHD) and schizophrenia (Bradshaw 2001). As such, executive dysfunction theory aligns with the notion that neurodevelopmental disorders are primarily, although not exclusively, disorders of the frontostriatal system (Bradshaw 2001).

Similar to the *cognitive* theory of executive dysfunction, Minshew and Goldstein (1998) proposed a *neurobehavioral* model specific to ASD, which describes it as a disorder of complex information processing across multiple neuropsychological domains. Empirical studies supporting this model have found that individuals with ASD perform equivalently to cognitively matched peers on simple tasks, but exhibit impaired performances on more complex tasks within the same cognitive domain, including the motor domain (Williams et al. 2006). Indeed, the complexity of motor tasks is suggested as a critical factor influencing the overall performance in ASD (Green et al. 2009).

Weak central coherence theory proposes that in ASD there is a bias toward local processing over global processing (Frith 1989). This bias is suggested to underpin difficulties with motor coordination and differences in motor sequencing styles (Booth et al. 2003; Fabbri-Destro et al. 2009).

Importantly, weak central coherence is commonly interpreted as a *difference* or *variation* in cognitive style, rather than a cognitive deficit, and is not necessarily a universal feature of the disorder (Jarrold and Russell 1997; Happé 1999; Happé and Frith 2006). This reflects the common heterogeneity found in ASD and suggests that central coherence may be best interpreted from a continuum approach (Happé and Frith 2006). Support for weak central coherence in ASD has been established in some studies (Rinehart et al. 2000; Noens and van Berckelaer-Onnes 2008) but not in others (López and Leekam 2003; Hoy et al. 2004; Burnette et al. 2005).

Theory of mind (also referred to as mentalizing theory) refers to an individual's ability to understand the thoughts and feelings of others, that is, to understand one's beliefs or mental states (Baron-Cohen 2000). Theory of mind has typically been explored in relation to the characteristic social impairments in ASD (Korkmaz 2011); however, it is also an important factor in regard to motor functioning. Motor acts are typically performed in social settings and initiated in response to other people's actions (Schmidt et al. 2011). Furthermore, motor learning is often achieved through observation and imitation. Understanding the social and emotional context underlying other people's behaviors will therefore facilitate an individual's ability to engage with his or her environment in a socially appropriate and meaningful way.

MOVEMENT ORGANIZATION AND SEQUENCING

Every purposeful motor act, such as throwing a ball, can be conceptualized as a sequence of discrete motor units that give rise to an overall movement (Fogassi et al. 2005). The fluidity, accuracy, and coordination of a movement are determined by an individual's capacity to appropriately plan, modulate, and execute each stage of the movement sequence. In the initial stage of movement organization, an individual plans his or her movement based on his or her intended action (Fogassi and Luppino 2005). This requires an individual to accurately interpret and incorporate the underlying goal and trajectory of the movement (Forti et al. 2011). After a motor program has been selected, the execution phase ensues. During movement execution, an individual is consistently engaged in the monitoring of his or her movement based on visual and proprioceptive feedback (on-line control), as well as past experience (off-line control) (Sosnik et al. 2009; Sacrey et al. 2015). At times, an individual may need to correct and/or adjust his or her movement while it is being executed, and this often arises due to errors in an individual's initial motor plan, neuromuscular noise, spatial errors, and/or changes in the environment (e.g., changing position of a target) (Forti et al. 2011). This interplay between planning and control processes aims to optimize overall movement time (Forti et al. 2011).

HOW DO CHILDREN WITH ASD SEQUENCE THEIR MOVEMENTS?

Upper-limb kinematic studies have consistently identified differences in overall consistency and organization of movement (Mari et al. 2003; Glazebrook et al. 2008), despite an overall ability to complete a particular motor act seemingly equivalently to age-matched peers. While atypical motor sequencing and coordination of motor units is well supported by empirical research, the nature of these difficulties is not well understood, and mixed findings regarding motor planning, execution, and control processes are reported (Sacrey et al. 2015). In addition to the common limitations associated with ASD research (heterogeneity and small sample sizes), this variability has been attributed to differences in tasks, measurement, and participant groups (e.g., broad age range and range of intellectual functioning) employed across motor sequencing studies (Glazebrook et al. 2008; Stoit et al. 2013; Sacrey et al. 2015). For example, when considering studies of motor control, each tends to employ different experimental paradigms that require an individual to modify and reprogram his or her initial motor plan, such as incorporating visual distractors (Dowd et al. 2010) or changes in end-point target characteristics (e.g., shape and size) (Fabbri-Destro et al. 2009).

Empirical studies have identified both atypical (Rinehart et al. 2006a; Dowd et al. 2012) and spared (Forti et al. 2011; Stoit et al. 2013) motor planning abilities across both child and adult ASD populations. Of those studies showing atypical planning profiles, movements in the ASD groups have typically been characterized by longer and more variable timing in the initial planning stages than in matched controls (Glazebrook et al. 2006, Rinehart et al. 2006b; 2008; Nazarali et al. 2009; Dowd et al. 2012). Poorer advanced planning has also been identified in precued tasks (Hughes 1996; Rinehart et al. 2001). Similarly, studies examining the execution phases of movement have identified equivalent motor execution in some instances (Rinehart et al. 2001, 2006a) but significantly slowed execution time in others (Glazebrook et al. 2006, 2008; Nazarali et al. 2009; Forti et al. 2011; Stoit et al. 2013). With regard to motor control, studies have consistently proposed impairments in on-line, feed-forward control in children (Mari et al. 2003; Schmitz et al. 2003; David et al. 2012; Dowd et al. 2012; Papadopoulos et al. 2012a) and young adults (Glazebrook et al. 2006; Nazarali et al. 2009) with ASD.

CAN MOTOR SEQUENCING PATTERNS IN ASD BE INTERPRETED IN THE CONTEXT OF COGNITIVE THEORY?

Consistent with the broader ASD literature, there is increasing focus on the interplay between the social, cognitive, and motor characteristics of ASD (Dowd et al. 2010; Papadopoulos et al. 2012b). While these associations remain theoretically based, they encourage further research directly exploring these links. Specifically, the approach to movement organization in ASD has been increasingly interpreted within the framework of existing ASD cognitive theories. While none of these interpretations are considered to account for the neuromotor profile of ASD in isolation, they encourage an alternative way of thinking about motor functioning in ASD using an integrative approach. This aligns with the multiple-deficits model (Pennington 2006) and may ultimately influence a more well-defined neuromotor profile, as well as more holistic and targeted intervention approaches.

When performing a motor act, an individual will typically incorporate the final goal or intention of the movement into his or her initial motor plan (Fogassi et al. 2005; Cattaneo et al. 2007; Fabbri-Destro et al. 2009). In children with ASD, studies have identified a failure to organize their movement in this way and, rather, to adjust for the intention of the movement later in the movement sequence (Cattaneo et al. 2007). Importantly, this indicates intact intention understanding (i.e., the ability to identify the overall goal of the movement). This is further supported by the fact that these children are able to complete the task accurately, albeit in a less organized and coordinated manner relative to age-matched peers. For example, studies identifying intact motor execution have identified poor anticipatory action planning, whereby children with ASD fail to incorporate visual distractors when planning, reprogramming, and executing their movements (Hughes 1996; Rinehart et al. 2006b; Dowd et al. 2012).

Several interpretations have been identified concerning why individuals with ASD appear to organize their movement differently to typically developing groups. In line with weak central coherence theory, children with ASD demonstrate a piecemeal approach to motor sequencing, whereby they treat each motor unit or chain as an isolated sequence and/or each trial as a discrete entity (Fabbri-Destro et al. 2009; Dowd et al. 2010; Forti et al. 2011). Specifically, there is a failure to incorporate the final, global motor action into the initial motor plan (Booth et al. 2003; Fabbri-Destro et al. 2009). This has been suggested to underpin difficulties with movement scaling (Glazebrook et al. 2006), consistency across tasks (Glazebrook et al. 2008) and anticipatory or advanced planning (Hughes 1996; Rinehart et al. 2001; Mari et al. 2003; Dowd et al. 2012).

Movement differences have also been proposed to arise from executive dysfunction, possibly due to impaired frontostriatal circuitry (Hughes 1996; Pennington 2006). Executive control has been proposed as an essential feature required to perform a proficient, goal-directed movement (Hughes 1996). For example, motor control is suggested to rely heavily on sensory integration, a process that is mediated by attention and requires higher-order cognitive processing (Rinehart et al. 2001). Indeed, difficulties in planning and control processes have been suggested to reflect impaired use of external feedback (e.g., visual cues) in ASD (Hughes 1996; Mari et al. 2003). Further to this, executive difficulties, such as perseveration, poor planning, and an inflexible thinking style, have been proposed to underlie some of the atypical motor sequencing observed in ASD, specifically difficulties with reprogramming movements (Glazebrook et al. 2008; Dowd et al. 2012; Papadopoulos et al. 2012a).

Consistent with executive dysfunction and complex information processing theory (Minshew and Goldstein 1998), an increased requirement for multilevel processing in a given motor task may impact overall motor proficiency (Sacrey et al. 2015). While there is some support for the notion that increased task difficulty is associated with greater motor planning difficulties (Hughes 1996; Glazebrook et al. 2008; Fabbri-Destro et al. 2009; Nazarali et al. 2009), conflicting findings have been reported. Most notably, a significant distinction between children with ASD and those *with* and *without* a history of language delay was identified in a manual aiming task across three levels of complexity. Level 1 was the most basic condition and involved no manipulation of the target and an instruction to move toward the target, and level 2 involved manipulation of the target and a similar instruction to move toward the target, whereas level 3 involved manipulation of the target as well as instructions to move to the opposite side of the target. Interestingly, cognitively able children with ASD showed equivalent motor planning difficulties across the three different task levels; however, children with ASD without a history of language delay showed a trend toward more impaired performance in the most simple task level, possibly reflective of *kinesia paradoxa* (Rinehart et al. 2006a). These findings suggested that the severity of ASD symptoms and cognitive ability may play a significant role in movement organization, particularly for motor planning. Specifically, the authors noted that while children with ASD both with and without a history of language delay may present with commonalities in functional motor impairment, the underlying processes responsible for these difficulties may be distinct between groups. Indeed, discriminant motor profiles have been reported in ASD groups with different cognitive ability, specifically between cognitively able children with ASD and children with both ASD and intellectual impairment (Mari et al. 2003; Green et al. 2009). For example, Mari et al (2003) identified impaired motor execution in children with full-scale IQ scores below 80 but not in cognitive able children with ASD.

VISUOMOTOR INTEGRATION

Another significant, but often overlooked aspect of motor control is the contribution of vision and eye movements to planning, accuracy, and timing of fine and gross motor actions. Motor actions are heavily reliant eye movements to guide planning of movement trajectory, provide on-line information about limb position in addition to proprioceptive evidence, and provide feedback about the accuracy of the movement end point (Glazebrook et al. 2009). It is often stated that ASD is associated with significant impairments in eye–hand coordination; however, ocular motor control is an often overlooked aspect of motor function (Gowen and Miall 2005), and it is rare for the relationship between eye movements and hand movements to be examined concomitantly in ASD.

Inaccuracies in eye movement may conceivably have detrimental, downstream consequences for ASD, such as language acquisition, attention, or visuomotor coordination (Brenner et al. 2007). There are several lines of evidence that support there being significant impairment to visuomotor integration (Annaz et al. 2010; Takarae et al. 2014) and ocular motor control in ASD (Mosconi et al. 2013; Johnson et al. 2013c; Schmitt et al. 2014).

Eye movements serve to maintain objects of interest on the fovea, the region of the retina that provides the greatest acuity and color detection (Leigh and Zee 2015). Accurate eye movements are essential for on-line regulation of fine and gross motor accuracy, in addition to proprioceptive signals, and also for providing visual feedback to refine movement accuracy over the long term. Saccades are semiballistic eye movements that shift the eye toward an object of interest, while smooth pursuit eye movements help us to track moving objects, while either an object or ourselves (or both) are in motion (Leigh and Zee 2015). These two main types of eye movements help us to plan actions and coordinate our whole-body movements, and give us visual information about our changing environment to enable us to adapt our actions *on the fly*. There are a number of known visual processing and ocular motor disturbances in ASD that are likely to impact these processes, which include impaired motion detection (Manning et al. 2013; Takarae et al. 2014), inaccurate eye movements (Takarae et al. 2004a, 2004b; Johnson et al. 2012; Schmitt et al. 2014), and inefficient timing of ocular motor with fine motor actions (Crippa et al. 2013).

Several studies have found that motion perception thresholds are much higher in ASD (Koldewyn et al. 2009; Annaz et al. 2010; Takarae et al. 2014). Active, closed-loop pursuit requires updating from visual area 5 (V5) to vermal lobules VI and VII. Gepner and Mestre (2002) explored postural reactivity in response to visual motion, and similarly reported "visuopostural detuning" in children with ASD, which is consistent with slower detection and updating of visual motion signals, and their integration with other motor systems. Bertone et al. (2003) found that motion processing was particularly impaired when more complex motion stimuli were used, requiring higher-level visual integration. This indicates inefficient integrative functioning of networks that mediate visuoperceptual processing in ASD. Indeed, this is supported by recent functional magnetic resonance imaging (fMRI) evidence from Takarae and colleagues (2014), who found that ASD showed greater activation and faster hemodynamic decay in V5 (area MT), the region responsible for motion detection, when passively viewing motion stimuli, yet reduced frontal and V5 activation when performing pursuit eye movements. The results reveal that the mechanisms that give rise to disturbances in motion processing and visually tracking a moving object are complex, and are likely due to intrinsic abnormalities in V5 and disruption of frontoparietal ocular motor networks.

In addition to impaired motion perception, there are consistent reports that ASD is associated with impairments in tracking moving objects. Eye movement tracking tends to be sluggish, as indicated by reduced eye velocity relative to the target, and needing to make additional catch-up saccades to maintain focus on a moving object. Numerous studies have now consistently demonstrated that pursuit eye movements are disrupted in ASD (Takarae et al. 2004a, 2007, 2008, 2014). Difficulty detecting motion, as well as impaired tracking of moving targets, may help to explain the reported difficulties with aiming and catching skills (Johnson et al. 2012; Papadopoulos et al. 2012b); if the ability to maintain eye movement trajectory with target trajectory is impaired, then this is likely to be detrimental to planning appropriate timing and placement of the body and limbs for catching a ball. Takarae et al. (2014) suggest that it is likely that a combination of bottom-up and top-down factors mediate this impairment.

Saccadic eye movements, which are associated with attentional shifts and are coupled with planning and initiating new attentional goals, are *dysmetric* in ASD. That is, although average saccade accuracy is no different from that of controls, eye movements of individuals with ASD are significantly more likely to overshoot or undershoot a target (Takarae et al. 2004b; Nazarali et al. 2009; Johnson et al. 2012; Schmitt et al. 2014). It is likely that saccade dysmetria would have important downstream effects on the motor planning and refining accuracy of fine motor actions if the ocular motor and visual system is unable to accurately and rapidly integrate visual cues from the environment, and provide feedback on motor accuracy. Children with ASD also have difficulty utilizing visual information to correct errors in motor accuracy over time (Mosconi et al. 2013; Johnson et al. 2013c).

Lastly, the ability of individuals with ASD to utilize visual feedback and integrate this with other motor actions is also disrupted. As we move our limbs toward a target that we are looking at, visual information is relayed back for adjustments to be made on line (Starkes et al. 2002; Crippa et al. 2013). However for very rapid movements, such as fine motor actions, it is rare for visual feedback to directly monitor performance of the effector (the limb or joint), but rather, our visual system is updating our motor system about global changes in the environment or stimuli we are interacting with. Instead, however, the role of eye movements in guiding handwriting is to maintain overall movement trajectory and monitor for errors in the writing. The study by Glazebrook and colleagues (2009) directly examined eye and hand coordination simultaneously. They found that greater variability in ocular motor control was associated with greater variability in the end point of their fine motor (hand) movements, and longer response times. Crippa and colleagues (2013) also explored the relationship between eye and hand coupling in ASD. Their findings indicated impaired synchrony of eye and hand movements during a task requiring them to both look and point.

Although the research in this space has been relatively limited, they indicate that ocular motor abnormalities in tracking both objects and fixed targets, impairment in utilizing visual feedback in refining motor error, and successfully integrating eye and hand actions contribute to impaired motor coordination in ASD. This is particularly relevant when evaluating motor tasks, such as handwriting, which are heavily reliant on intact eye–hand coordination and visual feedback.

HANDWRITING IN ASD

The following section offers a review of handwriting, which is well documented as a specific task that children with ASD encounter difficulty with as a function of their overarching motor impairment. Importantly, in school-aged children, handwriting represents an everyday, well-practiced skill that becomes relatively automated by grade 3 (age 8) and has been shown to be important for academic achievement and the development of social communication skills (Karlsdottir and Stefansson 2002; Feder and Majnemer 2007). Assessment of handwriting therefore provides an ecologically valid and clinically useful measure of motor proficiency in school-aged children.

In ASD, handwriting difficulties are commonly reported in school-aged children, and a high proportion of these individuals are referred for occupational therapy intervention (Cartmill et al. 2009; Rodger and Polatajko 2014). Handwriting is a complex and dynamic process that relies on the interactive processing of perceptual-motor and cognitive functions. Importantly, handwriting sequences can be easily broken down to examine different aspects of movement sequencing, such as motor planning and control, and can therefore illuminate which motor processes may underlie common functional motor impairment observed in ASD populations.

Poor handwriting was first identified as a clinical feature of ASD in the original description of the disorder by Hans Asperger in 1944. Clinically, it is common for children with ASD to be referred for occupational therapy for fine motor difficulties, specifically relating to handwriting impairment. In 2009, a survey of occupational therapists in two districts in Australia found children with ASD comprised 40% of their caseload, with 86% these referrals related to handwriting difficulties and/or fine motor impairment (Cartmill et al. 2009). Similarly in the United States, Church et al. (2000) established that 58% of young boys with ASD in their study received occupational therapy intervention for fine motor difficulties, including handwriting.

ASSESSMENT OF HANDWRITING PROFICIENCY

Historically, handwriting has been assessed using qualitative measures focused on the legibility of writing, typically indexed by quality and speed (Volman et al. 2006; Rosenblum and Livneh-Zirinski 2008; Kushki et al. 2011). While this has provided useful information about the overall writing *product*, this approach has been criticized by its failure to identify *where* in the handwriting process difficulties arise (Rosenblum and Livneh-Zirinski 2008; Falk et al. 2011). More recently, the introduction of digitizer-based technology has provided the opportunity for quick, quantitative, and objective measurement of handwriting *processes*, which produce precise and objective measures of spatial and temporal features, as well as force, planning, and control of movement (Rosenblum et al. 2006; Di Brina et al. 2008; Falk et al. 2011).

Features of Poor Handwriting

Studies of handwriting in typically developing children have shown that poor writers produce more variable movement profiles and a lack of spatial consistency than proficient writers (Smits-Engelsman and Van Galen 1997). Poor writers have also been found to have larger trajectories, reduced smoothness of movement (poor letter formation), and neuromotor noise (Van Galen et al. 1993; Smits-Engelsman and Van Galen 1997; Kushki et al. 2011). While faster movements are known to be associated with poor handwriting quality and legibility (Smits-Engelsman and Van Galen 1997), inconsistent findings have been reported in regard to speed of writing. Indeed, poor writers have been found to perform movements more slowly (Volman et al. 2006), more quickly (Karlsdottir and Stefansson 2002; Kushki et al. 2011), and more variably (Wann and Jones 1986) than matched controls.

Despite the high prevalence of handwriting difficulties in children with ASD, there remains a dearth of studies characterizing these impairments and variable findings are reported. Similarly to the broader ASD literature, studies are limited by their small sample sizes, heterogeneous clinical presentations, differing inclusion and diagnostic criteria, and lack of uniformity between both tasks and measures employed (e.g., task duration and cognitive and motor complexity) (Kushki et al. 2011).

Characterizing Handwriting Difficulties in ASD

Distinct handwriting profiles have been identified in both ADHD and cognitively able ASD populations, both in comparison with each other and typically developing (TD) populations, suggesting that the pattern of handwriting deficits evident in ASD may be unique to this population (Johnson et al. 2013a). While studies of handwriting in children with ASD are limited, they have identified difficulties with poor letter formation and legibility of text (; Myles et al. 2003; Cartmill et al. 2009; Fuentes et al. 2009; Kushki et al. 2011), more *variable* movement trajectories, and greater neuromotor noise (Johnson et al. 2013b). While some studies have identified slow writing speed (Hellinckx et al. 2013; Johnson et al. 2013c), others have found no significant differences in speed compared with matched controls (Cartmill et al. 2009). Similarly, while some studies have identified an impaired ability in children with ASD to correctly size, space, and align their letters (Cartmill et al. 2009; Hellinckx et al. 2013; Johnson et al. 2013a, 2013b), others have reported no differences (Fuentes et al. 2009; Johnson et al. 2015).

Predictors of Handwriting Impairment in ASD

Increasingly, attempts are being made to address the possible associations between general motor skills, age, IQ, and handwriting performance. Indeed, within the broader ASD-motor literature, significant differences in movement planning and execution have been identified between low- and high-functioning groups (Mari et al. 2003; Glazebrook et al. 2006). Despite a lack of consensus, studies have suggested that motor skills (Fuentes et al. 2009), perceptual reasoning (Fuentes et al. 2010), and age, gender, and visuomotor integration (Hellinckx et al. 2013) may predict handwriting *quality*, whereas verbal comprehension (Johnson et al. 2013a), age, reading abilities, and fine motor coordination (Hellinckx et al. 2013) may predict handwriting *speed*.

Can Handwriting Impairment Be Explained within Cognitive Theoretical Frameworks?

As explored earlier in this chapter, differences in motor planning and sequencing in ASD may reflect the underlying cognitive styles thought to present in this population. Indeed, theoretical links have been drawn between cognitive and handwriting styles in ASD in an attempt to characterize the possible difficulties in their planning, sequencing, and control of movement. Smaller and irregular spacing between words in cognitively able children with ASD was suggested to reflect a piecemeal planning approach to movement sequencing, consistent with weak central coherence theory (Johnson et al. 2013a). Indeed, this would differ from the global planning approach in typically developing children who have been shown to plan their writing sequences in advance using syllables as functional units (Kandel et al. 2006a, 2006b). Theory of mind has also been positively associated with writing quality and text length in adults with ASD without a history of language delay (Brown and Klein 2011). While there remains a paucity of empirical data, theoretically, it seems plausible that the variable handwriting profiles identified in children with ASD may reflect differing cognitive, perceptual, and motor demands inherent within certain tasks. Indeed, Cartmill et al. (2009) highlighted the significant overlay between cognition, perception, and action in their "sequential handwriting model" developed specifically for an ASD population. In a recent study by Johnson et al. (2015), children with ASD showed comparable sizing, movement consistency, and motor control relative to age-matched peers in a simplistic handwriting task. Consistent with complex information processing theory (Minshew and Goldstein 1998), this suggests that commonly observed handwriting difficulties in ASD may be moderated by the cognitive (e.g., attention, working memory, and language) and/or motor sequencing demands of a given task (Williams et al. 2006; Johnson et al. 2015). Further, with increased demand on an already vulnerable motor system, increasingly complex tasks (e.g., length and duration) may lead to greater fatigue of the muscular system and result in poorer legibility and control of movement (Johnson et al. 2013a; Prunty et al. 2014). More empirical studies focused on predictors of poor handwriting and establishing links between cognitive and handwriting or motor styles are needed to further progress our knowledge in this field.

CONCLUSION

Motor functioning is a critical component of how an individual experiences and behaves within his or her environment. In childhood, impaired motor functioning can impede opportunities for social play and academic achievement, as well as reduce confidence and self-esteem. Over the past several decades, there has been increased awareness that a significant proportion of children with ASD experience atypical motor functioning compared with age-matched peers. This often translates to significant functional difficulties, such as handwriting impairment, and requirement for therapeutic intervention, such as occupational therapy.

As the current review highlights, there appears to be a close interplay between motor and cognitive theory in ASD. There is a need to continue to understand motor functioning alongside the core social and communicative symptoms to achieve a more integrative approach to both research and clinical practice. Importantly, greater understanding of cognitive theory may assist in guiding evidence-based approaches to treating motor difficulties in ASD. Currently, there is an absence of translation between research and practice. Importantly, there is strong evidence to suggest that motor difficulties in specific domains, such as handwriting, may be unique and therefore require different intervention programs for TD individuals with similar functional impairment.

The current review demonstrates the value of assessing motor functioning within the framework of a meaningful and practical motor task, such as handwriting. While there is consensus regarding the presence of handwriting impairment in ASD, the nature of these impairments remains unclear (Kushki et al. 2011). It remains to be determined whether the processes underlying handwriting impairment in ASD are comparable to those seen in a purely dysgraphic population or if a distinct profile exists. Indeed, the current literature does provide support for the latter (Johnson et al. 2013a). The introduction of digitizer-based technology provides a practical and objective method of assessing handwriting in school-aged children and an opportunity to evaluate not only handwriting styles and ability, but also the efficacy of intervention programs.

Overall, given the large proportion of children who experience motor dysfunction, developing evidence-based motor interventions targeted at children with ASD appears to be an important goal of future research. Additionally, as many families already seek intervention for motor impairment, establishing the efficacy of existing treatments currently being used is critical.

REFERENCES

Annaz, D., A. Remington, E. Milne, M. Coleman, R. Campbell, M. S. C. Thomas, and J. Swettenham. 2010. Development of motion processing in children with autism. *Dev Sci* 13 (6):826–38.

Baron-Cohen, S. 2000. Theory of mind and autism: A review. *Int Rev Res Ment Retard* 23:169–84.

Bertone, A., L. Mottron, P. Jelenic, and J. Faubert. 2003. Motion perception in autism: A "complex" issue. *J Cogn Neurosci* 15 (2):218–25.

Booth, R., R. Charlton, C. Hughes, and F. Happé. 2003. Disentangling weak coherence and executive dysfunction: Planning drawing in autism and attention–deficit/hyperactivity disorder. *Philos Trans R Soc B Biol Sci* 358 (1430):387–92.

Bradshaw, J. L. 2001. *Developmental Disorders of the Frontostriatal System: Neuropsychological, Neuropsychiatric, and Evolutionary Perspectives*. New York: Psychology Press.

Brenner, L. A., K. C. Turner, and R.-A. Müller. 2007. Eye movement and visual search: Are there elementary abnormalities in autism? *J Autism Dev Disord* 37 (7):1289–309.

Brown, H. M., and P. D. Klein. 2011. Writing, Asperger syndrome and theory of mind. *J Autism Dev Disord* 41 (11):1464–74.

Brunsdon, V. E. A., and F. Happé. 2014. Exploring the 'fractionation' of autism at the cognitive level. *Autism* 18 (1):17–30.

Burnette, C. P., P. C. Mundy, J. A. Meyer, S. K. Sutton, A. E. Vaughan, and D. Charak. 2005. Weak central coherence and its relations to theory of mind and anxiety in autism. *J Autism Dev Disord* 35 (1):63–73.

Cartmill, L., S. Rodger, and J. Ziviani. 2009. Handwriting of eight-year-old children with autistic spectrum disorder: An exploration. *J Occup Ther Schools Early Interv* 2 (2):103–18.

Cattaneo, L., M. Fabbri-Destro, S. Boria, C. Pieraccini, A. Monti, G. Cossu, and G. Rizzolatti. 2007. Impairment of actions chains in autism and its possible role in intention understanding. *Proc Natl Acad Sci USA* 104 (45):17825–30.

Church, C., S. Alisanski, and S. Amanullah. 2000. The social, behavioral, and academic experiences of children with Asperger syndrome. *Focus Autism Other Dev Disabil* 15 (1):12–20.

Crippa, A., S. Forti, P. Perego, and M. Molteni. 2013. Eye-hand coordination in children with high functioning autism and Asperger's disorder using a gap-overlap paradigm. *J Autism Dev Disord* 43 (4):841–50.

David, F. J., G. T. Baranek, C. Wiesen, A. Miao, and D. E. Thorpe. 2012. Coordination of precision grip in 2–6 years-old children with autism spectrum disorders compared to children developing typically and children with developmental disabilities. *Front Integr Neurosci* 6:122.

Di Brina, C., R. Niels, A. Overvelde, G. Levi, and W. Hulstijn. 2008. Dynamic time warping: A new method in the study of poor handwriting. *Hum Mov Sci* 27 (2):242–55.

Dowd, A. M., J. L. McGinley, J. R. Taffe, and N. J. Rinehart. 2012. Do planning and visual integration difficulties underpin motor dysfunction in autism? A kinematic study of young children with autism. *J Autism Dev Disord* 42 (8):1539–48.

Dowd, A. M., N. J. Rinehart, and J. McGinley. 2010. Motor function in children with autism: Why is this relevant to psychologists? *Clin Psychol* 14 (3):90–6.

Fabbri-Destro, M., L. Cattaneo, S. Boria, and G. Rizzolatti. 2009. Planning actions in autism. *Exp Brain Res* 192 (3):521–5. doi: 10.1007/s00221–008–1578–3.

Falk, T. H., C. Tam, H. Schellnus, and T. Chau. 2011. On the development of a computer-based handwriting assessment tool to objectively quantify handwriting proficiency in children. *Comput Methods Programs Biomed* 104 (3):e102–11.

Feder, K. P., and A. Majnemer. 2007. Handwriting development, competency, and intervention. *Dev Med Child Neurol* 49 (4):312–7.

Fogassi, L., and G. Luppino. 2005. Motor functions of the parietal lobe. *Curr Opin Neurobiol* 15 (6):626–31.

Fogassi, L., P. F. Ferrari, B. Gesierich, S. Rozzi, F. Chersi, and G. Rizzolatti. 2005. Parietal lobe: From action organization to intention understanding. *Science* 308 (5722):662–7.

Forti, S., A. Valli, P. Perego, M. Nobile, A. Crippa, and M. Molteni. 2011. Motor planning and control in autism. A kinematic analysis of preschool children. *Res Autism Spectr Disord* 5 (2):834–42.

Fournier, K. A., C. J. Hass, S. K. Naik, N. Lodha, and J. H. Cauraugh. 2010. Motor coordination in autism spectrum disorders: A synthesis and meta-analysis. *J Autism Dev Disord* 40 (10):1227–40.

Freitag, C. M., C. Kleser, M. Schneider, and A. von Gontard. 2007. Quantitative assessment of neuromotor function in adolescents with high functioning autism and Asperger syndrome. *J Autism Dev Disord* 37 (5): 948–59.

Frith, U. 1989. *Autism: Explaining the Enigma*. Oxford: Basil Blackwell.

Fuentes, C. T., S. H. Mostofsky, and A. J Bastian. 2009. Children with autism show specific handwriting impairments. *Neurology* 73 (19):1532–7.

Fuentes, C. T., S. H. Mostofsky, and A. J Bastian. 2010. Perceptual reasoning predicts handwriting impairments in adolescents with autism. *Neurology* 75 (20):1825–9.

Gepner, B., and D. Mestre. 2002. Rapid visual-motion integration deficit in autism. *Trends Cogn Sci* 6 (11):455.

Glazebrook, C. M., D. Elliott, and J. Lyons. 2006. A kinematic analysis of how young adults with and without autism plan and control goal-directed movements. *Motor Control* 10 (3):244.

Glazebrook, C. M., D. Elliott, and P. Szatmari. 2008. How do individuals with autism plan their movements? *J Autism Dev Disord* 38 (1):114–26.

Glazebrook, C., D. Gonzalez, S. Hansen, and D. Elliott. 2009. The role of vision for online control of manual aiming movements in persons with autism spectrum disorders. *Autism* 13 (4):411–33.

Gowen, E., and R. C. Miall. 2005. Behavioural aspects of cerebellar function in adults with Asperger syndrome. *Cerebellum* 4 (4):279–89.

Green, D., T. Charman, A. Pickles, S. Chandler, T. Loucas, E. Simonoff, and G. Baird. 2009. Impairment in movement skills of children with autistic spectrum disorders. *Dev Med Child Neurol* 51 (4):311–6.

Happé, F. 1999. Autism: Cognitive deficit or cognitive style? *Trends Cogn Sci* 3 (6):216–22.

Happé, F., and U. Frith. 2006. The weak coherence account: Detail-focused cognitive style in autism spectrum disorders. *J Autism Dev Disord* 36 (1):5–25.

Hellinckx, T., H. Roeyers, and H. Van Waelvelde. 2013. Predictors of handwriting in children with autism spectrum disorder. *Res Autism Spectr Disord* 7 (1):176–86.

Hilton, C., L. Wente, P. LaVesser, M. Ito, C. Reed, and G. Herzberg. 2007. Relationship between motor skill impairment and severity in children with Asperger syndrome. *Res Autism Spectr Disord* 1 (4):339–49.

Hoy, J. A., C. Hatton, and D. Hare. 2004. Weak central coherence: A cross-domain phenomenon specific to autism? *Autism* 8 (3):267–81.

Hughes, C. 1996. Brief report: Planning problems in autism at the level of motor control. *J Autism Dev Disord* 26 (1):99–107.

Jarrold, C., and J. Russell. 1997. Counting abilities in autism: Possible implications for central coherence theory. *J Autism Dev Disord* 27 (1):25–37.

Johnson, B. P., J. G. Phillips, N. Papadopoulos, J. Fielding, B. Tonge, and N. J. Rinehart. 2013b. Understanding macrographia in children with autism spectrum disorders. *Res Dev Disabil* 34 (9):2917–26.

Johnson, B. P., J. G. Phillips, N. Papadopoulos, J. Fielding, B. Tonge, and N. J. Rinehart. 2015. Do children with autism and Asperger's disorder have difficulty controlling handwriting size? A kinematic evaluation. *Res Autism Spectr Disord* 11:20–6.

Johnson, B. P., N. J. Rinehart, O. White, L. Millist, and J. Fielding. 2013c. Saccade adaptation in autism and Asperger's disorder. *Neuroscience* 243:76–87.

Johnson, B. P., N. Papadopoulos, J. Fielding, B. Tonge, J. G. Phillips, and N. J. Rinehart. 2013a. A quantitative comparison of handwriting in children with high-functioning autism and attention deficit hyperactivity disorder. *Res Autism Spectr Disord* 7 (12):1638–46.

Johnson, B., N. Rinehart, N. Papadopoulos, B. Tonge, L. Millist, O. White, and J. Fielding. 2012. A closer look at visually guided saccades in autism and Asperger's disorder. *Front Integr Neurosci* 6:99.

Kandel, S., C. J. Alvarez, and N. Vallée. 2006a. Syllables as processing units in handwriting production. *J Exp Psychol* 32 (1):18.

Kandel, S., O. Soler, S. Valdois, and C. Gros. 2006b. Graphemes as motor units in the acquisition of writing skills. *Read Writ* 19 (3):313–37.

Karlsdottir, R., and T. Stefansson. 2002. Problems in developing functional handwriting. *Percept Mot Skills* 94 (2):623–62.

Kimhi, Y. 2014. Theory of mind abilities and deficits in autism spectrum disorders. *Top Lang Disord* 34 (4): 329–43.

Koldewyn, K., D. Whitney, and S. M. Rivera. 2009. The psychophysics of visual motion and global form processing in autism. *Brain*:awp272.

Korkmaz, B. 2011. Theory of mind and neurodevelopmental disorders of childhood. *Pediatr Res* 69: 101R–8R.

Kushki, A., T. Chau, and E. Anagnostou. 2011. Handwriting difficulties in children with autism spectrum disorders: A scoping review. *J Autism Dev Disord* 41 (12):1706–16.

Leary, M. R., and D. A. Hill. 1996. Moving on: Autism and movement disturbance. *Ment Retard* 34 (1):39.

Leigh, R. J., and D. S. Zee. 2015. *The Neurology of Eye Movements*. Vol. 90. Oxford: Oxford University Press.

López, B., and S. R. Leekam. 2003. Do children with autism fail to process information in context? *J Child Psychol Psychiatry* 44 (2):285–300.

Manning, C., T. Charman, and E. Pellicano. 2013. Processing slow and fast motion in children with autism spectrum conditions. *Autism Res* 6 (6):531–41.

Mari, M., U. Castiello, D. Marks, C. Marraffa, and M. Prior. 2003. The reach-to-grasp movement in children with autism spectrum disorder. *Philos Trans R Soc Lond B Biol Sci* 358 (1430):393–403.

Minshew, N. J., and G. Goldstein. 1998. Autism as a disorder of complex information processing. *Ment Retard Dev Disabil Res Rev* 4 (2):129–36.

Mosconi, M. W., B. Luna, M. Kay-Stacey, C. V. Nowinski, L. H. Rubin, C. Scudder, N. Minshew, and J. A. Sweeney. 2013. Saccade adaptation abnormalities implicate dysfunction of cerebellar-dependent learning mechanisms in autism spectrum disorders (ASD). *PLoS One* 8 (5):e63709.

Myles, B. S., A. Huggins, M. Rome-Lake, T. Hagiwara, G. P. Barnhill, and D. E. Griswold. 2003. Written language profile of children and youth with Asperger syndrome: From research to practice. *Educ Train Dev Disabil* 38:362–9.

Nazarali, N., C. M. Glazebrook, and D. Elliott. 2009. Movement planning and reprogramming in individuals with autism. *J Autism Dev Disord* 39 (10):1401–11.

Noens, I. L. J., and I. A. van Berckelaer-Onnes. 2008. The central coherence account of autism revisited: Evidence from the ComFor study. *Res Autism Spectr Disord* 2 (2):209–22.

Pan, C.-Y., C.-L. Tsai, and C.-H. Chu. 2009. Fundamental movement skills in children diagnosed with autism spectrum disorders and attention deficit hyperactivity disorder. *J Autism Dev Disord* 39 (12):1694–705.

Papadopoulos, N., J. McGinley, B. Tonge, J. Bradshaw, K. Saunders, A. Murphy, and N. Rinehart. 2012a. Motor proficiency and emotional/behavioural disturbance in autism and Asperger's disorder: Another piece of the neurological puzzle? *Autism* 16 (6):627–40.

Papadopoulos, N., J. McGinley, B. J. Tonge, J. L. Bradshaw, K. Saunders, and N. J. Rinehart. 2012b. An investigation of upper limb motor function in high functioning autism and Asperger's disorder using a repetitive Fitts' aiming task. *Res Autism Spectr Disord* 6 (1):286–92.

Pellicano, E., M. Maybery, K. Durkin, and A. Maley. 2006. Multiple cognitive capabilities/deficits in children with an autism spectrum disorder: "Weak" central coherence and its relationship to theory of mind and executive control. *Dev Psychopathol* 18 (1):77.

Pennington, B. F. 2006. From single to multiple deficit models of developmental disorders. *Cognition* 101 (2): 385–413.

Prunty, M. M., A. L. Barnett, K. Wilmut, and M. S. Plumb. 2014. An examination of writing pauses in the handwriting of children with developmental coordination disorder. *Res Dev Disabil* 35 (11):2894–905.

Rajendran, G., and P. Mitchell. 2007. Cognitive theories of autism. *Dev Rev* 27 (2):224–60.

Rinehart, N. J., B. J. Tonge, J. L. Bradshaw, R. Iansek, P. G. Enticott, and K. A. Johnson. 2006b. Movement-related potentials in high-functioning autism and Asperger's disorder. *Dev Med Child Neurol* 48 (4): 272–7.

Rinehart, N. J., J. L. Bradshaw, A. V. Brereton, and B. J. Tonge. 2001. Movement preparation in high-functioning autism and Asperger disorder: A serial choice reaction time task involving motor reprogramming. *J Autism Dev Disord* 31 (1):79–88.

Rinehart, N. J., J. L. Bradshaw, S. A. Moss, A. V. Brereton, and B. J. Tonge. 2000. Atypical interference of local detail on global processing in high-functioning autism and Asperger's disorder. *J Child Psychol Psychiatry* 41 (06):769–78.

Rinehart, N. J., M. A. Bellgrove, B. J. Tonge, A. V. Brereton, D. Howells-Rankin, and J. L. Bradshaw. 2006a. An examination of movement kinematics in young people with high-functioning autism and Asperger's disorder: Further evidence for a motor planning deficit. *J Autism Dev Disord* 36 (6):757–67.

Rodger, S., and Polatajko, H. 2014. Occupational therapy for children with autism. In *Comprehensive Guide to Autism*, ed. V. Patel, 2297–314. New York: Springer Science and Business Media.

Rosenblum, S., A. Y. Dvorkin, and P. L. Weiss. 2006. Automatic segmentation as a tool for examining the handwriting process of children with dysgraphic and proficient handwriting. *Hum Mov Sci* 25 (4):608–21.

Rosenblum, S., and M. Livneh-Zirinski. 2008. Handwriting process and product characteristics of children diagnosed with developmental coordination disorder. *Hum Mov Sci* 27 (2):200–14.

Sacrey, L.-A. R., T. Germani, S. E. Bryson, and L. Zwaigenbaum. 2015. Reaching and grasping in autism spectrum disorder: A review of recent literature. *Front Neurol* 5 (6):40.

Schmidt, R. C., P. Fitzpatrick, R. Caron, and J. Mergeche. 2011. Understanding social motor coordination. *Hum Mov Sci* 30 (5):834–45.

Schmitt, L. M., E. H. Cook, J. A. Sweeney, and M. W. Mosconi. 2014. Saccadic eye movement abnormalities in autism spectrum disorder indicate dysfunctions in cerebellum and brainstem. *Mol Autism* 5 (1):1.

Schmitz, C., J. Martineau, C. Barthélémy, and C. Assaiante. 2003. Motor control and children with autism: Deficit of anticipatory function? *Neurosci Lett* 348 (1):17–20.

Sipes, M., J. L. Matson, and M. Horovitz. 2011. Autism spectrum disorders and motor skills: The effect on socialization as measured by the Baby and Infant Screen for Children with aUtIsm Traits (BISCUIT). *Dev Neurorehabil* 14 (5):290–6.

Smits-Engelsman, B. C. M., and G. P. Van Galen. 1997. Dysgraphia in children: Lasting psychomotor deficiency or transient developmental delay? *J Exp Child Psychol* 67 (2):164–84.

Sosnik, R., F. Polyakov, and T. Flash. 2009. Motor Sequences A2—Squire, Larry R. In *Encyclopedia of Neuroscience*, 1047–56. Oxford: Academic Press.

Starkes, J., W. Helsen, and D. Elliott. 2002. A menage a trois: The eye, the hand and on-line processing. *J. Sports Sci* 20 (3):217–24.

Stoit, A. M. B., H. T. van Schie, D. I. E. Slaats-Willemse, and J. K. Buitelaar. 2013. Grasping motor impairments in autism: Not action planning but movement execution is deficient. *J Autism Dev Disord* 43 (12): 2793–806.

Takarae, Y., B. Luna, N. J. Minshew, and J. A. Sweeney. 2008. Patterns of visual sensory and sensorimotor abnormalities in autism vary in relation to history of early language delay. *J Int Neuropsychol Soc* 14 (6):980.

Takarae, Y., B. Luna, N. J. Minshew, and J. A. Sweeney. 2014. Visual motion processing and visual sensorimotor control in autism. *J Int Neuropsychol Soc* 20 (1):113.

Takarae, Y., N. J. Minshew, B. Luna, and J. A. Sweeney. 2004b. Oculomotor abnormalities parallel cerebellar histopathology in autism. *J Neurol Neurosurg Psychiatry* 75 (9):1359–61.

Takarae, Y., N. J. Minshew, B. Luna, and J. A. Sweeney. 2007. Atypical involvement of frontostriatal systems during sensorimotor control in autism. *Psychiatry Res* 156 (2):117–27.

Takarae, Y., N. J. Minshew, B. Luna, C. M. Krisky, and J. A. Sweeney. 2004a. Pursuit eye movement deficits in autism. *Brain* 127 (12):2584–94.

Van Galen, G. P., S. J. Portier, B. C. M. Smits-Engelsman, and L. R. B. Schomaker. 1993. Neuromotor noise and poor handwriting in children. *Acta Psychol* 82 (1–3):161–78.

Volman, M. J. M., B. M. van Schendel, and M. J. Jongmans. 2006. Handwriting difficulties in primary school children: A search for underlying mechanisms. *Am J Occup Ther* 60 (4):451–60.

Wann, J. P., and J. G. Jones. 1986. Space-time invariance in handwriting: Contrasts between primary school children displaying advanced or retarded handwriting acquisition. *Hum Mov Sci* 5 (3):275–96.

Williams, D. L., G. Goldstein, and N. J. Minshew. 2006. Neuropsychologic functioning in children with autism: Further evidence for disordered complex information-processing. *Child Neuropsychol* 12 (4–5): 279–98.

Concluding Remarks to Section I

Top-Down versus Bottom-Up Approaches to Connect Cognition and Somatic Motor Sensations

Elizabeth B. Torres

Chapter 3 highlighted the contributions of cognitive theories to autism research. The cognitivist ideas reviewed in the chapter provide a *top-down* approach to the possible relations between cognition and movements. Despite its relevance to help us formulate questions regarding motor control differences in autism spectrum disorder (ASD), the top-down approach tends to obstruct our ability to bridge cognition and action in neurodevelopment. This is, in part, due to a reliance on descriptions of a system that, although still young and growing, has already reached a steady-state rate of development. The system of a 5-year-old child or that of a young adolescent is physically growing at a steadier pace than that of a newborn baby. Indeed, the steady-state growth of a child stands in stark contrast to the rapid rate of growth of the nascent nervous systems of a newborn baby. The latter is changing on a daily basis at highly accelerated rates (Figure I.1). To better appreciate this difference, consider, for example, the rate of physical growth of a newborn baby. In 30 days, the body gains weight at a nonlinear rate of change that varies from 0.02 kg/day to nearly no change to actual weight loss in the first week (Figure I.1). If we were to apply such rates to the body of a 5-year-old child, the changes would be, even overnight, so appreciable to the child's brain that a total "recalibration" of all bodily and sensory maps would be required for that brain to be able to control that body from one day to the next. Indeed, Figure I.1c shows that the typical 5-year-old child (1825 days) changes weight at a rather slower rate per day in relation to the newborn baby.

None of the theoretical cognitive attempts to describe motor coordination, motor sequencing, or any type of inference about the actions of the child used to guess his or her mental states or the mental states of others (i.e., as in theory of mind [Baron-Cohen et al. 1985]) would work in this rapidly changing physical body scenario. Cognitive theories merely describe the observer's perception of a physical body in motion (i.e., producing behavior) without considering the evolution of the physical parameters that intervene in motor control and the sensations that their consequences produce. They describe an intermediate final end product of a body that reaches some stable configuration before it goes on to another major physiological change (e.g., puberty). This semisteady state of being is only a local window into more global developmental phenomena along the human life span. Zooming out of this local window (as in Figure I.1 examining the changes in weight and their rates of change for the first 5 years of life) underscores the fact that the cognitivist description needs to reconsider longitudinal change using a nonlinear, stochastic lens, rather than a locally linear, static, deterministic one.

The cognitivist researcher describes the individual performing a socially oriented or purposeful behavior that has already matured to some extent. The top-down inferences that cognitive theories make about the functioning of the mind are not based on evolving physical bodies with embedded evolving nervous systems, developing from the bottom up (Figure I.2). As such, the cognitivist could never see the need for understanding the mechanisms necessary to control a body in motion as basic ingredients required to construct predictive behavior underlying the description of the (presumed) mental intentions of others and their social consequences.

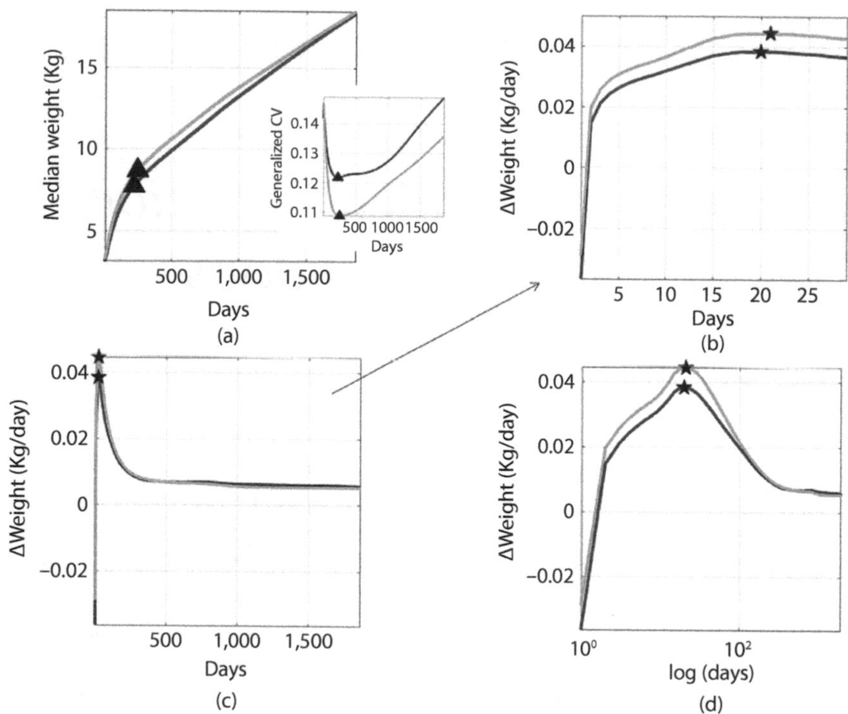

FIGURE I.1 The rate of change in weight is much more accelerated in the early days of the neonate than at 5 years of age. (a) The course of daily weight gain and its variability (inset) during the first 5 years of life show the marked nonlinear nature of these processes. The body steadily gains weight around 5 years of age, but in the first year of life the changes are accelerated. (b) Indeed, the baby gains an average of 0.5–1 kg/month for the first 6 months, but this rate slows down after 5 years (c and d). (d) Similar plot as (c) in log scale for better visualization. The stars mark a critical point of change from positive to negative slope in the gain (rate). The triangles mark a critical point of change in the generalized coefficient of variation (the estimated ratio of mean weight to variance) separating males (cyan) reaching the point at 252 days from females (magenta) reaching the point at 224 days (almost a month earlier). (Data obtained from 26,985 breast-fed babies per summary point [13,623 females and 13,362 males] available from public records accompanying the methods to produce the World Health Organization and Centers for Disease Control growth charts (Reproduced with permission from Torres et al., *Front Pediatr* 4(121):1–15, 2016.)

The rather disembodied approach of the cognitivists' theories fails to consider that the rapid physical changes that a newborn baby experiences while gaining autonomy over the body are also characterized by changes in the rates of growth of the peripheral nerves innervating the face, trunk, and limbs (Figure I.2). Such nerves ought to establish proper synapses to build networks that effectively communicate activity from the end effectors back to the also fast-growing brain. This brain will eventually have to develop deliberate autonomy over the body. Without this closed loop properly in placed between the peripheral nervous systems (PNSs) and the central nervous systems (CNSs), it will be very hard for the baby's nascent nervous systems to self-discover controllable change, i.e., to self-discover a self-corrective code that enables the prediction of sensory consequences from self-directed actions, i.e., beyond simpler stimulus–response associations.

Indeed, the error in the current conceptualization of cognitivist approaches is the disembodied notion of cognition understood as an information processing digital machine (more recently attempting to predict or anticipate the future using, e.g., Bayesian inference and other machine learning methods [e.g., Yufick and Friston 2016] to try to define intelligence). The fact that self-produced movements continuously affect our ongoing sensations is used by other contemporary approaches that have partly emerged in response to the impossibility of the cognitivist theories to connect body and mind. The new approaches (e.g., enacted cognition or embodied cognition [Varela et al. 2016]) try to bridge abstract thoughts to

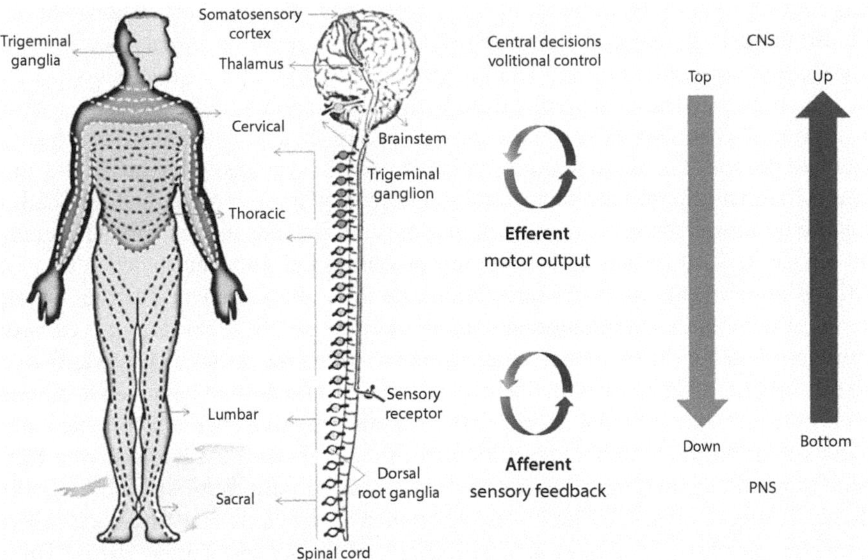

FIGURE I.2 Sensory-motor maps, nerves, and ganglia across the body and face project to cortical maps. The development of these underlying systems scaffold bottom-up and top-down interactions that enable subsequent cognitive decisions and sociomotor behaviors.

physical action. Yet these views tend to operate in the "here and now," whereby the sensory-motor loops are conceived as directly dependent on each other's currently experienced or enacted activity: the organism senses its self-produced motions and the self-produced motions affect the organism's sensations. The overall idea is in tune with the original principle of reafference by Von Holst (Von Holst and Mittelstaedt 1950), which we mentioned in Chapter 1: "Voluntary movements show themselves to be dependent on the returning stream of afference which they themselves cause." Without a doubt, the concept is a powerful one, but to direct the sensory organs to optimally sample the external world for successful purposeful and social behaviors, and to integrate that information in a timely manner with the continuous internal flow of somatic motor information, the organism will necessarily have to be a step ahead of the self-produced and self-sensed movements. Internal sensory-motor transduction and transmission delays vary with the stimuli. These variations forcedly require anticipating the sensory-motor consequences of impending actions, decisions, and thoughts. Compensating for such delays are among the tenets of contemporary internal models for action (IMAs) (e.g., Kawato and Wolpert 1998; Wolpert et al. 1998). However, such models have yet to provide appropriate statistical frameworks to track the unfolding of these processes in real time, and to account for their neurodevelopmental evolution (as discussed in Torres 2016). As in the above-mentioned cognitive approaches, the proposition of the IMA refers to the by-product of a maturation process, a process already taking place within a steady-state system. This formulation of the problem leaves out an avenue for the discovery of self-emergent phenomena in the nascent nervous systems of the newborn infant, developing adaptable interfaces to connect the fast-changing brain and body.

Throughout this book, we will introduce the notion of measuring, through the multilayered historicity of self-produced biophysical rhythms, the very sensory consequences that impending activity may have on the organism's experience of the world. It is our proposition that the evolving balance between this uncertainty of predicted consequences and the self-confirmation the developing organism attains over time is what forms the self-discovered notion of cause and effect. This important notion in turn leads to body ownership and agency, required ingredients to bridge physical volition to the type of mental intent that the above-mentioned cognitivist, enacted cognition, and neuromotor control approaches already take for granted.

The emergence of motor intent and its mental formulation require a maturation process that we can witness surfacing in the neurodevelopmental arena of a newborn infant (Torres et al. 2016). Part of this process includes attaining a proper balance between the actual consequences of the actions and those that the organism learns to predict from both spontaneous activity and active trial-and-error statistical sampling. When successful, these processes are then conducive of neurodevelopment oriented to embed the social medium in the organism's nervous systems and to project the organism's nervous systems' signatures onto the social medium. Such a mapping, when attained, leads to social life, whereby the organism becomes an integral part of the collective and the collective embraces the organism as one of its kind. When these evolving processes fail to occur, or when they derail, we come to witness impairments in social interactions between the organism's nervous systems and the social environment, but such impairments (as in the case of ASD) develop as well between the social environment and the organism's nervous systems, which the social medium fails to embrace.

We close this section of the book with the proposition that a *bottom-up* approach to neurodevelopment at the early stages may be more appropriate to capture the dynamic and variable nature of the nervous systems in transition to deliberate autonomy of the brain over the body (Figure I.2). Indeed, the emergence of an intentional brain that finds a way to deliberately control the body at will, a body that it gradually learns to own, may be better captured with methods that first track this emergent property from the periphery (Torres et al. 2013, 2016; Brincker and Torres 2013). The question then is how the autonomic nervous systems contribute in the early stages of life to the eventual maturation of the cognitive systems that these *top-down* cognitivist theories make reference to? How are affect, emotion, and logical reasoning gradually acquired, maintained, and modified through sensory, somatic motor loops?

To begin this line of inquiry, we need tools, and new data types, to quantify *change*, its rate, and the relationship between physical growth and the emergence of the balance between autonomous and voluntary neuromotor control (e.g., Torres et al. 2016). The quantification of such change in the organism as part of a group, and of the group as a whole operating organismic entity, is a new challenge for the social sciences to explore. In the next sections, we invite some thoughts along these lines in view of the critical need for early detection of stunting of neurodevelopment at large and of the consequences this may have for social exchange.

REFERENCES

Baron-Cohen, S., A. M. Leslie, and U. Frith. 1985. Does the autistic child have a "theory of mind"? *Cognition* 21 (1): 37–46.

Brincker, M., and E. B. Torres. 2013. Noise from the periphery in autism. *Front Integr Neurosci* 7:34.

Kawato, M., and D. Wolpert. 1998. Internal models for motor control. *Novartis Found Symp* 218:291–304; discussion 304–7.

Torres, E. B. 2016. Rethinking the study of volition for clinical use. In *Progress in Motor Control: Theories and Translations*, ed. J. Lazcko and M Latash. New York: Springer.

Torres, E. B., B. Smith, S. Mistry, M. Brincker, and C. Whyatt. 2016. Neonatal diagnostics: Toward dynamic growth charts of neuromotor control. *Front Pediatr* 4 (121):1–15.

Torres, E. B., M. Brincker, R. W. Isenhower, P. Yanovich, K. A. Stigler, J. I. Nurnberger, D. N. Metaxas, and J. V. Jose. 2013. Autism: The micro-movement perspective. *Front Integr Neurosci* 7:32.

Varela, F. J., E. Thompson, and E. Rosch. 2016. *The Embodied Mind: Cognitive Science and Human Experience.* Rev. ed. Cambridge, MA: MIT Press.

Von Holst, E., and H. Mittelstaedt. 1950. The principle of reafference: Interactions between the central nervous system and the peripheral organs. In *Perceptual Processing: Stimulus Equivalence and Pattern Recognition*, ed. P. C. Dodwell, 41–72. New York: Appleton-Century-Crofts.

Wolpert, D. M., R. C. Miall, and M. Kawato. 1998. Internal models in the cerebellum. *Trends Cogn Sci* 2 (9): 338–47.

Yufick, Y. M., and K. Friston. 2016. Life and understanding: The origins of "understanding" in self-organizing nervous systems. *Front Syst Neurosci* 10 (98).

Section II

Basic Research

Movement as a Social Model

4 Dissecting a Social Encounter from Three Different Perspectives

Elizabeth B. Torres

CONTENTS

Introduction ... 63
Dissecting a Social Encounter through the Eyes of Different Research Areas ... 64
Behaviorist Account from a Psychological Perspective ... 65
Physiologist Account ... 66
Computational Neuroscientist Account ... 67
Guessing Mental States of the Other Party Is Hard and Highly Subjective ... 68
Integrating All Three Accounts to Explore Deeper Layers of Detail ... 70
References ... 70

Chapter 2 closed with the question, is it time for a new model of autism spectrum disorder (ASD)? The psychological and psychiatric constructs defining ASD today describe issues with social interactions in very narrow ways. The methods of inquiry about social and cognitive issues are more an art than a science. They have turned into a stumbling block in scientific advancement, preventing progress toward the discovery of possible causes linking early sensory-motor issues in neurodevelopment with differences in social exchange that emerge later in life. This chapter uses a seemingly simple social encounter to illustrate how, by adopting different perspectives, one can better appreciate and objectively quantify the complexity of the social dyad. Using the hypothetical accounts of a behaviorist, a physiologist, and a computational neuroscientist as they each describe the same encounter, we show that indeed there is more than meets the eye.

INTRODUCTION

Our physical bodies are in constant motion from conception. Even when we are seemingly at rest, our heart is beating, our lungs breathing, and our physiological systems are processing all sorts of electrochemical reactions involving, among other measurable biophysical processes, the transduction and transmission of information across many layers of our nervous systems. And yet, at rest all these motions occur largely without our awareness. We do not see them, and as such, we do not describe them as part of our movements; we do not associate them with what we more generally call behavior. The continuous stream of minute fluctuations in our subtle inner motions, together with our overt actions, may have a profound impact on how we behave, socially or otherwise. Certainly, if you have a stomachache caused by a bad chemical reaction from some spoiled food you ate, you would not be talking about poetry or concocting some clever joke to amuse a crowd of friends. Most likely, you just rather be left alone until it passes.

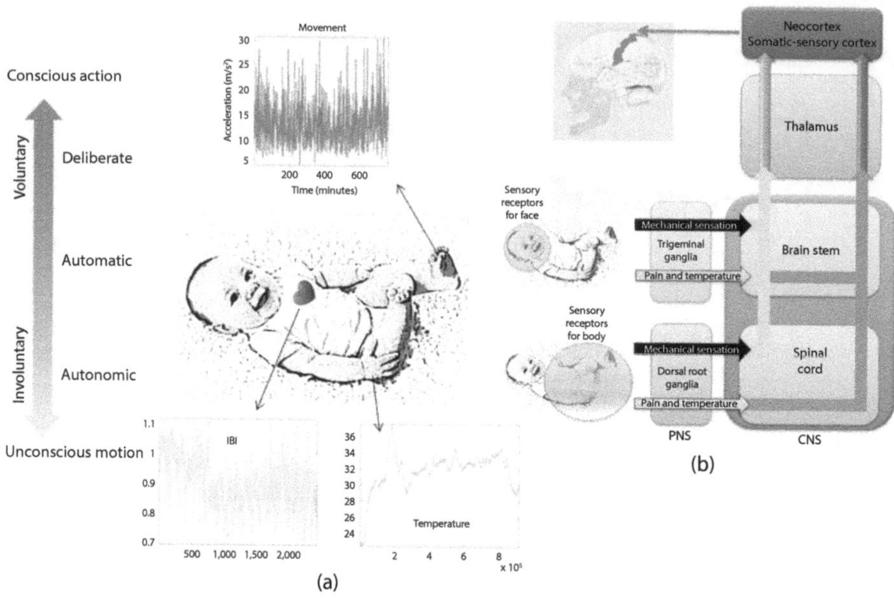

FIGURE 4.1 Extraction of micromovements is possible across different biophysical signals from physiological states registered in different body parts using wearable sensors. (a) Taxonomy of control levels involving different layers of micromovements mapping to different stochastic signatures. (b) Division of labor from early infancy during neurodevelopment impact different somatic motor networks in the face- and body-relevant dimensions of the social axes. (Reproduced with permission from Torres, E. B. et al., *Front. Pediatr.* 4:121, 2016.)

It must be terrible to not have that option, for example, as when having the physiology of your nervous systems in some continuous state of disarray that confines you to a lonesome existence in such a way you do not even realize, while others around you—perhaps unintentionally—interpret it as your being "antisocial" or having "low empathy." Conceivably, if they knew of your actual physiological state of disarray, they would try to assist you. But how would they know that your physiological systems are out of whack? They cannot see that in any way, unless they wore some kind of "special glasses" allowing them to see beyond what their naked eyes can naturally capture.

The minute fluctuations that occur in the motions that are sensed throughout the nervous systems can be measured with contemporary instrumentation and provide new lenses into subtle nervous systems' phenomena. We have coined the waveform representing these fluctuations in biophysical rhythms *micromovements* (Figure 4.1 and refer back to Chapter 1), as we extract them from bodily and mental rhythms and turn them into quantifiable data output by the nervous systems of the person. Paired with proper analytics, the micromovements can provide a new kind of special glasses to see beyond the obvious and inform us of central nervous system (CNS) and peripheral nervous system (PNS) interactions. To illustrate their use, let us first walk through a simple social situation as described by different (hypothetical) researchers, and then examine some social dyadic interactions using the micromovement perspective.

DISSECTING A SOCIAL ENCOUNTER THROUGH THE EYES OF DIFFERENT RESEARCH AREAS

Let us attempt to deconstruct the social encounter depicted in Figure 4.2. The encounter in question takes place between two people who may have seen each other once before. Through the length of time they sustain eye contact as they approach each other, they may admit to each other recalling their first fortuitous encounter sometime in the past, or they may right there and then decide to

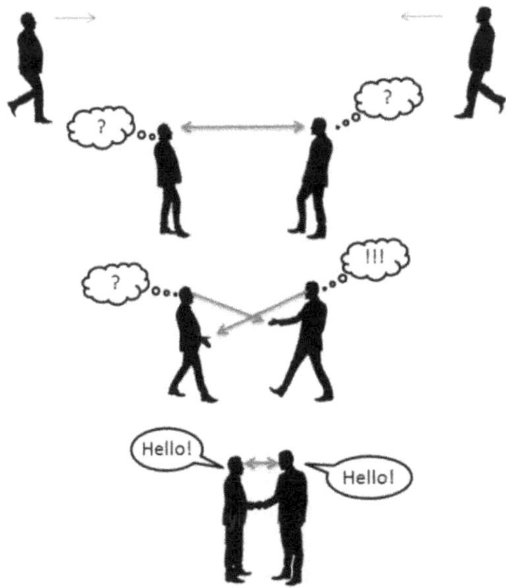

FIGURE 4.2 Genesis of a brief social encounter. Two fellows walking toward each other recognize their acquaintance from the distance and try to discern whether the other person is willing to admit to this mutual memory and engage in a brief social exchange, like a salutation and small talk. Body language involving sustained eye contact and facial microexpressions, including a smile, may give away the mutual willingness to stop, shake hands, and say hello. Alternatively, even a brief gesture like turning the body away from the interlocutor's body midline and avoiding eye contact, perhaps accompanied by spontaneous (flat) facial microexpressions denoting an unwillingness to engage, will determine the fate of this brief encounter.

make the eye contact so brief that there is no ambiguity in their unwillingness to proceed with a social exchange. Notice here that this is a deliberate decision, rather than a spontaneously occurring event.

If their eye contact was sustained long enough to go on with the social exchange, they may further provide mutual evidence for their willingness to proceed by orienting their body toward each other and extending their hands to prompt a handshake—we will safely assume here that this is an acceptable social form of salutation in the culture where these two individuals developed. And finally, they will execute the handshake and say hello to each other, perhaps going on to initiate some social chat.

This is a very hypothetical situation. We shall dissect that social encounter using the lens of a researcher whose area of expertise has to do with social behaviors, another researcher whose area of expertise focuses on the physiology of the nervous systems underlying that social behavior, and yet another view through the lens of a researcher whose area of expertise is modeling the types of sensory-motor integration processes and sensory-motor transformations that may underlie that social behavior through the use of mathematical and computational tools.

Finally, let us examine examples of dyadic social interactions using a research program that integrates all three accounts through an interdisciplinary collaborative approach.

Behaviorist Account from a Psychological Perspective

To study this seemingly simple social exchange, the behavioral psychologist will most likely draw a discrete set of events and assign a discrete (ordinal) scale to each event unambiguously detected by the naked eye. The account may go as follows (for example): (1) eye contact, (2) smile, (3) handshake, (4) word exchange ("Hello!"), and (5) initiate chat. Each one of these five events may have a subscale, say from 1 to 10, with 1 signifying poor and 10 excellent, and some other considerations in between. The researcher will go on and collect data on each of these events (1–5) according to each of the numbers coded by hand to "quantify" the overall behavior. The behaviorist may then use traditional statistical tools and analyze the cross-sectional data by averaging scores across large numbers of subjects. This will build a normative data set with the potential to help identify atypical patterns in the future based on what is "normally" expected in such a social encounter (as defined by the inventory). Examples of such approaches abound in the fields of clinical psychology and psychiatry. In fact, these types of structured inventories are commonly used to gather criteria to diagnose disorders that involve social deficits as mental illnesses, as well as to treat them through behavior-reshaping methods or prescribed psychotropic medications (Lord et al. 1989, 2001; Lord et al.; American Psychiatric Association 2013). Notably, none of these clinical inventories ever characterized normative data, so they feature absolute ordinal values of some arbitrary scale. As such, they are not properly standardized.

Physiologist Account

The physiologist will set up high-grade instrumentation using a variety of sensors to register signals throughout the nervous systems. Today's technological advances allow for noninvasive methods of data registration. Using contemporary (e.g., wireless) instrumentation, the physiologist will attempt to continuously register every detail of this exchange. She may track the eye motions to assess the length of time on a millisecond timescale that person-to-person foveation was sustained, quantify the saccades and the smooth pursuit eye motions throughout the exchange, and record (for example) heat activity from the facial muscles using thermal cameras strategically positioned to capture various facial configurations and detect universal signatures describing microexpressions of the face (Ekman and Rosenberg 1997). Then these data will be used to automatically infer possible emotional states. The physiologist may also record neck motions (perhaps with wearable inertial measurement units and wearable electromyographic sensors). Neck position and orientation will reveal trajectories of the head in the body, and eye tracking technology will reveal the position and orientation of the eyes in the head. This information will enable assessment of the system's use of different frames of references during sensory-motor transformations required in simple goal-directed saccades and hand motions. Simultaneously, bodily rhythms from all movable joints will also provide important information from each individual in the dyad and from their interactions as the multiple degrees of freedom in both participants coarticulate and the synergies dynamically fall in and out of synchrony. As the bodily rhythms fluctuate, so do the speech rhythms that the physiologist can record with a microphone.

The speech, generated by the sensory-motor apparatus from orofacial structures, will provide a rich body of data to—in concert with the face data—further help assess emotional components of the encounter. Likewise, sensors coregistering electrocardiograms and electrodermal activity (EDA) will provide several layers of data to assess inter-beat-interval time variability and to help estimate sympathetic and parasympathetic states of the autonomic nervous systems, along with skin surface temperature, respiration patterns, and other physiological signals.

This formidable amount of data will then be analyzed under a variety of statistical frameworks, machine learning and pattern recognition algorithms that will permit the physiologist to unveil easy-to-interpret self-emerging patterns. Such patterns will have statistical power because very likely the sensors have high sampling resolution and collect a large number of measurements for each motion parameter of the eyes, face, speech, neck, head, body, and limbs. To help the interpretation of the results, it is very likely that the physiologist will aim at mapping functional outcomes to anatomical structures along the nervous systems. This will help her situate the results in relation to known neuroscientific principles and add new information to that body of knowledge. As the behaviorist, the physiologist will try and collect all the data in neurotypical individuals in order to create a normative set to reference atypical patterns to. This concert of multi-sensory-motor data will provide the underpinnings of the behaviorist's account and further reveal information that escapes the naked eye. At a glance, the account of the social encounter by the physiologist seeks different layers of understanding from that of the behaviorist. Yet they are not at odds. They just study phenomena using different lenses and as such can provide different levels of description and interpretation. Without a doubt, both accounts are important, but to understand the underlying neurophysiology of the social encounter, the behavioral psychologist account falls rather short.

Computational Neuroscientist Account

The behaviorist's approach affords many possible interpretations and open-ended questions about this social encounter. It serves as a brainstorming phase of a research project, perhaps to begin formulating high-level questions about possible principles ultimately governing the encounter, with the caveat of never considering some of the phenomena that take place beneath awareness. The physiologist's approach, however, can provide the type of data conducive of objective criteria to complement, help verify, or expand the hypotheses that the behaviorist may formulate solely based on the obvious phenomena one can consciously perceive. Arguably, the above-described behaviorist's approach is often handcrafted to accommodate a priori defined criteria conforming to socioeconomic constraints. In the context of autism, these may include the availability of treatments (e.g., early intervention programs in the United States) or criteria for insurance coverage of prescribed psychotropic medications (also in the United States). The physiologist's approach can instead be centered on the patient to help provide outcome measures of physiological performance, so as to track the effectiveness or risk of treatments on the nervous systems of the patient, but also to help science develop new ways to uncover principles of the nervous systems' functions.

There is a third set of criteria to help dissect the social encounter in Figure 4.2. This involves that of a computational researcher. Here the goal is to go beyond hypothetical guesses or massive data gathering so as to analytically simulate aspects of the behavior potentially present in the encounter. The modeler will be able to obtain, via computer simulations, theoretical bounds on the data parameters empirically generated by the behaviors taking place during the social encounter. Once the simulations and boundary conditions are determined, the computational researcher can empirically verify parameter values from sensors directly measuring nervous systems' outputs that fall within typical or atypical ranges.

These analytical simulations will make predictions that the computational researcher will try to empirically challenge so as to be able to modify the model and make it as biologically plausible as possible. For example, visual processing by individual A of the approaching individual B is very complex to model, but current computational models of motion perception and motion recognition can be used to predict whether the motion is biological (Lange and Lappe 2006), as well as to predict the time to contact between the two approaching individuals (Lee 1980). Further, the modeler will have to address differences between biological motions of humans and nonhumans in order to flag that the encounter about to occur is likely to be with another person.

To assess the identity of the approaching individual B, the modeler will have to design the study of the processes following the above-mentioned highly complex visual recognition task. This will also include facial recognition and recognition of emotional states (Zhong et al. 2015). As individual B approaches observer A, a series of distance-based estimation will have to take place to assess the unfolding dynamics of motion and the time to close the gap of the encounter (Lee et al. 1999, 2001). These estimations will be required to transform the external retinotopic-based signals into internal kinesthetically based representations (Zipser and Andersen 1988; Torres and Zipser 2002). Such transformations from sensory to motor sensing coordinates will enable individual A to discern (1) the speed of the approaching person B, (2) an estimation of the awareness of the approaching person B about observer A, and (3) an estimation of the willingness of the approaching person B to facilitate or halt the encounter.

Models of facial recognition and recognition of emotional content in facial expressions (Ekman 2007) will necessarily have to be combined with models of foveation (Itti et al. 2005) and saccadic (Robinson 1973; Sparks and Mays 1990; Ron et al. 1994; Sparks 2002) and eye pursuit (Lisberger et al. 1987) motions so as to assess the likelihood that individual B will want to engage in a brief salutation. Assessment of that willingness entails probabilistic models to make predictions and gain confirmation of those predictions with variable degrees of certainty (Friston 2012a, 2012b). Most likely, they will entail Bayesian estimation models and neuroeconomic models of decision making (Glimcher and Fehr 2014). These models will enable balancing possible outcomes of anticipatory codes upon identification of "human individual whom I may have seen before is moving toward me." These may include "Should I sustain eye contact and say hello? Or should I turn my body and my face away from the incoming direction to give the signal that the brief encounter is not desirable at my end? What if I am OK with the encounter but the approaching party is not?" among other possibilities.

GUESSING MENTAL STATES OF THE OTHER PARTY IS HARD AND HIGHLY SUBJECTIVE

The computational researcher would need additional simulations to represent person A modeling possible mental states of the incoming person B. But unlike the portion of the decision-making process directly based on the person's internal sensory integrations and forward-and-inverse transformations to arrive at the conclusion of "I will willingly facilitate this encounter," the other set of integrations and transformation processes to estimate whether the other party B is interested in the encounter will be totally subjective and based on theorizing constructs about the other person's mind. That is, self-based assessments have the objective element of directly sensing, predicting, and inferring future actions and their sensory consequences based on one's own physical body and mental experiences. In marked contrast, when such assessments are based on the guesses of what the external stimuli (person B) may want to do, they carry large uncertainty. That externally based estimation process is far more difficult than the previously mentioned internally based process. And that level of uncertainty must be terrifying to a nervous system that cannot resolve such ambiguities internally in the first place, so as to anchor the world to a proper self-frame of reference. Without a frame of reference, all relative computations necessary to estimate distances and error correction codes will be impeded. Importantly, if supporting peripheral information necessary to help distinguish signal from noise is also compromised, the person will not be able to make timely decisions either. We will return to these aspects of the problem shortly for the cases of neurodevelopmental disorders on a spectrum, as they give rise to atypical social exchange. In this sense, conclusions about social deficits are currently reached without objective assessment, much less computational analytics of the types mentioned above. They are based on theoretical guesses about the other person's mental states, employing data-gathering techniques that are plagued with confirmation bias, severely incomplete due to the natural limited processing and information transmission capacities of sensory systems, and built on a foundation rather characterized by the accumulation of "scientific" evidence using a paradigm that does not admit to any of these caveats in the first place.

In the context of actual human social exchange, it is truly remarkable that despite the high uncertainties of mental theories people have about others, these types of social encounters take place. If one were to be conservative about possible outcomes and try to minimize uncertainty, most such social exchanges would not happen. And yet, they do happen. Implicitly, the nervous system takes such risk, an intriguing feature that may be possible to model using the neuroeconomics framework to balance error-driven versus reward-driven decision-making processes.

On this note, an entire subfield of psychology devoted to "theory of mind" (ToM) emerged some time ago (Baron-Cohen et al. 1985; Perner et al. 1989). In due time, this psychological construct also found a brain network seemingly devoted to ToM using the functional magnetic resonance imaging (fMRI) framework (Saxe and Kanwisher 2003), a framework that (sadly) shapes almost entirely the field of cognitive neuroscience. The fundamental flaws of the analytical techniques employed in this field and the interpretations of the handcrafted stories that emerge from their use and abuse have been eloquently described in various publications (Deen and Pelphrey 2012; Eklund et al. 2016). Yet, just as people in social encounters take the risk of guessing the mental states of others, so does the scientific community of cognitive neuroscience. They risk being wrong while making inferences on incomplete data and guessing their interpretations of how the brain may work out such complex social dynamics. Unfortunately, there seems to be more reward in the immediate outcome of publishing many papers under some black-box approach to data analyses, or gaining peer recognition and subsequent fame, than in unveiling basic principles with explanatory power. Perhaps being more conservative in the interpretations of those a priori handcrafted results will help open new questions, given that current questions are based on theoretical assumptions that for the most part, have not been empirically verified.

One of the problems here is that such bad science has had a direct impact in the lives of those affected by neurodevelopmental disorders that eventually affect social interactions. The claimed "hallmark" of cognitivists that the autistic person lacks a ToM is rather unfair. Likewise, the claims of their lacking empathy, being antisocial, and more generally purposefully lacking any type of interest in social exchange are rather troubling given that they are based on ordinal data from rather biased, made-up inventories that follow a self-fulfilling prophesy paradigm (Baron-Cohen et al. 1985; Leekam and Perner 1991; Sicotte and Stemberger 1999). Upon examination of the biophysical rhythms output by the nervous systems of the person with an observational diagnosis of autism spectrum disorder (ASD), we have learned that the statistical approaches and methods used in the above-mentioned body of work are severely incomplete and fundamentally flawed. And yet, in the absence of a neutral observer to reexamine such methods in light of new empirical evidence, such theories continue to be based more on art than science. They continue to have a negative impact in the lives of those families and contribute to the alienation and social rejection of the person affected by these heterogeneous sets of conditions.

Unlike the observational behaviorist and the guessing cognitivist, the computational modeler will have several additional layers of complexity to simulate once the encounter in Figure 4.2 takes place. Such simulations may involve, among other aspects, the neuromotor control of the face and body.

The face–body complex has well over 700 degrees of freedom (Evans 2015), including muscles, joints, and end effectors to carry out the necessary actions in this seemingly simple social encounter. How is the audiovisual information capturing the motions of the other person to be mapped onto the body of the viewer such as to create proper targets to spontaneously recruit and coordinate bodily joints and muscle groups? How can the potential affordances of the upcoming theoretical situation be anticipated to effectively steer the other person's attention (rather willingly) to our own desired outcomes? Seemingly trivial nuances could prematurely dissolve the potential social encounter. Among these are the tones of voice, speed and rhythms of the speech, inevitable facial expressions or bodily motions that fall largely beneath the person's awareness to be able to control them, and poor estimation of interlocutor distances.

A computational researcher trying to model the situation in Figure 4.2 would have to necessarily design various architectures considering hierarchical structures to cover multiple possible scenarios involving many layers of explicit and implicit information. Among these are cultural nuances (e.g., while Italians gesture abundantly during social exchange, and may speak simultaneously and loudly among a group, these practices would all be considered socially rude in British culture; likewise, many Asian cultures would consider it rude to look into the eyes of the interlocutor, whereas this is expected in U.S. culture, to the extent that not doing so is considered pathological).

Upon deploying computer simulations based on mathematical models of these multiple layers of interrelated motions from the eyes, the face, and the mouth (generating speech), accompanied by bodily rhythms, and so forth, the computational scientist would have to come up with proper models for entrainment and spontaneous versus controlled desynchronization of these elements. These would have to be designed in order to capture self-emerging nonstationary fluctuations during the exchange interleaved with steady-state segments. Such simulated behavior will have to give rise to multiple layers of temporal dynamics, as these are a hallmark of realistic social exchange. Indeed, concomitant processes will have different temporal scales demanding different strata of physical and mental dynamics with dynamically shifting priorities during the potential brief exchange to take place.

Designing models of motor control to simulate the motions of one single person has been an extremely difficult problem in computational motor neuroscience. Designing models of dyadic social exchange will surely be much more difficult. And yet, some aspects of sensory-motor transformations and the continuous internal dynamics of bodily actions may necessarily transfer to the dance of the social dyad. In particular, an attempt has been made to translate the notions of internal models for action (IMAs) from an individual system to a dyadic interaction setting (Wolpert et al. 2003), but the oversimplifications and assumptions of that proposed model are much too stringent to allow for a realistic outcome in typical scenarios, much less to capture critical aspects of atypical social exchanges.

Integrating All Three Accounts to Explore Deeper Layers of Detail

In an ideal world, the behaviorist, the physiologist, and the computational neuroscientist would join forces and try to integrate all three accounts under some unifying framework. Interdisciplinary collaboration is not always easy, though. More often than not, each body of knowledge is built independently. Integration of knowledge may be a challenge when an atypical nervous system is under study. It may take some time before multiple disciplines can unanimously agree on how to gather data to form a normative model. Then it may be even more challenging to gather data conducive of automatically unveiling systematic differences from normative data and to propose logical explanations based on first principles.

This section of the book provides different accounts from a behavioral-psychological perspective, a physiological characterization of behavior, and a computational approach to simple problems embedded in social exchange. These accounts are by no means exhaustive. They serve as mere illustration of the formidable complexity we scientists face when studying social phenomena.

REFERENCES

American Psychiatric Association. 2013. *Diagnostic and Statistical Manual of Mental Disorders.* 5th ed. Washington, DC: American Psychiatric Association.

Baron-Cohen, S., A. M. Leslie, and U. Frith. 1985. Does the autistic child have a "theory of mind"? *Cognition* 21 (1):37–46.

Deen, B., and K. Pelphrey. 2012. Perspective: Brain scans need a rethink. *Nature* 491 (7422):S20.

Eklund, A., T. E. Nichols, and H. Knutsson. 2016. Cluster failure: Why fMRI inferences for spatial extent have inflated false-positive rates. *Proc Natl Acad Sci USA* 113 (28):7900–5. doi: 10.1073/pnas.1602413113.

Ekman, P. 2007. *Emotions Revealed: Recognizing Faces and Feelings to Improve Communication and Emotional Life.* 2nd ed. New York: Owl Books.

Ekman, P., and E. L. Rosenberg. 1997. *What the Face Reveals: Basic and Applied Studies of Spontaneous Expression Using the Facial Action Coding System (FACS).* Series in Affective Science. New York: Oxford University Press.

Evans, N. 2015. *Bodybuilding Anatomy.* 2nd ed. Champaign, IL: Human Kinetics.

Friston, K. 2012a. The history of the future of the Bayesian brain. *Neuroimage* 62 (2):1230–3. doi: 10.1016/j.neuroimage.2011.10.004.

Friston, K. 2012b. Predictive coding, precision and synchrony. *Cogn Neurosci* 3 (3–4):238–9. doi: 10.1080/17588928.2012.691277.

Glimcher, P. W., and E. Fehr. 2014. *Neuroeconomics: Decision Making and the Brain.* 2nd ed. Amsterdam: Elsevier/Academic Press.

Itti, L., G. Rees, and J. K. Tsotsos. 2005. *Neurobiology of Attention.* Amsterdam: Elsevier/Academic Press.

Lange, J., and M. Lappe. 2006. A model of biological motion perception from configural form cues. *J Neurosci* 26 (11):2894–906. doi: 10.1523/JNEUROSCI.4915-05.2006.

Lee, D. 1980. Visuo-motor coordination in space-time. In *Tutorials in Motor Behavior*, ed. G. E. Stelmach and J. Requin, 281–95. Amsterdam: North-Holland.

Lee, D. N., A. P. Georgopoulos, M. J. Clark, C. M. Craig, and N. L. Port. 2001. Guiding contact by coupling the taus of gaps. *Exp Brain Res* 139 (2):151–9.

Lee, D. N., C. M. Craig, and M. A. Grealy. 1999. Sensory and intrinsic coordination of movement. *Proc Biol Sci* 266 (1432):2029–35. doi: 10.1098/rspb.1999.0882.

Leekam, S. R., and J. Perner. 1991. Does the autistic child have a metarepresentational deficit? *Cognition* 40 (3): 203–18.

Lisberger, S. G., E. J. Morris, and L. Tychsen. 1987. Visual motion processing and sensory-motor integration for smooth pursuit eye movements. *Annu Rev Neurosci* 10:97–129. doi: 10.1146/annurev.ne.10.030187.000525..

Lord, C., B. L. Leventhal, and E. H. Cook Jr. 2001. Quantifying the phenotype in autism spectrum disorders. *Am J Med Genet* 105 (1):36–8.

Lord, C., M. Rutter, P. C. DiLavore, S. Risi, and Western Psychological Services. *Autism Diagnostic Observation Schedule ADOS Manual*. Torrance, CA: Western Psychological Services.

Lord, C., M. Rutter, S. Goode, J. Heemsbergen, H. Jordan, L. Mawhood, and E. Schopler. 1989. Autism diagnostic observation schedule: A standardized observation of communicative and social behavior. *J Autism Dev Disord* 19 (2):185–212.

Perner, J., U. Frith, A. M. Leslie, and S. R. Leekam. 1989. Exploration of the autistic child's theory of mind: Knowledge, belief, and communication. *Child Dev* 60 (3):688–700.

Robinson, D. A. 1973. Models of the saccadic eye movement control system. *Kybernetik* 14 (2):71–83.

Ron, S., A. Berthoz, and S. Gur. 1994. Model of coupled or dissociated eye-head coordination. *J Vestib Res* 4 (5): 383–90.

Saxe, R., and N. Kanwisher. 2003. People thinking about thinking people. The role of the temporo-parietal junction in "theory of mind." *Neuroimage* 19 (4):1835–42.

Sicotte, C., and R. M. Stemberger. 1999. Do children with PDDNOS have a theory of mind? *J Autism Dev Disord* 29 (3):225–33.

Sparks, D. L. 2002. The brainstem control of saccadic eye movements. *Nat Rev Neurosci* 3 (12):952–64. doi: 10.1038/nrn986.

Sparks, D. L., and L. E. Mays. 1990. Signal transformations required for the generation of saccadic eye movements. *Annu Rev Neurosci* 13:309–36. doi: 10.1146/annurev.ne.13.030190.001521.

Torres, E. B., and D. Zipser. 2002. Reaching to grasp with a multi-jointed arm. I. Computational model. *J Neurophysiol* 88 (5):2355–67. doi: 10.1152/jn.00030.2002.

Wolpert, D. M., K. Doya, and M. Kawato. 2003. A unifying computational framework for motor control and social interaction. *Philos Trans R Soc Lond B Biol Sci* 358 (1431):593–602. doi: 10.1098/rstb.2002.1238.

Zhong, L., Q. Liu, P. Yang, J. Huang, and D. N. Metaxas. 2015. Learning multiscale active facial patches for expression analysis. *IEEE Trans Cybern* 45 (8):1499–510. doi: 10.1109/TCYB.2014.2354351.

Zipser, D., and R. A. Andersen. 1988. A back-propagation programmed network that simulates response properties of a subset of posterior parietal neurons. *Nature* 331 (6158):679–84. doi: 10.1038/331679a0.

5 More Than Meets the Eye
Redefining the Role of Sensory-Motor Control on Social Skills in Autism Spectrum Disorders

Caroline Whyatt

CONTENTS

What are Social Skills? 73
Social Skills in Autism Spectrum Disorders 75
The Origins of Social Skills 75
  Social Dialogue: Content Interdependence 75
  Definition and Conceptualization of the Mirror Neuron System 77
  The Social Dance: Temporal Interdependence 78
  Role of Active Movement in Development 78
How Do We Measure Social Interaction? 80
  Specialized Techniques to Examine Microlevel Evolving Social Dyadic Interactions (i.e., Synchronicity) 81
The Motor Perspective: A New Model to Examine Levels of Social Exchange in ASD 82
Conclusion 83
References 83

The previous chapters have begun to outline the power of utilizing kinematic analysis as a route to noninvasively profile levels of neurophysiological control, while illustrating the potential role of the "movement perspective" in autism. Specifically, these chapters intimate the cascading effects of this level of control on higher-level functions, such as cognition and social skills. This chapter aims to further discuss and elucidate what underpins our conceptualization of social skills—a key area of inquiry in autism spectrum disorder (ASD) research—and the potential role of sensory-motor control.

WHAT ARE SOCIAL SKILLS?

As a fundamental element of autism spectrum disorder (ASD) symptomatology (American Psychiatric Association 2013), social skills have long been a focus of ASD research and intervention programs (White et al. 2007). Yet our definition and understanding of social skills is complex and diverse, reflecting the subtle nuances of the social world in which we live. Social skills refer to the ability to navigate the social environment through interactions with others. We are primed for such interactions from birth, with a preference for the human voice and face (Fantz 1961; DeCasper et al. 1994). However, as altricial organisms we are also born unable to formulate and engage in verbal communication—initially interacting with our surroundings and others using physical motor behavior. Indeed, motor behavior, as a form of social communication or skill, continues past the acquisition of verbal language—accounting for a disproportionately large amount of human communication (Mehrabian and Ferris 1967; Mehrabian and Wiener 1967). As such, social skills consist of both verbal and nonverbal (motor behavior) forms of social interaction.

Through verbal and nonverbal social interactions, members of a dyad influence each other at two distinct levels—content and temporal interdependence (Figure 5.1). While content interdependence involves each member influencing the substance and outcome of an interaction, temporal interdependence refers to the timing and response of interactions—the "social dance."

These forms of interdependence can be deconstructed further to encompass macro- and microlevel analyses (Figure 5.2). Macrolevel behaviors are readily identifiable using observational data via standardized tools. Indeed, the use of communicative gestures and the concept of "turn taking" provide macrolevel measures of content and temporal interdependence, respectively—measures used within the fields of clinical psychology and psychiatry to profile social dyadic exchange. While these macrolevel behavioral outcomes are underpinned by microlevel fluctuations in content and temporal interdependence, a reliance on behavioral observational data lacks the precision to quantify this scaffolding layer. An inability to deconstruct performance to consider microlevel variability thus artificially limits our computational understanding—and the etiological model—of dyadic exchange. Indeed, this "dark matter" of neuroscience remains largely illusive, a difficulty that is particularly evident in the examination and consideration of ASD.

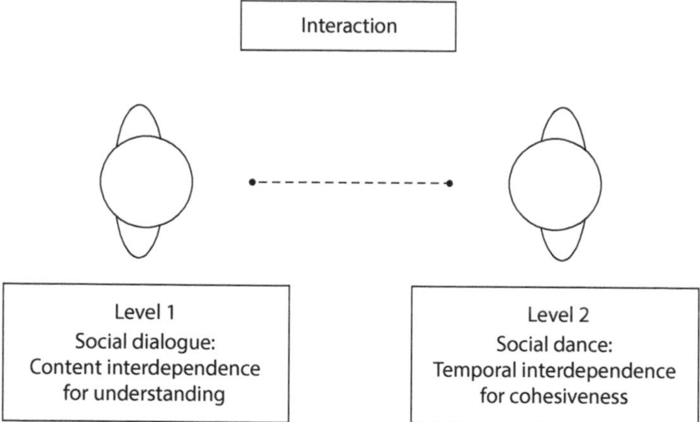

FIGURE 5.1 Schematic of an interaction illustrating the two levels of interdependence characterizing exchange.

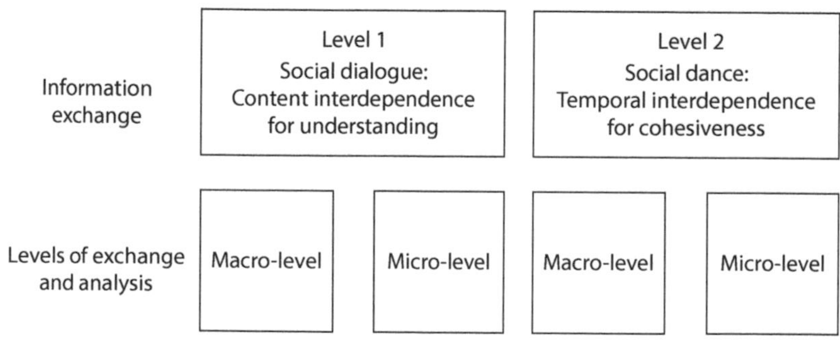

FIGURE 5.2 Schematic illustrating further deconstruction of content and temporal interdependence to macro- and microlevels of exchange.

SOCIAL SKILLS IN AUTISM SPECTRUM DISORDERS

ASD is an umbrella term for a spectrum of disorders often characterized by impaired social and cognitive ability. This spectrum is further compounded by the heterogeneous nature of ASDs, with no individual displaying a similar makeup of symptoms. Reflecting this complexity, ASD has no known etiology, resulting in an interpretation and classification within the fields of psychiatry and psychology. As a field of study, psychiatry serves a clinical purpose, facilitating the timely provision of diagnosis and treatment. As such, this area often relies on the use of easily administered inventories that utilize subjective interpretation of reported symptomology and observed behaviors. These behaviors are typically classified using standardized tools of social interaction—at the macrolevel of exchange. However, the scientific endeavor endorses the use of a detailed, thorough methodology that can provide replicable results and insight into underlying etiology. Unfortunately, such standardized tools lack the precision to objectively profile macro- and microlevels of social interaction to enrich our understanding of social exchange, or lack thereof, from a computational perspective. Many individuals with ASD are often considered unfazed or disconnected from others within their social environment. Conversely, others may appear distressed and unsettled. This dichotomy may be a by-product of the individual's response to social sensory information. Through the examination of microlevel fluctuations and interactions across a social dyad, levels of unconscious coupling at the content and temporal levels may be revealed—and viewed in light of sensory context. Indeed, recent evidence suggests that individuals prepare to "mirror" the actions of another's contagious social response before they are consciously aware of this (Lundqvist 1995)—a microlevel beyond the scope of subjective reporting or behavioral observation. Thus, it is proposed that an examination of social interaction at *both* the macro- and microlevels may facilitate a richer computational understanding of social dynamics in individuals with ASD. This insight may further facilitate an understanding of how best to design and develop therapeutic intervention for a range of disorders—within the remit of "precision psychiatry."

This chapter thus conceptualizes social skills as a form of interaction, mediated by both content and temporal interdependence across a dyad. Focusing on nonverbal communication (i.e., motor behavior), these concepts are discussed in light of developmental theories and underlying etiology, facilitating the design of a computational model of social skills. In addition, the chapter highlights the neglected role of microlevel temporal interdependence in the understanding of social dynamics. Specifically, the limited ability of current theories and discrete methodologies to examine and profile temporal interdependence during naturalistic social exchange—due to difficulties in objectively profiling this level of interaction—is illustrated. A new model that considers motor behavior as a form of continuous sensory feedback is proposed—and expanded upon in Chapter 7—broadening our understanding of social development and interaction. Discussing new methods to examine macro- and microlevels of content and temporal interdependence, through the use of empirically derived continuous data, the routes to profile social interaction are diversified and objectified.

THE ORIGINS OF SOCIAL SKILLS

Social Dialogue: Content Interdependence

The development of social skills begins in early infancy. As discussed in Chapter 6, one of the earliest forms of interpersonal interactive ability is infant imitation—the ability to mimic or repeat an action of another. This form of content-interdependent social behavior is complex and can take many forms, including manual and facial imitation. Basic imitation can be elicited from newborn infants as young as 32 hours old and provides the foundations for social knowledge, learning, and communication (Hanna and Meltzoff 1993; Sebanz et al. 2006; Bekkering et al. 2009). This early imitative ability has been further considered central to the development of a theory of mind (ToM) (Baron-Cohen et al. 1985; Rogers and Pennington 1991)—an influential cognitive perspective first coined by Premack and Woodruff (1978).

ToM, the ability to infer separate mental states in others, is considered a cornerstone of ASD developmental difficulty (Baron-Cohen et al. 1985). Coupled with the fact that social difficult form core elements of ASD symptomatology, it is perhaps social difficulties forming core elements of ASD symptomatology, it is perhaps unsurprising that imitation has been extensively examined in ASD research. Evidence repeatedly points to difficulties with imitation in individuals with ASD (Smith and Bryson 1994; Williams et al. 2001; Vivanti and Hamilton 2014), which is thought to then contribute to the underdevelopment of ToM (Baron-Cohen et al. 1985; Rogers and Pennington 1991; Meltzoff and Gopnik 1993). However, despite having a strong foothold in ASD research to date, a growing body of evidence is questioning the validity of the ToM perspective. Questions have been raised regarding the neurological location of the ToM module (Gallese 2006), the methods used to test ToM (Bloom and German 2000; Peterson et al. 2005), and its ability to reliably differentiate between a range of developmental difficulties (Russell et al. 1998; Yirmiya et al. 1998). Yet the presence of early imitative difficulty remains core to a growing area of inquiry in ASD research—in the form of the "broken mirror neuron" theory (Williams et al. 2001; Gallese 2001, 2006).

Given the presence of imitation in newborn infants, it has been considered an inherent nativist skill (Meltzoff and Moore 1977, 1983, 1992, 1997). However, this infers an impressive level of knowledge during infancy, including an inbuilt schema or map of the face or body, an understanding of basic action capabilities, and good visual or proprioception to guide and control motor output (Jones 2009). The mirror neuron system (MNS) removes the need for this nativist cognitive ability (Rizzolatti and Craighero 2004). First identified in the F5 area of the macaque monkey premotor cortex, the MNS refers to a subset of neurons that respond to both action production and observation (Rizzolatti et al. 1988, 1996; Di Pellegrino et al. 1992;). Facilitating action recognition, including "gestures made by other individuals," the MNS provides a physiological explanation for the presence and understanding of imitation (Di Pellegrino et al. 1992). Indeed, the ability to engage in successful social communication relies heavily on the interpretation and integration of social cues from a partner. From a nonverbal motor perspective, social cues can range in complexity, but rely on a fundamental ability to extrapolate meaning from a partner's motor actions (e.g., gestures). Thus, the MNS provides a simple and intuitive physiological basis for action understanding during interpersonal interaction. The broken mirror neuron theory of ASD thus proposes that difficulties with imitation and socialization are due to a physiological abnormality in the region of the MNS—providing a framework of ASD development from a perspective of content interdependence (Figure 5.3).

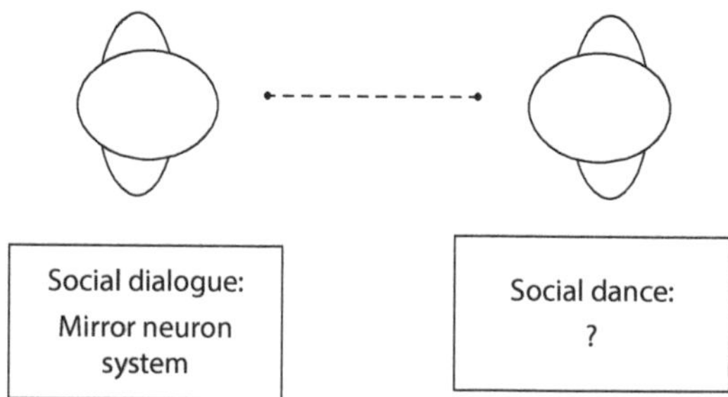

FIGURE 5.3 Difficulties with social dialogue, i.e., content interdependence—the ability to extract meaning from one another's actions, have been repeatedly tied to the underlying MNS. This hypothesis has been hailed as a potential explanation for ASD symptomatology, including difficulties with early imitation, empathy, and general social exchange. However, questions are raised over the view of the MNS, in particular its ability to account for difficulties with the social dance, i.e., temporal interdependence.

Despite a prevalent application in academia, the broken mirror neuron theory faces a number of difficulties. Most notably, evidence illustrates that some individuals with ASD have preserved levels of action understanding mediated by action type—meaningful or meaningless (Hamilton et al. 2007; Hobson and Hobson 2008; Rogers et al. 2010). With such evidence that impaired action understanding is not a ubiquitous feature of ASD, one may question whether mirror neurons can truly explain the myriad social symptoms associated with a diagnosis.

Definition and Conceptualization of the Mirror Neuron System

The consideration of action type and end-goal outcome on acquiring action understanding has been a characteristic feature of MNS activation from its first discovery (Rizzolatti et al. 1988; Rizzolatti and Sinigaglia 2010). Resonating with the coding of action in terms of perceptual outcome (Descartes 1984) and the ideomotor perspective (James 2013), this arguably abstract view limits the versatility and applicability of the MNS hypothesis. Specifically, an interpretation whereby the MNS codes for, and is activated by, a discrete end goal removes the ability of the system to fully program the motor response to stimuli by negating the impact of the unfolding kinematics. Thus, the MNS codes for a motor "vocabulary" (Rizzolatti et al. 1988; Rizzolatti and Arbib 1998) or general motor schema, rather than specifying feed-forward levels of kinematic control. While informative from a cognitivist perspective of action understanding—facilitating content interdependence during social interaction—this interpretation restricts the perspective of the MNS to the visual domain. This results in a view of the motor and perceptual systems as interwoven, yet functionally independent (Brincker 2010). Within a context of social learning, development, and communication, this interpretation of the MNS from a perceptual, visual perspective may be intuitive. With no physical connection to facilitate social communication and interaction, one is reliant upon the interpretation of visual signals or cues from others. As noted by Schmidt, coordination and interaction at a social level can only occur "via the visual systems" (Schmidt et al. 2011). However, more recent evidence illustrates the potential role of movement in both action understanding and imitation—implying significant levels of system cross talk.

The role of movement in action understanding is twofold. First, the movement or action capabilities of the individual appear central to their ability to identify and understand action through observation—one must be able to perform an action to reliably understand it (Calvo-Merino et al. 2005). Second, in a departure from a focus on the discrete end goal to facilitate action understanding, the unfolding or continuous movement kinematics of the observed action also facilitate prediction (Shim and Carlton 1997; Hayes et al. 2007, 2008; Ambrosini et al. 2011; Stapel et al. 2012). In line with evidence that individuals with ASD are less likely to imitate actions without a clear goal (Hobson and Hobson 2008; Rogers et al. 2010), evidence also suggests difficulty in using action kinematics to extrapolate information regarding action intention (Boria et al. 2009; Cossu et al. 2012; Gowen 2012). Combined, these difficulties spanning the use of both content (discrete end-goal) and temporal (continuous kinematics) levels of social information question the role of the MNS in ASD etiology and development. Specifically, the current understanding and conceptualization of the MNS fails to account for the apparent role of temporal, kinematic information in action understanding and replication. Despite evidence for neural population coding for actions that are orientation specific (Georgopoulos et al. 1986) and task or object specific (i.e., canonical neurons [Rizzolatti et al. 1988]), questions remain over the coding of external temporal characteristics. These include the ability to translate allocentric observations into egocentric levels of temporal control (the frame of reference used to prescribe and translate spatial and temporal dynamics between and across individuals). A range of neurons within the posterior parietal cortex are known to code for retinotopic to body transformations (Buneo et al. 2002), facilitating translation of spatial dynamics anchored to the individual or allocentrically to sensory information (Andersen and Zipser 1988; Zipser and Andersen 1988; Snyder 2000). Yet, little is known about temporal sensory-spatial transformations into egocentric levels of scaled kinematic control, and the preservation of temporal dynamics (Torres et al. 2010). Indeed, the MNS to date does not account for our innate ability to both extrapolate accurate temporal information from external events and create a level of synergistic temporal coordination or interdependence across a social dyad (Riley et al. 2011).

The Social Dance: Temporal Interdependence

Successful social interactions rely on an ability to extrapolate meaning from a partner's actions (i.e., content interdependence—perhaps driven by the MNS), but also on an ability to synchronize with a partner (i.e., temporal interdependence). Effective interpersonal synchronization is defined as "the dynamic and reciprocal adaptation of the temporal structure of behaviors between interactive partners" (Delaherche et al. 2012). For instance, during an interaction, social cues and prompts must be "read," but these cues must also be responded to in an adequate time frame, when such cues remain "valid." This temporal coupling is a characteristic feature of social interaction—the social dance.

Temporal organization and perception is core to everyday behavior. Actions, whether relatively simple or skilled, appear to require the coupling of spatial demands to temporal control. The empirical examination of natural, coordinated reaching movements implies that spatial trajectories follow a nearly straight path—minimizing redundancy, thus ensuring the retention of spatially accurate goal-directed behaviors. Moreover, this level of spatial consistency is mirrored in levels of temporal consistency, namely, the use of a bell-shaped temporal profile. This coupling has been modeled, for instance, in the minimum torque change model (Uno et al. 1989; Nakano et al. 1999), and the minimum jerk model (Flash and Hogan 1985). Such computational theories of motor control assume that knowledge of the temporal profile is acquired and programmed a priori. However, upon closer examination such studies often harness paradigms whereby participants are required to repeatedly respond to prespecified stimuli. Under such conditions, the acquisition of a coupled stable spatial and temporal profile of motor control is perhaps unsurprising. Indeed, studies have illustrated that the geometrical principles of motor output are potentially acquired prior to (Torres and Zipser 2002), and display independence from (Atkeson and Hollerbach 1985; Boessenkool et al. 1998; Nishikawa et al. 1999), temporal characteristics, implying that these levels of planning are decoupled. Furthermore, levels of spatial and temporal variation accompany learning processes underpinning the acquisition of motor coordination (von Hofsten 1991, 2007; Torres and Andersen 2006; Whyatt and Craig 2013b). Taken in conjunction, such findings question the assumption that a temporal profile of a given movement is known a priori.

Within the domain of social interactions, knowledge of the temporal dynamics, specifically those of a new partner, are highly unlikely to be preprogrammed a priori; rather, the dyadic synergy must evolve. However, despite the prevalence of the MNS theory of socialization (and ASD), this perspective fails to adequately explain the acquisition and evolution of such temporal synchronization. Therefore, how can the temporal characteristics of others' actions be understood within the framework of MNS? And how can members of a dyad create a unified framework for temporal synchronization? It is proposed that this can be achieved through a reconceptualization of the MNS to integrate the role of active movement in the understanding of others' actions, the properties of the environment, and the dynamics between these.

Role of Active Movement in Development

Active explorations of the environment through the use of early intrapersonal (infant–environment) interactions are vital for the development of the visual system (Singer 1985) and subsequent levels of motor coordination (Held 1965). From both a dynamic systems approach (Thelen 1979) and an ecological perspective (Gibson 1969), early active explorative behavior shapes development through the refinement of the perceptual system (Fajen 2005), and the creation of action or behavioral understanding (DeCasper and Carstens 1981; Thelen and Smith 1994, 1996; Libertus and Needham 2010). Within this framework, infant behavioral development is considered an emergent and self-organizing consequence of recursive interactions with the environment. Specifically, behavior is viewed as a consequence of multimodal correspondences, with afferent feedback from closely occurring events (i.e., multimodal experiences) producing or strengthening associations within the neural pathways (Edelman 1987). Through repeated exposure and the strengthening of neural connections in response to afferent feedback, the infant gradually acquires stable, generalizable patterns of behavior (synergy)—in what Thelen and colleagues term an "attractor state" (Thelen et al. 1991; Thelen and Smith 1996). This attractor state is achieved through actively sampling the degrees of freedom available (permutations) for the completion of the behavior, allowing for these variations to be assimilated into the behavioral understanding for future predictive judgments. Importantly, Thelen and colleagues note that this afferent information can take many forms including visual and auditory; yet it can also be "kinesthetic sensation" (Thelen and Smith 1996), or rather, from another stance, this may be considered "kinesthetic reafference" (Holst and Mittelstaedt 1950; Holst et al. 1971). Within this framework, active exploratory behavior results in behavioral modification through the strengthening of neural pathways in response to both external feedback and concomitant kinesthetic reafference.

By conceptualizing movement as a form of direct sensory feedback (kinesthetic reafference), it is proposed that this form of active behavior provides a spatial and temporal framework to understand the dynamics of the environment. Specifically, introduced by E. Torres and colleagues (Torres 2011; Torres et al. 2015, 2016)—and harmonizing with theoretical models of ecological psychology of movement guiding action (e.g., Lee et al. 1999; Lee 2009; Gibson 2014)—this role of movement as a form of sensory feedback can be expanded to consider how active movement facilitates identification of one's own action capabilities, the development of prospective control, and the identification of active feedback. In particular, the underlying stochastic signature of exploratory behaviors provides a framework in which to build a predictive model to facilitate prospective control, allowing an infant or individual to consider the consequences of sensory information prior to action. This would suggest that individuals use their own bodily movements to generate a frame of reference to extrapolate a representation of external temporal dynamics—assimilated into the "attractor" or predictive state. Thus, visual information and kinesthetic reafference provide a grounding of afferent information in which to translate action outcome and understanding, resulting in a broader interpretation of the MNS. This suggests that both the perceptual and motor systems are interwoven and functionally dependent, as opposed to functionally independent. This functional dependence builds on foundational concepts of motor development, whereby active exploratory motor behavior provides a basis for perceptual refinement (i.e., identification of invariant properties) and action understanding. Moreover, viewed within the context of phylogenetic development, a taxonomy of motor control has been proposed (Torres 2011), spanning from macrolevel goal-directed and spontaneous actions through to microlevel fluctuations. These auxiliary movements will be "fed" into the system, providing further scaffolding information for ongoing control and insight into the functioning of the nervous systems. By viewing motor progression and skill acquisition within the context of development—spontaneity giving way to goal-directed actions—and the ongoing role of microfluctuations, the role of the MNS in motor development and acquisition may be refined. Furthermore, under this perspective, an individual's movement or action capabilities will directly impact his or her perceptual awareness and understanding of observed actions—in line with previous evidence for the role of kinematics in action understanding.

Functional dependence and cross talk between the perceptual and motor systems thus suggests that each member of the dyad will draw upon their own action capabilities and frame of spatial and temporal reference to engage in coordinated actions and interaction. This reconceptualization enables the examination of social interaction through motor coordination, as opposed to the visual quantification of behavioral states. Moreover, drawing on this perspective, the role of each individual's impact on the interaction outcome can be profiled. In light of sensory-motor difficulties associated with a diagnosis of ASD (e.g., Whyatt and Craig 2012, 2013a), how does this lower-level difficulty impact higher-level social interaction? Individuals with perceivable sensory-motor irregularities, such as bradykinesia (a perceivable slowing of voluntary motor control) or tremor (uncontrollable rhythmical back-and-forth movements), may experience difficulty using their own motor profile as a framework to translate the actions of others. In this instance, the "corrupted" sensory-motor output is fed back into the system as kinesthetic reafference, which may impede an individual's ability to reach a predictive state (Torres et al. 2013). This closed system may reinforce motor difficulties and prevent an individual from reliably interpreting temporal signals from the environment or, in this instance, another individual, thus impeding his or her ability to engage successfully within a social dyad. As such, profiling social interaction at both the individual and dyadic levels may provide additional insight into both the stability and quality of the dyad, in addition to the relative impact of each individual on social outcomes. However, this requires an ability to precisely profile or measure microlevel temporal synchronicity and exchange across a social dyad.

HOW DO WE MEASURE SOCIAL INTERACTION?

Despite the complex dynamics characterizing social interactions, methods to examine and assess these myriad skills are limited. Current standardized psychological and psychiatric methods designed to profile social interaction include assessment tools such as the Coding Interactive Behavior (Feldman 1998, 2003) and the Infant and Maternal Regulatory Scoring Systems (IRSS and MRSS) (Tronick and Weinberg 1990). Each is reliant on subjective visual quantification of macrolevel observed behaviors, such as turn taking (temporal interdependence) and social affect (content interdependence), by trained coders or examiners (Figure 5.4). While effective for providing surface-level measurement, these tools have inherent levels of examiner bias, and lack the precision to quantify microlevel fluctuations in interdependence that characterizes social interaction.

Both verbal and nonverbal social skills are restricted in quantity and quality in individuals with ASD—forming a central theme to diagnosis and intervention—as outlined in the *Diagnostic and Statistical Manual of Mental Disorders* (American Psychiatric Association 2013). The Autism Diagnostic Observation Schedule (ADOS & ADOS-2) (Lord et al. 2000, 2012) reflects this symptomatology by measuring levels of social affect, and repetitive and stereotyped behaviors. This standardized assessment tool is considered the gold standard in diagnostic measures and provides a unique opportunity to assess features of ASD within the context of controlled social interactions. Through engagement in play, the examiner uses a number of social "presses" to elicit a naturalistic response from the individual. The quality of response, or lack thereof, provides an insight into aspects of ASD, which is used to assess the presence and severity of symptoms. Comprising modules that vary in complexity, the ADOS-2 examines both verbal (where appropriate) and nonverbal social interaction at

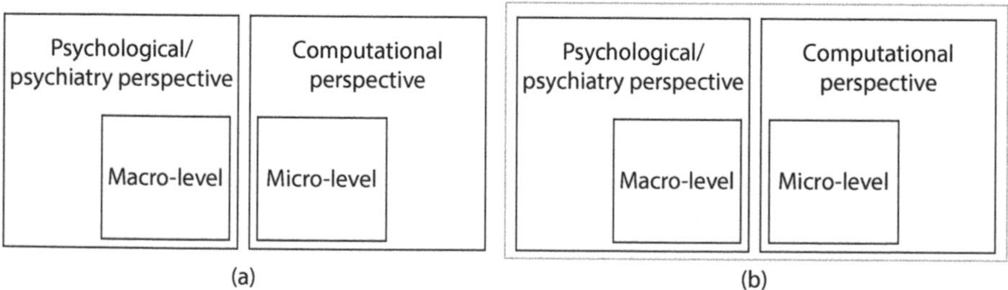

FIGURE 5.4 (a) Schematic illustrating the areas of examination of standardized psychological and psychiatric tools of social exchange. As noted, these remain focused at the level of observational behavioral analysis, and thus are restricted to macrolevel outcome measures. Conversely, as discussed below, computational methods designed to overcome inherent limitations using such subjective, behavioral data focus on microlevel outcome metrics; however, they often fail to consider higher-level macrolevel outcomes—despite often being calibrated by subjective measures. (b) Schematic illustrating the proposed framework, encompassing both macro- and microlevel examination.

levels of content and temporal interdependence. For instance, components such as "anticipation of a social routine," "joint attention," and "communication" provide measures of temporal interdependence, while "quality of response to the examiner" and "communicative gestures" provide content-level assessment. However, despite examining social affect through response to an examiner's social presses or prompts, the ADOS-2 fails to consider interactions at a dyadic level. Instead, the ADOS-2 limits assessment to the examinee, neglecting the impact of the examiner in this complex exchange. Moreover, in line with traditional measures of socialization, this diagnostic tool relies on static "snapshots" at a macrolevel of observational quantification. This quantification of continuous dynamic social behavior using a discrete scale is artificially limiting, while assessment metrics that depend on the expertise of the examiner or coder result in a tool that is prone to subjective bias and error, lacking the precision to quantify microlevel behaviors.

Specialized Techniques to Examine Microlevel Evolving Social Dyadic Interactions (i.e., Synchronicity)

Turn taking and temporal synchronicity provide a foundation for socialization and communication. Synchronicity has been examined from a range of perspectives across psychological, physiological, and computer sciences. A recent review by Delaherche and colleagues (2012) provides a comprehensive overview of the attempts to measure and objectively profile interpersonal synchrony using both noncomputational and computational methods. In particular, this review illustrates the dominance of recurrent analysis and correlational models across a total of 34 studies. Despite promising methods, the 34 studies are limited in scope with a mode number of social dyads of six—a relatively small number to provide robust metrics of socialization, irrespective of methodology applied. A summative overview of these current methodologies is provided below, followed by the introduction of a new platform for future implementation and the design of social metrics—illustrated further in Chapter 7.

Recurrent analytical techniques are prominent in the field of coordination dynamics (Kugler et al. 1982; Turvey et al. 1982; Kelso 1984), with a focus on the synchronization of oscillatory movements (such as interlimb rhythmical coordination). Building on the Haken–Kelso–Bunz model, the "relative phase" of these movements has been examined in light of controlling variables (Haken et al. 1985)—mapping transitions from anti- to in-phase action. Such studies illustrate the potency of joint action coordination, with members of a dyad gradually shifting toward rhythmical in-phase (i.e., synchronized) attractor states (Schmidt et al. 2011). These provide compelling mathematical modeled evidence for the transition and emergence of stable, in-phase rhythmical coordination across a social dyad. However, these studies often rely on laboratory-stereotyped actions (Schmidt et al. 1994, 2011; Amazeen et al. 1995, 1998; Richardson et al. 2005, 2007), with explicit timing constructs, as opposed to naturalistic interactive behaviors. Indeed, preliminary work characterizing interaction synergies under naturalistic conditions, using a knock-knock paradigm, illustrates the difficulty in systematically deconstructing this level of behavior (Schmidt et al. 2011), resulting in a reliance on "observed entrainment" as measured using traditional, subjective coder ratings.

In addition, correlational methods, such as cross-correlational models and regression models, are regularly employed to examine levels of interpersonal temporal synchronicity. These models examine linear or nonlinear relations between two variables coding for social behavior. However, such models are often founded on an assumption of "stationarity" for temporal relations over time (Boker et al. 2002). This core concept infers that similar patterns of temporal dynamics will be witnessed between variables *X* and *Y* over time, with the assumed mean and variance of the signal properties holding across the entire duration of the analysis (Shao and Chen 1987; Hendry and Juselius 2000; Boker et al. 2002). This assumption is limiting in a number of domains, specifically, in relation to temporal synchronicity within naturalistic behaviors across a social dyad—wherein the exchange and interdependence are assumed to be dynamic, and thus nonstationary. As such, a sliding window for a "windowed cross-correlational analysis," profiling the relations between intervals of the data, may be preferred (Boker et al. 2002; Ashenfelter et al. 2009). Unfortunately, despite promising techniques, these methods have been restricted in their implementation, including the profiling of temporal synchronicity by a single body part, for example, head rotation (Boker et al. 2002; Ashenfelter et al. 2009), and through use in an unstructured environment, minimizing inferences at a macrolevel (Boker et al. 2002; Campbell 2008; Ashenfelter et al. 2009). Moreover, such studies often fail to provide a unified method of data for representation of parameters of synchronicity (Delaherche et al. 2012), restricting implementation and interpretation.

In the area of artificial intelligence, there is growing interest in the dynamics of naturalistic social interactions within the field of computer science. "Social signal processing" aims to circumvent difficulties associated with the aforementioned noncomputational models for naturalistic interpersonal synchrony. Through the use of computational, automatic analogues, these studies aim to profile and systematically "capture" the complexities of naturalistic interactions (Delaherche et al. 2012; Vinciarelli et al. 2009). As outlined by Delaherche and colleagues, this area of research is reexamining the quality and quantity of interactions using sequential learning models, such as hidden Markov models (HMMs) and conditional random fields (CRFs). Applying a maximum likelihood approach, these models produce probability distributions to predict the outcome metrics of social signals across a dyad. However, these comprehensive mathematical models and learning techniques are often underpinned by subjective coding measures of social interaction. For instance, a recent analysis of social signals across a parent–infant exchange in children diagnosed with ASD or an intellectual disability, and typically developing children, utilized an integrative methodology (Saint-Georges et al. 2011). This methodology focused on the application of a Markovian model to characterize predictive relations between each member of the dyad. However, upon closer inspection, these results are based on the coding of home videos using the Infant Caregiver Behavior Scale, as rated by four human coders (Saint-Georges et al. 2011). This use of "traditional" observation-based coding metrics to calibrate computational algorithms is repeatedly demonstrated (Messinger et al. 2010; Sravish et al. 2013; Avril et al. 2014; Provenzi et al. 2015).

Therefore, throughout this field there is a continuing trend for the application of sophisticated methodologies and mathematical models that are underpinned by subjectively derived data. Difficulty in extrapolating and objectifying naturalistic social behaviors may reflect this overreliance on subjectively profiling naturalistic social interactions. Despite complex models, the use of metrics produced by standardized tools, such as the Coding Interactive Behavior (Feldman 1998, 2003), the ADOS (Lord et al. 2000, 2012), and the IRSS and MRSS (Tronick and Cohn 1987; Tronick and Weinberg 1990), arguably undermines the strength of this area. Computational models derived from subjective macrolevel behavioral outcomes, such as those utilized in psychology and psychiatry, raise questions over the objectivity and utility of such sophisticated metrics. Moreover, the use of such observational tools for initial "calibration" results in a reliance on discrete measures of social interactions, such as turn taking and joint attention. By using epoched data, the evolution of this complex dynamic process is thus neglected. Indeed, social interactions are considered nonlinear, with the dynamics of the dyad occurring on a nonlinear scale. Enforcing measurements using a discrete model artificially limits the understanding of this fluid construct, and hinders the resulting computational models. A continuous metric, which can be sequentially deconstructed into time intervals, may better reflect the interaction and provide additional insight into this complex construct. As such, a new model is proposed to examine levels of social exchange in ASD using continuous, empirically driven data.

THE MOTOR PERSPECTIVE: A NEW MODEL TO EXAMINE LEVELS OF SOCIAL EXCHANGE IN ASD

As introduced at the opening of this section, there are three potential methods to approach the question "What are social skills?" Perspective, and research background, will inevitably guide our approach in attempting to quantify, and empirically examine, these underlying skills. As presented, there is a gradual shift toward computational methodologies and approaches, yet the complex nature of social interactions requires a systematic, thorough method to precisely quantify social skills. Viewed from a motor perspective, with social interactions composed of macro- and microlevel exchange between individuals, a multilayered framework may be achievable. Building on the developmental models of sensory-motor control and cognition, it is suggested that future methods draw on lower-level processes of motor control. Harnessing modern motion capture technology, such an approach enables the objective quantification of synchronicity with high levels of temporal precision, facilitating a macro- and microanalysis. In addition, this objective methodology can provide results for a multilayered analysis from metrics in line with the psychological and physiological perspectives, through to those in line with computational modeling techniques. However, the first task is to identify a method to objectively profile levels of motor control: specifically, what variables should be extracted to facilitate the design of a computational model? The following chapters provide insight into the various approaches for the examination and deconstruction of social dynamics—including those specific to the classification of ASD symptomatology. These are drawn together toward a multilayered approach that is briefly introduced and discussed in Chapter 7.

CONCLUSION

This chapter has discussed social interaction and the development of social skills within the framework of sensory-motor control. Initially, the predominant perspective of social interaction was discussed: content interdependence. This initial level of exchange, easily profiled using standardized tools, reflects behavioral outcomes within social interactions, and forms a key—and vital—area of focus within ASD research. Specifically, the role of early imitative behaviors has been extensively examined and established as a foundational component of content interdependence—thus social skills. This traditional level of examination was discussed in light of the discovery of the MNS, leading to speculation over its potential role in ASD development. However, this underlying physiological mechanism faces scrutiny—in particular, the retention of a solely top-down perspective, that fails to adequately consider the role and impact of movement, and self-emerging temporal dynamics in synergistic social exchange. Indeed, microlevels of temporal interdependence (i.e., the social dance) are notoriously difficult to profile, particularly within naturalistic social interactions. New mathematical methodologies to profile this subtle level of interaction—both computational and noncomputational—face a number of challenges, leading to an overreliance on the use of subjective scoring metrics—such as those achieved through the use of standardized tools. Building on developmental theories of motor control, this chapter illustrates the potential of movement, as a form of bottom-up feedback (kinesthetic reafference), to provide a framework to extract temporal information from our environment, and thus enable social coupling. Utilizing principles of the micromovement perspective, this approach endorses the systematic and objective profiling of social interactions using kinematic data—a model that is further introduced in Chapter 7. As will be demonstrated throughout this section, under this new interpretation of ASD, and considering the impact of movement, our understanding of social dynamics may be enriched, but more specifically, we may provide new computational routes to better define and model fundamental symptomatology of ASD.

REFERENCES

Amazeen, P. G., E. L. Amazeen, and M. T. Turvey. 1998. Dynamics of human intersegmental coordination: Theory and research. In *Timing of Behavior: Neural, Psychological, and Computational Perspectives*, ed. D. A. Rosenbaum and C. E. Collyer, 237–59. Cambridge, MA: MIT Press.

Amazeen, P. G., R. C. Schmidt, and M. T. Turvey. 1995. Frequency detuning of the phase entrainment dynamics of visually coupled rhythmic movements. *Biol Cybern* 72 (6):511–8.

Ambrosini, E., M. Costantini, and C. Sinigaglia. 2011. Grasping with the eyes. *J Neurophysiol* 106 (3):1437–42.

American Psychiatric Association. 2013. Diagnostic and Statistical Manual of Mental Disorders. 5th ed. Washington, DC: American Psychiatric Association.

Andersen, R. A., and D. Zipser. 1988. The role of the posterior parietal cortex in coordinate transformations for visual-motor integration. *Can J Physiol Pharmacol* 66 (4):488–501.

Ashenfelter, K. T., S. M. Boker, J. R. Waddell, and N. Vitanov. 2009. Spatiotemporal symmetry and multifractal structure of head movements during dyadic conversation. *J Exp Psychol Hum Percept Perform* 35 (4):1072.

Atkeson, C. G., and J. M. Hollerbach. 1985. Kinematic features of unrestrained vertical arm movements. *J Neurosci* 5 (9):2318–30.

Avril, M., C. Leclère, S. Viaux, S. Michelet, C. Achard, S. Missonnier, M. Keren, D. Cohen, and M. Chetouani. 2014. Social signal processing for studying parent–infant interaction. *Front Psychol* 5:1437.

Baron-Cohen, S., A. M. Leslie, and U. Frith. 1985. Does the autistic child have a "theory of mind"? *Cognition* 21 (1):37–46.

Bekkering, H., E. R. A. De Bruijn, R. H. Cuijpers, R. Newman-Norlund, H. T. Van Schie, and R. Meulenbroek. 2009. Joint action: Neurocognitive mechanisms supporting human interaction. *Top Cogn Sci* 1 (2): 340–52.

Bloom, P., and T. P. German. 2000. Two reasons to abandon the false belief task as a test of theory of mind. *Cognition* 77 (1):B25–31.

Boessenkool, J. J., E.-J. Nijhof, and C. J. Erkelens. 1998. A comparison of curvatures of left and right hand movements in a simple pointing task. *Exp Brain Res* 120 (3):369–76.

Boker, S. M., J. L. Rotondo, M. Xu, and K. King. 2002. Windowed cross-correlation and peak picking for the analysis of variability in the association between behavioral time series. *Psychol Methods* 7 (3):338.

Boria, S., M. Fabbri-Destro, L. Cattaneo, L. Sparaci, C. Sinigaglia, E. Santelli, G. Cossu, and G. Rizzolatti. 2009. Intention understanding in autism. *PloS One* 4 (5):e5596.

Brincker, M. 2010. *Moving Beyond Mirroring—A Social Affordance Model of Sensorimotor Integration during Action Perception*. New York: City University of New York.

Buneo, C. A., M. R. Jarvis, A. P. Batista, and R. A. Andersen. 2002. Direct visuomotor transformations for reaching. *Nature* 416 (6881):632–6.

Calvo-Merino, B., D. E. Glaser, J. Grezes, R. E. Passingham, and P. Haggard. 2005. Action observation and acquired motor skills: An FMRI study with expert dancers. *Cereb Cortex* 15 (8):1243–9.

Campbell, N. 2008. Multimodal processing of discourse information; the effect of synchrony. Presented at 2008 Second International Symposium on Universal Communication, Osaka, Japan, December 15–16.

Cossu, G., S. Boria, C. Copioli, R. Bracceschi, V. Giuberti, E. Santelli, and V. Gallese. 2012. Motor representation of actions in children with autism. *PLoS One* 7 (9):e44779.

DeCasper, A. J., and A. A. Carstens. 1981. Contingencies of stimulation: Effects on learning and emotion in neonates. *Infant Behav Dev* 4:19–35.

DeCasper, A. J., J.-P. Lecanuet, M.-C. Busnel, C. Granier-Deferre, and R. Maugeais. 1994. Fetal reactions to recurrent maternal speech. *Infant Behav Dev* 17 (2):159–64.

Delaherche, E., M. Chetouani, A. Mahdhaoui, C. Saint-Georges, S. Viaux, and D. Cohen. 2012. Interpersonal synchrony: A survey of evaluation methods across disciplines. *IEEE Trans Affect Comput* 3 (3):349–65.

Descartes, R. 1984. *The Philosophical Writings of Descartes*, trans. J. Cottingham, R. Stoothoff, and D. Murdoch. Vol. I. Cambridge: Cambridge University Press.

Di Pellegrino, G., L. Fadiga, L. Fogassi, V. Gallese, and G. Rizzolatti. 1992. Understanding motor events: A neurophysiological study. *Exp Brain Res* 91 (1):176–80.

Edelman, G. M. 1987. *Neural Darwinism: The Theory of Neuronal Group Selection*. New York: Basic Books.

Fajen, B. R. 2005. Perceiving possibilities for action: On the necessity of calibration and perceptual learning for the visual guidance of action. *Perception* 34 (6):717–40.

Fantz, R. L. 1961. The origin of form perception. *Sci Am* 20466–72.

Feldman, R. 1998. Coding interactive behavior manual. Unpublished. Bar-Ilan University, Israel.

Feldman, R. 2003. Infant–mother and infant–father synchrony: The coregulation of positive arousal. *Infant Ment Health J* 24 (1):1–23.

Flash, T., and N. Hogan. 1985. The coordination of arm movements: An experimentally confirmed mathematical model. *J Neurosci* 5 (7):1688–703.

Gallese, V. 2001. The 'shared manifold' hypothesis. From mirror neurons to empathy. *J Conscious Stud* 8 (5–6): 33–50.

Gallese, V. 2006. Intentional attunement: A neurophysiological perspective on social cognition and its disruption in autism. *Brain Res* 1079 (1):15–24.

Georgopoulos, A. P., A. B. Schwartz, and R. E. Kettner. 1986. Neuronal population coding of movement direction. *Science* 233 (4771):1416–9.

Gibson, E. J. 1969. *Principles of Perceptual Learning and Development.* New York: Appleton-Century-Crofts.

Gibson, J. J. 2014. *The Ecological Approach to Visual Perception: Classic Edition.* New York: Psychology Press.

Gowen, E. 2012. Imitation in autism: Why action kinematics matter. *Front Integr Neurosci* 6:117.

Haken, H., J. A. S. Kelso, and H. Bunz. 1985. A theoretical model of phase transitions in human hand movements. *Biol Cybern* 51 (5):347–56.

Hamilton, A. F. de C., R. M. Brindley, and U. Frith. 2007. Imitation and action understanding in autistic spectrum disorders: How valid is the hypothesis of a deficit in the mirror neuron system? *Neuropsychologia* 45 (8):1859–68.

Hanna, E., and A. N. Meltzoff. 1993. Peer imitation by toddlers in laboratory, home, and day-care contexts: Implications for social learning and memory. *Dev Psychol* 29 (4):701.

Hayes, S. J., D. Ashford, and S. J. Bennett. 2008. Goal-directed imitation: The means to an end. *Acta Psychol* 127 (2):407–15.

Hayes, S. J., N. J. Hodges, R. Huys, and A. M. Williams. 2007. End-point focus manipulations to determine what information is used during observational learning. *Acta Psychol* 126 (2):120–37.

Held, R. 1965. Plasticity in sensory-motor systems. *Sci Am* 213 (5):84–94.

Hendry, D. F., and K. Juselius. 2000. Explaining cointegration analysis: Part 1. *Energy J* 1–42.

Hobson, R. P., and J. A. Hobson. 2008. Dissociable aspects of imitation: A study in autism. *J Exp Child Psychol* 101 (3):170–85.

Holst, E., and H. Mittelstaedt. 1950. Das reafferenzprinzip. *Naturwissenschaften* 37 (20):464–76.

Holst, E. V., H. Mittelstaedt, and P. C. Dodwell. 1971. The principle of reafference: Interactions between the central nervous system and the peripheral organs. In *Perceptual Processing: Stimulus Equivalence and Pattern Recognition*, ed. P. C. Dodwell, 41–71. New York: Appleton-Century-Crofts.

James, W. 2013. *The Principles of Psychology.* Worcestershire: Read Books Ltd.

Jones, S. S. 2009. The development of imitation in infancy. *Philos Trans R Soc Lond B Biol Sci* 364 (1528): 2325–35.

Kelso, J. A. 1984. Phase transitions and critical behavior in human bimanual coordination. *Am J Physiol Regul Integr Comp Physiol* 246 (6):R1000–4.

Kugler, P. N., J. A. S. Kelso, and M. T. Turvey. 1982. On the control and coordination of naturally developing systems. In *The Development of Movement Control and Coordination*, ed. J. A. S. Kelso and J. E. Clark, 5–78. New York: Wiley.

Lee, D. N. 2009. General tau theory: Evolution to date. *Perception* 38 (6):837.

Lee, D. N., C. M. Craig, and M. A. Grealy. 1999. Sensory and intrinsic coordination of movement. *Proc R Soc Lond B Biol Sci* 266 (1432):2029–35.

Libertus, K., and A. Needham. 2010. Teach to reach: The effects of active vs. passive reaching experiences on action and perception. *Vision Res* 50 (24):2750–7.

Lord, C., P. C. DiLavore, and K. Gotham. 2012. *Autism Diagnostic Observation Schedule.* Torrance, CA: Western Psychological Services.

Lord, C., S. Risi, L. Lambrecht, E. H. Cook Jr., B. L. Leventhal, P. C. DiLavore, A. Pickles, and M. Rutter. 2000. The Autism Diagnostic Observation Schedule—Generic: A standard measure of social and communication deficits associated with the spectrum of autism. *J Autism Dev Disord* 30 (3):205–23.

Lundqvist, L.-O. 1995. Facial EMG reactions to facial expressions: A case of facial emotional contagion? *Scand J Psychol* 36 (2):130–41.

Mehrabian, A., and M. Wiener. 1967. Decoding of inconsistent communications. *J Pers Soc Psychol* 6 (1):109.

Mehrabian, A., and S. R. Ferris. 1967. Inference of attitudes from nonverbal communication in two channels. *J Consult Psychol* 31 (3):248.

Meltzoff, A. N., and A. Gopnik. 1993. The role of imitation in understanding persons and developing a theory of mind. In *Understanding Other Minds: Perspectives from Autism*, ed. S. Baren-Cohen, H. Tager-Flusberg, and D. J. Cohen, 335–66. New York: Oxford University Press.

Meltzoff, A. N., and M. K. Moore. 1977. Imitation of facial and manual gestures by human neonates. *Science* 198 (4312):75–8.

Meltzoff, A. N., and M. K. Moore. 1983. Newborn infants imitate adult facial gestures. *Child Dev* 54 (3): 702–9.

Meltzoff, A. N., and M. K. Moore. 1992. Early imitation within a functional framework: The importance of person identity, movement, and development. *Infant Behav Dev* 15 (4):479–505.

Meltzoff, A. N., and M. K. Moore. 1997. Explaining facial imitation: A theoretical model. *Early Dev Parent* 6 (3–4):179.

Messinger, D. M., P. Ruvolo, N. V. Ekas, and A. Fogel. 2010. Applying machine learning to infant interaction: The development is in the details. *Neural Netw* 23 (8):1004–16.

Nakano, E., H. Imamizu, R. Osu, Y. Uno, H. Gomi, T. Yoshioka, and M. Kawato. 1999. Quantitative examinations of internal representations for arm trajectory planning: Minimum commanded torque change model. *J Neurophysiol* 81 (5):2140–55.

Nishikawa, K. C., S. T. Murray, and M. Flanders. 1999. Do arm postures vary with the speed of reaching? *J Neurophysiol* 81 (5):2582–6.

Peterson, C. C., H. M. Wellman, and D. Liu. 2005. Steps in theory-of-mind development for children with deafness or autism. *Child Dev* 76 (2):502–7.

Premack, D., and G. Woodruff. 1978. Does the chimpanzee have a theory of mind? *Behav Brain Sci* 1 (04): 515–26.

Provenzi, L., R. Borgatti, G. Menozzi, and R. Montirosso. 2015. A dynamic system analysis of dyadic flexibility and stability across the face-to-face still-face procedure: Application of the state space grid. *Infant Behav Dev* 38:1–10.

Richardson, M. J., K. L. Marsh, and R. C. Schmidt. 2005. Effects of visual and verbal interaction on unintentional interpersonal coordination. *J Exp Psychol Hum Percept Perform* 31 (1):62.

Richardson, M. J., K. L. Marsh, R. W. Isenhower, J. R. L. Goodman, and R. C. Schmidt. 2007. Rocking together: Dynamics of intentional and unintentional interpersonal coordination. *Hum Mov Sci* 26 (6):867–91.

Riley, M. A., M. Richardson, K. Shockley, and V. C. Ramenzoni. 2011. Interpersonal synergies. *Front Psychol* 2:38.

Rizzolatti, G., and C. Sinigaglia. 2010. The functional role of the parieto-frontal mirror circuit: Interpretations and misinterpretations. *Nat Rev Neurosci* 11 (4):264–74.

Rizzolatti, G., and L. Craighero. 2004. The mirror-neuron system. *Annu Rev Neurosci* 27:169–92. doi: 10.1146/annurev.neuro.27.070203.144230.

Rizzolatti, G., and M. A. Arbib. 1998. Language within our grasp. *Trends Neurosci* 21 (5):188–94.

Rizzolatti, G., L. Fadiga, V. Gallese, and L. Fogassi. 1996. Premotor cortex and the recognition of motor actions. *Cogn Brain Res* 3 (2):131–41.

Rizzolatti, G., R. Camarda, L. Fogassi, M. Gentilucci, G. Luppino, and M. Matelli. 1988. Functional organization of inferior area 6 in the macaque monkey. *Exp Brain Res* 71 (3):491–507.

Rogers, S. J., and B. F. Pennington. 1991. A theoretical approach to the deficits in infantile autism. *Dev Psychopathol* 3 (2):137–62.

Rogers, S. J., G. S. Young, I. Cook, A. Giolzetti, and S. Ozonoff. 2010. Imitating actions on objects in early-onset and regressive autism: Effects and implications of task characteristics on performance. *Dev Psychopathol* 22 (01):71–85.

Russell, P. A., J. A. Hosie, C. D. Gray, C. Scott, N. Hunter, J. S. Banks, and M. C. Macaulay. 1998. The development of theory of mind in deaf children. *J Child Psychol Psychiatry* 39 (6):903–10.

Saint-Georges, C., A. Mahdhaoui, M. Chetouani, R. S. Cassel, M.-C. Laznik, F. Apicella, P. Muratori, S. Maestro, F. Muratori, and D. Cohen. 2011. Do parents recognize autistic deviant behavior long before diagnosis? Taking into account interaction using computational methods. *PloS One* 6 (7):e22393.

Schmidt, R. C., N. Christianson, C. Carello, and R. Baron. 1994. Effects of social and physical variables on between-person visual coordination. *Ecol Psychol* 6 (3):159–83.

Schmidt, R. C., P. Fitzpatrick, R. Caron, and J. Mergeche. 2011. Understanding social motor coordination. *Hum Mov Sci* 30 (5):834–45.

Sebanz, N., H. Bekkering, and G. Knoblich. 2006. Joint action: Bodies and minds moving together. *Trends Cogn Sci* 10 (2):70–6.

Shao, X., and P. Chen. 1987. Normalized auto- and cross-covariance functions for neuronal spike train analysis. *Int J Neurosci* 34 (1–2):85–95.

Shim, J., and L. G. Carlton. 1997. Perception of kinematic characteristics in the motion of lifted weight. *J Motor Behav* 29 (2):131–46.

Singer, W. 1985. Activity-dependent self-organization of the mammalian visual cortex.

Smith, I. M., and S. E. Bryson. 1994. Imitation and action in autism: A critical review. *Psychol Bull* 116 (2):259.

Snyder, L. H. 2000. Coordinate transformations for eye and arm movements in the brain. *Curr Opin Neurobiol* 10 (6):747–54.

Sravish, A. V., E. Tronick, T. Hollenstein, and M. Beeghly. 2013. Dyadic flexibility during the face-to-face still-face paradigm: A dynamic systems analysis of its temporal organization. *Infant Behav Dev* 36 (3):432–7.

Stapel, J. C., S. Hunnius, and H. Bekkering. 2012. Online prediction of others' actions: The contribution of the target object, action context and movement kinematics. *Psychol Res* 76 (4):434–45.

Thelen, E. 1979. Rhythmical stereotypies in normal human infants. *Anim Behav* 27:699–715.

Thelen, E., and L. B. Smith. 1994. *A dynamic systems approach to the development of cognition and action*. MIT Press/Bradford books series in cognitive psychology. Cambridge, MA: MIT Press, pp. xxiii, 376.

Thelen, E., and L. B. Smith. 1996. *A Dynamic Systems Approach to the Development of Cognition and Action*. Cambridge, MA: MIT Press.

Thelen, E., B. D. Ulrich, and P. H. Wolff. 1991. Hidden skills: A dynamic systems analysis of treadmill stepping during the first year. *Monogr Soc Res Child Dev* i–103.

Torres, E. B. 2011. Two classes of movements in motor control. *Ex Brain Res* 215 (3–4):269–83.

Torres, E. B., A. Raymer, L. J. Gonzalez Rothi, K. M. Heilman, and H. Poizner. 2010. Sensory-spatial transformations in the left posterior parietal cortex may contribute to reach timing. *J Neurophysiol* 104 (5): 2375–88.

Torres, E. B., and D. Zipser. 2002. Reaching to grasp with a multi-jointed arm. I. Computational model. *J Neurophysiol* 88 (5):2355–67.

Torres, E. B., M. Brincker, R. W. Isenhower, P. Yanovich, K. A. Stigler, J. I. Nurnberger, D. N. Metaxas, and J. V. José. 2013. Autism: The micro-movement perspective. *Front Integr Neurosci* 7:32.

Torres, E. B., P. Yanovich, and D. N. Metaxas. 2015. Give spontaneity and self-discovery a chance in ASD: Spontaneous peripheral limb variability as a proxy to evoke centrally driven intentional acts. *Front Integr Neurosci* 7:46

Torres, E. B., R. W. Isenhower, J. Nguyen, C. Whyatt, J. I. Nurnberger, J. V. Jose, S. M. Silverstein, T. V. Papathomas, J. Sage, and J. Cole. 2016. Toward precision psychiatry: Statistical platform for the personalized characterization of natural behaviors. *Front Neurol* 7:8.

Torres, E., and R. Andersen. 2006. Space–time separation during obstacle-avoidance learning in monkeys. *J Neurophysiol* 96 (5):2613–32.

Tronick, E. Z., and Cohn, J. E. 1987. *Revised Monadic Phases Manual*. Unpublished manuscript.

Tronick, E. Z., and M. K. Weinberg. 1990. The infant regulatory scoring system (IRSS). Unpublished. Boston, MA: Children's Hospital/Harvard Medical School.

Turvey, M. T., H. L. Fitch, and B. Tuller. 1982. The Bernstein perspective. I. The problems of degrees of freedom and context-conditioned variability. In *Human Motor Behavior: An Introduction*, ed. J. A. S. Kelso, 239–52. Hillsdale, NJ: Erlbaum.

Uno, Y., M. Kawato, and R. Suzuki. 1989. Formation and control of optimal trajectory in human multijoint arm movement. *Biol Cybern* 61 (2):89–101.

Vinciarelli, A., M. Pantic, and H. Bourlard. 2009. Social signal processing: Survey of an emerging domain. *Image Vision Comput* 27 (12):1743–59.

Vivanti, G., and A. Hamilton. 2014. Imitation in autism spectrum disorders. In *Handbook of Autism and Pervasive Developmental Disorders*, ed. F. R. Volkmar, R. Paul, S. J. Rogers, and K. A. Pelphrey, 278–301. 4th ed. Hoboken, NJ: Wiley.

von Hofsten, C. 1991. Structuring of early reaching movements: A longitudinal study. *J Motor Behav* 23 (4): 280–92.

von Hofsten, C. 2007. Action in development. *Dev Sci* 10 (1):54–60.

White, S. W., K. Keonig, and L. Scahill. 2007. Social skills development in children with autism spectrum disorders: A review of the intervention research. *J Autism Dev Disord* 37 (10):1858–68.

Whyatt, C., and C. M. Craig. 2013a. Sensory-motor problems in autism. Front Integr Neurosci 7:51.

Whyatt, C., and C. M. Craig. 2013b. Interceptive skills in children aged 9–11 years, diagnosed with autism spectrum disorder. *Res Autism Spectr Disord* 7 (5):613–23.

Whyatt, C. P., and C. M. Craig. 2012. Motor skills in children aged 7–10 years, diagnosed with autism spectrum disorder. *J Autism Dev Disord* 42 (9):1799–809.

Williams, J. H. G., A. Whiten, T. Suddendorf, and D. I. Perrett. 2001. Imitation, mirror neurons and autism. *Neurosci Biobehav Rev* 25 (4):287–95.

Yirmiya, N., O. Erel, M. Shaked, and D. Solomonica-Levi. 1998. Meta-analyses comparing theory of mind abilities of individuals with autism, individuals with mental retardation, and normally developing individuals. *Psychol Bull* 124 (3):283.

Zipser, D., and R. A. Andersen. 1988. A back-propagation programmed network that simulates response properties of a subset of posterior parietal neurons. *Nature* 331 (6158):679–84.

6 Action Evaluation and Discrimination as Indexes of Imitation Fidelity in Autism

Justin H. G. Williams

CONTENTS

Introduction.......89
Investigating the Relationship between Imitation and Autism.......91
Measuring Imitation.......92
Using Kinematics.......92
Object Movement Reenactment.......93
An Investigation in Autism.......93
Outcome Variables.......93
Facial Imitation.......95
Investigating the Relationship between Imitation and Autism: Copying Values.......98
Conclusions.......99
References.......100

This chapter introduces kinematics-based assessment tools to quantify imitation in general. The work is presented as part of a research program that aims at unveiling possible links between motor dysfunction and impairments in social interactions. Several examples of the use of these kinematic metrics and accompanying paradigms are presented that involve important components of the social exchange. These examples and methods are discussed in light of diagnostics tools, such as the Autism Diagnostic Observation Schedule and Autism Diagnostic Interview–Revised, that openly disregard sensory-motor issues in autism spectrum disorder. Paradoxically, these observational tools provide ordinal scores of social tasks that inherently require proper sensory-motor integration and both overt and covert forms of imitation for their successful completion. As such, the tools provided in this chapter may pave the way toward combining such observational tests with objective methods to eventually link subsets of imitation tasks inherently present in sociomotor behavior with the types of communication exchange such tasks inevitably require.

INTRODUCTION

Much of this book concerns itself with the existence of impaired motor function in autism spectrum disorder (ASD). The implication is that sensorimotor development is critical for the development of social behavior. However, while there is much overlap between impaired motor function and impaired social development, the mapping is far from straightforward. Many children with developmental coordination disorder are socially quite able, and many children with ASD have quite typical or advanced motor skills. Therefore, there are many unanswered questions about the relationship between motoric development and social cognition.

If we consider what makes for the motoric differences between typical development and autism, then an obvious place to start is to examine those features of behavior that are diagnostic using the standard research tools: the Autism Diagnostic Interview (ADI) and Autism Diagnostic Observation Schedule (ADOS) (Lord et al. 2000; Rutter et al. 2003). While many aspects of motor skills, such as poor balance or handwriting, may be impaired in autism, they may also be impaired in other developmental disorders. Those identified by the algorithms of the diagnostic tools are those motor skills that are linked specifically to the other diagnostic features of autism, and which are therefore directly related to impaired social cognition. If you look through the algorithmic items in the Autism Diagnostic Interview–Revised (ADI-R) and ADOS, you see that significant proportions of the items reflect motor behavior. Within the ADI-R, items asking about gaze control, facial expression, actions used for social overture, gesture, and imitation make up 10 of 29 items in the first two domains, while those asking about repetitive actions make up 3 out of 8 items in the third domain. For the ADOS, the number of action-based items becomes less as verbal development progresses across the modules and language becomes the dominant mediator of social interaction, but it remains the case that the use of actions in communication is central to the diagnosis across all modules. Again, this concerns the use of gesture, gaze, and facial expression to communicate.

At this point, a valid question might be to ask if gesture, facial expression, and gaze control are really motor skills. I would strongly argue that they are motor skills, being acquired through learning from others, and which improve through practice. Yet, I also suggest that this is a question well worth exploring because the difference between these forms of motor skills and traditional motor skills, such as handwriting, bicycle riding, and knot tying, can inform us about developmental relationships between motoric and social cognitive development.

The next step is to ask just how these discriminative patterns of behavior differ between those children with autism and those who are typically developing. While there is considerable value in examining the quantity of socially communicative action observed when diagnosing autism, much information also comes from examining the quality. For example, a person with autism may show an absence of descriptive gesture during interpersonal interaction, but more likely it will be poorly formed and vague. Therefore, during the demonstration task in the Autism Diagnostic Observation Schedule–Generic (ADOS-G), when participants are asked to mime tooth brushing, the gestures are quite likely to be vague and quite general, such as just bringing a loosely formed grip action to the side of the mouth and moving it up and down. Some children with autism may show an absence of declarative pointing (pointing out something to show it) but many will point but fail to coordinate the pointing action with an appropriate gaze shift. Few people with autism will show a complete lack of facial expression, but most will show a diminished range. Parents will report that simple expressions like a smile and anger are expressed, but there is a lack of the subtle modulation of facial expression typically seen in both children and adults during social communication. In some cases, expressions and gestures are exaggerated and poorly modulated, perhaps being used inappropriately in some situations. So typically, social actions in autism are not just diminished in frequency, but they are also different in quality. They lack the detail, breadth, and complexity of typical socially communicative actions, and tend to be poorly integrated with one another or their context.

These differences imply a failure to acquire an action-based knowledge of social communication. Social communication is a culturally acquired skill, which means that we acquire it by watching how others do it—in other words, through imitation. Facial expressions are a very good example of socially communicative actions. Earlier perspectives on facial expressions considered them to be "universals." Darwin (2009), in writing about facial expression, described them as being constant across cultures and even across species. While this may be true for basic facial expressions, recent research has thrown light on the cross-cultural variability of expression (Jack et al. 2012). Furthermore, even if basic emotional expressions are quite constant across cultures, there are well-recognized variations and culturally specific facial gestures, which demonstrate that they are acquired by learning from others, that is, through imitation.

INVESTIGATING THE RELATIONSHIP BETWEEN IMITATION AND AUTISM

This brings us to the core of the matter: the hypothesis that imitation is core to the psychopathology of autism, and that while general motor skills are a nonspecific feature of impaired neurodevelopment, imitation is specifically impaired in autism. Almost every study examining imitation in autism that has not been marred by floor or ceiling effects has found group differences (for reviews, see Rogers and Williams 2006; Smith and Bryson 1994; Williams et al. 2004). Highly significant group differences can be found with only 10–20 individuals per group and in all populations, including adolescents and adults with IQs in the normal range (Rogers et al. 1996; Avikainen et al. 2003), and across a wide variety of tasks. Most recently, a meta-analysis of 53 studies (Edwards 2014) found that those with ASD performed an average of 0.81 standard deviations (SDs) below individuals without ASD on imitation tasks, that the impairment was specific to ASD, and that ADOS scores (but not IQ scores) correlated negatively, significantly, and strongly with imitation abilities. Furthermore, group differences were not affected by factors such as study setting, novelty of actions, format of imitation tasks (live vs. not), number of actions to imitate, or verbal prompts. In addition, when imitation performance was defined by both form and end point, it showed deficits, but not when it was defined only by an end point.

The evidence for a specific deficit therefore appears to be somewhat conclusive. A problem with imitation in autism has been clearly and unequivocally documented, and so we have identified a social learning deficit that lies at the base of the cascade of social cognitive development and can result in autism. However, three big questions remain to be answered:

1. If imitation impairment caused autism, then impaired imitation would be a discriminative and diagnostic feature. However, there remains less than 1 SD of difference between groups in performance of imitation tasks, and many children with autism do not have imitation impairment. Furthermore, enhanced mimicry is a feature of ASD, indicating that some children are excellent at copying, and the imitation items in the ADOS (module 1) and ADI-R are not discriminatory. How can autism occur with intact imitation if imitation impairment underlies autism?
2. Imitation may underpin impairments in the development of gesture and facial expression, but how does it relate to repetitive behaviors and low social motivation? Is there a causative relationship between imitation impairment and consequent development of those ASD symptoms that reflect poor social motivation or repetitive behavior?
3. Is imitation part of a causal pathway in the manifestation of autism, or is it just a correlate of other cognitive impairment? In other words, are the cognitive mechanisms specific to imitation necessary for the development of those abilities that are impaired in autism? Imitation is a complex ability that relies on motor skills, memory, and attention. There is widespread evidence for deficits in all these capacities in autism (Kanner 1943; Wing 1981; Mundy and Neal 2000; Dawson et al. 2002; Dziuk et al. 2007). Indeed, Asperger described general impairment of motor skills in his original clinical descriptions, and motoric problems are recognized as an associated feature in the 10th revision of the International Classification of Diseases (ICD-10). Green et al. (2002) found developmental coordination disorder to be an almost ubiquitous feature of autism. Deficits in episodic memory and working memory are similarly well documented, as are abnormalities in attention. The imitation problem may simply reflect a failure of children with autism to attend to relevant social stimuli and practice the appropriate motor skills. The question may be framed in more biological terms. Autism is widely considered to be a neurodevelopmental disorder that is heavily dependent on genetic variation. Therefore, it is quite likely that the genes that are associated with the autism phenotype have pleiotropic effects, which have effects on motor skills, memory, and attention, and also consequences for imitation skills. It can therefore be easily argued that an association between autism and imitation ability is no more than a nonspecific association

because of genetic pleiotropy, resulting in commonly comorbid deficits in memory, motor skills, and attention.

We need to do a lot more to understand the relationship between imitation and ASD, and the hypothesis needs to be more specific. "Imitation" may cover a broad range of action types and forms of learning, and may require a much tighter specification of parameters. In this chapter, I argue that two studies that we have conducted provide two lines of argument in support of a narrower hypothesis. The first argues that there is a specific impairment of imitation in autism, while the other shows that between-individual variance in capacity to imitate affective values through the imitation of facial expression is linked to empathy, a social cognitive ability. I then outline a methodological approach for the measurement of imitation ability, by defining it in terms of a capacity to discriminate between actions of similar form, before discussing how this may provide a fruitful research direction for understanding the neurocognitive basis of autism, and its assessment and treatment.

MEASURING IMITATION

To my knowledge, all the studies in the meta-analysis by Edwards commonly rely on a qualitative scoring approach. This means that actions are modeled and a participant is asked to copy them. In the do-as-I-do approach (Hayes and Hayes 1952), which is the most commonly used, models show participants a series of actions and participants are asked to repeat them. The do-as-I-do indexes the degree of similarity between observed and enacted actions. If done properly, two raters establish interrater reliability and observe an imitated action blind to the participant's group status. Nevertheless, scoring remains necessarily crude, as the coding remains subjective, and rates an act of imitation on a limited scale (e.g., 0, 1, 2, or 3). It also provides a single summary rating that combines accuracy across all the elements, including the speed and coordination. The method imposes no presumptions on the ways in which the copied action may differ from the modeled action and does not credit the imitator's ability to take into account the relative importance of different aspects. In this way, the do-as-I-do method supports "blind copying" as the preferred method of imitation, rather than action understanding. In addition, the scoring is also blind to the way in which a copied action may differ from the modeled action. In theory, the susceptibility of imitation in autism to certain specific aspects of cognition, for example, dexterity or memory, might be examined by altering the specific cognitive demands of the tasks. However, the degree to which it is possible to show that some types of task are more affected than others, for example, gestural versus action on object, or sequential versus single, is limited. This is because introduction of changes to one set of cognitive demands of the task, for example, the memory demands, is difficult to do without altering others, such as the attentional or motoric demands. Consequently, Edwards (2014) was not able to find that the characteristic of the task in terms of action content or experimental design had any consistent effect on effect size. However, as mentioned, research points to impaired imitation of force and speed (or style) (Hobson and Lee 1999; Perra et al. 2008; Wild et al. 2012), whereas clinical observation of impaired gesture in the ADOS (assuming gesture is learned through imitation) implies impaired copying of form. One way to further our understanding of the imitation impairment would be to show that some aspects of imitation are affected differently than others, which means that different parameters of imitation need to be varied and then measured separately from one another.

USING KINEMATICS

An alternative approach may be to use kinematic measures, which can accurately measure properties of actions and describe them using a range of parameters. Although this approach limits the measurements to a few specific parameters, these can be measured with a high level of accuracy and reliability, and so may facilitate a systematic approach to testing specific hypotheses about the imitation deficit in autism. The first studies to explore the use of kinematics to study imitation in autism

(Wild et al. 2010, 2012) report that participants with autism were poorer at imitating the speed of actions than controls, which they suggest may stem from different patterns of visual attention. While this constitutes a step forward in (1) providing quantitative evidence for an imitation deficit and (2) showing a specific deficit for copying speed, the link to visual attention remains correlative, and so the possibility remains that the deficit could stem from impaired motor function, visual attention, or working memory.

OBJECT MOVEMENT REENACTMENT

Certain types of observational learning are superficially similar, yet theoretically distinct from imitation. Whiten (2006) describes an experiment (Custance et al. 1999) with capuchin monkeys that observe other monkeys opening containers of prize food items. The monkeys might learn to operate the opening mechanism (e.g., removal of a bolt) by observing another monkey, but they would not use the same technique to achieve it (e.g., they would push the bolt out instead of pulling it). This is a form of emulation that is concerned with copying the object movements but not the actions. They termed this "object movement reenactment" (OMR), which requires the recreation of object movements caused by an action without necessarily requiring the action to be copied (Custance et al. 1999) This distinction was introduced by Heyes et al. (1994), who compared an imitation condition where the subject observed an action with an object (a rat pressing a lever to obtain a reward) with one where the object underwent identical movements with no actor (lever depression only—also leading to reward), as if controlled by a ghost.

This method makes it possible to create two tasks with exactly the same demands in terms of measured motor output, but where one requires imitation and the other only requires reenactment of the action end point. If the imitation problem in autism is specific to imitation, we would expect to see worse performance in the imitation task in autism, relative to possible additional impairment on the OMR task, which is nonspecifically related to motor impairment.

AN INVESTIGATION IN AUTISM

This was the study described by Stewart et al. (2013). It required the creation of two types of stimuli in the form of video recordings. First, an actor was videoed while drawing shapes on the screen of a tablet (three shapes, three sizes, and three speeds). We used some software developed in our laboratory for recording the movements made by the stylus on the surface of a tablet computer (Kinematic Assessment Tool [Culmer et al. 2009]—described below). After these videos were recorded, we then created a further set, using the recorded trajectories to drive the movement path of a red dot. Then the actor sat in front of the tablet but did not move, while a red dot could be seen to move on the tablet tracing out the same shapes at different speeds and sizes. Another critical difference between the two sets of stimuli was the camera angle. In the imitation stimuli, the camera was angled so that the action could be seen but not the end point of the action or the object being drawn on the screen. In the OMR stimuli, the object end point was visible. For this study, the parameters that could be readily extracted were the path length of a movement and the duration of an action. We were therefore able to design an imitation task where we specifically set the performance parameters in terms of the variables that we could quantitatively measure (action speed and size), and could therefore scaffold it by asking participants to pay particular attention to these parameters. We hypothesized that imitation would be worse among adolescents with ASD than among their Typically Developing (TD) peers.

OUTCOME VARIABLES

Williams et al. (2014) developed two approaches to analysis of the data, which may be considered comparable to the two-way method or the do-as-I-do method. The two-way method is essentially a measure of the correlation between the model and participant's behavior. If imitation occurs, then the copied behavior is more likely to occur following a seen behavior than an unseen behavior, and therefore imitation can be operationally defined as the statistical dependence of the acted behavior on the seen behavior, that is, as a correlation between observed and enacted behaviors. We therefore conducted correlative analyses between the model and participant data, which ask about the strength of the statistical dependency of the parameters of the participants' action on those of the model. Figure 6.1 shows that the slopes were greater than 1 for both groups, but more so for the ASD group. This was because as the model values got larger (i.e., the shapes drawn got bigger), participants failed to increase the size of object drawn at the same rate. This is an example of contraction bias—a well-recognized phenomenon whereby we all have a tendency to be biased toward the mean when asked to estimate a variable that is continuously distributed. The bias demonstrates a feature of the correlative method for examining imitation in that error can be distinguished from bias, and it would be possible to have a perfect correlation, that is, complete statistical dependency of one action upon another, but without the action kinematics matching, due to a bias. Another feature of the correlative method is that it can be applied to determine whether an individual is copying, rather than just looking at group differences. Stewart et al. (2013) reported that more children with autism than controls failed to reach a statistically significant level of correlation between model and participant, specifically for imitation of action duration, indicating that those children had not imitated.

The second approach to analysis corresponds to the do-as-I-do method and simply measures the degree of error between participant and model. Error measures then lend themselves to parametric analysis and a repeat measures analysis of variance (ANOVA) experimental design. Stewart et al. (2013) were able to show a marked group effect and a further group X task interaction, while controlling for IQ and age. This showed that there was a general motoric problem in the ASD group, but on top of this, there was also a specific imitation impairment.

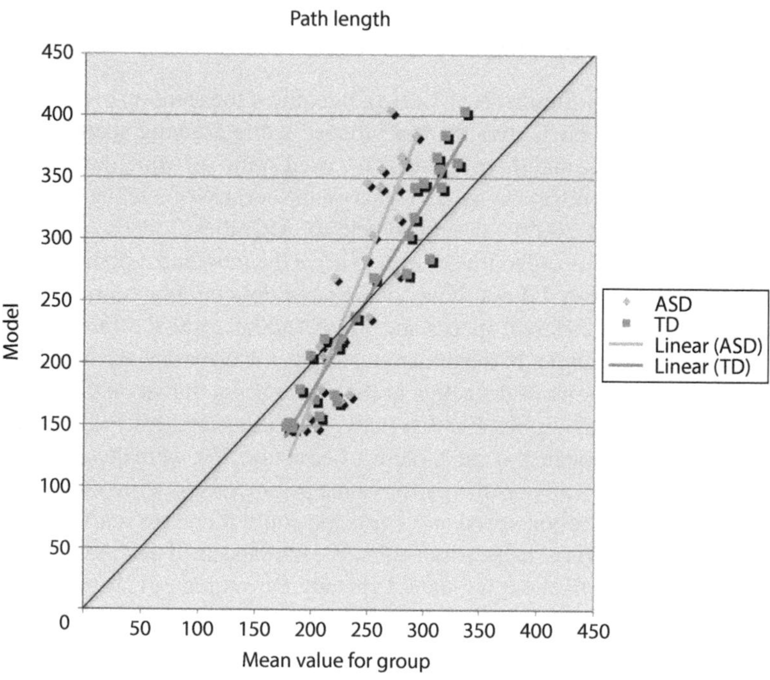

FIGURE 6.1 For each of the 27 trials, the mean value of the path length for the whole group is plotted against that of the model. In both groups, the slope is greater than 1, but more so for the ASD group, indicative of greater contraction bias in the ASD group.

FACIAL IMITATION

These manual imitation studies established the feasibility, a methodology, and an analytic approach for the measurement of imitation fidelity in typical development and autism. However, this relies on the measurement of one parameter at a time, and as mentioned earlier, the clinical impairments in autism suggest a problem in collating the distinctive features of actions in relation to their context during imitation. For example, while it is the case that a lack of descriptive gesture and declarative pointing are important diagnostic features of autism, it is not usually single parameters that are not learned, but the correct form or context in which they are applied. Furthermore, it is possible that the learning of those aspects of actions that are particularly relevant to social communication might be more specifically impaired in autism. In particular, imitation of actions such as those used in the facial expression of emotion may be particularly impaired. Facial expressions offer a particularly good model because they involve collating multiple actions (e.g., mouth, forehead, and jaw muscles) to achieve configurations that are distinctly linked to specific mental states.

Perhaps curiously, facial imitation has been relatively little researched. Indeed, studies of facial imitation in autism have been characterized by significant methodological limitations, as well as being low in number. Much interest has been shown in neonatal imitation (Meltzoff and Moore 1977), but many argue that this is simply mimicry (Jones 2009). Studies of facial imitation in older populations utilizing basic emotions (Carr et al. 2003; Dapretto et al. 2006; Tardif et al. 2007) would seem to be crude tests of empathy given that recognition of basic emotion is achieved by 1-year-olds (McClure 2000). For previously learned expressions, these tasks require only recognition and then execution of a stereotyped behavior. Other tasks involving novel sequences or novel facial actions may seem to be stronger tests of imitative ability (Rogers et al. 1996; Bernier et al. 2007; Tardif et al. 2007) but do not seem relevant for the purpose of facial expression, which is usually to communicate emotion, and are not good tests of the capacity to generate complex or subtly different expressions.

In order to test the ability to imitate an emotional expression, we sought to determine whether a methodology similar to that used with manual imitation could be applied to facial emotion. That would require us to take a single parameter as an outcome measure, vary it systematically across a series of trials, and see how closely the participant's copy correlates with it. For the purposes of facial emotion, it is possible to parametrically control the amount of a specific emotion expressed in a face. Standardized facial expressions have been generated by a few labs (e.g., the Eckman faces and the Karolinska faces) that can be considered to represent basic expressions at the 100% level. By identifying the landmark features of a face, it is possible to move these landmarks to alter the expression that is projected. For example, if the positions of landmark features are determined for a face that is neutral and one that is completely sad ("100% sad"), then when the landmark features are halfway between the two, the expression will be 50% sad. It is also possible to blend facial images in predetermined amounts. It would therefore be possible to blend two emotions by systematically varying amounts to create a linear arrangement whereby as one moves along the line, the emotion changes from one to another. Similarly, one could blend three emotions to increase the novelty of the expression and increase task demands further.

We elected to divide the six basic emotions into two sets of three emotions: (1) fear, happy, and disgust and (2) surprise, anger, and sad. These are the two sets where the emotions in each set are thought to be most dissimilar to each other. For each set, we constructed a triangular array of 15 expressions. To calculate the amount of each emotion in each expression, we first considered each emotion to be on an axis perpendicular to the other two. The extreme emotions at the apexes were slightly caricatured at 110% the basic emotion. The proportion of each emotion in the triangular array would then be calculated according to its Euclidean distance from the apex. Those along the edge were only a blend of two emotions, while those in the center were blends of all three emotions. The array of expressions is shown in Figure 6.2.

The principle of the two-way method is that imitation will be evidenced by a behavior that corresponds to the one being shown. If we apply that principle here, then perfect imitation will be

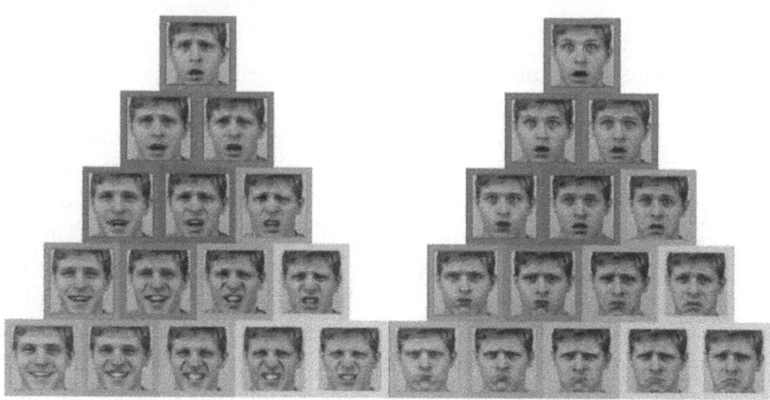

FIGURE 6.2 Stimuli used for the facial expression experiment. Each facial stimulus is displayed individually, but they are shown here as an array to illustrate the structure of variation across the repertoire. Original stimuli were obtained from the Karolinska Facial Expression Database and used with their permission.

evidenced by facial expressions, which can be seen to correspond to the model expressions more than those that are similar. The more similar the expressions, the harder it will be to evidence discrimination in imitation. To test that, we asked a group of young people to imitate the two arrays of facial expressions. Each expression was shown individually, and the participant was given 5 seconds and a countdown ("3, 2, 1") before a shutter sound was heard and the image was captured. For each expression, photographs were then printed. We then asked two raters to try to match an individual's set of photographs to the model set of photographs. After matching, we unblinded them and looked at the accuracy of the matching. Error was measured for each photograph as the number of steps it was away from the model photograph to which it corresponded.

Some points are worth noting about this "sorting" method. Earlier ideas that we considered in thinking about measuring facial imitation were along "do-as-I-do" lines, meaning that we would measure changes in landmark position for expressions and see how well they corresponded to those of the model. This approach would present several challenges. In the first place, the positioning of landmarks and consequent measurement for each stimulus would be impractically time-consuming and laborious. Second, because landmark positions change according to facial identity, it is hard to know how we would go about comparing them. As humans, we are experts in looking at human faces. We are generally sensitive to a change of about 20% in facial expression (e.g., Law-Smith et al. 2010). In sorting the expressions, using our novel approach, we are not asking about the degree of correspondence between each individual's expression and each modeled expression and then taking an average. Rather, we are looking at a single individual's pattern of variance of facial expression and looking at how the structure of that variance corresponds to that of a synthetic standardized model's repertoire. Furthermore, because the blends are of emotional expressions, the synthesized expressions are a repertoire of emotional expressions. The task is therefore one of motoric control over emotional expression within a context of imitation, which means identifying and being able to enact those characteristics of emotional expressions that make them distinctive from one another. The error score generated for each individual is a measure of this ability.

In our initial study (Williams et al. 2013), we aimed to test the methodology by testing three hypotheses—whether there was a practice effect, whether visual feedback improved performance, and whether individual differences correlated with social cognitive function (measured by self-reported "empathic quotient" [EQ]). We found a trend toward an effect of practice: no effect of visual feedback, but a significant effect of EQ, with higher-scoring, more empathic individuals showing more accurate imitation. There was no sex effect.

The relationship between EQ and facial imitation was exciting, not least because of its potential strength, being evident within a sample of just 24 individuals. One criticism was that it might just reflect differences in capacity to recognize emotions, but the literature on emotion recognition and empathy shows a far weaker relationship than we were showing in this study. It seemed much more likely that the method was revealing evidence for a direct relationship between imitation and empathic development. Nevertheless, this initial study clearly required replication and, furthermore, begged the important question as to what neurocognitive mechanism might be implicated in linking facial imitation to empathy.

In the second study (Braadbaart et al. 2014), we sought to conduct the imitation task during functional magnetic resonance imaging (fMRI). In order to specifically examine the correlates of imitation, we introduced a control, "instruction" task, whereby exactly the same images were viewed, but participants were told to execute a preinstructed nonimitation response to a letter cue. Therefore, participants saw the same facial images for each trial, but above each image was an I, an O, or a T, instructing them to imitate, make an O with their mouth, or protrude their tongue, respectively. The study differed from the previous one in using new images constructed from the Karolinska database rather than the Eckman faces. Participants performed the task outside of the scanner first to provide behavioral measures. Inside the scanner, a camera mounted on a head coil allowed compliance to be monitored, but we could not obtain images to measure fidelity.

We were interested in three types of outcomes measure—the effects of imitation compared with instruction, neural correlates of individual differences in EQ, and neural correlates of accuracy. Finally, the areas where accuracy and EQ correlates overlapped would illustrate the neural mechanism that mediates the relationship between accuracy and EQ.

First, the behavioral study replicated the finding of the previous study, showing that EQ correlated with imitation accuracy. An interesting point to note here is that once again, we found no sex differences in imitation ability, despite the correlation with EQ, which does show a sex difference. This could well be because the studies are both underpowered to detect it. For the purposes of this chapter, I combined the results from these two studies. On a combined sample of 19 males and 24 females, a significant difference in EQ is found (male = 35.4, SD = 9.5; female = 42.4, SD = 11.6; $t = 2.14$, $p = 0.038$), but no suggestion of any difference in imitation error (male = 12.5, SD = 4.0; female = 11.4, SD = 3.9; $t = 0.90$, $p = 0.373$). Similarly, a logistic regression showed marked effects of study (the second scored higher errors than the first) and EQ, but clearly no effects of sex (empathy: beta 95% CI = –0.209–0.050, $p = 0.002$; study: beta 95% CI = 3.65–7.08, $p < 0.001$; sex: beta 95% CI = –2.30–1.30).

With respect to the fMRI results, the overall effects of imitate over mismatch revealed few effects, but most interestingly, these were located in the occipital face area (OFA). The OFA has been implicated in facial emotion recognition (Winston et al. 2003), and application of transcranial magnetic stimulation to OFA has been shown to impair emotion recognition (Pitcher et al. 2008). Furthermore, the occipital cortex has been shown to be sensitive to motor activity (Astafiev et al. 2004) and have mirror neuron properties using multivoxel pattern analysis (Oosterhof et al. 2013). These latter studies have identified a slightly more lateral and rostral region with these properties but have focused on manual actions. It is predicted that OFA will be sensitive to motor input, but studies have not yet been directed specifically to that question (Pitcher et al. 2011). Conversely, it also seems quite possible that the OFA could be sensitive to input from other areas concerned with emotional processing, including the orbitofrontal cortex and inferior frontal gyrus. The study by Braadbart et al. also suggests that many of the effects of imitation over mismatch are relatively small and only become detectable when sample sizes are sufficiently large.

Much larger effects of condition were seen for the instruction > imitate contrast. These were centered on the insula, middle temporal gyrus, and precuneus. The insula is well-recognized to become active during conflict, and the data suggest that imitate is a default condition, while to act in a nonimitative way to a facial stimulus, to inhibit a tendency to imitate and enact a prelearned response to a secondary stimulus, is more cognitively demanding.

However, the main purpose of the study was to identify the neural mechanisms that mediated the relationship between EQ and accuracy. Correlations with facial imitation accuracy occurred in both dorsal premotor and parietal regions, while correlations with EQ occurred in the somatosensory cortex, hippocampus, and dorsal premotor cortex. A conjunction analysis using strict criteria identified a region of dorsal premotor cortex, as correlating with both EQ and facial imitation accuracy. A review of the literature found that this area did not correspond to premotor area for facial activity as one might have predicted, but to locations identified as being active during visual imagery of motor actions. Therefore, the critical link between empathic traits and imitation accuracy appears to be mediated by the capacity for motor imagery—to imagine what face is being made during facial imitation. Also, those with more empathic traits show more activity in areas of somatosensory and aspects of parietal cortex during imitation, associated with action encoding and attention to the experience of emotion (Straube and Miltner 2011). These two observations raise the possibility that facial imitation ability and empathy may both be associated with levels of emotional awareness. Emotional awareness would seem to be quite an amorphous concept and one that is difficult to measure. The Levels of Emotional Awareness Scale (Lane et al. 1990) scores the degree of complexity and differentiation that participants ascribe to emotional experiences. It is based on the theory of Lane and Schwartz (1987) that emotional awareness develops from experience of the body in action and bodily sensations, which lead to increasingly complex representations of emotions in the form of blends of different feelings. Lindquist and Feldman-Barrett refer to this as "emotional granularity." By measuring the ability of participants to differentiate between increasingly similar emotions, the measure of facial imitation may therefore provide a measure of emotional granularity, which, according to the theory of Lane and Schwartz, will correspond to emotional awareness.

INVESTIGATING THE RELATIONSHIP BETWEEN IMITATION AND AUTISM: COPYING VALUES

Our studies of facial imitation in autism are as yet unpublished, and further data on manual imitation are also still to be published. Unsurprisingly, we find the capacity for facial imitation and manual imitation to be diminished in ASD. Data therefore point to a diminished capacity in autism to specifically differentiate actions from one another, whether they are emotional expressions or measured as single action parameters. I finish the chapter by hypothesizing two mechanisms by which the capacity to differentiate between actions in imitation might be impaired in autism, and how this might result in alternative patterns of clinical symptoms.

The affective-sharing or motivational and representational theories provide two alternative mechanisms that explain the link between imitation and the social cognitive impairment in autism. The representational model considers the theory of mind deficit to result from a failure to attribute mental states to an observed behavior. A developmental model argues for a hierarchical structure of goal attribution to observed actions, which leads to the generation of "metarepresentations," whereby thoughts are inferred to lie behind other thoughts. At the level of secondary representation (Perner 1991; Suddendorf and Whiten 2001), an action may be observed and the purpose of that action (which can be described as the "goal," "intention," or "motor plan") can be inferred or simulated. Imitation involves the attribution of intention to associate the form of the action with its purpose (or goal). The representational (or mentalizing) theory of autism argues that a failure to develop secondary representations would explain the imitation problem in autism (as well as things like pretend play), but evidence has been problematic. No problems have been found in tests of intentional attribution in autism, and the theory of mind deficit is only seen to be delayed in development. I suggest that the failure does not occur at any *level* of representation, or even rest on certain *levels* being achieved at specific ages. Rather, I suggest that the complexity (or granularity) of an action's representation increases with age and development of motor skills, and it is the *granularity* of that representation that is impaired in autism, resulting is impaired quality of gesture and facial expression.

The affect-sharing or motivational hypothesis (Bachevalier and Loveland 2006; Chevallier et al. 2012) argues that autism is characterized by a deficit of socially motivated behavior. According to this idea, social behaviors are not experienced as rewarding and so are not positively reinforced, resulting in an imitation deficit. The orbitofrontal–amygdala circuit lies at the heart of the social motivational theory. Much emphasis has been placed in recent years on the ventromedial prefrontal cortex (vmPFC) as a location where actions or, more accurately, the outcomes of actions become reinforced (Amodio and Frith 2006). More recently, the vmPFC has been shown to play a role in encoding action-specific values and is necessary for the differentiation of action values from one another (FitzGerald et al. 2012). If these findings are applied to the social motivational theory of autism, it may not therefore be so much that there is a specific failure to reinforce social behaviors in autism, as a problem differentiating between behaviors at the level of their action-specific values, and therefore between social actions in terms of their reinforcement values or associations with outcomes. To learn the contextual role of an action through imitation (including the role of an action within a sequence of other actions) requires specific outcome values to be attached to specific actions. Interestingly, one study has suggested that value encoding in the vmPFC is based on the GABA-glutamate excitation–inhibition balance (Jocham et al. 2012). This is of interest because it is a popular theory that a GABA-glutamate imbalance results in autism (Rojas et al. 2015).

The motivational and representational theories therefore both share a common property. In both theories, there is a failure in autism to differentiate between actions at the representational level. In representational theory, the complexity of action representation within the somatosensory, parietal, and motor cortex is diminished in autism, and impacting on granularity of actions that communicate emotion. The dependence of emotional representation on sensorimotor representation means that coarse granularity of communicative action affects emotional representation, resulting in reduced discrimination between emotions at a level of emotional awareness. Taking the perspective of a motivational framework, the capacity to differentiate between actions of different reinforcement values will be problematic in a different way, affecting a capacity to learn the role of an action in context. Once again, coarse granularity of action representation will result in failure to attribute different reinforcement values to different actions, with the result that different actions will have similar socioemotional reinforcement values, and one action will not be learned in preference to another as being appropriate for social communication. However, the same problem may arise if neural mechanisms in vmPFC for flexible attribution of values to actions are developmentally impaired.

Quantitative measures of imitation using the paradigms we have developed provide an approach to investigating both of these models by measuring the capacity of sensorimotor learning systems to differentiate between similar actions, whether in terms of their kinematic parameters or their socioemotional reinforcement values. A value-based model of imitation also provides a unifying hypothesis for both representational and motivational theories, since the capacity for the orbitofrontal–amygdala circuit to differentiate between actions will depend on both how well those actions are differentiated at the level of encoding and the resolution of the system to differentiate them. Furthermore, we have shown that the values of actions to be copied can be parametrically varied to reflect either the meaning of the actions or their kinematic values.

A further hypothesis is that while poor quality of action representation might be broadly associated with autism, different sources of impaired action representation will affect the clinical picture in different ways. If the problem is primarily within action reinforcement systems, autism might be characterized by largely intact motor skills but more emotional difficulties and rigid behavior, as well as abnormal or even exaggerated gesture (as is sometimes seen in autism). In contrast, if the problem lies in action-encoding systems primarily affecting the granularity of action representation, it will be more likely to be associated with motor clumsiness and poor emotional representation.

CONCLUSIONS

In conclusion, impaired imitation has been repeatedly demonstrated to be associated with autism, and action expression in social behavior has a diminished range and complexity (or *granularity*) in autism. A study using quantitative methodology and a closely matched motor control has shown that imitation is a specific impairment that cannot be accounted for by general motor impairment or attentional problems. A novel method examining the imitation of emotional expressions suggests that the capacity to differentiate between subtly different emotional expressions predicts empathic ability. This is in keeping with theory that suggests that emotional awareness depends on the granularity of emotional representation in motor and sensory systems. I also suggest that the capacity to differentiate actions at the level of reinforcement learning is integral to discriminating between actions in terms of their associated outcomes, and therefore the representation of complex action. Quantitative measures of action imitation fidelity measure a capacity to discriminate between actions, in terms of their associated reinforcement values or representational meanings. Importantly, this relies on measuring the actions executed rather than the capacity for perceptual distinction. Our current research suggests that these measures may provide valuable markers for both identification and assessment, as well as possible targets for the remediation of social cognitive impairment in development.

REFERENCES

Amodio, D. M., and C. D. Frith. 2006. Meeting of minds: The medial frontal cortex and social cognition. *Nat Rev Neurosci* 7 (4):268–77.

Astafiev, S. V., C. M. Stanley, G. L. Shulman, and M. Corbetta. 2004. Extrastriate body area in human occipital cortex responds to the performance of motor actions. *Nat Neurosci* 7 (5):542–8.

Avikainen, S., A. Wohlschläger, S. Liuhanen, R. Hänninen, and R. Hari. 2003. Impaired mirror-image imitation in Asperger and high-functioning autistic subjects. *Curr Biol* 13 (4):339–41.

Bachevalier, J., and K. A. Loveland. 2006. The orbitofrontal–amygdala circuit and self-regulation of social–emotional behavior in autism. *Neurosci Biobehav Rev* 30 (1):97–117.

Bernier, R., G. Dawson, S. Webb, and M. Murias. 2007. EEG mu rhythm and imitation impairments in individuals with autism spectrum disorder. *Brain Cogn* 64 (3):228–37.

Braadbaart, L., H. De Grauw, D. I. Perrett, G. D. Waiter, and J. H. G. Williams. 2014. The shared neural basis of empathy and facial imitation accuracy. *Neuroimage* 84:367–75.

Carr, L., M. Iacoboni, M.-C. Dubeau, J. C. Mazziotta, and G. L. Lenzi. 2003. Neural mechanisms of empathy in humans: A relay from neural systems for imitation to limbic areas. *Proc Natl Acad Sci USA* 100 (9): 5497–502.

Chevallier, C., G. Kohls, V. Troiani, E. S. Brodkin, and R. T. Schultz. 2012. The social motivation theory of autism. *Trends Cogn Sci* 16 (4):231–9.

Culmer, P. R., M. C. Levesley, M. Mon-Williams, and J. H. G. Williams. 2009. A new tool for assessing human movement: The Kinematic Assessment Tool. *J Neurosci Methods* 184 (1):184–92.

Custance, D., A. Whiten, and T. Fredman. 1999. Social learning of an artificial fruit task in capuchin monkeys (*Cebus apella*). *J Comp Psychol* 113 (1):13.

Dapretto, M., M. S. Davies, J. H. Pfeifer, A. A. Scott, M. Sigman, S. Y. Bookheimer, and M. Iacoboni. 2006. Understanding emotions in others: Mirror neuron dysfunction in children with autism spectrum disorders. *Nat Neurosci* 9 (1):28–30.

Darwin, C. 1872. The *Expression of the Emotions in Man and Animals*. London: John Murray.

Dawson, G., S. Webb, G. D. Schellenberg, S. Dager, S. Friedman, E. Aylward, and T. Richards. 2002. Defining the broader phenotype of autism: Genetic, brain, and behavioral perspectives. *Dev Psychopathol* 14 (03): 581–611.

Dziuk, M. A., J. C. Larson, A. Apostu, E. M. Mahone, M. B. Denckla, and S. H. Mostofsky. 2007. Dyspraxia in autism: Association with motor, social, and communicative deficits. *Dev Med Child Neurol* 49 (10):734–9.

Edwards, L. A. 2014. A meta-analysis of imitation abilities in individuals with autism spectrum disorders. *Autism Res* 7 (3):363–80.

FitzGerald, T. H. B., K. J. Friston, and R. J. Dolan. 2012. Action-specific value signals in reward-related regions of the human brain. *J Neurosci* 32 (46):16417–23.

Green, D., G. Baird, A. L. Barnett, L. Henderson, J. Huber, and S. E. Henderson. 2002. The severity and nature of motor impairment in Asperger's syndrome: A comparison with specific developmental disorder of motor function. *J Child Psychol Psychiatry* 43 (5):655–68.

Hayes, K. J., and C. Hayes. 1952. Imitation in a home-raised chimpanzee. *J Comp Physiol Psychol* 45 (5):450.

Heyes, C. M., E. Jaldow, T. Nokes, and G. R. Dawson. 1994. Imitation in rats (*Rattus norvegicus*): The role of demonstrator action. *Behav Proc* 32 (2):173–82.

Hobson, R. P., and A. Lee. 1999. Imitation and identification in autism. *J Child Psychol Psychiatry* 40 (4): 649–59.

Jack, R. E., O. G. B. Garrod, H. Yu, R. Caldara, and P. G. Schyns. 2012. Facial expressions of emotion are not culturally universal. *Proc Natl Acad Sci USA* 109 (19):7241–4.

Jocham, G., L. T. Hunt, J. Near, and T. E. J. Behrens. 2012. A mechanism for value-guided choice based on the excitation-inhibition balance in prefrontal cortex. *Nat Neurosci* 15 (7):960–1.

Jones, S. S. 2009. The development of imitation in infancy. *Philos Trans R Soc Lond B Biol Sci* 364 (1528): 2325–35.

Kanner, L. 1943. Autistic disturbances of affective contact. *Nerv Child* 2:217–50.

Lane, R. D., and G. E. Schwartz. 1987. Levels of emotional awareness: A cognitive-developmental theory and its application to psychopathology. *Am J Psychiatry* 144 (2):133–43.

Lane, R. D., D. M. Quinlan, G. E. Schwartz, P. A. Walker, and S. B. Zeitlin. 1990. The Levels of Emotional Awareness Scale: A cognitive-developmental measure of emotion. *J Pers Assess* 55 (1–2):124–34.

Lindquist, K. A and L Feldman-Barrett. 2008. Emotional Complexity. In *The Handbook of Emotions*, 3rd Edition M. Lewis, J. M. Haviland-Jones, and L. F. Barrett (Eds.). New York: Guilford, pp 513–530.

Lord, C., S. Risi, L. Lambrecht, E. H. Cook Jr., B. L. Leventhal, P. C. DiLavore, A. Pickles, and M. Rutter. 2000. The Autism Diagnostic Observation Schedule—Generic: A standard measure of social and communication deficits associated with the spectrum of autism. *J Autism Dev Disord* 30 (3):205–23.

McClure, E. B. 2000. A meta-analytic review of sex differences in facial expression processing and their development in infants, children, and adolescents. *Psychol Bull* 126 (3):424.

Meltzoff, A. N., and M. K. Moore. 1977. Imitation of facial and manual gestures by human neonates. *Science* 198 (4312):75–8.

Mundy, P., and A. R. Neal. 2000. Neural plasticity, joint attention, and a transactional social-orienting model of autism. *Int Rev Res Ment Retard* 23:139–68.

Oosterhof, N. N., S. P. Tipper, and P. E. Downing. 2013. Crossmodal and action-specific: Neuroimaging the human mirror neuron system. *Trends Cogn Sci* 17 (7):311–8.

Perner, J. 1991. *Understanding the Representational Mind*. Cambridge, MA: MIT Press.

Perra, O., J. H. G. Williams, A. Whiten, L. Fraser, H. Benzie, and D. I. Perrett. 2008. Imitation and 'theory of mind' competencies in discrimination of autism from other neurodevelopmental disorders. *Res Autism Spectr Disord* 2 (3):456–68.

Pitcher, D., L. Garrido, V. Walsh, and B. C. Duchaine. 2008. Transcranial magnetic stimulation disrupts the perception and embodiment of facial expressions. *J Neurosci* 28 (36):8929–33.

Pitcher, D., V. Walsh, and B. Duchaine. 2011. The role of the occipital face area in the cortical face perception network. *Exp Brain Res* 209 (4):481–93.

Rogers, S. J., and J. H. G. Williams. 2006. *Imitation and the Social Mind: Autism and Typical Development*. New York: Guilford Press.

Rogers, S. J., L. Bennetto, R. McEvoy, and B. F. Pennington. 1996. Imitation and pantomime in high-functioning adolescents with autism spectrum disorders. *Child Dev* 2060–73.

Rojas, D. C., K. M. Becker, and L. B. Wilson. 2015. Magnetic resonance spectroscopy studies of glutamate and GABA in autism: Implications for excitation-inhibition imbalance theory. *Curr Dev Disord Rep* 2 (1): 46–57.

Rutter, M., A. Le Couteur, and C. Lord. 2003. Autism diagnostic interview-revised, 29–30. Los Angeles, CA: Western Psychological Services.

Smith, I. M., and S. E. Bryson. 1994. Imitation and action in autism: A critical review. *Psychol Bull* 116 (2):259.

Smith, M. J. L.., B. Montagne, D. I. Perrett, M., Gill, and L. Gallagher. 2010. Detecting subtle facial emotion recognition deficits in high-functioning autism using dynamic stimuli of varying intensities. *Neuropsychologia* 48 (9):2777–781.

Stewart, H. J., R. D. McIntosh, and J. H. G. Williams. 2013. A specific deficit of imitation in autism spectrum disorder. *Autism Res* 6 (6):522–30.

Straube, T., and W. H. R. Miltner. 2011. Attention to aversive emotion and specific activation of the right insula and right somatosensory cortex. *Neuroimage* 54 (3):2534–8.

Suddendorf, T., and A. Whiten. 2001. Mental evolution and development: Evidence for secondary representation in children, great apes, and other animals. *Psychol Bull* 127 (5):629.

Tardif, C., F. Lainé, M. Rodriguez, and B. Gepner. 2007. Slowing down presentation of facial movements and vocal sounds enhances facial expression recognition and induces facial–vocal imitation in children with autism. *J Autism Dev Disord* 37 (8):1469–84.

Whiten, A. 2006. The dissection of imitation and its 'cognitive kin' in comparative and developmental psychology. In *Imitation and the Social Mind: Autism and Typical Development*, ed. S. J. Rogers and J. H. G. Williams, 227–50. New York: Guilford Press.

Wild, K. S., E. Poliakoff, A. Jerrison, and E. Gowen. 2010. The influence of goals on movement kinematics during imitation. *Exp Brain Res* 204 (3):353–60.

Wild, K. S., E. Poliakoff, A. Jerrison, and E. Gowen. 2012. Goal-directed and goal-less imitation in autism spectrum disorder. *J Autism Dev Disord* 42 (8):1739–49.

Williams, J. H. G., A. T. A. Nicolson, K. J. Clephan, H. de Grauw, and D. I. Perrett. 2013. A novel method testing the ability to imitate composite emotional expressions reveals an association with empathy. *PloS One* 8 (4):e61941.

Williams, J. H. G., A. Whiten, and T. Singh. 2004. A systematic review of action imitation in autistic spectrum disorder. *J Autism Dev Disord* 34 (3):285–99.

Williams, J. H. G., J. M. Casey, L. Braadbaart, P. R. Culmer, and M. Mon-Williams. 2014. Kinematic measures of imitation fidelity in primary school children. *J Cogn Dev* 15 (2):345–62.

Wing, L. 1981. Asperger's syndrome: A clinical account. *Psychol Med* 11 (01):115–29.

Winston, J. S., J. O'Doherty, and R. J. Dolan. 2003. Common and distinct neural responses during direct and incidental processing of multiple facial emotions. *Neuroimage* 20 (1):84–97.

7 ADOS

The Physiology Approach to Assess Social Skills and Communication in Autism Spectrum Disorder

Caroline Whyatt and Elizabeth B. Torres

CONTENTS

Introduction 103
Definition and Working Conceptualization of Social Skills 104
Multilayered, Bidirectional Approach to Social Dynamics in Autism Spectrum Disorder 106
Combining the Psychological and Physiological Perspectives: An Objective Exploration into the Social Dyad 107
SPIBA and the Micromovement Data Type 110
Affect versus Motor Control? 113
Conclusion: What Can This Tell Us? 115
References 116

This section of the book has provided an outline of research aimed at exploring the development and refinement of social skills, social cognition, and communication—a core area of inquiry of autism research. Yet, as noted, an individual's background and training will guide research—in terms of both the questions posed and the approaches adopted for analyses, the inferences made, and the interpretation of data. This chapter aims to provide a concrete working example of social dynamics in autism spectrum disorder as decomposed and considered from the perspective of a physiologist and computational neuroscientist. In particular, this chapter illustrates the role of dyadic exchange within the framework of closed feedback loops, which consider reentrant information from sensations of self-generated motion—an element currently missing from the working conceptualization of social exchange. Further, the exchange of volitional and spontaneously co-occurring social motions across a dyad will be objectively quantified, and examined as evolving levels of entrainment. Through this new multidisciplinary movement sensing perspective, we demonstrate the potential utility of such metrics to inform and reshape a diagnostic tool—the Autism Diagnostic Observation Schedule (Lord et al. 2000, 2012), from a *monologue* to a *social dyad*.

INTRODUCTION

Clinically defined and characterized by "classical" behavioral symptomatology, autism spectrum disorder (ASD) (APA 2013) continues to be largely classified as a psychological or psychiatric disorder (see Chapter 2). This classification, prominent across academic, clinical, and public arenas, is reflected in *definitions*—that draw on broad symptomatology, including impaired social and communicative ability, and restricted and repetitive behaviors—and methods of *diagnosis*. Within this framework—and as part of the coarse symptomatology of ASD—social skills play a critical role.

Specifically, easily identified through observational techniques, and a core feature of ASD, social skills provide an intuitive step toward diagnosis, and offer insight into underlying psychological processes and neurological underpinnings (e.g., see Chapter 5). However, our approach to the use of, and understanding of, such higher-level skills is dependent on the perspective that we adopt (see Chapter 4). One's research background and training will inevitably shape our conceptualization and understanding of what social skills are, and thus how these may be harnessed, quantified, and remedied. This chapter aims to illustrate the benefit of each perspective while highlighting the potential of a multidisciplinary lens to reshape our often modular, one-sided, or isolated conceptualization.

DEFINITION AND WORKING CONCEPTUALIZATION OF SOCIAL SKILLS

Encompassing concepts such as social reciprocity or interaction, and language or communication skills, the underlying construct of social skills is largely conceptualized as the ability of an individual to engage in a meaningful interpersonal interaction within a dyad (or larger) setting. Traditionally conceived of as verbal in nature, social skills and communication exist on a continuum of *both* verbal and nonverbal interactions. Further, as outlined in Chapter 5, through these verbal and nonverbal interactions, members of a dyad influence each other at two levels—*content* and *temporal* interdependence at both *micro-* and *macrolevels*. This multilayered deconstruction of social skills and communication provides initial insight into the complexity of these higher-level dynamics. However, the level of examination—and thus how these are harnessed—varies.

From the *psychological perspective*, social skills are core to infant development, and remain prominent in adult existence, facilitating the building of cultural beliefs and shared understanding, and the development of stable relationships. Seminal work empirically deconstructing this early dyadic exchange demonstrates subtle levels of content and temporal entrainment across the infant–caregiver dyad in the macrolevel feeding patterns of new mothers and microlevel suck-burst patterns of infants (Kaye 1977, Schaffer 1996), cycled infant–caregiver gaze on–off patterns (Beebe, Jaffe et al. 2010), and early "vocal" exchanges (Wolff 1969, Schaffer and Liddell 1984). Illustrative of the first levels of sociocommunication skills, this work demonstrates macrolevel behavioral organization of dyadic exchange by profiling the microlevel temporal entrainment, that is, the underlying periodicity of exchange (Schaffer 1977, Kaye and Fogel 1980, Lester, Hoffman et al. 1985, Cohn and Tronick 1987). Yet, despite the pivotal role of social dynamics—particularly during development—quantifying social skills and interpersonal relationships within the psychological or psychiatric remit is arguably limited. Indeed, current standardized psychological and psychiatric methods designed to profile social interaction rely heavily on observational assessment tools, such as the Coding Interactive Behavior (Feldman 1998, Feldman 2003) and the Infant and Maternal Regulatory Scoring Systems (IRSS and MRSS) (Tronick and Weinberg 1990). Although designed to consider the *bidirectional* relationship—that is, both members of the dyad—on behavioral outcomes, such tools are reliant on descriptive methods, via the use of visual quantification of macrolevel observed behaviors by trained coders or examiners. Indeed, despite employing analytical methods to examine the bidirectionality of early dyadic interactions through time and frequency metrics, and the isolation of stochastic versus periodic cycles of exchange e.g. Cohn and Tronick (1987), such seminal work relies on the primary quantification of exchange through subjective measures—via the monadic phases manual (Tronick 1987). This reliance on visual metrics restricts our interpretation of microdynamics to those that are at a substantial level so as to be observed.

The *physiologist* may aim to provide a more concrete, objective method to record and profile levels of social skills, social cognition, and communication, by making precise recordings of physiological (bodily) control. A growing area of inquiry, perhaps in part due to advances in technology, this is akin to the initial level of a motor or movement perspective. Indeed, studies have employed eye-tracking technology in an attempt to further quantify traditionally psychological metrics of social dynamics, such as early infant–caregiver joint attention, through an examination of synchronized and sustained fixation on joint regions of interest (ROIs) (e.g. Yu and Smith 2013). Furthermore, by recording physiological landmarks of members of a dyad (or larger), attempts to deconstruct the internal dynamics for social synchronization and coordination—that is, temporal interdependence—have been made. As discussed in Chapter 5, this field of "coordination dynamics" utilizes high-speed motion capture technology, and draws prominently from recurrent analytical techniques, to objectively profile the potency of joint action coordination and entrainment (Kugler, Kelso et al. 1982, Turvey, Fitch et al. 1982, Kelso 1984; Schmidt, Fitzpatrick et al. 2011). However, despite providing evidence of coordination dynamics at an underlying temporal level that can impact macrolevel behaviors, such work is limited to artificial paradigms (Schmidt, Christianson et al. 1994; Amazeen, Schmidt et al. 1995; Amazeen, Amazeen et al. 1998; Richardson, Marsh et al. 2005; Richardson, Marsh et al. 2007; Schmidt, Fitzpatrick et al. 2011) (also see Chapter 5). Indeed, in more naturalistic contexts such physiologist perspectives revert back to a reliance on underlying psychological coding techniques of entrainment to guide the analytical methods (Schmidt et al. 2011). Thus, despite attempts to provide impartial, objective metrics to quantify macro- and microlevels of social dyadic exchange, the physiological perspective faces a number of inherent limitations, including an inability to extrapolate findings generalizable to a broader naturalistic contextual setting.

Building from the physiologist methodology, the *neuroscience perspective* aims to isolate areas of the brain that are responsible for social cognition and thus social skills. Neurological areas vital in the identification of socially relevant facial stimuli and characteristics (e.g. Morris, Frith et al. 1996, Phillips, Young et al. 1997, Winston, O'Doherty et al. 2007), the detection and utilization of biologically relevant motion information (e.g. Allison, Puce et al. 2000), and action understanding (e.g. Rizzolatti 2005) have been isolated. Yet, despite advances in brain imaging techniques, such metrics are restricted to an artificial examination during an experimental—or medically—restricted scan. Such an approach constrains our understanding to considering the impact of socially relevant information on an *individual*—that is, a unidirectional approach—rather than a neurological conceptualization of bidirectional interaction. Further, movement—an inherent part of dyadic exchange, particularly at the nonverbal level—is a well-documented limiting factor in the use of modern brain imaging and scanning technology, including functional magnetic resonance imaging (fMRI) and electroencephalogram (EEG), and even ocular (Friston, Williams et al. 1996, Croft and Barry 2000, Gwin, Gramann et al. 2010). Thus, current *computational neuroscience* models of social cognition, skills, and communication focus heavily on the level of the central nervous system (CNS), as characterized by underlying neural activity. However, as discussed throughout this book, this arguably restricted interpretation—artificially removing contributions of movement as a form of sensing and the role of the *peripheral nervous system* (PNS)—from computational models, limits our understanding of the global social environment, including the impact of motor control and sensory processing. Attempts to integrate motor control and social interaction have been made in recent years (Frith and Wolpert 2003), yet difficulties extrapolating such information to a broader context remain. Indeed, despite drawing heavily on forward planning models of action control, such theoretical constructs place an assumption of a priori information in one's ability to "decode" such socially and biologically relevant information. Potential limitations of such an approach have been discussed in Chapter 5, demonstrating the complexity of this "dark matter" of neuroscience (Schilbach, Timmermans et al. 2013).

Combined, the psychological, physiological, and computational neuroscience perspectives, although informative, are arguably restricted in their approach. Indeed, the challenge posed by a "second person of neuroscience"—the dark matter of neuroscience today (Schilbach, Timmermans et al. 2013)—has been repeatedly raised in an attempt to open dialogue regarding methodology and assumptions. Despite this, inherent limitations and preconceived conceptualizations based on one's background and field of study pose a tangible barrier. Indeed, reflecting the complexity of natural human behaviors, particularly those such as social exchange, we argue that this modular approach is outdated. Rather, we propose a multilayered, multidisciplinary approach to quantify, examine, and thus understand social exchange in *complex systems* (Figure 7.1). In our inquiry, we

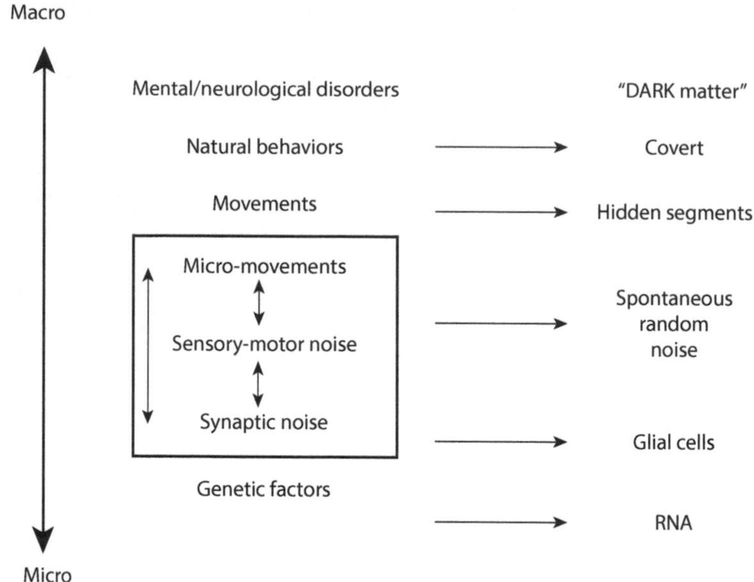

FIGURE 7.1 Multilayered system of inquiry from macro- to microlevels—inevitably, information is neglected at each level, information that falls largely beneath our awareness. For example, observational metrics that rely on the description of behavior focus on overt aspects, while the study of movements that make up such behaviors omit incidental segments that supplement goal-directed actions (Torres, 2011). Further, traditional kinematics-parameter averaging removes minute fluctuations within the amplitude and timing of movements as "noise"—information that may contain important signals (Brincker and Torres, 2013; Torres et al. 2013). Finally, recent discoveries regarding the underlying role of glial cells and RNA are also examples of data that were previously omitted.

will incorporate new elements of behavior at the macro- and microlevels across different spatial and temporal scales. As noted, these components of the social exchange have been traditionally overlooked due to both limitations in observational (psychological and physiological) metrics, and the a priori assumptions placed on such complex phenomena in an attempt to simplify, or reduce, the research condition. The remainder of this chapter thus presents an overview of a multilayered approach to examining social dynamics. This model integrates new elements—previously overlooked due to a priori assumptions—in an attempt to objectively quantify the "social dance" for a population with known social difficulties: ASD.

MULTILAYERED, BIDIRECTIONAL APPROACH TO SOCIAL DYNAMICS IN AUTISM SPECTRUM DISORDER

Current psychological and psychiatric tools for the diagnosis and characterization of ASD draw heavily on the role of social skills as a fundamental axis of symptomatology (APA, 2013). The Autism Diagnostic Observation Schedule (ADOS*) (Lord et al. 2012) is considered the "gold standard" assessment tool currently available to assist in diagnosis† (Ozonoff, Goodlin-Jones et al. 2005, Kanne, Randolph et al. 2008). The ADOS is thus equipped with a range of measures to assess the quality of *spontaneous* socialization in ASD, including the use of communicative gestures, joint attention, and quality of response to the examiner. Drawing on these traditionally *psychological* metrics that tap into

* ADOS will be used to refer to all versions of the ADOS, including the generic and second edition.

† The ADOS is typically used in conjunction with additional tools for contextual information, such as the Autism Diagnostic Interview–Revised (ADI-R) (Lord, C., et al. 1994).

the diagnostic conceptualization of ASD, the ADOS provides a unique opportunity to measure social cognition and skills from the broader macrolevel from the standpoint of an observer. Specifically, the ADOS provides a structured, controlled social environment, and *attempts* to simultaneously harness naturalistic—spontaneous—*bidirectional* dyadic exchange. However, upon closer examination, the metrics extracted from this observational psychological model rely on a *unidirectional* approach. Indeed, through the use of a semistructured controlled social environment, the ADOS targets a range of symptomatic features of ASD, with an examiner using a number of social "presses" to illicit a response from the individual through age-appropriate play-like behaviors. The quality of social response, or lack thereof, provides an insight into aspects of autism, which is used to assess the presence and severity of symptoms. Yet, no information is recorded as to the potential impact of the clinician on the outcomes of this social exchange—a cornerstone of a dyad—artificially restricting outcome metrics to the "performance" of the participant or examinee. Further, such observational scoring metrics face inherent limitations with subjective coder bias and error, and exist on ordinal scales that neglect subtle aspects of behavior occurring at timescales beyond conscious awareness (Figure 7.1). In particular, the observer or clinician is explicitly looking for spontaneous overtures —in response to the social presses that they present. Combined, such a platform results in potential levels of confirmation bias, and an artificial restriction to the inclusion of discrete behaviors that exist at an observational level so as to be "coded." As such, we need to (1) adopt an approach that examines the social *dyad* rather than the child in isolation (a dyadic ADOS rather than an ADOS monologue); (2) integrate an "objective neutral observer" provided by data-driven methods and statistical frameworks that can span across, and integrate between, the multiple macro- and microlevels of inquiry to include "hidden" movement classes; and (3) provide metrics that can encapsulate the *continuous flow* of evolving social dyadic exchange between both members of the dyad to examine entrainment and synchronicity. By coupling this standardized psychological tool with in-depth objective methods to quantify microlevel coordination, higher-level psychological metrics of social interaction may be sequentially deconstructed, proving a model and method to address these limitations. Further, drawing on core principles founded in mathematics, this objective exploration may facilitate a computational modeling approach—vital in the autism endeavor.

Combining the Psychological and Physiological Perspectives: An Objective Exploration into the Social Dyad

The following provides an overview of an ongoing research study currently being completed at the Sensory-Motor Integration Laboratory of Rutgers University—funded by the New Jersey Governors Council for Medical Research and Treatment of Autism.

This project initially draws on the concrete and controlled environment of the ADOS platform, to examine constructs defining social skills, cognition, and communication from a macropsychological level. As such, the ADOS is administered and scored according to a standardized protocol by a trained clinical team member. Outcome metrics using ordinal data are scored for subsequent consideration, yet of most importance, the order and controlled administration of social presses is tracked, for subsequent targeted analysis and decomposition. Through this sequential deconstruction, the project aims to examine the relationship between higher-macro-level observed psychological constructs of social dynamics and underlying microlevel forms of temporal and content interdependence as measured using objective metrics. Indeed, through this method, the project aims to isolate and identify tasks presented within the global psychological tool that are particularly informative of underlying dyadic exchange and social skills. To incorporate this nuanced understanding of social dynamics, and at the level of dyadic interaction, high-end wireless motion capture technology is integrated. Specifically, lightweight inertial measurement units (IMUs) (APDM) are positioned on key anatomical landmarks of *both* the clinician and the examinee or participant—six positioned on each member, as demonstrated in Figure 7.2.

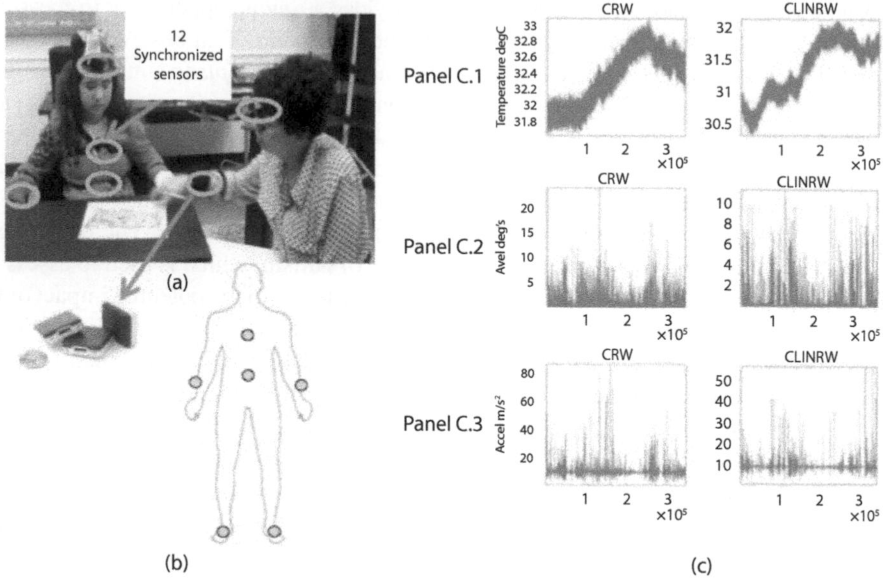

FIGURE 7.2 Experimental setup with sensors and example data. (a) Image of a typical paradigm for the administration of the ADOS, whereby a clinician creates a standardized social environment to elicit a spontaneous response. As indicated, 12 IMUs are strategically positioned across the dyad—6 on each member—at key anatomical landmarks, as demonstrated in (b). (c) Synchronously sampling at 128 Hz, these IMUs provide temperature (c.1), angular velocity (c.2), and acceleration (c.3) metrics, on which underlying kinematic analysis can be performed.

Sampling at 128 Hz, these sensors provide *synchronized* measurements of temperature, angular velocity, and acceleration from across *both* members of the dyad. These synchronized signals, harnessed from the output of the nervous systems, are subsequently examined at the microlevel of somatic sociomotor coordination. Specifically, recorded motor output is also considered within the framework of reentrant kinesthetic sensory input—"kinesthetic reafference" (Holst and Mittelstaedt 1950). As discussed below, the lead–lag information of each body part of each member of the dyad is considered to understand how the motoric biorhythm of one system guides the other—that is, levels of entrainment and temporal interdependence—during the ADOS exchange. Mirroring the multilayered approach of Figure 7.1 to the study of social interactions, kinematic research in the specific area of autism also exists on a layered continuum of analysis (e.g., Torres et al. 2013; Torres 2011)—as such, the first question to consider is what form of kinematic analysis is most informative?

In the case of individuals with ASD, higher macrolevel observations of kinematic control imply a general level of motor difficulty (Green, Charman et al. 2009, Whyatt and Craig 2012), which has been objectively profiled using standard microlevel kinematic methods to confirm levels of motoric irregularity that can be directly linked to macrolevel behavioral outcomes (Whyatt and Craig 2013). However, both of these "traditional" levels of kinematic, physiological analysis rely on the examination of goal-directed behaviors across discrete timescales (an epoch) to examine specific overt behaviors at the expense of larger timescales—that is, those of continuous, evolving motor output. Indeed, similar to the difficulties encountered by the examination of unfolding coordination dynamics (e.g. Schmidt, Christianson et al. 1994, Amazeen, Schmidt et al. 1995), the longitudinal profiling of evolving nonlinear motor control, a characteristic of continuous social interaction, negates the use of handpicked epochs in discrete methods of analysis.

Consider, for example, the complex sports routines of boxing (jab, cross, hook, and uppercut) (Figure 7.3). The hand trajectories and speed profiles derived from these complex motions reveal hidden segments that the athlete is unaware of. For each alternating hand punch, the athlete focuses on

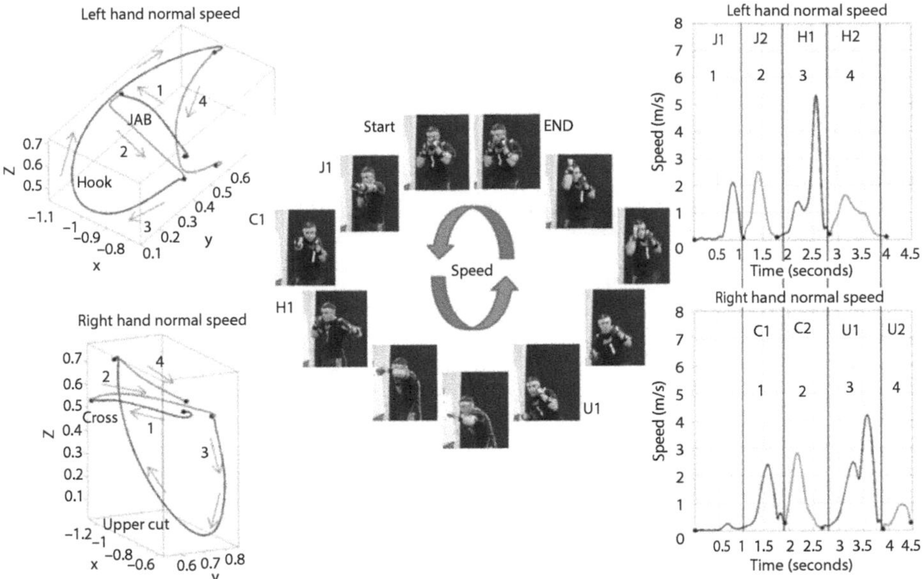

FIGURE 7.3 Hidden movement segments of boxing behavior. The jab–cross–hook–uppercut routine is decomposed here for the right and left hand (end points of the upper-body kinematic linkage). The center picture shows the athlete from start to end performing the routine at variable speeds on command (fast or slow called at random by a computer program). The traces correspond to a slow-motion case. (a) Trajectories with the segments delineating the start and end of each subroutine in the order in which they occurred, marked by arrows. (b) Temporal speed profiles of the positional trajectories shown in (a). The J2, H2, C2 and U2 marks the hidden movement segments of this complex boxing behavior. While the athlete attends to the forward punches with one hand (J1, H1, C1 and U1), the other hand is simultaneously retracting. These supplementary (incidental) motions co-occurring with the staged (deliberate) ones the athlete directs to a goal (the opponent) are the hidden segments that "glue" our complex behaviors along a continuum and make the fluid. The supporting role of these actions was previously unknown, as we had not yet quantified them and had no way to distinguish them from the goal-directed (forward) ones. The athlete was also unaware of them. The experimenter was therefore surprised by the resulting plots of these motions (see Figure 7.4). (Reproduced from Torres, E. B. *Exp Brain Res* 215 (3–4):269–83, 2011. With permission.)

the forward, goal-directed segment of the hand aiming at the opponent, while the retracting segment of the other hand is co-occurring. Despite overt focus on the forward movement, the athlete's nervous systems also attend to these "hidden" segments, such as the retraction. Yet, an external observer "coding" the dyadic behavior between the athlete and his opponent may only "see" overt segments of the action—those directed to the very dynamically moving target (opponent). When empirically quantified at a high resolution, this example from sports science illustrates the additional layers of complexity embedded within our actions—with different "classes" of hidden movements isolated (Torres 2011). Utilizing a third "neutral objective observer," a quantitative approach can be adopted that automatically separates the effect of changes in motion dynamics (e.g., speed) from the geometry of the motion trajectory (Figure 7.4). A computational model (Torres 2002) guided by a mathematical equation can then be harnessed to identify levels of intent from the signatures of deliberateness, or spontaneity, in the motions (Torres 2011). Interestingly, this distinction which is obvious in neuro-typical systems does not occur, or is less obvious in systems with ASD (Figure 7.5). Namely, this approach detected the presence of the memoryless exponential distribution, denoting a "here and now" statistical code characterizing ASD—a code with no certainty in the reliance of past events to predict future events (Figure 7.5). In other words, the peripheral signal that is echoed back to the brain bears information on the moment, yet each moment is experienced anew. This discovery can be appreciated in

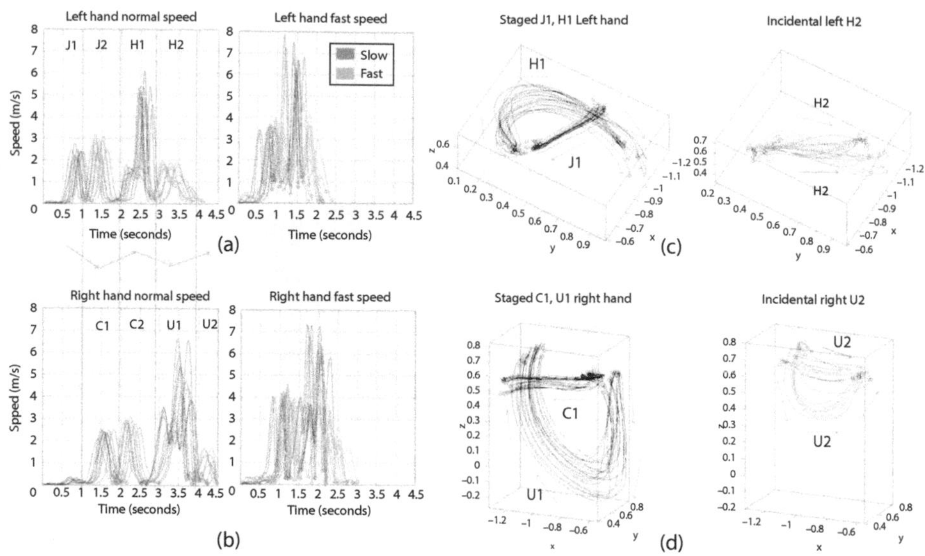

FIGURE 7.4 Automatic distinction of staged (deliberate) and incidental (spontaneous) movement classes coexisting in complex behaviors performed by systems with redundant degrees of freedom (DoF). (a, b) Speed profiles of the left- and right-hand trajectories alternating staged and incidental motions from the full boxing routine performed many times along a continuous flow. The athlete followed the random call of "slow" or "fast." The trials are then grouped by speed, with the lighter segments denoting the hidden movements and black segments denoting the ones the athlete and the experimenter were attending to. Note that the speed profiles remain similar in structure while contracting in time. (c, d) This time contraction does not affect the geometry of the staged-segment trajectories of each subroutine. However, it changes the geometry of the incidental segments. For example, take the incidental uppercut U2 and compare it with the staged uppercut U1. While the fast U2 follows a rather curved trajectory, the slow U2 follows a nearly straight one. Keep in mind that these segments were performed in randomly called order. This speed invariance in the geometry of staged behavioral segments is a signature of deliberateness that contrasts with the variations in spontaneous behavioral segments escaping the naked eye. (Reproduced from Torres, E. B. *Experimental brain research*, 215(3-4), 269-283, 2011. With permission.)

Figure 7.5, which further explores the boxing routines of Figure 7.3 in an adolescent individual with ASD (e.g., Torres 2011).

This example further illustrates levels of trial-to-trial variation in the amplitude and timing of kinematics—parameters that are extracted from the supplementary and goal-directed segments, and that can be further assessed using the statistical platform for individualized behavioral analysis (SPIBA). It is this overarching methodology that can be translated to empirically examine social dyadic interactions in the clinical arena.

SPIBA AND THE MICROMOVEMENT DATA TYPE

The micromovement perspective, introduced by Torres and colleagues, provides a new level of kinematic analysis, whereby minute fluctuations within the sensory-motor signature are captured to characterize neurophysiological control (Torres et al. 2013). Within this framework, the continuous profiling of behaviors is endorsed and the stochastic signature of variation within this signature is empirically estimated (Figure 7.4).

This method serves as a departure from traditional methodologies that rely on discrete metrics, and thus lends itself to the precise profiling of naturalistic (continuously flowing) social interactions. Further, as discussed throughout this book, the use of underlying variability within this signal (micromovements) can be empirically profiled at the individual level, providing insight into the predictability (or likely future "states") of the system, based on prior registered states. Importantly, as

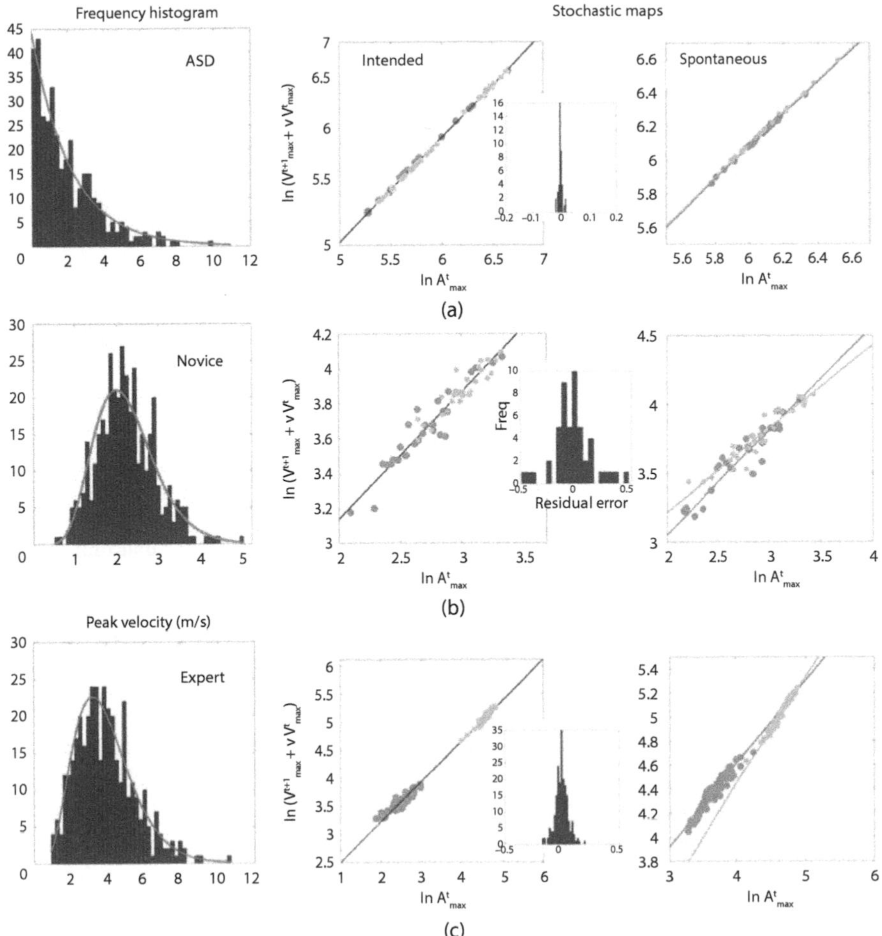

FIGURE 7.5 Signatures of intended and spontaneous behaviors differ between participants with ASD and neurotypical controls. (a) Linear speed micromovements from the peak velocity along the hand trajectories of the jab segments (in Figures 7.3 and 7.4) manifest an exponential-like distribution in ASD, while controls (b, c) are skewed to symmetric. Stochastic maps from a first-order rule that anticipates the variations in future speed from the combination of variations in past speed and acceleration differ between ASD and neurotypical controls in very precise ways. Notably, the intended segments do not distinguish the different speeds, and unlike controls, the ASD's spontaneous movement segments lack the variations to predict the motion dynamics. The memoryless exponential distribution of their variations suggests that the movements are performed in the here and now, in marked contrast to the anticipatory signature of the neurotypical performance.

noted above, the micromovement approach has uncovered a "special" stochastic signature present across multiple biorhythms of ASD motions. Such results illuminate the potential difficulties of "movement sensing" in autism—thus the movement sensing perspective.

The central tenet of the new methodology proposed here is to examine levels of coherence across the bodily rhythms of participants within a dyad in search for entrainment and synergies within (Figure 7.6a) and across (Figure 7.6b) the bodies in motion. As such, this method can provide insight into, *first*, the underlying state of the sensory-motor system of each individual. Through this method, the state of the sensory-motor system can be empirically profiled along a continuum of predictive states: from those with a low noise-to-signal ratio (as characterized by a symmetric distribution with low dispersion) through to a highly variable state with a high noise-to-signal ratio and

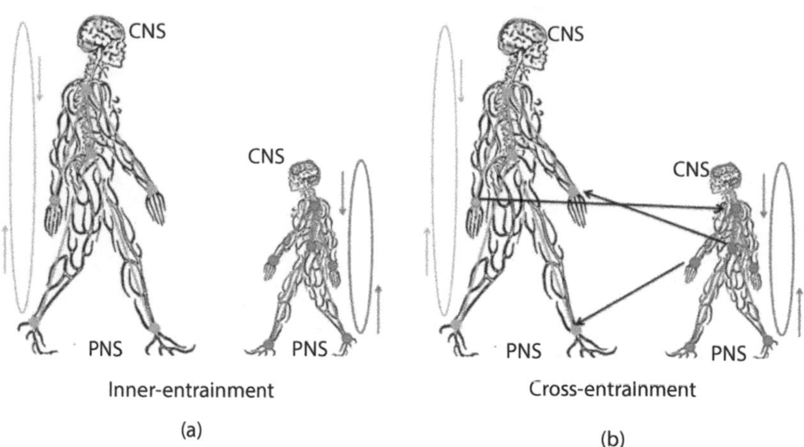

FIGURE 7.6 Schematic representation of the dyadic networks and their coupled activities across CNS-PNS interactions. (a) Intranetwork activity of each dyad participant for one state configuration per unit time. (b) Cross-network coupling with lead–lag network coherence state configuration per unit time. Colored arrows denote the closed-loop intranetwork activity for each dyad participant, while black arrows denote the coupled activity across the two networks. In a dynamic setting, these configurations change (activities evolve as in a movie). As such, they provide a temporal profile of the networks' states. Each contributing node of the overall dyad network provides biorhythms for the continuous tracking of the PNS activity as dictated by the CNS.

randomness (the latter characterized by the memoryless exponential distribution). By empirically estimating the state of an individual's system, SPIBA provides an objective characterization of an individual's neurophysiological control of self-generated movements.

To achieve this level of precision, bundled somatic motor information is collated, minute by minute, from each IMU for a participant (and clinician) across each session. Underlying variability or micromovements (Torres et al. 2013)—moments of maximal deviation—within the acceleration signal are extracted and normalized to control for allometric variation, providing a time series or "spike train" of underlying kinematic fluctuations. This normalized time series is subsequently profiled, empirically establishing the probability distribution function that best characterizes this stochastic process—with four moments utilized (mean, variance, skewness, and kurtosis). This level of processing provides insight into the underlying level of neurophysiological control (Torres et al. 2016)—a level that can be subsequently considered in light of further outcome metrics (see below and Figure 7.8).

Second, this framework can facilitate precise examination of nonlinear evolving synchronicity across the social network—that is, members of the dyad. Information exchange is thus examined within the synergistic coordination of individual anatomical landmarks across each member of the dyad, but also extended to the interconnected synergies across the dyad as a whole. As such, the bodily nodes of both participants (i.e., sensors on anatomical landmarks) are treated as interconnected nodes of a large network (analogous to a network of nerves (Figure 7.6), given that the data readout from the peripheral bodily network is controlled by the central networks of the brain). Then mathematical tools from network analyses are adapted to the analyses of the dyad elements in isolation, and of those in tandem (see Whyatt & Torres 2017 for methodological information). Figure 7.6 provides a schematic representation of these networks, while Figure 7.7 provides an example of network connectivity metrics extracted across the network recorded during an ADOS session. Specifically, these metrics (Figure 7.7) provide information regarding the direction of the interaction—that is, who leads the interaction and when considered in the global framework of the controlled ADOS administration—for what tasks (Figure 7.7b). For instance, despite administration of the ADOS taking (on average) 30–50 minutes to complete per session, core metrics draw heavily on key tasks and critical moments of exchange. Viewing this objective underlying metric of dyadic synergy or entrainment, one can

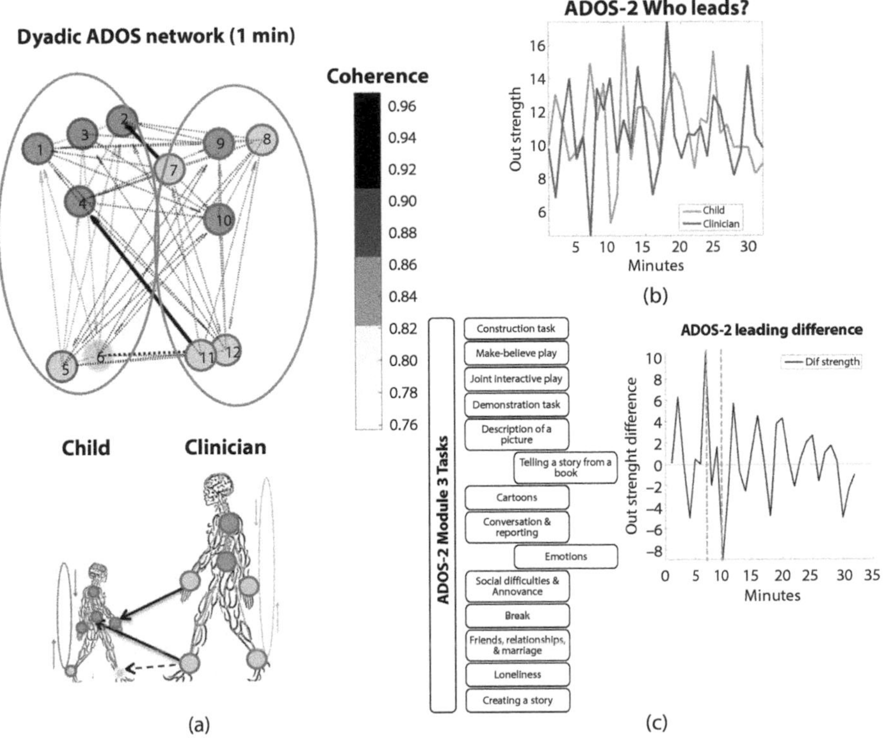

FIGURE 7.7 Dyadic ADOS network and its dynamic temporal profiles. (a) Network analyses of the two dyad participants for 1 minute (out of 40 minutes) of the dyadic ADOS exchange. Different colors of the circles denote different modules denoting cross-network coupled synergies, while the circles' "edge" denotes the coherence level of the nodes connected to other nodes in the network. Arrows denote the connection and the direction of leading activity according to phase lead profiles. Black arrows are internetworks' coupled activity denoting cross-entrainment levels. (b) Illustrative example of leading information across the ADOS-2 administration. Specifically, leading information derived from a pairwise cross coherence analysis across the dyad is summed to result in node-out strength for each member across the session. (c) The difference in out-strength between each member of the dyad is subsequently calculated, and isolated within the framework of the ADOS-2 administration - highlighting the importance of the Telling a Story (TS) task and Emotion (EMO) competent.

blindly isolate elements of the ADOS administration in which the clinician or participant or child was leading the exchange. As demonstrated in Figure 7.7b and c, the weight of outgoing leading information across all nodes (i.e., sensors) for each member of the dyad can be summed to provide a total metric (outstrength metric; see Figure 7.7b). This can be profiled across the course of the session —and the difference between the outstrength of both member of the dyad examined in light of overarching ADOS tasks. This examination can thus illustrate who out of the dyad is leading the exchange for each task (see Figure 7.7c), and which are most informative.

AFFECT VERSUS MOTOR CONTROL?

The leading–lagging profiles, and their critical points, can provide information regarding important differences in task demands, differences that may not be obvious to the most experienced examiner, or even to the designers of the observational tools, such as the ADOS. Indeed, examination of critical points of difference in the strength of leading information for both the clinician and participants - isolate two core tasks: the Telling-a-story (TS) task and the Emotional component (EMO). While the design and requirements of the tell-a-story (TS) task denote a motorically demanding activity, the

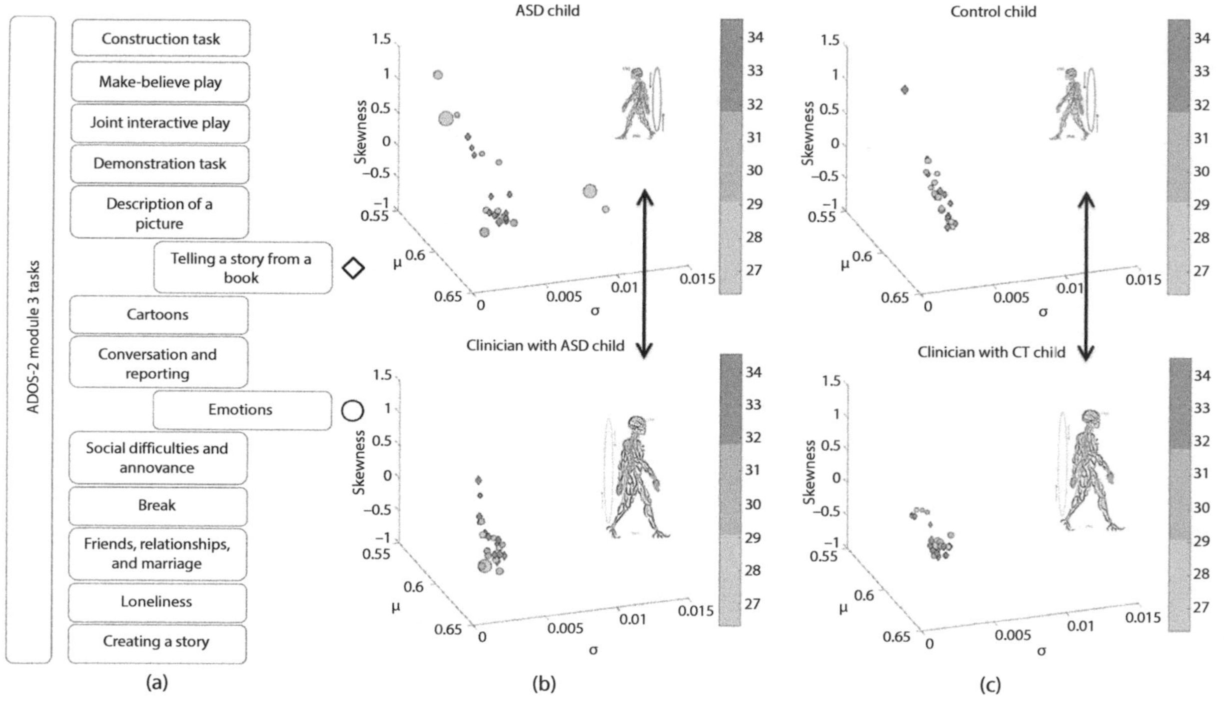

FIGURE 7.8 Affect versus motor control? Quantifying marked differences in the signatures of micromovements during the EMO and TS tasks. Using the aforementioned method, critical points in leading information during the administration of the ADOS were examined – blindly isolating two primary tasks: Telling a story, and the Emotion Component (Panel A). Automatic distinction between the motoric demands of each task is evident in the estimated gamma moments and the temperature profiles (Panel B). The EMO outcome measure shows high levels of involuntary micromovements (lighter circles), defined by the lower-temperature profiles of the motions during the emotionally demanding task. In marked contrast, the motorically demanding TS task outputs more activity (darker diamonds) with a higher-temperature profile from higher battery drainage during actively self-generated voluntary motions (see color bar). The ASD profile (top left panel) is also more variable and differs in the shapes of the estimated probability distribution functions (skewness and kurtosis moments denoted by the z-axis and the size of the marker, respectively).

emotional (EMO) task lacks this motor element. Specifically, the former requires the child to enact and tell a story to the examiner—a form of social exchange, while the latter requires the participant to answer a range of emotionally salient questions—targeting elements such as loneliness, relationships, and emotions. The amount of uncertainty and emotional distress such questions elicited in each child (see also Chapter 26 on bullying) is reflected in a very different stochastic landscape in ASD than that uncovered in the typically developing age- and sex-matched controls (CT). This unexpected signature of an increase in the spontaneous involuntary micromovements served to characterize this emotional component. While the constituent components of the EMO task would imply no involvement of motion, the sensor technology has output a level of lower-temperature motion (implying involuntary actions) statistically different from that of the TS task. Figure 7.8 provides this contrast in results for representative children, with both ASD and age-matched control participants (completing the same ADOS module). Further, as performance is examined in a truly dyadic nature, the examiner's or clinician's motions are also profiled per session (in the corresponding bottom panels). The ASD population demonstrates a spread of the gamma moments in space, particularly for the circles that represent motions across the body recorded during the EMO task. These parameters clearly contrast with those of the control population, but also with those of the examiner in both contexts. Indeed, the motoric demands of the TS task and the affect demands of the EMO task are automatically uncovered in the stochastic profile of the micromovements extracted from these bodily rhythms.

The results raise the question—have these metrics tapped into a level of affect that is currently beyond the scope of traditional psychological tools? As noted, the emotional component contains a range of questions that are designed to target emotional constructs, such as loneliness, friendships, and sadness. Although often stereotyped as experiencing difficulties with emotional regulation, expression, and empathy (Cohn and Tronick 1987)—largely a by-product of the psychological perspective interpretation of social skills and cognition—such work may give voice to those feelings. Currently being examined at a larger group level, and considered in light of psychological outcomes, these underlying microlevel metrics may provide novel insight into the underlying coping systems of individuals with ASD and may speak to a level of empathy—or discomfort—beyond our current scope.

CONCLUSION: WHAT CAN THIS TELL US?

Combined, this multilayered approach to the deconstruction of social skills demonstrates the importance of considering microlevels of exchange—a level currently beyond psychological metrics alone. Indeed, by coupling standardized psychological tools with objective, precise kinematic measurements of physiological control, novel insight into levels of dyadic entrainment may be achieved. Such objectives, informative in a variety of arenas, are particularly useful for individuals and populations living under the stereotype of poor social skills, social cognition, and communication. With the ADOS adopted as a framework, this model has provided a controlled social environment in which to deconstruct complex naturalistic social dynamics, while maintaining direct links to clinically relevant behavioral metrics, and simultaneously illustrating perceived difficulties with such restricted tools. Through the use of objective metrics, connections beyond the macrolevel—that is, subtle attempts to engage—may be identified. If so, such tools may demonstrate that rather than characterizing individuals with ASD as unable to communicate and engage, it may be time to consider how such an interpretation may be artificially enforced by *our inability* to perceive such attempts. By viewing performance during the ADOS through an alternative lens, we may identify the impact of the clinician on this dyadic process, and consider the possibility that we are simply out of step with individuals on the autism spectrum. Indeed, it may be argued that the ADOS of today is merely an instrument that serves to highlight the child's social deficits (arguably as induced, in part, by the examiner's style of prompting). It gives us a one-sided account of the severity of the problem, but social exchange is not one-sided. Under the sensory and somatic motor umbrella, the ADOS of tomorrow could be an instrument that serves a different purpose—to highlight the potential and best capabilities of the child in a truly dyadic context.

REFERENCES

Allison, T., A. Puce, and G. McCarthy. 2000. Social perception from visual cues: Role of the STS region. *Trends Cogn Sci* 4 (7):267–78.

Amazeen, P. G., E. L. Amazeen, and M. T. Turvey. 1998. Dynamics of human intersegmental coordination: Theory and research. In *Timing of Behavior: Neural, Psychological, and Computational Perspectives*, ed. D. A. Rosenbaum and C. E. Collyer, 237–59. Cambridge, MA: MIT Press.

Amazeen, P. G., R. C. Schmidt, and M. T. Turvey. 1995. Frequency detuning of the phase entrainment dynamics of visually coupled rhythmic movements. *Biol Cybern* 72 (6):511–18.

APA (American Psychiatric Association). 2013. *Diagnostic and Statistical Manual of Mental Disorders*. 5th ed. Washington, DC: APA.

Beebe, B., J. Jaffe, S. Markese, K. Buck, H. Chen, P. Cohen, L. Bahrick, H. Andrews, and S. Feldstein. 2010. The origins of 12-month attachment: A microanalysis of 4-month mother–infant interaction. *Attach Hum Dev* 12 (1–2):3–141.

Bowlby, J. 2008. *A Secure Base: Parent-Child Attachment and Healthy Human Development*. New York: Basic Books.

Brincker, M., and E. B. Torres. 2013. Noise from the periphery in autism. *Front Integr Neurosci* 7:34.

Cohn, J. F., and E. Z. Tronick. 1987. Mother–infant face-to-face interaction: The sequence of dyadic states at 3, 6, and 9 months. *Dev Psychol* 23 (1):68.

Croft, R. J., and R. J. Barry. 2000. Removal of ocular artifact from the EEG: A review. *Neurophysiol Clin* 30 (1):5–19.

Feldman, R. 1998. Coding interactive behavior manual. Unpublished. Bar-Ilan University, Israel.

Feldman, R. 2003. Infant–mother and infant–father synchrony: The coregulation of positive arousal. *Infant Ment Health J* 24 (1):1–23.

Friston, K. J., S. Williams, R. Howard, R. S. J. Frackowiak, and R. Turner. 1996. Movement-related effects in fMRI time-series. *Magn Reson Med* 35 (3):346–55.

Frith, C. D., and D. M. Wolpert. 2003. *The Neuroscience of Social Interaction: Decoding, Imitating, and Influencing the Actions of Others*. Oxford: Oxford University Press.

Gidley Larson, J. C., A. J. Bastian, O. Donchin, R. Shadmehr, and S. H. Mostofsky. 2008. Acquisition of internal models of motor tasks in children with autism. *Brain* 131 (Pt 11):2894–903. doi: 10.1093/brain/awn226.

Green, D., T. Charman, A. Pickles, S. Chandler, T. Loucas, E. Simonoff, and G. Baird. 2009. Impairment in movement skills of children with autistic spectrum disorders. *Developmental Medicine & Child Neurology* 51 (4): 311–316.

Gwin, J. T., K. Gramann, S. Makeig, and D. P. Ferris. 2010. Removal of movement artifact from high-density EEG recorded during walking and running. *J Neurophysiol* 103 (6):3526–34.

Haswell, C. C., J. Izawa, L. R. Dowell, S. H. Mostofsky, and R. Shadmehr. 2009. Representation of internal models of action in the autistic brain. *Nat Neurosci* 12 (8):970–2. doi: 10.1038/nn.2356.

Hertz-Picciotto, I., and L. Delwiche. 2009. The rise in autism and the role of age at diagnosis. *Epidemiology (Cambridge, Mass.)* 20 (1):84.

Holst, E., and H. Mittelstaedt. 1950. Das reafferenzprinzip. *Naturwissenschaften* 37 (20):464–76.

Kanne, S. M., J. K. Randolph, and J. E. Farmer. 2008. Diagnostic and assessment findings: A bridge to academic planning for children with autism spectrum disorders. *Neuropsychol Rev* 18 (4):367–84.

Kaye, K. 1977. Toward the origin of dialogue. In *Studies in Mother-Infant Interaction*, ed. H. R. Schaffer, 89–117. London: Academic Press.

Kaye, K., and A. Fogel. 1980. The temporal structure of face-to-face communication between mothers and infants. *Dev Psychol* 16 (5):454.

Kelso, J. A. 1984. Phase transitions and critical behavior in human bimanual coordination. *Am J Physiol Regul Integr Comp Physiol* 246 (6):R1000–4.

Kugler, P. N., J. A. S. Kelso, and M. T. Turvey. 1982. On the control and coordination of naturally developing systems. In *Development of Movement Control and Coordination*, ed. J. A. S. Kelso and J. E. Clark, 5–78. New York: John Wiley & Sons.

Lester, B. M., J. Hoffman, and T. B. Brazelton. 1985. The rhythmic structure of mother-infant interaction in term and preterm infants. *Child Dev* 56 (1):15–27.

Lord, C., M. Rutter, and A. Le Couteur. 1994. Autism Diagnostic Interview-Revised: a revised version of a diagnostic interview for caregivers of individuals with possible pervasive developmental disorders. *Journal of autism and developmental disorders* 24 (5):659–685.

Lord, C., P. C. DiLavore, and K. Gotham. 2012. *Autism Diagnostic Observation Schedule*. Torrance, CA: Western Psychological Services.

Lord, C., S. Risi, L. Lambrecht, E. H. Cook Jr., B. L. Leventhal, P. C. DiLavore, A. Pickles, and M. Rutter. 2000. The Autism Diagnostic Observation Schedule–Generic: A standard measure of social and communication deficits associated with the spectrum of autism. *J Autism Dev Disord* 30 (3):205–23.

Morris, J. S., C. D. Frith, D. I. Perrett, and D. Rowland. 1996. A differential neural response in the human amygdala to fearful and happy facial expressions. *Nature* 383 (6603):812.

Ozonoff, S., B. L. Goodlin-Jones, and M. Solomon. 2005. Evidence-based assessment of autism spectrum disorders in children and adolescents. *J Clin Child Adoles Psychol* 34 (3):523–40.

Phillips, M. L., A. W. Young, C. Senior, M. Brammer, C. Andrew, A. J. Calder, E. T. Bullmore, D. I. Perrett, D. Rowland, and S. C. R. Williams. 1997. A specific neural substrate for perceiving facial expressions of disgust. *Nature* 389 (6650):495–8.

Richardson, M. J., K. L. Marsh, and R. C. Schmidt. 2005. Effects of visual and verbal interaction on unintentional interpersonal coordination. *J Exp Psychol Hum Percept Perform* 31 (1):62.

Richardson, M. J., K. L. Marsh, R. W. Isenhower, J. R. L. Goodman, and R. C. Schmidt. 2007. Rocking together: Dynamics of intentional and unintentional interpersonal coordination. *Hum Mov Sci* 26 (6): 867–91.

Rizzolatti, G. 2005. The mirror neuron system and its function in humans. *Anat Embryol* 210 (5):419–21.

Schaffer, H. R. 1996. *Social Development*. Oxford: Blackwell Publishing.

Schaffer, H. R. 1977. Early interactive development. In *Studies in Mother-Infant Interaction*, ed. H. R. Schaffer, 3–16. London: Academic Press.

Schaffer, H. R., and C. Liddell. 1984. Adult-child interaction under dyadic and polyadic conditions. *Br J Dev Psychol* 2 (1):33–42.

Schilbach, L., B. Timmermans, V. Reddy, A. Costall, G. Bente, T. Schlicht, and K. Vogeley. 2013. Toward a second-person neuroscience. *Behav Brain Sci* 36 (4):393–414.

Schmidt, R. C., N. Christianson, C. Carello, and R. Baron. 1994. Effects of social and physical variables on between-person visual coordination. *Ecol Psychol* 6 (3):159–83.

Schmidt, R. C., P. Fitzpatrick, R. Caron, and J. Mergeche. 2011. Understanding social motor coordination. *Hum Mov Sci* 30 (5):834–45.

Torres, E. B. 2001. Theoretical framework for the study of sensory-motor integration. PD, Cognitive Science, University of California, San Diego.

Torres, E. B. 2011. Two classes of movements in motor control. *Exp Brain Res* 215 (3–4):269–83. doi: 10.1007/s00221-011-2892-8.

Torres, E. B. 2012. Atypical signatures of motor variability found in an individual with ASD. *Neurocase* 1:1–16. doi: 10.1080/13554794.2011.654224.

Torres, E. B. 2013. Signatures of movement variability anticipate hand speed according to levels of intent. *Behav Brain Funct* 9:10.

Torres, E. B., and D. Zipser. 2002. Reaching to grasp with a multi-jointed arm. I. Computational model. *J Neurophysiol* 88 (5):2355–67. doi: 10.1152/jn.00030.2002.

Torres, E. B., and K. Denisova. 2016. Motor noise is rich signal in autism research and pharmacological treatments. *Sci Rep* 6:37422. doi: 10.1038/srep37422.

Torres, E. B., M. Brincker, R. W. Isenhower, P. Yanovich, K. A. Stigler, J. I. Nurnberger, D. N. Metaxas, and J. V. Jose. 2013. Autism: The micro-movement perspective. *Front Integr Neurosci* 7:32. doi: 10.3389/fnint.2013.00032.

Torres, E. B., R. W. Isenhower, J. Nguyen, C. Whyatt, J. I. Nurnberger, J. V. Jose, S. M. Silverstein, T. V. Papathomas, J. Sage, and J. Cole. 2016. Toward precision psychiatry: Statistical platform for the personalized characterization of natural behaviors. *Front Neurol* 7:8. doi: 10.3389/fneur.2016.00008.

Trevarthen, C. 1979. Communication and cooperation in early infancy: A description of primary intersubjectivity. In *Before Speech: The Beginning of Interpersonal Communication*, ed. M. Bullowa, 530–71. Vol. 1. Cambridge: Cambridge University Press.

Trevarthen, C. 2001. Intrinsic motives for companionship in understanding: Their origin, development, and significance for infant mental health. *Infant Ment Health J* 22 (1–2):95–131.

Tronick, E. Z., and M. K. Weinberg. 1990. The infant regulatory scoring system (IRSS). Unpublished. Boston: Children's Hospital/Harvard Medical School.

Turvey, M. T., H. L. Fitch, and B. Tuller. 1982. The Bernstein perspective. I. The problems of degrees of freedom and context-conditioned variability. In *Human Motor Behavior: An Introduction*, ed. J. A. S. Kelso, 239–52. Hillsdale, NJ: Erlbaum.

Whyatt, C. P., and C. M. Craig. 2012. Motor skills in children aged 7–10 years, diagnosed with autism spectrum disorder. *J Autism Dev Disord* 42 (9):1799–809. doi: 10.1007/s10803–011–1421–8.

Whyatt, C. P., and C. M. Craig. 2013. Sensory-motor problems in autism. *Front Integr Neurosci* 7:51.

Whyatt, C. P., and E. B. Torres. 2017. *The social-dance: decomposing naturalistic dyadic interaction dynamics to the 'micro-level'*. In Fourth International Symposium on Movement and Computing, MOCO'17, 28–30 June. London, UK: ACM.

Winston, J. S., J. O'Doherty, J. M. Kilner, D. I. Perrett, and R. J. Dolan. 2007. Brain systems for assessing facial attractiveness. *Neuropsychologia* 45 (1):195–206.

Wolff, P. H. 1969. The natural history of crying and other vocalizations in early infancy. In *Determinants of Infant Behavior*, ed. B. M. Foss, 81–109. Vol. 4. London: Methuen & Co.

Yu, C., and L. B. Smith. 2013. Joint attention without gaze following: Human infants and their parents coordinate visual attention to objects through eye-hand coordination. *PloS One* 8 (11):e79659.

8 On the Brainstem Origin of Autism

Disruption to Movements of the Primary Self

Jonathan Delafield-Butt and Colwyn Trevarthen

CONTENTS

Introduction: Motor Control of the Embodied Self Mediates Autopoesis of Conscious Experience, and Its Consensual Sharing ... 120
Characteristics of Prospective Control of Movement ... 120
Disrupted Movements in Autism ... 121
Movement at the Root of Human Communication and Social Understanding ... 122
Locating Motor-affective Intelligence in the Integrative Work of the Brainstem ... 124
Central Role of Timing and Serial Ordering in Intelligent Moving ... 124
Brainstem Neurophysiological System for Motor Control and Communication of Motives ... 125
Neurological Evidence of Brainstem Abnormality Affecting Motor Timing in Autism: The Inferior Olive ... 126
Brainstem Center for Regulation of Social and Emotional Expressions: The Nucleus Ambiguus and Related Systems ... 127
Additional Evidence That Brainstem Disruption in ASD Also Affects Arousal and Social Engagement: The Locus Coeruleus and Related Systems ... 128
Intrinsic and Environmental Factors Affecting ASD through the Course of Development ... 129
Conclusions: Identifying and Supporting Problems Arising from Disruption of Motives for Development of Cognition and Interpersonal Relations ... 130
Methods of Therapy and Education That Support Hopes for Movement ... 130
Questions at the Forefront of Understanding How the Brain for Purposeful Movement Develops and How It Learns ... 131
Appendix: Case History of Case 1 (Reproduced From Bailey et al. 1998) ... 131
References ... 132

This chapter examines evidence for a disorder of the intrinsic motive processes of the purposeful self in autism spectrum disorder, which leads to weakening of shared experience in early childhood. Changed motor and affective regulations that identify autism are traced to faults in neurogenesis in the core brainstem systems of the fetus. These fundamental systems have evolved to serve the development of sensory guidance for motor activity and affective regulation of projects of thought and action, including communication of intentions and feelings with other human selves.

Affective neuroscience describes subcortical organs in mammals that are responsible for the coherence of a primary conscious self-as-agent, with emotions that communicate feelings for selective sociability with other individuals. In humans, this affective consciousness is adapted as the foundation for active engagement of an infant with a world of objects and people by expressions under the control of shared rhythms of an "intrinsic motive pulse." We give primary importance to the disorder in autism of the accuracy of timing in this resonant central nervous system, responsible for coordination of movement with companions. We relate this understanding of the disorder to problems in the monitoring of prospective regulation of actions of the conscious self by a body-related affective valence, which affects the arousal of personal satisfaction of purposes or anxiety at their failure, and engagement in affectionate or antagonistic relations. This leads to evaluation of participation in movements with shared feelings for therapy and teaching to help the socioemotional development and learning of children with autism, as well as provide advice for lifetime care.

In autism, the essential embodiment of early childhood experience for growth of knowledge, skill, and collaborative social understanding appears weakened by a sensorimotor deficit in motivation and its affective control. This has lifelong developmental consequences, affecting the intersubjective responses of family, and then cooperative attentions of companions and teachers in the community. Miscoordination of movements leads to frustration, distress, and anxiety, creating social withdrawal and avoidance, or overcompensations expressed as increased arousal and hyperactivity. Indeed, we propose that disabilities in cognitive intelligence and language are secondary to weakness in the prospective control of movements with affective appraisal of anticipated experiences.

We identify the origin of these symptoms in disorders of brainstem mechanisms that develop in the late embryo stage and that are essential for motor and affective regulations, as well as autonomic processing. In particular, data indicate an anatomical and functional disruption of the inferior olive, associated with control of motor timing by the cerebellum, and abnormal development of the neighboring nucleus ambiguus, involved in expressions of social engagement and speech. These nuclei appear to be critical components of the core neuropsychological system that develops abnormally to produce the varied autistic spectrum disorders.

We draw attention to the limitations of research methods in neuroscience and psychology that seek to identify a primary cognitive, information processing, and neocortically mediated disorder by testing the response of the individual in artificial situations. New research using microkinesic descriptive methods clarifies motor deficits that characterize autism. Furthermore, extensive imaging of brain activities supports a philosophical psychology of embodiment that elucidates how confusion in unconscious prospective control of actions from fetal stages impairs the child's developing subjective agency. Finally, we offer information on movement-based therapies that can help to facilitate learning, self-regulation, and pleasure in social interaction for individuals with autism spectrum disorder.

INTRODUCTION: MOTOR CONTROL OF THE EMBODIED SELF MEDIATES AUTOPOESIS OF CONSCIOUS EXPERIENCE, AND ITS CONSENSUAL SHARING

Characteristics of Prospective Control of Movement

Movement is the generator and regulator of animated experience. An animal can engage effectively with the world and explore its properties only through muscle activity that is regulated purposefully in body-related time and space (Llinás 2001), and with affective appraisal of its risks and benefits (Panksepp 2005; Packard and Delafield-Butt 2014).

Movement of the human body, with its elaborate adaptations for communication of interests and feelings, holds properties essential to the psychological well-being of the individual as a whole self, and for generating opportunities for social cooperation and affording perceptual information for learning, sharing, and elaboration of conscious skill and knowledge (Condon 1975b, 1979; Trevarthen 2001, 2014; Trevarthen et al. 2014). Two essential life functions defined by the systems theorist Humberto Maturana as "autopoesis," or "self-making," and "consensuality," the constructive collaboration of vital individuals, be they cells in tissues and organs, or individuals in viable social or cultural groups (Maturana and Varela 1980; Maturana et al. 1995; Packard and Delafield-Butt 2014), are affected in varying degrees by changed brain development in individuals with autism spectrum disorder (ASD).

Normal human movements are prospectively controlled (von Hofsten 2007; Lee 2009) to constitute a basic subjective intentionality or core mental state of the individual-as-agent from early fetal life (Delafield-Butt and Trevarthen 2013; Delafield-Butt and Gangopadhyay 2013). Passive, reactive reflex corrections only occur in an unanticipated emergency. Accumulated evidence in prenatal stages of human development demonstrates that fetal movements are controlled in body-related time and space as prereflective intentions—active generators and regulators of experience and expressive of emotions (Piontelli 1992; Lecanuet et al. 1995; Zoia et al. 2007; Delafield-Butt and Gangopadhyay 2013; Reissland et al. 2013, 2014). Movement, as the physical expression of our psychological being, manifests our intentions and expresses our feelings in the nuances of body posture, composure, and composition, and in the "forms of its vitality" of gestures in shared social space (Stern 2010). Whether we wish them to do so or not, movements communicate our intentions to others in gesture, speech, symbols, and the imaginative projects that we create in any activity, privately, in intimate relations, or in public (Baldwin 1895; Trevarthen et al. 2011). They convey the "human seriousness of play" (Turner 1982), sharing the passions by which we regulate social cooperation and the creation of cultural conventions of education, religion, art, and technique (Trevarthen 2014; Delafield-Butt and Adie 2016).

Disrupted Movements in Autism

It has become increasingly clear over the last decade that ASD is characterized by a disruption to motor coordination and timing (Trevarthen et al. 1998; Trevarthen 2000; Trevarthen and Daniel 2005; Trevarthen and Delafield-Butt 2013a). Since Teitelbaum and colleagues' paper in 1998 (Teitelbaum et al. 1998) that showed poor posture and coordination of the limbs in a retrospective video analysis of newborns who later developed autism, a growing field of research is measuring and characterizing motor deficits (Fournier et al. 2010; Torres and Donnellan 2013). Motor skills are disrupted in toddlers with autism, not simply delayed, and this motor disturbance becomes exacerbated over the first years of life (Lloyd et al. 2013). The cause of this deficit in motor kinesics and its place in the development of autism is fundamental for understanding the etiology of the condition, and for planning treatment (Condon and Ogston 1966; Condon 1975a).

Motor control research in the last decade demonstrates that the kinematics of components of action in tasks as varied as making simple horizontal arm movements (Cook et al. 2013), reaching (Sacrey et al. 2014), reaching and grasping (Stoit et al. 2013), making arm movements to goals (Dowd et al. 2012), and handwriting (Kushki et al. 2011) are disturbed in individuals with autism. These are disturbances in goal-directed tasks that serve the intentions of the agent. Postural adjustments during load-shift tasks (Schmitz et al. 2003) and during gait (Rinehart et al. 2006) are affected. And efficient prospective organization of movements in a series or chain of purposes is thwarted (Fabbri-Destro et al. 2009). Prospective, or feed-forward, mechanisms of motor timing appear fundamentally disrupted in autism (David et al. 2012). Perceptual awareness of others' intentions conveyed in body movement or in eye gaze is also weakened (Pierno et al. 2006; Cattaneo et al. 2007). A comprehensive meta-analysis of all motor data in autism revealed substantial motor coordination deficits pervasive across the spectrum of ASD diagnoses (Fournier et al. 2010). Motor disruption can be considered a core feature of autism.

The psychological upshot of the motor disruption in autism is a disruption to a principal form of *prospective motor agency*—the capacity to efficiently enact desired intentions through actions of the body (Delafield-Butt and Gangopadhyay 2013; Trevarthen and Delafield-Butt 2013a; Trevarthen 2016). Disruption to prospective motor timing leads to a disruption in successfully completing a desired intention, which in turn leads to anxiety and distress, and can create social isolation with its consequent autistic emotional avoidance and rejection as compensation. However, the subtle nature of the disruption in autism to prospective motor control and the means by which these features may be observed do not as yet allow for their inclusion in standard clinical diagnostic criteria (American Psychiatric Association 2013). We believe this will change as principles and methods of motor assessment become more accessible to clinicians (Anzulewicz et al. 2016) and the motor disruption in autism becomes better understood by the clinical community.

Movement at the Root of Human Communication and Social Understanding

Efficient control of purposeful movement is necessary to communicate, to share intentions, and to generate shared meaning about the world. Human meaning is first co-created nonverbally in shared projects of discovery, before words or language develop (Condon 1975b; Trevarthen and Delafield-Butt 2013b; Delafield-Butt and Trevarthen 2015). Shared embodied intersubjective intelligence remains a foundation for social understanding throughout life, giving individuals in cooperative engagement a "second-person perspective," before rational and abstract "theories of mind" develop, and the capacities to share these using words (Reddy 2008).

The brain systems that subserve this second-person perspective are becoming increasingly clear, and recognized as the "mirror neuron" systems that resonate between individuals to allow a shared understanding of another's intentions as they are acted out through movements of the body (Rizzolatti and Sinigaglia 2008; Gallese et al. 2009; Schilbach et al. 2013). This presents an embodied social understanding conveyed through movements, which becomes the foundation for the capacity to reflect on this knowledge of the other for a more abstract, rational social understanding. But any cortically mediated mirror neuron system depends on regulations from subcortical motivations that establish fundamental resonances between individuals. These include the brainstem-mediated polyvagal systems of expressive movement responsible for the coordination of gesture, speech, intentional action, and importantly, autonomic visceral activity controlling heart rate, breathing, blood oxygenation, and metabolism (Porges 2011; Porges and Furman 2011).

These two systems sustaining vitality, for the individual and consensually, are part of a larger brainstem integration of proprioceptive information across the body into a coherent plan for effective sequences of motor action, which Jaak Panksepp identifies as the "primary SELF" or "simple ego-type life form" (Panksepp 1998, 2005; Panksepp and Biven 2012). The acquired capacities of the neocortex to discriminate and remember perceptual information reflectively, and to respond adaptively with refined movements of manipulation or speech, are animated and developed by motives and emotions of this primary self (Merker 2007, 2013). This fundamental experience of living, perceiving, and acting purposefully in the world appears to be disrupted in autism.

Embedded Hierarchy of Conscious Purpose, Adapted for Communication

Nobel laureate Roger Sperry reminds us that "the sole product of brain function is motor coordination" (Sperry 1952, p. 297). Moving purposefully and in communication with each other lies at the heart of what we do, and its form of action is a direct reflection of one's neurological and psychological integrity. The generation and action plan of movements is informed by a sense of self in relation with others from the beginning of life, even in the first motor actions of the fetus *in utero* (Delafield-Butt and Gangopadhyay 2013; Trevarthen 2016). At this early age, the conscious scope and understanding of actions is limited by lack of experience, but the movements of the fetus are shaped and timed to explore sensations within the body and in the accessible world, and to test the responses of the world contingent on motor intentions. These are sensitive for intimacy with the mother's expressions of life, or those of a twin. In social interaction with newborn infants, movements of the hands and feet, face and voice, touch and engage another person to communicate the interest and excitement of human life, understood and reciprocated by imitation (Kugiumutzakis and Trevarthen 2015; Trevarthen and Delafield-Butt 2013b).

The individual movements of fetuses or infants are organized in hierarchies of purpose that develop in complexity through infancy and childhood (Figure 8.1). These begin as simple, single movements to goals, such as the reach of the arm to touch or of the leg to kick, and progress to small projects of serially organized single movements that perform more distal and more ambitious tasks, such as reach to grasp or a reach–grasp–place (Delafield-Butt and Gangopadhyay 2013).

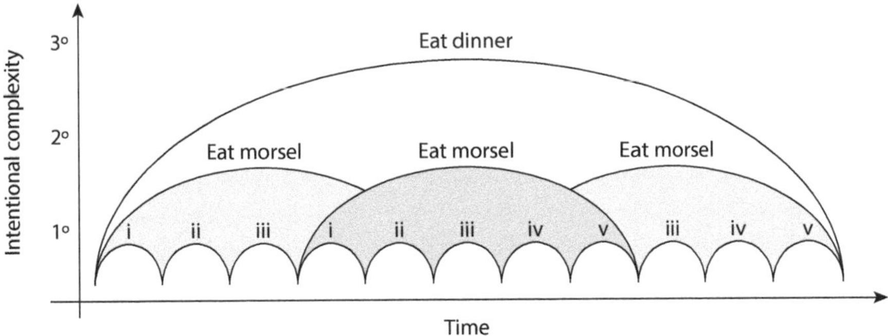

FIGURE 8.1 Developmental hierarchy of intentional action. Schematic of the nested organization of three levels of complexity of sensorimotor intentionality: (1) a primary sensorimotor intentionality operative in individual action units and evident in early fetal life; (2) a higher-order, secondary sensorimotor intentionality that structures and coordinates the primary actions into small projects with a common goal, evident in late fetal life; and (3) a tertiary intentionality that organizes the ones below it, emerging in late infancy and toddlerhood and elaborated throughout human life. In the example illustrated, the distal tertiary intention to "eat dinner" is enacted by a sequence of repeated secondary levels of sensorimotor intentionality, with each "eat morsel" itself composed of a sequence of more proximal actions. The primary level is the action units themselves, sequentially ordered here: (i) moving the arm to the food, (ii) grasping the food, (iii) moving the food to the mouth, (iv) releasing the food into the mouth, and finally, one link to represent (v) mastication and swallowing. The overlapped primary and secondary levels represent simultaneous activity. In autism, the primary level of action organization is disrupted in early development, which transmits disorder up the levels to affect motor projects (reach–grasp–place) and also the integration and coherence of higher-order purpose and understanding. Each level of motor organization matches its counterpart levels of conscious process described in Figure 9.2 (see also Delafield-Butt and Gangopadhyay 2013).

A fetus in the last 10 weeks of gestation makes a movement to suck the thumb with anticipatory opening of the mouth as the hand approaches (Reissland et al. 2014). Such intentional serial organization of movement arguably shares the same foundation as that of logic (Lashley 1951), giving an embodied motor origin of higher cognition (Pezzulo 2011).

As development proceeds, small projects, as are seen in the newborn, are themselves serially organized to perform skilled tasks with more abstract goals and distal reach, such as putting on a shoe to go outdoors, dressing for dinner, or cooking dinner before guests arrive. This final, tertiary level of abstract processing is free of the contingencies of the present movement, achieving higher-order imaginary ambitions to act, rather than primary process intentions in action with prospects of immediate satisfaction. Higher-order abstractions involve what is called "mentalizing," and a rational understanding of what has happened in the world that is familiar, and what is likely to happen in the future (Delafield-Butt and Gangopadhyay 2013; Delafield-Butt and Trevarthen 2013).

The tertiary processes are cortically-mediated, whereas the primary and secondary processes evident at birth are brainstem- and limbic-mediated ones (Figure 8.2) (Solms and Panksepp 2012; Trevarthen and Delafield-Butt 2017). And it is here, in the brainstem at the site of primary process consciousness, that we find signs of the motor deficit in autism with evidence of significant neurological disruptions (Trevarthen et al. 1998; Trevarthen 2000; Rodier and Arndt 2005; Welsh et al. 2005; Trevarthen and Delafield-Butt 2013a).

These primary process conscious acts are the buildings blocks on which social understanding is made meaningful in life stories (Bruner 1990, 2003; Delafield-Butt and Trevarthen 2013; Trevarthen and Delafield-Butt 2013b). Brought to life in shared, serially organized projects with another person, either directly in face-to-face intersubjective engagement or in shared attention to an object or task, these motor projects form the foundation for experience of narratives that unfolds over time, rich with personal meaning and delivering insight into the values of a culture

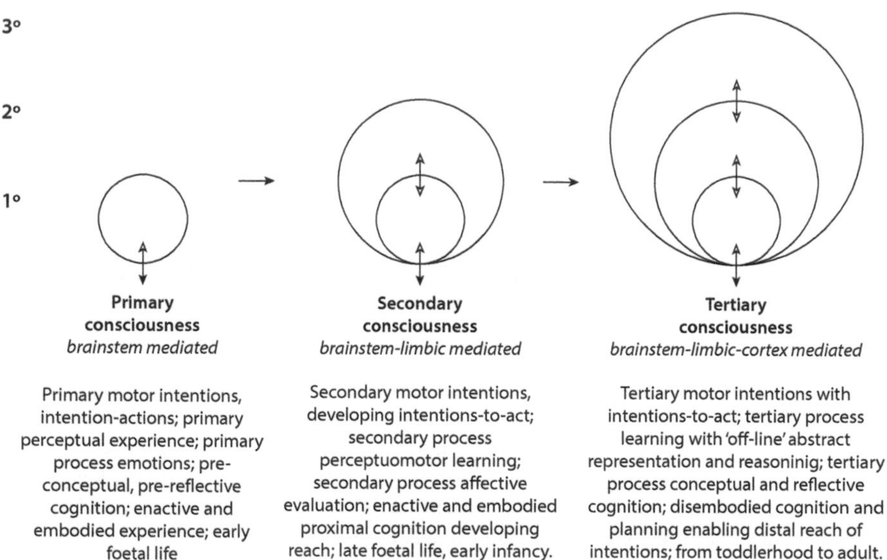

FIGURE 8.2 Development of human consciousness. Primary conscious function evident in early fetal life later structures secondary process limbic function as these mature in late fetogenesis. Secondary processes in turn regulate primary processes. As development proceeds and neocortical function comes to the foreground in late infancy and early childhood, these exert control over the activity of secondary process emotions and intentions. A nested hierarchy of top-down and bottom-up regulation ensures coherence across the system, each level conscious and fully functional, contributing to an integrated conscious experience in the present moment. In autism, disturbance to primary consciousness disrupts development of secondary and tertiary consciousness. Arrows represent bottom-up and top-down information flow. Filled arrowheads represent engagement with the external world. Expansion of knowledge and affective and perceptual discrimination through learning, reflection, and reasoning made in active engagement with the world, both with social others and in the world of concrete and abstract objects, is remembered and expands the content of tertiary consciousness from early childhood throughout life. The capacity of tertiary knowledge to increase enables a rich, projected future of imagined possibilities that come to dominate adult consciousness, and can leave the secondary and primary levels neglected in rational discourse (see also Trevarthen and Delafield-Butt 2016).

(Delafield-Butt and Trevarthen 2015; Delafield-Butt and Adie 2016). The origins of primary intersubjective narratives between an infant and a caring other are dependent on the precise timing and rhythms of two motor systems operating in time and in tune with one another, generating a "communicative musicality" in mutual acts of imagination with poetic rhythm and tone (Malloch 2000; Malloch and Trevarthen 2009; Daniel and Trevarthen 2017). And it is this sensory-motor timing with interpersonal awareness that appears to be fundamentally disrupted in autism, preventing social understanding, shared narrative meaning making, and natural growth in the rhythms and patterns of a family culture (St. Claire et al. 2007; Trevarthen and Delafield-Butt 2013a). Children with autism do not perceive the vitality inherent in the subsecond timing and form of action—its vitality dynamic—as other children do (Rochat et al. 2013).

LOCATING MOTOR-AFFECTIVE INTELLIGENCE IN THE INTEGRATIVE WORK OF THE BRAINSTEM

Central Role of Timing and Serial Ordering in Intelligent Moving

Analysis of the literature on autism motor deficits identifies three types of error evident in individuals with autism, each affecting *prospective motor timing and integration* (Trevarthen and

Delafield-Butt 2013a): (1) generation of *single actions*, such as when extending the hand to touch, or indicate, an object of interest; (2) organization of a *series of actions* to perform more complex tasks or projects, including speaking; and (3) simultaneous *coordination of multiple action units* across the body to achieve coherent purpose, as in postural accommodations when standing, walking, or running.

To perform a movement well, the timing of every part must be made in precise coordination with all the muscle states of the rest of the body, balancing all forces of inertia and momentum in synchrony so that the actions give spatial and temporal coherence of purpose to the task at hand (Bernstein 1967; Lee et al. 1999). Coordination of movement throughout the body, with autonomic integration of regulators of internal vital state or "energy," is the function of the central nervous system. This integrative action (Sherrington 1906) is generated and regulated first within the brainstem and hypothalamus, working tightly with time keeping of the cerebellum. Secondarily, more precise assimilation of environmental affordances is afforded with the adaptable circuits of the midbrain limbic system and both the limbic cortex and neocortex of the forebrain.

Coghill (1929), in his comparative analysis of the animal nervous system, called the brainstem the "head ganglion of the nervous system," recognizing that it is the primary integrative region of information from the senses and across the body. This information is organized along three principle perceptual axes: (1) *visceroception* of information from inside the body detailing its vital physiological needs; (2) *proprioception* of the body in motion, giving the physical dynamic state of forces in the body as it moves through the world; and (3) *exteroception* from the distance receptors (eyes, ears, and nose) and by touch receptors that put the active body and its vital needs within an external environment of people, places, and things (Sherrington 1906).

Each movement must be prospectively controlled (von Hofsten 1993, 2004, 2007; Lee 2005, 2009). To achieve their purpose, the outwardly directed forces of muscle action must be coupled with compensatory forces in the body to produce a smooth and efficient action, working synergistically with all the other movements across the body. This basic prospective knowledge of the proprioceptive and biomechanical consequences of a conceived action or intention forms the first essential intelligence on which a comprehensive and expanding consciousness of the effects of different actions in different circumstances can be built by learning. As development proceeds, knowledge of the contingencies of the world forms a rich conceptual understanding built on the basic template of action and response.

The whole action–response system was identified by James Mark Baldwin as a set of "circular reactions" (Baldwin 1895). This theory of generative, agent-led learning stands in contrast to the passive stimulus–response paradigm of the laboratory experiment. The two paradigms address the same fundamental mechanism of learning—correlation of information between different occasions of life activity. However, the method of testing hypotheses about the mechanism of consciousness and its adaptation isolates the intelligence of a stationary subject in a set world, free of distractions. In normal circumstances, the human animal self-generates and selects sensory stimulation for its own, vital needs within a "speculative" reality, and in collaboration with other individuals whose manifestations of intentions and feelings are perceived as coregulators for engagement (Reddy 2008). Rarely is the animal passive and responsive, as experimental psychology requires for its tests. It is an active generator of the perceptual and affective experiences that make up what Jacob von Uexküll defined as its Umwelt, or the "life-world" it is "interested in" (von Uexküll 1926, 1957). Its intelligence is constructed by it and shared by gesture and sign with others' intelligences (Sebeok 1977).

Brainstem Neurophysiological System for Motor Control and Communication of Motives

The brainstem systems responsible for integration of the sensory and motor information required to perform a simple purposeful act of avoidance, orientation, or capture are now recognized to generate a basic psychological experience, called “primary process functions” (Panksepp and Northoff 2009; Panksepp and Biven 2012). Core feelings, senses of value, and intentions to act in movement are common to all mammals (Panksepp 2011). They are preconceptual and prereflective, but they are nonetheless fundamentally conscious, generating experiences of awareness that shape learning, and that influence the development of higher midbrain and cortical functional anatomy (Merker 2007, 2013; Vandekerckhove and Panksepp 2011). All lines of evidence—neuroanatomical, behavioral, and psychological—indicate that this core process of action with awareness and affective appraisal is disrupted in autism, and from early in development.

The brainstem takes up information from the senses of proprioception, hearing, touch, and taste that are needed for self-regulation of movements, and their use in communication. It responds to music and is a primary site for coordination of movements that engage with the rhythms and affective qualities of melody (Damásio 2010; Porges 2010). Individuals with autism have sensory problems affecting this intuitive awareness. The brainstem includes the autonomic nervous system, which controls levels of arousal and involuntary bodily functions, such as breathing and heart rate, and also regulates sleep, all of which can be irregular in people with autism (Goodwin et al. 2006; Richdale and Schreck 2009; Levine et al. 2012).

Brainstem anatomy and functions transform as the body becomes active in new ways in early childhood. Further changes in the volume of the brainstem and cerebellum between 8 and 16 years (Jou et al. 2009, 2013) suggest that in adolescence, motor-affective changes associated with ASD will be evident in new ways.

Neurological Evidence of Brainstem Abnormality Affecting Motor Timing in Autism: The Inferior Olive

Early postmortem histological studies indicated significant structural and morphological differences in brainstem nuclei of individuals with autism (see Welsh et al. 2005). Further, MRI scans of individuals with autism, although unable to resolve the individual nuclei, show consistent change in the overall size of the brainstem in individuals with autism (Jou et al. 2009, 2013). A recent meta-analysis of 1000 brain scans performed across 18 sites in Europe and North America shows that changes of brainstem volume are one of two significant differences across autistic brains compared with those developing normally (Haar et al. 2014). The other is a change in cortical thickness of the left superior temporal gyrus responsible for movements of speech, and for discriminating awareness of social expressions. These changes in the cortex will have developed as consequences of earlier changes in brainstem systems. In their comprehensive analysis of brain and behavior, Rodier and Arndt (2005) conclude, “There is no region but the brainstem for which so many lines of evidence indicate a role in autism” (p. 146).

Arndt et al.’s (2005) report of brain region–specific alterations of the trajectories of neuronal volume growth throughout the life span in autism suggests that cell–cell communication, adhesion, or migration factors in embryogenesis may be affected, and supports the conclusion that the neuroanatomy of the brainstem has been altered prior to birth in people with autism (Figure 8.3). Further, Bailey et al. (1998) report dysplastic configuration of the lamella of a central pacemaker organ, the *inferior olive*, and the presence of ectopic neurons lateral to the inferior olive. Efficient inferior olive function is necessary for the subsecond timing and integration required for efficient, skilled action (Welsh et al. 1995; Llinás 2001). Anatomical disruption to the inferior olive is known to lead to a corresponding functional disruption in sensorimotor timing and integration, due to its particular, tight structure–function relation, a product of dense cell body packing and a shared bioelectric field across cells that affects their combined electrophysiological properties (Welsh et al. 2005).

An anatomical growth error in the inferior olive appears to explain errors in sensorimotor timing and integration, which arise prenatally and will cause inefficiency of movement after birth. Inefficiency in early movement leads to distress and frustration in simple motor tasks and in communication, and an increasing compensatory cognitive load as development proceeds. “Abnormal

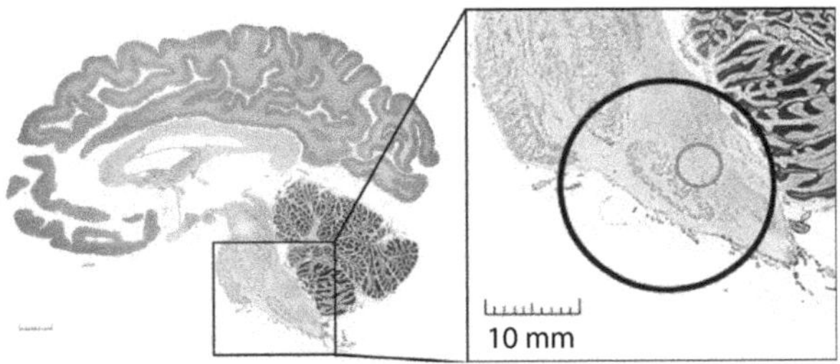

FIGURE 8.3 Parasagittal section of whole brain (left side) showing the significant structure of the inferior olivary nucleus with its gyrated layer of cell bodies (right side, circled black) and adjacent nucleus ambiguus (right side, circled gray). (Adapted with permission from http://www.brains.rad.msu.edu and http://brainmuseum.org, supported by the U.S. National Science Foundation.)

patterns of motor learning in children with autism spectrum disorder, showing an increased sensitivity to proprioceptive error and a decreased sensitivity to visual error, may be associated with abnormalities in the cerebellum" (Marko et al. 2015), for which the inferior olive directly serves as the principle pacemaker. Subsecond motor timing and integration of skilled movement expand with the development of new cerebellar regulations for fast manual and oral movements that are essential for efficient communication of knowledge and skills in hominids (Hoffman and Falk 2012). We conclude that a growth error in inferior olive morphogenesis will disturb timing and integration of intentions and lead to frustration, social withdrawal, and subsequent cognitive processes of compensation identified as autistic (Welsh et al. 2005; Delafield-Butt and Gangopadhyay 2013; Trevarthen and Delafield-Butt 2013a) (Figure 8.4).

The inferior olive is responsible for high-speed sensory and motor integration with rhythms in the range of 7–13 Hz, or one pulse every 50–150 μs, which corresponds to the upper limit of consciously regulated rhythmic movements, as in eye saccades, fast finger tapping, and rapid speech (Welsh et al. 1995; Osborne 2009; Delafield-Butt and Trevarthen 2015; Trevarthen 2016). Abnormal morphogenesis in early development will lead to mistimed integration of muscle contractions across the body and distortion of the kinematics of very fast movement, as reported for persons with autism. In consequence, the actor's comprehension of intended goals and motor timing to achieve them will be complicated (Whyatt and Craig 2012, 2013a, 2013b; Torres et al. 2013, 2016), as well as how the units of movement are chained together in complex projects and in synchronized messages for communication (Boria et al. 2009; Fabbri-Destro et al. 2009; Cattaneo et al. 2007).

Interestingly, kinematic data from a three-dimensional motion-tracking study of simple horizontal sinusoidal (back-and-forth) right arm movements (Cook et al. 2013) reveal those movements of individuals with autism to be fast and jerky—lacking efficient regulation of acceleration and velocity and showing an increase in amplitude of the jerk (rate of change of acceleration) as they swung their arms back and forth. Strikingly, the reported increase in jerk amplitude occurred at a rate of 12 Hz, indicative of disturbed inferior olive function (Welsh et al. 2005). The autistic subjects were also unable to discriminate differences between representations of normal and abnormal movement displays, as well as normal subjects. It was concluded that for subjects with autism, "developmental experience of their own atypical kinematic profiles may lead to disrupted perception of others' actions" (Cook et al. 2013, p. 2816).

Brainstem Center for Regulation of Social and Emotional Expressions: The Nucleus Ambiguus and Related Systems

Close to the inferior olive is the nucleus ambiguus, of particular interest because of its role in the regulation of arousal and expressive movements in social engagement. The ambiguus is the nucleus of origin of motor fibers of the glossopharyngeal, vagus, and cerebral portion of the spinal accessory

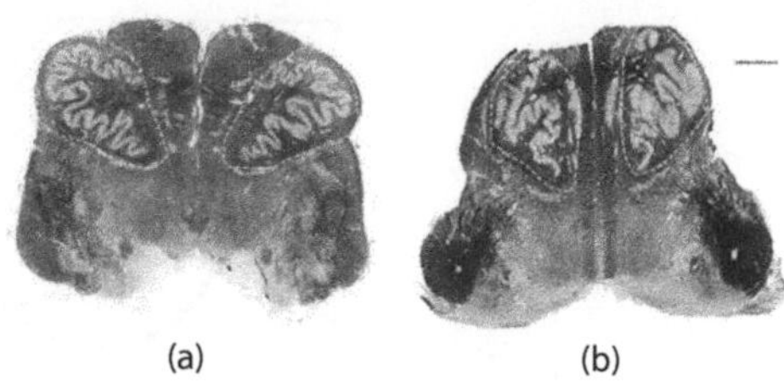

FIGURE 8.4 Transverse section through the medulla oblongata showing the dense gyrations of the inferior olive (dotted lines) in (a) a neurotypical individual and (b) an individual with autism. Note the regular, unbroken, cell-dense gyrations of the inferior olive in (a), but in (b) the inferior olives show an abnormal outline; the band of neurons is irregular and broken up, indicating failure of the neurophysiological coherence for fast, skilled movement timing and integration. This particular individual suffered from severe autism with notable disruption to motor control (see case report reproduced in the appendix). Luxol fast blue and cresyl violet; bar represents 2.5 mm. (Reproduced from Bailey et al. 1998. With permission of Oxford University Press.)

nerve, important in the control of speech, vagal regulation of arousal, and transmission to higher cortical regions. It is intimately connected and forms a part of the "social engagement system." A growth error in this nucleus would appear to offer an explanation for the flat tone of vocal expression and reluctance to engage in expressive talk, which is a characteristic of children or adults with ASD, although studies investigating disruption of development in the ambiguus are lacking. Variations in the vital state mediated by the nucleus ambiguus as part of the polyvagal system, which governs output from the brainstem to the viscera, provide a neuromotor and neurophysiological substratum for "primary-process instinctual emotions" (Porges and Furman 2011; Panksepp and Biven 2012).

The core integrative pathways of the autonomic or visceral brain have been elaborated through evolution to give an instinctive evaluative foundation for formulating ambitious engagements with a world sensed through movement. They are essential regulators of the development of the most highly developed organs of conscious animal life, culminating in the culture-creating human mind. Secondary-process and tertiary-process emotions expand the capacity of the neocortex to learn. Their emotional evaluations and representations in thoughts influence free will and intentions to act (Panksepp and Biven 2012; Solms and Panksepp 2012). They become confused and weakened in emotional illness, including in ASD, requiring therapy that supports regulation of life and its habits by constructive emotions (Panksepp and Biven 2012).

We find clear evidence that the inferior olive and the nucleus ambiguus, which together mediate motor timing and integration of the polyvagal systems to sustain the vital state, enable simultaneous social coregulations of embodied agency and autopoesis that begin to be active early in prenatal development, before the neocortex is functional in recording refined skills of action and awareness of a world to be richly discovered. Before birth, the fetus develops a cooperative "amphoteronomic" sharing of vital resources with the mother. After birth, a developing neocortex and cerebellum record mastery of refined skills of action and awareness of a world to be richly discovered with new sensory powers, as the infant and toddler participate in actions and experiences "synrhythmically" with affectionate companions before accepting tools and disciplined practices of a defined culture (Trevarthen et al. 2006). Every step in this growth of adaptive understanding is sensitive to any abnormality of initiative and awareness, and is critical for the developmental trajectory of the child.

Additional Evidence That Brainstem Disruption in ASD Also Affects Arousal and Social Engagement: The Locus Coeruleus and Related Systems

In agreement with Welsh et al. (2005), we identify the inferior olive as a likely primary source of disruption of the mind in early prenatal stages by affecting subsecond timing and integration of motor impulses. We propose that information on the development of this system and the neighboring brainstem nuclei that participate in developing emotions, including the nucleus ambiguus responsible for control of expressions for social engagement, will advance our understanding of ASD pathogenesis, and advise us how best to respond to it. Moreover, two other tightly related brainstem systems are thought to be affected in autism: those for regulation of arousal to conscious activity, and sensory-motor organs of expression for social signaling.

The "arousal crescent," extending from the lower brainstem to the hypothalamus, is sensitive to multimodal information and becomes excited by "unpredictability and uncertainty" (Pfaff 2006, p. 55). This basic perceptual and affective discrimination forms a core feature in the identification, and thus use, of information from experience—facilitating the generation of a sense of meaning of a stimulus set within its environment, producing generalized brain states. The locus coeruleus, a group of cells at the lower brainstem of all mammalian animals, responds to sudden, salient information important for contextualizing the meaning of this information in terms of heightening arousal. Heightened sensitivity to multimodal sensory stimuli and inappropriate or decontextualized responses are regular features of autism (Donnellan et al. 2013; Kushki et al. 2013). These inappropriate responses will have a profound effect on the ability of individuals with ASD to formulate generalizable brain states, creating strain, and may lead to so-called "weakened central coherence" with compensatory attention to local detail and repetitive movement (Happé and Frith 2006).

The polyvagal social engagement system identified by Porges (2011), with its lynchpin centered on the nucleus ambiguus, is an emotional expressive system mediating insight into feelings within another's experience and intentions. Uniquely developed in humans and social mammals (Porges 1995, 2001, 2007; Porges and Furman 2011), this system provides the foundation for a body language of signs that refer to objects and their practical uses. The system also provides direct neurophysiological coupling between autonomic self-regulation of the visceral state and social cooperation, by communication via facial expression, voice, and manual gesture. Evolutionary adaptation in vagal regulation of the autonomic nervous system, together with the evolutionary emergence of an integrated social signaling system, enables complex visceral regulations of self-awareness or "being alive" to be shared socially:

> Phylogenetic transitions resulted in brainstem areas regulating the vagus becoming intertwined with the areas regulating the striated muscles of the face and head. The result of this transition was a dynamic social engagement system with social communication features (e.g., facial expression, head movements, vocalizations, and listening) interacting with visceral state regulation. (Porges 2011, p. 203)

Abnormal excitability or indifference to threatening stimuli, combined with flattening or narrowing of expressive behaviors in communication, may explain symptoms identified with autism in childhood. Specifically, these will affect the way in which a child cooperates and shares feelings with family and teachers, requiring special sensibility in response.

INTRINSIC AND ENVIRONMENTAL FACTORS AFFECTING ASD THROUGH THE COURSE OF DEVELOPMENT

The cause of these growth errors that we have identified as the initial cause of ASD is likely any combination of genetic (Aitken 2010), environmental (viral or stress related), or naturally occurring spontaneous errors of epigenetic regulation. A considerable portion of the genes that have been implicated in autism pathogenesis are found to be expressed in the brainstem (Nolan, personal communication). Yet, the story is complex. ASD pathogenesis results from some significant interaction between genetic and environmental factors, with genetic factors accounting for less than half of its etiology, demonstrating that the environment, including the social environment, is a significant factor (Hallmayer et al. 2011; Sandin et al. 2014).

It is important, for both understanding of the atypical behaviors of young children with ASD and provision of beneficial treatment or therapy, to recognize that the response of other persons, especially parents in early years, may contribute to their difficulties in self-regulation and in communication and learning. There is evidence from videos of interactions between a parent and an infant who is later diagnosed with autism that the disordered attention, reduced expressive behavior and play, and repetitive motor activities recognized by parents as deviant (Saint-Georges et al. 2010) led them or other carers to use exciting, distracting, controlling, or restraining behaviors, which confuse the child (St. Claire et al. 2007). In their affectionate efforts to help the child, caregivers may contribute to the child's difficulties. This problem may be assisted by professional advice that demonstrates to the caregivers how the child responds better with less persuasive attentions.

CONCLUSIONS: IDENTIFYING AND SUPPORTING PROBLEMS ARISING FROM DISRUPTION OF MOTIVES FOR DEVELOPMENT OF COGNITION AND INTERPERSONAL RELATIONS

Once one accepts that the organization, control, and structure of human movement are fundamental for our intelligent behavior, as the primate with the most advanced motor intelligence (Graziano 2009), not only in single acts to reach identified goals using the experience of objects that excite interest in the present moment, but also for the mental composition of imaginative purposes and the coherence of complex projects that develop through a lifetime of learning cultural habits (Donaldson 1992), then the role of the motor deficit identified in autism pathogenesis becomes clear. Levels of cooperative awareness and the sharing of cultural meaning depend on affective and cooperative social engagement of imaginative movement. Children with autism find it difficult to sustain more complex purposes in activity, with sure appreciation of what the environment affords now and what the future may hold. They are also confused by instruction, especially if it is imperative and unreceptive, which leads them to "fall behind" in the attainment of "common sense."

Research shows that the degree of motor skill and coordination in young children is correlated with their academic skill and attainment in school. There is a tight link between the development of movement in early childhood and the development of intelligence (Wassenberg et al. 2005; Davis et al. 2011; Pagani and Messier 2012), as the neurologist and pioneer therapist Geoffrey Waldon discovered (Solomon et al. 2012). Response to this developmental process requires adaptation of methods of assessment and education to appreciate basic motor processes of intention and communication (Teitelbaum et al. 1998; Acquarone 2007; Teitelbaum and Teitelbaum 2008; Delafield-Butt and Gangopadhyay 2013; Trevarthen and Delafield-Butt 2013a).

We propose that appreciation of difficulties from the point of view of a child with autism, with deliberate attention to his or her initiatives, is essential for optimal education and emotional support in companionship. Comprehending the feelings and awareness of children is made easier by a theory of learning that recognizes evidence that the human brain grows with regulations from brainstem functions that determine how knowledge and skills are acquired by activation and modification of forebrain cortical functions—regulations that are made apparent in pre-rational expressive movements from prenatal stages. Research on the foundations of motor intelligence that links studies of brainstem systems and the cerebellum with intrauterine studies of the maturation of movements in the fetus is particularly promising.

Methods of Therapy and Education That Support Hopes for Movement

Experienced therapists trained to attend to, and wait for, small positive initiatives of the child for progressive and enjoyable interaction can strengthen communication and shared enjoyment, as well as benefit confident states of self-regulation and fluency of movement (Amos 2013). In a remarkable study, parents assisted to engage with sensitive attunement to the feelings and intentions of their child with autism significantly improved their child's long-term socioemotional well-being and reduced symptom severity (Pickles et al. 2016). Sensitive psychoanalytically informed methods practiced for early intervention, and "art" therapies that support willing engagement in song, musical performance, or dance, have been shown to be helpful both for affected infants and toddlers and for their parents (Acquarone 2007). In the introduction to the second edition of his book *The Interpersonal World of the Infant*, which sought to focus the attention of psychoanalysts on nonverbal narratives of feelings and affect-loaded memories or habits, Daniel Stern appreciated the strong response that his account of the interpersonal world of the infant received from practitioners of dance, music, body, and movement and existential psychotherapies (Stern 2000, p. xv). His book on vitality dynamics (Stern 2010) pursued and greatly enriched this approach, which certainly has an application for individuals with ASD of all ages. Indeed, there are a great variety of methods aimed at supporting acting, thinking, and communication for cooperation in children with autism, for example, with encouragement to play (Daniel 2008), to respond to being imitated (Nadel 2014), or to participate in a form of dance movement therapy (Trevarthen and Fresquez 2015).

Questions at the Forefront of Understanding How the Brain for Purposeful Movement Develops and How It Learns

We now need improved knowledge of key components of the primary motor or affective systems in the brain, including the form and function of the inferior olive and associate nuclei, such as the ambiguous, using high-resolution brain scanning techniques or focused postmortem histological assessment. In the case of the former, preliminary data demonstrate that 7 T MRI can delineate the inferior olive brainstem nuclei with some precision, offering a precise technique for imaging the brainstem that was previously unavailable. Moreover, the neurological abnormalities discovered can be related to motor kinematic measures. On the other hand, postmortem histology offers the advantage of cellular and genetic resolution for detail at the molecular level of brainstem composition. Both routes offer promising and insightful new information into the etiology of autism.

Further, motor kinematic studies will benefit from this detailed account of the source of inefficiencies in a movement, whether measured as units of acceleration and deceleration in spontaneous movement (Whyatt and Craig 2012; Crippa et al. 2015) or as the jerk profile (Cook et al. 2013). Disruption to the inferior olive predicts the change in regulation of these characteristic features of motor inefficiency, yet this link has yet to be fully explored.

Finally, as the field as a whole comes to understand and characterize the particular motor deficit in autism, so we will begin to define its motor signature (Anzulewicz et al. 2016). Clarification of an autism-specific motor signature, with its affective regulations, will help to identify novel, noninvasive biobehavioral markers for autism and give resolution to specific neurological changes in autism in the brainstem responsible for generating the feelings and intentions of the primary self-expressed and formed through movement. Attention to these motor changes provides an exciting new route to improved practice for therapists and families that attends to the primary nature of the individual as embodied, emotional, intentional, and not necessarily verbal. The brainstem-mediated primary self is ontogenetically prior to, and generative of, a reflective, conceptual self-made richly communicative in language.

This primary self remains fundamental for social connection and meaning-making, and for attention in mental health and well-being. But its basic nature can be lost in our social world with its technical demands of prescribed behaviors and appropriate language.

APPENDIX: CASE HISTORY OF CASE 1 (REPRODUCED FROM BAILEY ET AL. 1998)

Aspects that involve movement are highlighted in *italics* (authors' own) to draw attention to the prevalence of movement and its putative underlying motor disruption in each act:

> As a baby he was a poor feeder who disliked being held. A clinical hearing test was failed at 7.5 months but the parents knew that he could hear soft sounds and was sensitive to vibrations. He had *persistent*

difficulties with gross motor control, was clumsy and did not chew. He could be propped to stand at 2 years of age but *could not move from this position*. He acquired *a few sounds but no speech*; he screamed frequently, especially if there was an echo. He did not turn to his name or speech, and never followed eye gaze or pointing. He could sometimes follow simple instructions, particularly if context bound. He did not imitate or copy, but would sometimes point to a picture in a book. In infancy he continued to dislike being held and sometimes urinated when picked up. He took no interest in people and would only look at his parents if they jumped and waved their arms. He appeared to focus on parts of people and was more interested in his parents' glasses and earrings than their faces; he was particularly interested in buckles and zips. He could spot small items such as milk bottle tops and paper clips but would ignore large objects in the environment. He would not seek comfort if hurt. He would *bite* his parents and other children, and appeared to enjoy the chaotic reaction that this provoked. He became increasingly destructive and overactive. He was interested in mechanical things and would spend most of the day in minute examination and manipulation of tiny objects; *his fine motor co-ordination appeared unimpaired, although he acquired few fine motor skills*. He liked to fiddle with bunches of keys, and would attempt to put these in locks. He enjoyed watching a spinning top, and would spin wheels for hours; he also liked watching credits at the end of television programs. He *flicked light switches repeatedly*. He would often *flap his arms and pant*, particularly if excited, and this could be *accompanied by rocking on his toes*. He liked to look at the ceiling and *spin*, and also enjoyed going on roundabouts. *In the 1st year he rubbed his feet together and clenched his hands together in the midline; when older he engaged in hand stereotypies close to his face. He gnawed at his fingers and nails, head-banged and pulled at his penis*. He appeared intrigued by pain; he went back repeatedly to an exposed mains socket to get a shock and he cut himself with a razor. He would occasionally cry if he hurt himself but appeared insensitive to temperature. He had marked pica and would drink the water in a paddling pool until sick.

REFERENCES

Acquarone, S. 2007. *Signs of Autism in Infants: Recognition and Early Intervention*. London: Karnac.

Aitken, K. J. 2010. *An A-Z of Genetic Factors in Autism*. London: Jessica Kingsley.

American Psychiatric Association. 2013. *Diagnostic and Statistical Manual of Mental Disorders*. 5th ed. Washington, DC: American Psychiatric Association.

Amos, P. 2013. Rhythm and timing in autism: Learning to dance. *Front Integr Neurosci* 7:27. doi: 10.3389/fnint.2013.00027.

Anzulewicz, A., K. Sobota, and J. T. Delafield-Butt. 2016. Toward the autism motor signature: Gesture patterns during smart tablet gameplay identify children with autism. *Sci Rep* 6:31107.

Arndt, T. L., C. J. Stodgell, and P. M. Rodier. 2005. The teratology of autism. *Int J Dev Neurosci* 23 (2–3): 189–99. doi: 10.1016/j.ijdevneu.2004.11.001.

Bailey, A., P. Luthert, A. Dean, B. Harding, I. Janota, M. Montgomery, M. Rutter, and P. Lantos. 1998. A clinicopathological study of autism. *Brain* 121:889–905.

Baldwin, J. M. 1895. *Mental Development in the Child and the Race*. New York: Macmillan Company.

Bernstein, N. A. 1967. *The Co-ordination and Regulation of Movements*. Oxford: Pergamon Press.

Boria, S., M. Fabbri-Destro, L. Cattaneo, L. Sparaci, C. Sinigaglia, E. Santelli, G. Cossu, and G. Rizzolatti. 2009. Intention understanding in autism. *PLoS One* 4 (5):e5596. doi: 10.1371/journal.pone.0005596.

Bruner, J. S. 1990. *Acts of Meaning*. Cambridge, MA: Harvard University Press.

Bruner, J. S. 2003. *Making Stories: Law, Literature, and Life*. New York: Farrar, Strauss, & Giroux.

Cattaneo, L., M. Fabbri-Destro, S. Boria, C. Pieraccini, A. Monti, G. Cossu, and G. Rizzolatti. 2007. Impairment of action chains in autism and its possible role in intentional understanding. *Proc Natl Acad Sci USA* 104: 17825–30. doi: 10.1073pnas.0706273104.

Coghill, G. E. 1929. *Anatomy and the Problem of Behaviour*. Cambridge: Cambridge University Press.

Condon, W. S. 1975a. Multiple response to sound in dysfunctional children. *J Autism Child Schizophr* 5 (1): 37–56.

Condon, W. S. 1975b. Speech makes babies move. In *Child Alive: New Insights into the Development of Young Children*, ed. R. Lewin, 81–90. London: Temple Smith.

Condon, W. S. 1979. Neonatal entrainment and enculturation. In *Before Speech: The Beginnings of Human Communication*, ed. M. Bullowa, 131–48. London: Cambridge University Press.

Condon, W. S., and W. D. Ogston. 1966. Sound film analysis of normal and pathological behavior patterns. *J Nerv Ment Dis* 143 (4):338–47.

Cook, J. L., S. J. Blakemore, and C. Press. 2013. Atypical basic movement kinematics in autism spectrum conditions. *Brain* 136 (Pt 9):2816–24. doi: 10.1093/brain/awt208.

Crippa, A., C. Salvatore, P. Perego, S. Forti, M. Nobile, M. Molteni, and I. Castiglioni. 2015. Use of machine learning to identify children with autism and their motor abnormalities. *J Autism Dev Disord* 45 (7): 2146–56. doi: 10.1007/s10803–015–2379–8.

Damásio, A. 2010. *Self Comes to Mind: Constructing the Conscious Brain*. New York: Pantheon Books.

Daniel, S. 2008. The therapeutic needs of children with autism: A framework for partners in non-directive play. *Br J Play Ther* 4:18–34.

Daniel, S., and C. Trevarthen, eds. 2017. *Rhythms of Relating: Stories from Children's Therapies*. London: Jessica Kingsley Publishers.

David, F. J., G. T. Baranek, C. Wiesen, A. F. Miao, and D. E. Thorpe. 2012. Coordination of precision grip in 2–6 years-old children with autism spectrum disorders compared to children developing typically and children with developmental disabilities. *Front Integr Neurosci* 6:122. doi: 10.3389/fnint.2012.00122.

Davis, E. E., N. J. Pitchford, and E. Limback. 2011. The interrelation between cognitive and motor development in typically developing children aged 4–11 years is underpinned by visual processing and fine manual control. *Br J Psychol* 102 (3):569–84. doi: 10.1111/j.2044–8295.2011.02018.x.

Delafield-Butt, J. T., and J. Adie. 2016. The embodied narrative nature of learning: Nurture in school. *Mind Brain Educ* 10 (2):117–31.

Delafield-Butt, J. T., and N. Gangopadhyay. 2013. Sensorimotor intentionality: The origins of intentionality in prospective agent action. *Dev Rev* 33 (4):399–425. doi: 10.1016/j.dr.2013.09.001.

Delafield-Butt, J. T., and C. Trevarthen. 2013. Theories of the development of human communication. In *Theories and Models of Communication*, ed. P. Cobley and P. Schultz, 199–222. Berlin: De Gruyter Mouton.

Delafield-Butt, J. T., and C. Trevarthen. 2015. The ontogenesis of narrative: From moving to meaning. *Front Psychol* 6:1157. doi: 10.3389/fpsyg.2015.01157.

Donnellan, M. 1992. *Human minds: An exploration*. London: Allen Lane.

Donnellan, A. M., D. A. Hill, and M. R. Leary. 2013. Rethinking autism: Implications of sensory and movement differences for understanding and support. *Front Integr Neurosci* 6:124. doi: 10.3389/fnint.2012.00124.

Dowd, A. M., J. L. McGinley, J. R. Taffe, and N. J. Rinehart. 2012. Do planning and visual integration difficulties underpin motor dysfunction in autism? A kinematic study of young children with autism. *J Autism Dev Disord* 42 (8):1539–48. doi: 10.1007/s10803–011–1385–8.

Fabbri-Destro, M., L. Cattaneo, S. Boria, and G. Rizzolatti. 2009. Planning actions in autism. *Exp Brain Res* 192: 521–25. doi: 10.1007/s00221–008–1578–3.

Fournier, K. A., C. J. Hass, S. K. Naik, N. Lodha, and J. H. Cauraugh. 2010. Motor coordination in autism spectrum disorders: A synthesis and meta-analysis. *J Autism Dev Disord* 40 (10):1227–40. doi: 10.1007/s10803–010–0981–3.

Gallese, V., M. Rochat, G. Cossu, and C. Sinigaglia. 2009. Motor cognition and its role in the phylogeny and ontogeny of action understanding. *Dev Psychol* 45:103–13.

Goodwin, M. S., J. Groden, W. F. Velicer, L. P. Lipsitt, M. G. Baron, S. G. Hofmann, and G. Groden. 2006. Cardiovascular arousal in individuals with autism. *Focus Autism Other Dev Disabil* 21 (2):100–23. doi: 10.1177/10883576060210020101.

Graziano, M. 2009. *The intelligent movement machine: An ethological perspective on the primate motor system.* New York: Oxford University Press.

Haar, S., S. Berman, M. Behrmann, and I. Dinstein. 2014. Anatomical abnormalities in autism? *Cereb Cortex* 26: 1440–52. doi: 10.1093/cercor/bhu242.

Hallmayer, J., S. Cleveland, A. Torres, et al. 2011. Genetic heritability and shared environmental factors among twin pairs with autism. *Arch Gen Psychiatry* 68 (11):1095–102. doi: 10.1001/archgenpsychiatry.2011.76.

Happé, F., and U. Frith. 2006. The weak coherence account: Detail-focused cognitive style in autism spectrum disorders. *J Autism Dev Disord* 36 (1):5–25. doi: 10.1007/s10803–005–0039–0.

Hoffman, M., and D. Falk. 2012. *Evolution of the Primate BraIn: From Neuron to Behavior, Progress in Brain Research*. Amsterdam: Elsevier.

Jou, R. J., N. J. Minshew, N. M. Melhem, M. S. Keshavan, and A. Y. Hardan. 2009. Brainstem volumetric alterations in children with autism. *Psychol Med* 39 (8):1347–54. doi: 10.1017/S0033291708004376.

Jou, R. J., T. W. Frazier, M. S. Keshavan, N. J. Minshew, and A. Y. Hardan. 2013. A two-year longitudinal pilot MRI study of the brainstem in autism. *Behav Brain Res* 251:163–7. doi: 10.1016/j.bbr.2013.04.021.

Kugiumutzakis, G., and C. Trevarthen. 2015. Neonatal imitation. In *International Encyclopedia of the Social and Behavioral Sciences*, ed. J. D. Wright, 481–88. Oxford: Elsevier.

Kushki, A., E. Drumm, M. Pla Mobarak, N. Tanel, A. Dupuis, T. Chau, and E. Anagnostou. 2013. Investigating the autonomic nervous system response to anxiety in children with autism spectrum disorders. *PLoS One* 8 (4):e59730. doi: 10.1371/journal.pone.0059730. PONE-D-12–20901 [pii]..

Kushki, A., T. Chau, and E. Anagnostou. 2011. Handwriting difficulties in children with autism spectrum disorders: A scoping review. *J Autism Dev Disord* 41 (12):1706–16. doi: 10.1007/s10803–011–1206–0.

Lashley, K. S. 1951. The problem of serial order in behavior. In *Cerebral Mechanisms in Behavior*, ed. L. A. Jeffress, 112–36. New York: Wiley.

Lecanuet, J.-P., W. P. Fifer, N. A. Krasnegor, and W. P. Smotherman, eds. 1995. *Fetal Development: A Psychobiological Perspective*. Hillsdale, NJ: Erlbaum.

Lee, D. N. 2005. Tau in action in development. In *Action as an Organiser of Learning*, ed. J. J. Rieser, J. J. Lockman and C. A. Nelson. Hillsdale, NJ: Erlbaum.

Lee, D. N. 2009. General tau theory: Evolution to date. *Perception* 38:837–58.

Lee, D. N., C. M. Craig, and M. A. Grealy. 1999. Sensory and intrinsic coordination of movement. *Proc R Soc Lond B* 266:2029–35.

Levine, T. P., S. J. Sheinkopf, M. Pescosolido, A. Rodino, G. Elia, and B. Lester. 2012. Physiologic arousal to social stress in children with autism spectrum disorders: A pilot study. *Res Autism Spectr Disord* 6 (1): 177–83. doi: http://dx.doi.org/10.1016/j.rasd.2011.04.003.

Llinás, R. 2001. *I of the Vortex: From Neurons to Self.* Cambridge, MA: MIT Press.

Lloyd, M., M. MacDonald, and C. Lord. 2013. Motor skills of toddlers with autism spectrum disorders. *Autism* 17 (2):133–46. doi: 10.1177/1362361311402230.

Malloch, S., and C. Trevarthen. 2009. *Communicative Musicality: Exploring the Basis of Human Companionship*. Oxford: Oxford University Press.

Malloch, S. N. 2000. Mothers and infants and communicative musicality. *Music Sci* 3 (1 Suppl):29–57.

Marko, M. K., D. Crocetti, T. Hulst, O. Donchin, R. Shadmehr, and S. H. Mostofsky. 2015. Behavioural and neural basis of anomalous motor learning in children with autism. *Brain* 138 (3):784–97. doi: 10.1093/brain/awu394.

Maturana, H., and F. Varela. 1980. *Autopoiesis and Cognition: The Realization of the Living*. Dordecht, the Netherlands: Reidel.

Maturana, H., J. Mpodozis, and J. Carlos Letelier. 1995. Brain, language and the origin of human mental functions. *Biol Res* 28 (1):15–26.

Merker, B. 2007. Consciousness without a cerebral cortex: A challenge for neuroscience and medicine. *Behav Brain Sci* 30:63–134.

Merker, B. 2013. The efference cascade, consciousness, and its self: Naturalizing the first person pivot of action control. *Front Psychol* 4:501. doi: 10.3389/fpsyg.2013.00501.

Nadel, J. 2014. *How Imitation Boosts Development: In Infancy and Autism Spectrum Disorder*. Oxford: Oxford University Press.

Osborne, N. 2009. Towards a chronobiology of musical rhythm. In *Communicative Musicality: Exploring the Basis of Human Companionship*, ed. S. Malloch and C. Trevarthen, 545–64. Oxford: Oxford University Press.

Packard, A., and J. T. Delafield-Butt. 2014. Feelings as agents of selection: Putting Charles Darwin back into (extended neo-) Darwinism. *Biol J Linn Soc* 112 (2):332–53.

Pagani, L. S., and S. Messier. 2012. Links between motor skills and indicators of school readiness at kindergarten entry in urban disadvantaged children. *J Educ Dev Psychol* 2 (1):95–107.

Panksepp, J. 1998. *Affective Neuroscience: The Foundations of Human and Animal Emotions*. New York: Oxford University Press.

Panksepp, J. 2005. Affective consciousness: Core emotional feelings in animals and humans. *Conscious Cogn* 14:30–80.

Panksepp, J. 2011. Cross-species affective neuroscience decoding of the primal affective experiences of humans and related animals. *PloS One* 6 (9):e21236.

Panksepp, J., and G. Northoff. 2009. The trans-species core SELF: The emergence of active cultural and neuro-ecological agents through self-related processing within subcortical-cortical midline networks. *Conscious Cogn* 18:193–215.

Panksepp, J., and L. Biven. 2012. *The Archaeology of Mind: Neuroevolutionary Origins of Human Emotions*. Norton Series on Interpersonal Neurobiology. New York: Norton.

Pezzulo, G. 2011. Grounding procedural and declarative knowledge in sensorimotor anticipation. *Mind Lang* 26: 78–114.

Pfaff, D. W. 2006. *Brain Arousal and Information Theory: Neural and Genetic Mechanisms*. Cambridge, MA: Harvard University Press.

Pickles, A., A. Le Couteur, K. Leadbitter, E. Salomone, R. Cole-Fletcher, H. Tobin, I. Gammer, J. Lowry, G. Vamvakas, and S. Byford. 2016. Parent-mediated social communication therapy for young children with autism (PACT): Long-term follow-up of a randomised controlled trial. *Lancet* 388 (10059): 2501–9.

Pierno, A. C., M. Mari, S. Glover, I. Georgiou, and U. Castiello. 2006. Failure to read motor intentions from gaze in children with autism. *Neuropsychologia* 44 (8):1483–8. doi: 10.1016/j.neuropsychologia.2005.11.013.

Piontelli, A. 1992. *From Fetus to Child*. London: Routledge.

Porges, S. W. 1995. Orienting in a defensive world: Mammalian modifications of our evolutionary heritage. A polyvagal theory. *Psychophysiology* 32 (4):301–18.

Porges, S. W. 2001. The polyvagal theory: Phylogenetic substrates of a social nervous system. *Int J Psychophysiol* 42 (2):123–46.

Porges, S. W. 2007. The polyvagal perspective. *Biol Psychol* 74:116–43.

Porges, S. W. 2010. Music therapy and trauma: Insights from polyvagal theory. In *Music Therapy & Trauma: Bridging Theory and Clinical Practice*, ed. K. Stewart, 3–15. New York: Satchnote Press.

Porges, S. W. 2011. *The Polyvagal Theory: Neurophysiological Foundations of Emotions, Attachment, and Communication*. New York: Norton & Co.

Porges, S. W., and S. A. Furman. 2011. The early development of the autonomic nervous system provides a neural platform for social behaviour: A polyvagal perspective. *Infant Child Dev* 20:106–18. doi: 10. 1002/icd.688.

Reddy, V. 2008. *How Infants Know Minds*. Cambridge, MA: Harvard University Press.

Reissland, N., B. Francis, and J. Mason. 2013. Can healthy fetuses show facial expressions of "pain" or "distress"? *PLoS One* 8 (6):e65530. doi: 10.1371/journal.pone.0065530.

Reissland, N., B. Francis, E. Aydin, J. Mason, and B. Schaal. 2014. The development of anticipation in the fetus: A longitudinal account of human fetal mouth movements in reaction to and anticipation of touch. *Dev Psychobiol* 56 (5):955–63. doi: 10.1002/dev.21172.

Richdale, A. L., and K. A. Schreck. 2009. Sleep problems in autism spectrum disorders: Prevalence, nature, & possible biopsychosocial aetiologies. *Sleep Med Rev* 13 (6):403–11. doi: 10.1016/j.smrv.2009.02.003.

Rinehart, N. J., B. J. Tonge, R. Iansek, J. McGinley, A. V. Brereton, P. G. Enticott, and J. L. Bradshaw. 2006. Gait function in newly diagnosed children with autism: Cerebellar and basal ganglia related motor disorder. *Dev Med Child Neurol* 48 (10):819–24. doi: 10.1111/j.1469–8749.2006.tb01229.x.

Rizzolatti, G., and C. Sinigaglia. 2008. *Mirrors in the BraIn: How Our Minds Share Actions and Emotions*. Oxford: Oxford University Press.

Rochat, M. J., V. Veroni, N. Bruschweiler-Stern, C. Pieraccini, F. Bonnet-Brilhault, C. Barthelemy, J. Malvy, C. Sinigaglia, D. N. Stern, and G. Rizzolatti. 2013. Impaired vitality form recognition in autism. *Neuropsychologia* 51 (10):1918–24. doi: 10.1016/j.neuropsychologia.2013.06.002.

Rodier, P. M., and T. L. Arndt. 2005. The brainstem in autism. In *The Neurobiology of Autism*, ed. M. L. Bauman and T. L. Kemper, 136–49. Baltimore: John Hopkins University Press.

Sacrey, L. A., T. Germani, S. E. Bryson, and L. Zwaigenbaum. 2014. Reaching and grasping in autism spectrum disorder: A review of recent literature. *Front Neurol* 5:6. doi: 10.3389/fneur.2014.00006.

Saint-Georges, C., A. Mahdhaoui, M. Chetaoani, R. S. Cassel, M.-C. Laznik, F. Apicella, P. Muratori, S. Maestro, F. Muratori, and D. Cohen. 2010. Do parents recognize autistic deviant behavior long before diagnosis? Taking into account interaction using computational methods. *PLoS One* 6 (78):e22393. doi: doi:10.1371/journal.pone.0022393.

Sandin, S., P. Lichtenstein, R. Kuja-Halkola, H. Larsson, C. M. Hultman, and A. Reichenberg. 2014. The familial risk of autism. *JAMA* 311 (17):1770–7. doi: 10.1001/jama.2014.4144.

Schilbach, L., B. Timmermans, V. Reddy, A. Costall, G. Bente, T. Schlicht, and K. Vogeley. 2013. Toward a second-person neuroscience. *Behav Brain Sci* 36 (4):393–414. doi: 10.1017/s0140525x12000660.

Schmitz, C., J. Martineau, C. Barthélémy, and C. Assaiante. 2003. Motor control and children with autism: Deficit of anticipatory function? *Neurosci Lett* 348:17–20. doi: 10.1016/S0304–3940(03)00644-X.

Sebeok, T. A. 1977. *How Animals Communicate*. Bloomington: Indiana University Press.

Sherrington, C. 1906. *The Integrative Action of the Nervous System*. New Haven, CT: Yale University Press.

Solms, M., and J. Panksepp. 2012. The "id" knows more than the "ego" admits: Neuropsychoanalytic and primal consciousness perspectives on the interface between affective and cognitive neuroscience. *Brain Sci* 2: 147–74. doi: 10.3390/brainsci2020147.

Solomon, W., C. Holland, and M. J. Middleton. 2012. *Autism and Understanding: The Waldon Approach to Child Development*. Thousand Oaks, CA: Sage.

Sperry, R. W. 1952. Neurology and the mind-brain problem. *Am Sci* 40:291–312.

St. Claire, C., L. Danon-Boileau, and C. Trevarthen. 2007. Signs of autism in infancy: Sensitivity for rhythms of expression in communication. In *Signs of Autism in Infants: Recognition and Early Intervention*, ed. S. Acquarone. 21–45. London: Karnac Books.

Stern, D. N. 2000. *The Interpersonal World of the Infant: A View from Psychoanalysis and Development Psychology*. 2nd ed. New York: Basic Books.

Stern, D. N. 2010. *Forms of Vitality*. Oxford: Oxford University Press.

Stoit, A. M., H. T. van Schie, D. I. Slaats-Willemse, and J. K. Buitelaar. 2013. Grasping motor impairments in autism: Not action planning but movement execution is deficient. *J Autism Dev Disord* 43 (12):2793–806. doi: 10.1007/s10803–013–1825–8.

Teitelbaum, O., and P. Teitelbaum. 2008. *Does Your Baby Have Autism? Detecting the Earliest Signs of Autism*. Garden City Park, NY: Square One Publishers.

Teitelbaum, P., O. Teitelbaum, O. Nye, J. Fryman, and R. G. Maurer. 1998. Movement analysis in infancy may be useful for early diagnosis of autism. *Proc Natl Acad Sci USA* 95:13982–7.

Torres, E. B., and A. M. Donnellan, eds. 2013. *Autism: The Movement Perspective*. Frontiers in Integrative Neuroscience Research Topic. London: Nature Frontiers Group.

Torres, E. B., M. Brincker, R. W. Isenhower, P. Yanovich, K. A. Stigler, J. I. Nurnberger, D. N. Metaxas, and J. V. Jose. 2013. Autism: The micro-movement perspective. *Front Integr Neurosci* 7:32. doi: 10.3389/fnint.2013.00032.

Torres, E. B., R. Isenhower, J. Nguyen, C. Whyatt, J. I. Nurnberger, J. V. Jose, S. Silverstein, T. V. Papathomas, J. Sage, and J. Cole. 2016. Towards precision psychiatry: Statistical platform for the personalized characterization of natural behaviors. *Front Neurol* 7:8. doi: 10.3389/fneur.2016.00008.

Trevarthen, C. 2000. Autism as a neurodevelopmental disorder affecting communication and learning in early childhood: Prenatal origins, post-natal course and effective educational support. *Prostaglandins Leukot Essent Fatty Acids* 63 (1–2):41–6. doi: 10.1054/plef.2000.0190.

Trevarthen, C. 2001. The neurobiology of early communication: Intersubjective regulations in human brain development. In *Handbook on Brain and Behavior in Human Development*, ed. A. F. Kalverboer and A. Gramsbergen, 841–82. Dordrecht, the Netherlands: Kluwer.

Trevarthen, C. 2016. The spiritual nature of the infant self: An imaginative actor in relations of affection. *J Conscious Stud* 23 (1–2):258–82.

Trevarthen, C., and C. Fresquez. 2015. Sharing human movement for well-being: Research on communication in infancy and applications in dance movement psychotherapy. *Body Mov Dance Psychother* 10 (4):194–210. doi: 10.1080/17432979.2015.1084948.

Trevarthen, C., and J. T. Delafield-Butt. 2013a. Autism as a developmental disorder in intentional movement and affective engagement. *Front Integr Neurosci* 7:49.

Trevarthen, C., and J. T. Delafield-Butt. 2013b. Biology of shared meaning and language development: Regulating the life of narratives. In *The Infant Mind: Origins of the Social Brain*, ed. M. Legerstee, D. Haley, and M. Bornstein, 167–99. New York: Guildford Press.

Trevarthen, C., and J. T. Delafield-Butt. 2017. Development of consciousness. In *Cambridge Encyclopedia of Child Development*, ed. B. Hopkins, E. Geangu, and S. Linkenauger. Cambridge: Cambridge University Press.

Trevarthen, C., and S. Daniel. 2005. Disorganized rhythm and synchrony: Early signs of autism and Rett syndrome. *Brain Dev* 27:S25–34.

Trevarthen, C., J. Robarts, D. Papoudi, and K. J. Aitken. 1998. *Children with Autism: Diagnosis and Intervention to Meet Their Needs*. London: Jessica Kingsley Publishers.

Trevarthen, C., J. T. Delafield-Butt, and B. Schögler. 2011. Psychobiology of musical gesture: Innate rhythm, harmony and melody in movements of narration. In *Music and Gesture II*, ed. A. Gritten and E. King, 11–43. Aldershot, UK: Ashgate.

Trevarthen, C., K. J. Aitken, E. Nagy, J. T. Delafield-Butt, and M. Vandekerckhove. 2006. Collaborative regulations of vitality in early childhood: Stress in intimate relationships and postnatal psychopathology. In *Developmental Psychopathology*, ed. D. Cicchetti and D. J. Cohen, 65–126. New York: John Wiley & Sons.

Trevarthen, C., M. Gratier, and N. Osborne. 2014. The human nature of culture and education. *Wiley Interdiscip Rev Cogn Sci* 5 (2):173–92. doi: 10.1002/wcs.1276.

Turner, V. W. 1982. *From Ritual to Theatre: The Human Seriousness of Play*. New York: Performing Arts Journal Publications.

Vandekerckhove, M., and J. Panksepp. 2011. A neurocognitive theory of higher mental emergence: From anoetic affective experiences to noetic knowledge and autonoetic awareness. *Neurosci Biobehav Rev* 35 (9): 2017–25.

von Hofsten, C. 1993. Prospective control—A basic aspect of action development. *Hum Dev* 36:253–70.

von Hofsten, C. 2004. An action perspective on motor development. *Trends Cogn Sci* 8:266–72.

von Hofsten, C. 2007. Action in development. *Dev Sci* 10 (1):54–60.

von Uexküll, J. 1926. *Theoretical Biology, International Library of Psychology, Philosophy, and Scientific Method*. London: Kegan Paul, Trench, Trubner, & Co.

von Uexküll, J. 1957. A stroll through the worlds of animals and men. In *Instinctive Behavior: The Development of a Modern Concept*, ed. C. H. Schiller, 5–80. New York: International Universities Press.

Wassenberg, R., F. J. Feron, A. G. Kessels, J. G. Hendriksen, A. C. Kalff, M. Kroes, P. P. Hurks, M. Beeren, J. Jolles, and J. S. Vles. 2005. Relation between cognitive and motor performance in 5- to 6-year-old children: Results from a large-scale cross-sectional study. *Child Dev* 76 (5):1092–103. doi: 10.1111/j.1467–8624.2005.00899.x.

Welsh, J. P., E. S. Ahn, and D. G. Placantonakis. 2005. Is autism due to brain desynchronization? *Int J Dev Neurosci* 23:253–63. doi: 10.1016/j.ijdevneu.2004.09.002.

Welsh, J. P., E. J. Lang, I. Suglhara, and R. Llinas. 1995. Dynamic organization of motor control within the olivocerebellar system. *Nature* 374:453–57.

Whyatt, C., and C. Craig. 2013a. Sensory-motor problems in autism. *Front Integr Neurosci* 7:51.

Whyatt, C., and C. M. Craig. 2013b. Interceptive skills in children aged 9–11 years, diagnosed with autism spectrum disorder. *Res Autism Spectr Disord* 7 (5):613–23.

Whyatt, C. P., and C. M. Craig. 2012. Motor skills in children aged 7–10 years, diagnosed with autism spectrum disorder. *J Autism Dev Disord* 42 (9):1799–809. doi: 10.1007/s10803–011–1421–8.

Zoia, S., L. Blason, G. D'Ottavio, M. Bulgheroni, E. Pezzetta, Al. Scabar, and U. Castiello. 2007. Evidence of early development of action planning in the human foetus: A kinematic study. *Exp Brain Res* 176:217–26.

9 The Gap between Intention and Action

Altered Connectivity and GABA-mediated Synchrony in Autism

*John P. Hussman**

CONTENTS

Introduction 139
Diagnostic Considerations 140
External Behavior versus Internal States of Mind 141
Connectivity and GABA-mediated Synchrony 142
  Altered Connectivity in Autism 142
  Altered GABA-mediated Synchrony in Autism 143
Perspectives 145
  Instructional Strategies: Playing to Strengths 145
  Presuming Competence 146
References 147

Identifying common molecular functions among autism-related genes, and common neurobiological correlates of autism-related behaviors, is essential to understanding the nature of autism. This chapter focuses on two such mechanisms that are suggested by a broad range of genetic, neuroanatomical, and clinical evidence in autism: (1) altered connectivity, at both anatomical and functional levels, and (2) altered excitatory–inhibitory balance, particularly affecting the properties of GABAergic circuits that regulate temporal synchrony and feedback. I review important work related to these two components of the basic research and argue that presuming competence is the most important ingredient to understand, research, and treat autism.

INTRODUCTION

Autism is a "spectrum" condition defined symptomatically and observationally, based on marked qualitative differences in two central domains:

1. Social communication and interaction, including reciprocity, use of nonverbal cues, and the initiation and maintenance of relationships (APA, 2013)

* This work was originally presented in a lecture entitled "Does Science Support Support?" at the MIT Media Lab during the 2011 Summer Institute of the Syracuse Institute on Communication and Inclusion. Additional material on altered synchrony in autism was presented in a 2016 lecture at the Hussman Institute for Autism entitled "Linking Neurobiology to the Observed Features of Autism."

2. Restricted or repetitive patterns of behavior, including echolalia, unusual object use, inflexibility of routines, circumscribed interests, and an altered response to sensory aspects of the environment

While significant and observable challenges in these core domains may be assigned the specific diagnosis of autism, it does not follow that the diagnosis of autism reflects a specific neurobiological mechanism. Large-scale population studies indicate that the majority of autism risk is rooted in genetic factors, but there is significant heterogeneity across individuals, with common, rare, inherited, and de novo variants in hundreds of individual genes contributing to liability for autism (De Rubeis and Buxbaum 2015). Similarly, functional MRI studies have demonstrated significant differences in cortical activation patterns in autism, compared with neurotypical controls, but these patterns are also characterized by greater "noise"—a tendency toward individualized variations in functional connectivity that may not be shared across individuals (Hahamy et al. 2015).

As a result, the question "What causes autism?" is ill-posed, as numerous distinct etiologies may produce the same broadly observable phenotype. Still, given that individuals on the autism spectrum demonstrate identifiable disruptions in the domains of social communication, interaction, and behavior, many of these etiologies may exert their effect through common pathways. For this reason, identifying common molecular functions among autism-related genes, and common neurobiological correlates of autism-related behaviors, is essential to understanding the nature of autism.

This chapter focuses on two such mechanisms that are suggested by a broad range of genetic, neuroanatomical, and clinical evidence in autism:

1. Altered connectivity, at both the anatomical and functional levels
2. Altered excitatory–inhibitory balance, particularly affecting the properties of GABAergic circuits that regulate temporal synchrony and feedback

These mechanisms contribute to an understanding of observed features in autism, as well as common features that are not well captured by current diagnostic criteria—particularly difficulties in motor initiation and praxis. Both mechanisms play a role in the integration of signals that are distributed across spatially distinct processing hubs involved in cognition, communication, social behavior, sensory processing, and motor function. This integration, in turn, has an impact on the ability to link intention to action, and ideation to execution, as well as the ability to demonstrate internal states through external behavior.

DIAGNOSTIC CONSIDERATIONS

The original characterization of autism by Kanner in 1943 was quite severe in comparison with current use of the same label (Kanner 1943). Kanner described individuals with autism as differing "markedly and uniquely from anything reported so far," "not responding to anything that comes to them from the outside world," and characterized by "extreme autism, obsessiveness, stereotypy, and echolalia." Prior to 1980, the estimated prevalence of autism was consistently reported below 1 in 2000 (Blaxill 2004). In 1980, the third edition of the *Diagnostic and Statistical Manual* of the American Psychiatric Association included autism as a subset of pervasive developmental disorders (PDDs) (APA 1980). In 2013, the DSM-5 definition of autism spectrum disorder (ASD) created a single umbrella to include conditions previously classified as autistic disorder, Asperger's syndrome, and all PDDs "not otherwise specified" by a distinct diagnosis (PDD-NOS). By 2016, the U.S. Centers for Disease Control and Prevention (CDC) estimated that 1 in 68 school-aged children were on the autism spectrum (CDC 2016). Most of the upward trend in autism diagnosis can be accounted for by such changes in diagnostic criteria, as well as greater service availability, public awareness, and ascertainment (Fombonne 2005).

Because the diagnostic threshold has become notably less extreme over time, the terms *autism spectrum condition* (ASC) or simply *autism* are used here, rather than *autism spectrum disorder*. Baron-Cohen et al. (2009) favor this term not only because it is less stigmatizing, but also because autism-related traits appear to be continuously distributed in the general population, with the diagnosis based on a clinical judgment about the point where these traits are significant enough to interfere with daily life functioning (Baron-Cohen et al. 2009). From this perspective, the 1 in 2000 prevalence associated with Kanner's original characterization of autism can be heuristically viewed as equivalent to setting the diagnostic threshold 3.29 standard deviations away from the mean of a normal distribution. By contrast, more recent CDC prevalence estimates of 1 in 88 (2012) and 1 in 68 (2016) correspond to thresholds of 2.28 and 2.18 standard deviations from the mean, respectively.

EXTERNAL BEHAVIOR VERSUS INTERNAL STATES OF MIND

Although ASC is defined observationally, the classification of symptoms relating to communication, social interaction, and behavior is often paired with inferences relating to intelligence and states of mind. Such inferences are problematic because the ability to *demonstrate* intelligence or thought may be directly affected by the symptoms of autism. For example, if speech and execution of intentional movement are affected by autism, tests of intelligence that rely on speech and movement will produce invalid results even in measures that may be valid among neurotypical individuals.

This distinction between observable features of autism and internal states of mind is consistently described by nonverbal or limited-verbal individuals with autism that later developed the ability to communicate independently using alternative and augmentative communication (AAC) methods:

> When I was growing up, speaking was so frustrating. I could see the words in my brain, but then I realized that making my mouth move [was needed to] get those letters to come alive, they died as soon as they were born. What made me feel angry was to know that I knew exactly what I was to say and my brain was retreating in defeat.
>
> **Jamie Burke**
> *(Biklen and Attfield 2005)*

> One of the biggest misunderstandings you have about us is your belief that our feelings aren't as subtle and complex as yours. Because how we behave can appear so childish in your eyes, you tend to assume that we're childish on the inside too. Stuck here inside these unresponsive bodies of ours, with feelings we can't properly express, it's always a struggle just to survive.
>
> **Naoki Higashida**
> *(Higashida 2013)*

Self-descriptions such as these indicate a perceived gap in autism between intention and action, between the ideation of speech and movement and its execution through motor plans. This concern is particularly relevant because motor difficulties are often the earliest observable signs of autism (Chawarska et al. 2007; Landa and Garrett-Mayer 2006; Teitelbaum et al. 1998). Motor skills at age 2 are highly correlated with later outcome measures (Sutera et al. 2007), and a robust correlation is observed between measures of motor function and measures of intelligence on standard tests (Green et al. 2009; Hartman et al. 2010; Vuijk et al. 2010; Wuang et al. 2008), which necessarily rely on verbal and motor skills.

While this correlation could be driven by some underlying feature of autism that jointly affects both intelligence and motor ability, individuals with ASC show discrepantly higher performance on nonverbal tests of intelligence (Dawson et al. 2007), processing speed (Scheuffgen et al. 2000), and inspection time (Wallace et al. 2009) than they do on standard intelligence tests. These alternate measures capture fundamental aspects of "fluid intelligence" (thinking, reasoning, and processing), but are poorly correlated with "crystallized intelligence," which is based on the accumulation of facts and experience (Osmon and Jackson 2002). Thus, standard measures of intelligence in autism may be confounded by challenges in verbal and motor ability, as well as restricted exposure to age-level curriculum, but may not be indicative of more general thinking, reasoning, or processing skills.

With respect to motor function, it is important to distinguish basic motor skill from praxis. Basic motor skill is assessed based on execution of straightforward axial and limb movements, including gait, balance, pointing, and repetitive tapping. Praxis, in contrast, relies on the translation of internal "action models" into the performance of skilled, multistep, goal-directed motor behaviors (Mostofsky and Ewen 2011). Thus, praxis requires not only basic motor skill, but also knowledge of representations of the movement, and translation of these representations into movement plans.

Individuals with autism demonstrate significant challenges in praxis, even after controlling for age, IQ, basic motor skill, and postural knowledge (Dowell et al. 2009). Notably, praxis in children with autism is a strong predictor of social, communicative, and behavioral characteristics, significantly correlated with these features, as measured using the Autism Diagnostic Observation Schedule. This correlation with praxis remains significant even after controlling for basic motor skill, suggesting that dyspraxia may represent a core feature of autism (Dziuk et al. 2007).

CONNECTIVITY AND GABA-MEDIATED SYNCHRONY

Convergent evidence in genomics, histology, neuroimaging, and electrophysiology suggests two related neurobiological mechanisms—connectivity and GABA-mediated synchrony—that can account for many of the observed features of autism. A central feature of both is the coordination of signals across multiple, spatially distinct processing hubs.

Altered Connectivity in Autism

The hypothesis of altered connectivity in autism was first proposed by Just et al. (2004, 2007) based on findings using functional magnetic resonance imaging (fMRI) (which measures the synchronization of activation across brain regions), as well as anatomical morphometry. This hypothesis views the difficulties observed in autism as nonlocalized: an "emergent property of the collaboration among brain centers," rather than a single "core deficit." From this perspective, difficulties are most likely to arise when a task requires the coordination and integration of multiple processing centers, including regions responsible for motor function, as well as the perceptual and affective processing of social stimuli. Social interaction, language, and behavior are viewed as particularly vulnerable to altered connectivity, because these are the domains that are most dependent on the synchronized integration of information from spatially discrete processing hubs (Wass 2011).

Convergent lines of evidence support the hypothesis of altered connectivity and circuit formation in autism. Applying noise reduction techniques to large-scale genome-wide association data, Hussman et al. (2011) demonstrated that high-confidence genes associated with autism show significant functional enrichment in processes governing regulation of the neuronal cytoskeleton and the outgrowth and guidance of axons and dendrites, with secondary enrichment in pathway-related excitatory–inhibitory neurotransmission. Conversely, the set of genes most correlated to neuroanatomic connectivity, which is enriched for genes involved in neuronal development and axon guidance, shows a significant overlap with genes implicated in autism (French and Pavlidis 2011).

Anatomically, a reduction of long-range fiber tracts is observed in autism, with more exuberant short-range connectivity potentially compensating for this reduction. Individuals with ASC show increased volume of radiate white matter (Herbert et al. 2004), particularly comprised of abundant short fibers in the primary motor cortex. This difference has a robust correlation with deficits in motor skill (Mostofsky et al. 2007). There is an observed reduction in the largest axons that communicate over long distances, with more abundant connections between neighboring areas (Zikopoulos and Barbas 2010). An abundance of short connective fibers is also observed in frontal and temporal regions, relative to long-range connections (Casanova et al. 2002b).

Evidence from fMRI studies demonstrates that individuals with ASC exhibit reduced long-range functional connectivity between frontal and posterior parietal brain regions (Just et al. 2004; Mostofsky and Ewen 2011; Solomon et al. 2009). High-resolution (dynamic) coherence also shows reduced long-range connections in ASC in frontal-occipital connections, and increased short-range connections in lateral-frontal connections, with differences correlated with the severity of observed symptoms (Barttfeld et al. 2011). By contrast, individuals who spontaneously recover language after stroke show increased frontal-parietal integration (Sharp et al. 2010).

Both imitation and praxis depend on frontal-parietal circuits for the execution of "action models." Specifically, skilled execution relies on connectivity between premotor regions responsible for selecting and sequencing intended motor programs, and posterior parietal regions that form and store these programs as spatial representations of movement (Mostofsky and Ewen 2011).

Take a moment to execute the following action: reach forward, pick up an imaginary grape, and place it into a bowl. Now, reach forward, pick up an imaginary grape, and bring it to your mouth to eat. Repeated execution of such action chains results in two distinct representations in the parietal lobe, one corresponding to the complete bowl sequence, and the other corresponding to the complete mouth sequence. Conceptually, the choice of the desired sequence occurs in frontal areas responsible for executive control, and the associated motor plan is retrieved from parietal areas. Once a given sequence is chosen, frontal-parietal circuits typically trigger muscle activation related to the entire sequence, at the very outset of the action. For example, when grasping to eat, activation of mouth-opening muscles is typically evident even during the grasping action. In ASC individuals, however, no activation of mouth-opening muscles is observed when grasping to eat until the food immediately approaches the mouth (Cattaneo et al. 2007).

Similarly, when several actions are combined to produce a single goal-directed motor plan, the kinematics of individual component movements are affected by the context and final goal of the sequence. However, in autism, this modulation does not occur, suggesting that individuals with autism experience difficulty chaining discrete motor acts into a global action (Fabbri-Destro et al. 2009). Indeed, children with ASC show less activation in the cerebellum, with relatively greater frontostriatal activation, a shift in activation patterns that is associated with an increased need for conscious execution of planned movements (Mostofsky et al. 2009).

This increased reliance on sequential execution of component movements is echoed in self-reports by individuals with autism describing their subjective experience (Biklen and Attfield 2005):

> To learn the technique of moving my right hand needed control over the ball and socket joint of the shoulder and then the hinge joint of my elbow and finally fold the other fingers and keep the point finger out. After that, focusing on the object which matched the word.
>
> **Tito Mukhopadhyay**

> It is hot; we should open the window.... I can describe the action: I must push the button with my finger. But my hesitation grows while I try to put the sequences to go through the action. I mentally review the necessary steps, but the first one simply doesn't come out. I'm trapped. To help the child with autism, verbally give me the sequences and facilitate me while I try to organize myself.
>
> **Alberto Frugone**

Altered GABA-mediated Synchrony in Autism

In 2001, Hussman first proposed the hypothesis that autism may reflect dysfunction in a single factor shared in common by many neural circuits: GABAergic inhibition and corresponding regulation of glutamate-induced excitation. A suppressed inhibitory tone was proposed to result in excitatory overstimulation of glutamate receptors on neurons, resulting in excessive neural activity and difficulties in "gating" sensory information. This loss of inhibitory control would then result in deterioration in the quality of sensory information due to the failure to suppress competing noise. The ability to process sensory information and learning tasks could then be overwhelmed (Hussman 2001). Rubenstein and Merzenich (2003) later restated this hypothesis in 2003 in terms of an increased ratio of excitation to inhibition in autism.

Loss of GABAergic influence (e.g., ketamine antagonism of NMDA receptor–bearing GABAergic neurons) and excessive stimulation of non-NMDA glutamate receptors generate pathology and neuroanatomical features that mirror what is observed in autism. Loss of inhibitory control can result in hyperexcitation of target neurons, with preferential damage to large and medium-sized pyramidal and multipolar neurons (Farber et al. 1998). Consistent with this mechanism, loss of Purkinje cells, multipolar GABAergic neurons located in the cerebellar cortex, remains one of the most consistent neuroanatomical findings in autism (Kemper and Bauman 1993). Individuals with autism also show significant alterations in GABAergic architecture of neocortical minicolumns (Casanova et al. 2002a). Blatt et al. (2001) provided the first direct evidence that the GABAergic system is altered in autism, reporting a significant reduction in benzodiazepine and GABA-A receptor density in the hippocampus, predominantly in the region of the pyramidal cell layer.

Importantly, the role of GABAergic circuitry extends beyond the general inhibition of excitatory impulses. GABAergic circuitry is indispensable in mediating "temporal binding" or "synchrony"—the time-sensitive coordination of disperse signals across multiple regions of the brain into coherent percepts. Social interaction, communication, and complex movements are all dependent on such coordinated activity. Reduced temporal binding has been suggested to contribute to symptoms observed in autism (Brock et al. 2002). Wallace and Stevenson (2014) provide a useful review of temporal binding and its relevance to developmental disabilities.

In addition to local connections among neurons, large numbers of cells are linked by a smaller set of "hub" neurons that orchestrate synchronization across the network. Analysis of network dynamics and physiology reveals that these hubs represent a subpopulation of GABAergic interneurons (Bonifazi et al. 2009). These interneurons regulate alternating periods of excitatory and inhibitory activity, which generate wavelike oscillations in local field potential that can be measured by an electroencephalogram (EEG).

Time-sensitive integration of cognitive, sensory, and motor information is achieved by binding action potentials that occur within the same "temporal binding window," much like passengers entering a train car, or pedestrians entering segments of a revolving door. Singer (1999) first proposed that neuronal oscillations in the gamma frequency band between 30 and 90 cycles per second (Hz) could enable temporal binding. When groups of neurons are entrained in synchronized oscillations, their joint signal is amplified, and "noise" is reduced. High-frequency oscillations appear well suited to the rapid, time-sensitive integration of sensory inputs. Neuronal oscillations in the gamma frequency band have widespread evidence of importance in feature integration, selective attention, associative learning, lexical processing, and other forms of perception (Bhattacharya et al. 2002).

Temporal binding of sensory inputs is well illustrated by the sound-induced flash illusion (Shams et al. 2000). When a single visual flash is accompanied by multiple auditory beeps, the single flash is perceived as multiple flashes. When beeps are separated by 57 ms, the strength of gamma band responses discriminates between trials where the illusion is perceived by neurotypical observers and those where it is not perceived (Bhattacharya et al. 2002). The sound-induced flash illusion is not discriminated by children with autism, and less precise temporal processing is observed with increasing stimulus complexity (Stevenson et al. 2014).

Optimal gamma oscillations are produced by delayed feedback and shunting inhibition by fast-spiking, soma-inhibiting, GABAergic basket cells expressing parvalbumin (PV), a robust marker for interneurons, and specialized for GABA-A-mediated conductance (Bartos et al. 2007). Notably, multiple mouse models of autism show a common circuit disruption in PV-positive GABAergic inhibitory interneurons (Gogolla et al. 2009).

Children and adolescents with autism demonstrate decreased gamma band activity as measured by EEG (Wilson et al. 2007). Gamma band oscillations are suggested to link structural connectivity with network synchronization, serving as a fundamental basis for the integration of cortical information flows (Fries 2009). Disruptions of network synchronization in autism, identified by EEG analysis, are consistent with deficient GABAergic inhibition, and suggest a reduction in the number and/or strength of thalamocortical connections. Moreover, the specific pattern of phase disruptions—reduced phase-shift duration and increased phase-lock duration in the occipital-parietal regions—is consistent with repetitive behavior and language difficulties observed in autism (Thatcher et al. 2009).

The superior temporal sulcus (STS) provides an informative model for the integration of information from spatially discrete processing hubs. The STS runs along the length of each temporal lobe, and is attuned to socially meaningful stimuli, for example, showing preferential activation to voices versus other sounds. This activation is less evident in autism, based on fMRI. When communication between STS across cortical hemispheres is required, neurotypical individuals show enhanced gamma band coherence, which is not observed in individuals with ASC (Peiker et al. 2015). Perhaps not surprisingly, GABA concentration in the STS predicts gamma power and perception in a sound-induced flash illusion (Balz et al. 2016).

Motor function is another domain that relies on the coherent integration of spatially discrete inputs in order to link intended movement to skilled execution. Motor control can be conceptualized as a feedback process whereby outgoing (efferent) motor commands are accompanied by an efference copy or "internal motor model." This copy provides an estimate of the sensory feedback or "corollary discharge" that is expected from the proper execution of the desired movement. In response to motor activation, the sensory system sends actual feedback, which is then compared with the estimate, and any discrepancy between these is accompanied by corrective responses to align the actual movement with the intended trajectory (Miall and Wolpert 1996).

Notably, GABA-mediated gamma band synchrony appears to facilitate the integration of sensorimotor feedback during motor execution. Specifically, postmovement cortical potentials (reafferent feedback signals) during movement execution are associated with highly focused gamma synchronization in the 40–60 Hz band, which always occurs in contacts located in the primary sensorimotor areas. This suggests that gamma event-related synchronization facilitates postmovement reafferent feedback from muscles and joints to the primary sensorimotor cortex, enabling the accuracy and ongoing control of movement (Szurhaj and Derambure 2006).

PERSPECTIVES

The foregoing results indicate that the observed features of autism are consistent with altered connectivity, at both anatomical and functional levels, and altered excitatory–inhibitory balance, particularly affecting the properties of GABAergic circuits that regulate temporal synchrony and feedback. Both mechanisms are central to the integration of signals that are distributed across spatially distinct processing hubs involved in cognition, communication, social behavior, sensory processing, and motor function. They also offer useful perspectives relating to instructional strategies, as well as the "presumption of competence" toward individuals with autism.

Instructional Strategies: Playing to Strengths

As noted previously, circuit formation in autism appears to compensate for reduced long-range connectivity with more exuberant short-range connectivity between adjacent processing regions. This suggests instructional strategies that leverage local connectivity (proprioceptive input for motor tasks and visualization for comprehension) to partially substitute for long-range connectivity.

For example, during sentence comprehension, individuals with ASC activate parietal and occipital brain areas (adjacent to Wernicke's area) for both low- and high-imagery sentences, suggesting they engage mental imagery in both conditions (Kana et al. 2006). However, when performing motor tasks, individuals with autism are less reliant on visual feedback than neurotypical individuals.

Instead, learning novel movements is more strongly reliant on proprioceptive feedback (Haswell et al. 2009). The formation of action models through proprioceptive feedback evidently plays to the strengths of individuals with autism, by placing greater reliance on abundant short-range connections between the adjacent somatosensory and motor cortices (Mostofsky and Ewen 2011).

Similarly, haptic feedback engages the sense of touch by applying opposing force, resistance, or other motion to provide proprioceptive feedback to the individual. Importantly, such feedback should be distinguished from guidance, which provides support in the same direction as the intended movement. Haptic feedback appears to facilitate the decoding of motor imagery, "closing the sensorimotor loop" (Gomez-Rodriguez et al. 2011) between intended and actual motor behaviors. In conjunction with visual feedback, haptic training may be an effective tool for teaching sensorimotor skills that have a force-sensitive component to them (Morris et al. 2007).

In many cases, even passive touch may enable individuals with autism to bridge the gap between intention and action. This observation is supported by self-reports of individuals with autism (Biklen and Attfield 2005):

> Touch is always a big help when an activity is new for me. Only through practice and through the gradual fading of touch the activity can be done independently. I needed to be touched on my right shoulder for doing any new skill. So I consider that the touch method is a vital step to speed up my learning skill.
>
> **Tito Mukhopadhyay**

> I take mechanical steps alone, but if taken by the hand or the arm, I walk regularly.
>
> **Alberto Frugone**

Touch given prior to action affects the integration of visual and proprioceptive body location information. The brain uses cues from passive touch and vision to update its own position and to experience self-location (Zopf et al. 2011). Passive tactile input can also improve stability. If passive input about posture is available, postural control adapts to this input, producing stabilizing reactions (Rogers et al. 2001).

Presuming Competence

Increasing evidence of altered connectivity and synchrony in autism suggests great caution against inferring internal states of mind from observed symptoms and behaviors. There may be a significant mismatch between thought, ideation, and intention, and the ability to *demonstrate* these internal states through behavior, which requires the ability to recruit and coordinate multiple systems necessary for their execution.

This potential mismatch between internal states and external behavior in autism has important implications in both social and intellectual domains. Difficulty demonstrating competence can easily result in the restriction of educational content to a simplistic or "functional" curriculum. Individuals with autism may also be deprived of social interaction on their own terms, as difficulty navigating social interaction may be misinterpreted as a lack of interest in human relationships:

> I can't believe that anyone born as a human being really wants to be left all on their own, not really. The truth is, we'd love to be with other people. But because things never, ever go right, we end up getting used to being alone, without even noticing this is happening. Whenever I overhear someone remark how much I prefer being on my own, it makes me feel desperately lonely.
>
> **Naoki Higashida**
> *(Higashida 2013)*

Donnellan (1984) has proposed the concept of the "least dangerous assumption" with respect to individuals with autism and other developmental conditions: in the absence of conclusive data, decisions should be based on assumptions that, if incorrect, will have the least harmful effect on the individual. This criterion suggests that access to age-level curriculum, social and educational inclusion, and engagement in community should not be conditioned on measures of "readiness" or the ability to pass a test that relies on verbal or motor ability. This view does not imply the abandonment of "functional" daily living skills as part of the information set provided to individuals with autism, but strongly questions common practices that lower the level of instruction to the level of comprehension demonstrated by testing, and that isolate individuals to segregated settings on the basis of assumed "low function."

Arguably, the least dangerous assumption toward individuals with autism is to adopt a presumption of competence with respect to internal states, including the capacity to learn, understand, enjoy social relationships, appreciate knowledge, and benefit from inclusion in school, family, and community life. Accordingly, the static labels "high functioning" and "low functioning" could be usefully replaced by first presuming competence, and focusing instead on creating opportunities, expanding abilities, and identifying ways for these individuals to *demonstrate* that competence.

REFERENCES

APA (American Psychiatric Association). 1980. *Diagnostic and Statistical Manual of Mental Disorders*. 3rd ed. Washington, DC: APA.

APA (American Psychiatric Association). 2013. *Diagnostic and Statistical Manual of Mental Disorders*. 5th ed. Washington, DC: APA.

Balz, J., J. Keil, Y. R. Romero, R. Mekle, F. Schubert, S. Aydin, B. Ittermann, J. Gallinat, and D. Senkowski. 2016. GABA concentration in superior temporal sulcus predicts gamma power and perception in the sound-induced flash illusion. *Neuroimage* 125:724–30.

Baron-Cohen, S., F. J. Scott, C. Allison, J. Williams, P. Bolton, F. E. Matthews, and C. Brayne. 2009. Prevalence of autism-spectrum conditions: UK school-based population study. *Br J Psychiatry* 194 (6):500–9.

Bartos, M., I. Vida, and Pe. Jonas. 2007. Synaptic mechanisms of synchronized gamma oscillations in inhibitory interneuron networks. *Nat Rev Neurosci* 8 (1):45–56.

Barttfeld, P., B. Wicker, S. Cukier, S. Navarta, S. Lew, and M. Sigman. 2011. A big-world network in ASD: Dynamical connectivity analysis reflects a deficit in long-range connections and an excess of short-range connections. *Neuropsychologia* 49 (2):254–63.

Bhattacharya, J., L. Shams, and S. Shimojo. 2002. Sound-induced illusory flash perception: Role of gamma band responses. *Neuroreport* 13 (14):1727–30.

Biklen, D., and R. Attfield. 2005. *Autism and the Myth of the Person Alone*. New York: NYU Press.

Blatt, G. J., C. M. Fitzgerald, J. T. Guptill, A. B. Booker, T. L. Kemper, and M. L. Bauman. 2001. Density and distribution of hippocampal neurotransmitter receptors in autism: An autoradiographic study. *J Autism Dev Disord* 31 (6):537–43.

Blaxill, M. F. 2004. What's going on? The question of time trends in autism. *Public Health Rep* 119 (6):536.

Bonifazi, P., M. Goldin, M. A. Picardo, I. Jorquera, A. Cattani, G. Bianconi, A. Represa, Y. Ben-Ari, and R. Cossart. 2009. GABAergic hub neurons orchestrate synchrony in developing hippocampal networks. *Science* 326 (5958):1419–24.

Brock, J., C. C. Brown, J. Boucher, and G. Rippon. 2002. The temporal binding deficit hypothesis of autism. *Dev Psychopathol* 14 (02):209–24.

Casanova, M. F., D. P. Buxhoeveden, A. E. Switala, and E. Roy. 2002a. Minicolumnar pathology in autism. *Neurology* 58 (3):428–32.

Casanova, M. F., D. P. Buxhoeveden, A. E. Switala, and E. Roy. 2002b. Neuronal density and architecture (gray level index) in the brains of autistic patients. *J Child Neurol* 17 (7):515–21.

Cattaneo, L., M. Fabbri-Destro, S. Boria, C. Pieraccini, A. Monti, G. Cossu, and G. Rizzolatti. 2007. Impairment of actions chains in autism and its possible role in intention understanding. *Proc Natl Acad Sci USA* 104 (45):17825–30.

CDC (U.S. Centers for Disease Control and Prevention). 2016. CDC estimates 1 in 68 school-aged children have autism; no change from previous estimate. Atlanta: CDC, March 31. http://www.cdc.gov/media/releases/2016/p0331-children-autism.html.

Chawarska, K., R. Paul, A. Klin, S. Hannigen, L. E. Dichtel, and F. Volkmar. 2007. Parental recognition of developmental problems in toddlers with autism spectrum disorders. *J Autism Dev Disord* 37 (1):62–72.

Dawson, M., I. Soulières, M. A. Gernsbacher, and L. Mottron. 2007. The level and nature of autistic intelligence. *Psychol Sci* 18 (8):657–62.

De Rubeis, S., and J. D. Buxbaum. 2015. Recent advances in the genetics of autism spectrum disorder. *Curr Neurol Neurosci Rep* 15 (6):1–9.

Donnellan, A. M. 1984. The criterion of the least dangerous assumption. *Behav Disord* 9:141–50.

Dowell, L. R., E. Mark Mahone, and S. H. Mostofsky. 2009. Associations of postural knowledge and basic motor skill with dyspraxia in autism: Implication for abnormalities in distributed connectivity and motor learning. *Neuropsychology* 23 (5):563.

Dziuk, M. A., J. C. Larson, A. Apostu, E. M. Mahone, M. B. Denckla, and S. H. Mostofsky. 2007. Dyspraxia in autism: Association with motor, social, and communicative deficits. *Dev Med Child Neurol* 49 (10): 734–9.

Fabbri-Destro, M., L. Cattaneo, S. Boria, and G. Rizzolatti. 2009. Planning actions in autism. *Exp Brain Res* 192 (3):521–5. doi: 10.1007/s00221–008–1578–3.

Farber, N. B., J. W. Newcomer, and J. W. Olney. 1998. The glutamate synapse in neuropsychiatric disorders: Focus on schizophrenia and Alzheimer's disease. *Prog Brain Res* 116:421–37.

Fombonne, E. 2005. Epidemiology of autistic disorder and other pervasive developmental disorders. *J Clin Psychiatry* 66:3.

French, L., and P. Pavlidis. 2011. Relationships between gene expression and brain wiring in the adult rodent brain. *PLoS Comput Biol* 7 (1):e1001049.

Fries, P. 2009. Neuronal gamma-band synchronization as a fundamental process in cortical computation. *Annu Rev Neurosci* 32:209–24.

Gogolla, N., J. J. LeBlanc, K. B. Quast, T. C. Südhof, M. Fagiolini, and T. K. Hensch. 2009. Common circuit defect of excitatory-inhibitory balance in mouse models of autism. *J Neurodev Disord* 1 (2):172.

Gomez-Rodriguez, M., J. Peters, J. Hill, B. Schölkopf, A. Gharabaghi, and M. Grosse-Wentrup. 2011. Closing the sensorimotor loop: Haptic feedback facilitates decoding of motor imagery. *J Neural Eng* 8 (3):036005.

Green, D., T. Charman, A. Pickles, S. Chandler, T. Loucas, E. Simonoff, and G. Baird. 2009. Impairment in movement skills of children with autistic spectrum disorders. *Dev Med Child Neurol* 51 (4):311–6.

Hahamy, A., M. Behrmann, and R. Malach. 2015. The idiosyncratic braIn: Distortion of spontaneous connectivity patterns in autism spectrum disorder. *Nat Neurosci* 18 (2):302–9.

Hartman, E., S. Houwen, E. Scherder, and C. Visscher. 2010. On the relationship between motor performance and executive functioning in children with intellectual disabilities. *J Intellect Disabil Res* 54 (5):468–77.

Haswell, C. C., J. Izawa, L. R. Dowell, S. H. Mostofsky, and R. Shadmehr. 2009. Representation of internal models of action in the autistic brain. *Nat Neurosci* 12 (8):970–2.

Herbert, M. R., D. A. Ziegler, N. Makris, P. A. Filipek, T. L. Kemper, J. J. Normandin, H. A. Sanders, D. N. Kennedy, and V. S. Caviness. 2004. Localization of white matter volume increase in autism and developmental language disorder. *Ann Neurol* 55 (4):530–40.

Higashida, N. 2013. *The Reason I Jump: The Inner Voice of a Thirteen-Year-Old Boy with Autism*. New York: Random House.

Hussman, J. P. 2001. Letters to the editor: Suppressed GABAergic inhibition as a common factor in suspected etiologies of autism. *J Autism Dev Disord* 31 (2):247–8.

Hussman, J. P., R.-H. Chung, A. J. Griswold, J. M. Jaworski, D. Salyakina, D. Ma, I. Konidari, P. L. Whitehead, J. M. Vance, and E. R. Martin. 2011. A noise-reduction GWAS analysis implicates altered regulation of neurite outgrowth and guidance in autism. *Mol Autism* 2 (1):1.

Just, M. A., V. L. Cherkassky, T. A. Keller, R. K. Kana, and N. J. Minshew. 2007. Functional and anatomical cortical underconnectivity in autism: Evidence from an FMRI study of an executive function task and corpus callosum morphometry. *Cereb Cortex* 17 (4):951–61.

Just, M. A., V. L. Cherkassky, T. A. Keller, and N. J. Minshew. 2004. Cortical activation and synchronization during sentence comprehension in high-functioning autism: Evidence of underconnectivity. *Brain* 127 (8): 1811–21.

Kana, R. K., T. A. Keller, V. L. Cherkassky, N. J. Minshew, and M. A. Just. 2006. Sentence comprehension in autism: Thinking in pictures with decreased functional connectivity. *Brain* 129 (9):2484–93.

Kanner, L. 1943. Autistic disturbances of affective contact. *Nerv Child* 2:217–50.

Kemper, T. L., and M. L. Bauman. 1993. The contribution of neuropathologic studies to the understanding of autism. *Neurol Clin* 11 (1):175–87.

Landa, R., and E. Garrett-Mayer. 2006. Development in infants with autism spectrum disorders: A prospective study. *J Child Psychol Psychiatry* 47 (6):629–38.

Miall, R. C., and D. M. Wolpert. 1996. Forward models for physiological motor control. *Neural Netw* 9 (8): 1265–79.

Morris, D., H. Tan, F. Barbagli, T. Chang, and K. Salisbury. 2007. Haptic feedback enhances force skill learning. Presented at the Second Joint EuroHaptics Conference and Symposium on Haptic Interfaces for Virtual Environment and Teleoperator Systems (WHC '07), March 22–24, Tsukuba, Japan.

Mostofsky, S. H., M. P. Burgess, and J. C. Gidley Larson. 2007. Increased motor cortex white matter volume predicts motor impairment in autism. *Brain* 130 (8):2117–22.

Mostofsky, S. H., and J. B Ewen. 2011. Altered connectivity and action model formation in autism is autism. *Neuroscientist* 17 (4):437–48.

Mostofsky, S. H., S. K. Powell, D. J. Simmonds, M. C. Goldberg, B. Caffo, and J. J. Pekar. 2009. Decreased connectivity and cerebellar activity in autism during motor task performance. *Brain*:awp088.

Osmon, D. C., and R. Jackson. 2002. Inspection time and IQ: Fluid or perceptual aspects of intelligence? *Intelligence* 30 (2):119–27.

Peiker, I., N. David, T. R. Schneider, G. Nolte, D. Schöttle, and A. K. Engel. 2015. Perceptual integration deficits in autism spectrum disorders are associated with reduced interhemispheric gamma-band coherence. *J Neurosci* 35 (50):16352–61.

Rogers, M. W., D. L. Wardman, S. R. Lord, and R. C. Fitzpatrick. 2001. Passive tactile sensory input improves stability during standing. *Exp Brain Res* 136 (4):514–22.

Rubenstein, J. L. R., and M. M. Merzenich. 2003. Model of autism: Increased ratio of excitation/inhibition in key neural systems. *Genes Brain Behav* 2 (5):255–67.

Scheuffgen, K., F. Happé, M. Anderson, and U. Frith. 2000. High "intelligence," low "IQ"? Speed of processing and measured IQ in children with autism. *Dev Psychopathol* 12 (01):83–90.

Shams, L., Y. Kamitani, and S. Shimojo. 2000. Illusions: What you see is what you hear. *Nature* 408 (6814):788.

Sharp, D. J., F. E. Turkheimer, S. K. Bose, S. K. Scott, and R. J. S. Wise. 2010. Increased frontoparietal integration after stroke and cognitive recovery. *Ann Neurol* 68 (5):753–6.

Singer, W. 1999. Neuronal synchrony: A versatile code for the definition of relations? *Neuron* 24 (1):49–65.

Solomon, M., S. J. Ozonoff, S. Ursu, S. Ravizza, N. Cummings, S. Ly, and C. S. Carter. 2009. The neural substrates of cognitive control deficits in autism spectrum disorders. *Neuropsychologia* 47 (12):2515–26.

Stevenson, R. A., J. K. Siemann, T. G. Woynaroski, B. C. Schneider, H. E. Eberly, S. M. Camarata, and M. T. Wallace. 2014. Evidence for diminished multisensory integration in autism spectrum disorders. *J Autism Dev Disord* 44 (12):3161–7.

Sutera, S., J. Pandey, E. L. Esser, M. A. Rosenthal, L. B. Wilson, M. Barton, J. Green, S. Hodgson, D. L. Robins, and T. Dumont-Mathieu. 2007. Predictors of optimal outcome in toddlers diagnosed with autism spectrum disorders. *J Autism Dev Disord* 37 (1):98–107.

Szurhaj, W., and P. Derambure. 2006. Intracerebral study of gamma oscillations in the human sensorimotor cortex. *Progr Brain Res* 159:297–310.

Teitelbaum, P., O. Teitelbaum, J. Nye, J. Fryman, and R. G. Maurer. 1998. Movement analysis in infancy may be useful for early diagnosis of autism. *Proc Natl Acad Sci USA* 95 (23):13982–7.

Thatcher, R. W., D. M. North, J. Neubrander, C. J. Biver, S. Cutler, and P. DeFina. 2009. Autism and EEG phase reset: Deficient GABA mediated inhibition in thalamo-cortical circuits. *Dev Neuropsychol* 34 (6): 780–800.

Vuijk, P. J., E. Hartman, E. Scherder, and C. Visscher. 2010. Motor performance of children with mild intellectual disability and borderline intellectual functioning. *J Intellect Disabil Res* 54 (11):955–65.

Wallace, G. L., M. Anderson, and F. Happé. 2009. Brief report: Information processing speed is intact in autism but not correlated with measured intelligence. *J Autism Dev Disord* 39 (5):809–14.

Wallace, M. T., and R. A. Stevenson. 2014. The construct of the multisensory temporal binding window and its dysregulation in developmental disabilities. *Neuropsychologia* 64:105–23.

Wass, S. 2011. Distortions and disconnections: Disrupted brain connectivity in autism. *Brain Cogn* 75 (1): 18–28.

Wilson, T. W., D. C. Rojas, M. L. Reite, P. D. Teale, and S. J. Rogers. 2007. Children and adolescents with autism exhibit reduced MEG steady-state gamma responses. *Biol Psychiatry* 62 (3):192–97.

Wuang, Y.-P., C.-C. Wang, M.-H. Huang, and C.-Y. Su. 2008. Profiles and cognitive predictors of motor functions among early school-age children with mild intellectual disabilities. *J Intellect Disabil Res* 52 (12): 1048–60.

Zikopoulos, B., and H. Barbas. 2010. Changes in prefrontal axons may disrupt the network in autism. *J Neurosci* 30 (44):14595–609.

Zopf, R., S. Truong, M. Finkbeiner, J. Friedman, and M. A. Williams. 2011. Viewing and feeling touch modulates hand position for reaching. *Neuropsychologia* 49 (5):1287–93.

Section III

Let's Get the Math Right to Improve Diagnosis, Research, and Treatment Outcomes

Preface to Section III
First Things First–Let Us Get the Math Right

Elizabeth B. Torres

Science follows the path of intuitive exploration—an endeavor to find answers to the unknown. Guided by, and founded upon, the use of mathematics, science tests and confirms the conjectures of creative scientific thinking, resulting in a corpus of collective knowledge that has been robustly examined and can be reproduced by a community following the scientific method. This scientific method is thus based on the systematic collection and scrutiny of empirical evidence attained through precise measurement. As such, the means employed to measure phenomena are as important as the methods used for analysis. Choosing an inappropriate mathematical framework to analyze our data or overconstraining the way in which data are gathered or measured can often derail the path of scientific inquiry. Constrained methodology and/or inappropriate methods of analysis are often reflected in a constrained, dogmatic one-sided view of a phenomenology that is ungeneralizable to the broader context—an inherent feature of the replication crisis now facing psychology (Francis 2012a, 2012b, 2012c, 2012d and see Chapter 11). This crisis has had a profound effect on the academic field of inquiry at large, leading to increased scrutiny and questioning of methodologies employed. Yet more importantly, this epidemic implies that psychological results are not conducive to generalizable knowledge that may benefit humanity at large—that is, they are unlikely to build toward lawlike findings that we can trust as general rules to integrate into the foundations for further inquiry. Indeed, building a core foundational corpus of knowledge to spawn further scientific inquiry and discovery is at the heart of the scientific method. Thus, modes of inquiry, the methods of data gathering, and analysis techniques in fields that deal with mental health and psychological phenomena, including those within a clinical setting, are arguably more an art than a science—as defined by the scientific method. This section aims to expose some of the issues that we need to address in the specific field of autism spectrum disorder (ASD) research if we are to make progress in posing proper lines of inquiry to begin defining the phenomena surrounding this constellation of disorders. Drawing on mathematical principles, these chapters aim to illustrate the importance of the concrete application of sound instrumentation to measure phenomena at all levels—including complex human behaviors. Methods to analyze and scrutinize data that can be applied within this broad context will be introduced in an attempt to showcase how the field can move toward applications that can invariably hold stable across different cultures and historical time periods for generalizable, replicable data.

Chapter 10 provides an overview of statistical considerations that should be made prior to choosing a framework for analyses. Chapter 11 provides concrete examples of inappropriate use of statistical methods. Chapter 12 then provides examples of this process when working with data collected from a group of individuals with ASD. This chapter discusses and illustrates these methods drawing contrasts with existing paradigms within the field of psychology and psychiatry—demonstrating known difficulties inherent with these fields, including the replication crisis (also discussed in Chapter 10), impeding generalizability (e.g., Gallistel 2009; Nickerson 2000).

Chapter 12 also provides an account of contemporary problems with data analyses owing to the complexities inherent in sensory-motor processes present in different "behaviors." The chapter discusses the inadequacy of current assumptions and analytical approaches to formulate problems and possible solutions in ASD behavioral analyses. Chapter 13 provides examples of new data types across different scales of noise-to-signal ratio that allow us to "zoom in and out" of the phenomena using different "lenses" and alternate between analytical formulations that simulate phenomena in a synthetic arena and hypotheses that are directly tested in the empirical arena. This chapter closes with an example of new methods to intervene in ASD while respecting the child's will and rights to spontaneous self-exploration and self-discovery.

REFERENCES

Francis, G. 2012a. The psychology of replication and replication in psychology. *Perspect Psychol Sci* 7 (6): 585–94.

Francis, G. 2012b. Publication bias and the failure of replication in experimental psychology. *Psychon Bull Rev* 19 (6):975–91.

Francis, G. 2012c. Replication initiative: Beware misinterpretation. *Science* 336 (6083):802.

Francis, G. 2012d. Too good to be true: Publication bias in two prominent studies from experimental psychology. *Psychon Bull Rev* 19 (2):151–6.

Gallistel, C. R. 2009. The importance of proving the null. *Psychol Rev* 116 (2):439–53.

Nickerson, R. S. 2000. Null hypothesis significance testing: A review of an old and continuing controversy. *Psychol Methods* 5 (2):241–301.

10 Non-Gaussian Statistical Distributions Arising in Large-Scale Personalized Data Sets from Biophysical Rhythms of the Nervous Systems

Jorge V. José

CONTENTS

Introduction 155
Gaussian Distribution 158
Poisson Random Process 158
Gamma Additive Distribution Function 159
Weibull Additive Distribution Function 160
General Additive Probability Distribution Function 161
Lognormal Multiplicative Distribution Function 161
Kolmogorov–Smirnov Test 161
Law of Large Numbers and the Central Limit Theorem 162
Conclusions 163
Acknowledgments 164
References 164

This chapter provides a review of some statistical concepts and mathematical background for a new type of behavioral analyses amenable to understanding the stochastic properties of biophysical rhythms harnessed from the human nervous systems. The proposed methods are part of a broader statistical platform for individualized behavioral analysis that makes no a priori assumptions about the inherent variability of the biophysical data. Further, some recommendations are provided on general strategies to derive personalized biometrics and to handle big data using new data types arising from wearable sensors useful to implement contemporary mobile-health concepts.

INTRODUCTION

We are presently living through a revolutionary period in the biomedical sciences. One of the reasons for this is the high-throughput data being produced, for example, in genomics and transcriptomic sequencing, in the proteome and metabolome, and in neuroscience. This is a consequence of recent technological advances that allow the measuring of biological quantities with ever higher precision, in particular for a single individual, fitting within the context of *personalized medicine*. These quantitative measurements generate large data sets with high complexity requiring careful statistical and theoretical modeling methods to extract relevant biological information. Theoretical and computational approaches in the biological areas of research mentioned above have made significant advances, but they still have not reached a significant level of understanding the basic processes that would ultimately lead to the central goal of being able to diagnose and develop appropriate corrective therapies.

This experimental and technological revolution is presently happening generally, but in particular in neuroscience. It needs by force to have proper theoretical and computational analytics tools to extract the relevant physiological and behavioral information contained in the data. This is particularly important after evidence that using canned programs without understanding their basic assumptions can lead to wrong results and interpretations (Eklund et al. 2016). The brain performs probabilistic computations when facing our everyday evolutionary challenges, following adaptive behavioral strategies that constantly demand making optimal decisions. Within this probabilistic framework, it is important to separate the physiological signal from the ever-present noise due to the inherent neuronal molecular or synaptic processes, as well as the noise generated by measuring devices, or computational algorithms that inherently make assumptions that may not bear relevance for the actual experimental data sets. Problems with analyzing the experimental data may also come from making a priori assumptions about the statistical model that may or may not agree with the intrinsic probabilistic nature of the measured data. Several theoretical models have been developed at the neuronal or synaptic level, like the Hodgkin–Huxley (HK) model (Hodgkin and Huxley 1952), which describes the action potentials' propagation, or the Hebbian plasticity memory modeling (Hebb 1949). These models have proven to be very informative in quantitatively connecting theory to experiment.

No equivalent theoretical modeling exists describing behavior at the peripheral nervous system level. Although limb movements are produced from signals coming from the central nervous system and effected from external sensory information, how to model going from neurons to limbs' behavior is not fully understood at the human level. Further, the theoretical modeling situation is even less advanced when considering the quantitative description of psychiatric problems. Clinicians base their diagnostics on qualitative narratives from patients and families that involve a set of heterogeneous symptoms and maladies with broad classifications described, in particular, in the fifth edition of the *Diagnostic and Statistical Manual of Mental Disorders* (DSM-5) (American Psychiatric Association 2013). There is, however, a recent effort to change this situation involving what is known as *precision psychiatry* (Insel 2014; Torres et al. 2016) and *computational psychiatry* (Friston et al. 2014; Wang and Krystal 2014; Torres et al. 2016). These new areas of quantitative research involve increasing close collaborations between quantitative scientists in the physical sciences, together with psychologists, psychiatrists, and health care clinicians. This is catalyzed by an attempt to try to utilize frontline technological advances in imaging techniques as, for example, with wearable devices. By developing the right analytics, based on bioinformatics, machine learning (including contemporary deep-learning-based approaches), and statistical data analyses, more quantitative and reliable, personalized, and precise clinical diagnoses might be produced. The expectation is then that clinicians will be able to make faster and better-informed assessments of a patient's medical conditions, leading to maximum-efficacy treatments based on precision and personalized medicine.

The real question then is, how do we rationally and successfully analyze the wealth of data produced by recent measuring tools, which by nature involve a competition between signal and noise? How do we develop proper statistical tools to analyze this large trove of personalized biomedical data? Hopefully, the results from this type of effort will produce more mathematical realistic models, within the same spirit as the HK model of action potential propagation, even if it has its own limitations.

The purpose of this chapter is to emphasize the need to be careful about what statistical techniques to use to analyze the data, in particular data that are specific to an individual and not an ensemble of individuals. These data are often produced by a very large number of trials and continuous measurements on each individual. This is very important since up to now, experts in biostatistics have had no guidance as to how to uniquely analyze single individual's statistical data. They have to resort to testing several a priori hypotheses, often assuming that they have *Gaussian distribution* probabilistic data to arrive at their conclusions. The question is then, what a priori statistical assumptions should one make from the start about the statistical properties of the measured data?

The main message from this short review is that one should make *no* a priori assumptions about the statistical nature of the signal's distribution data until after a proper separation between signals-to-noise ratios is carefully done. Only then will the signal statistical properties be properly determined from the filtered data: in particular, making evident the significant differences between analyzing individualized data from those of a large number of subjects. In the latter case, it is common to assume a priori that the data can be described by a Gaussian distribution. This is the case when doing analysis of variance (ANOVA) or calculations involving, for example, linear regression analysis (Limpert et al. 2001; Limpert and Stahel 2011). The situation is different when the data analyzed come from one particular individual. It has recently been found empirically by studying different neurological disorders that the usual Gaussian assumption is not fulfilled (Torres 2011, 2012; Torres et al. 2013). Empirical distributions are not always found to be bell-shaped Gaussian, but instead asymmetric, that is, *having small means and large variances*.

In this chapter, I discuss the properties of some of those alternative distributions, like the Poisson, gamma, Weibull, and general distributions, which have the last distributions as special cases. I also discuss the lognormal (LN) distribution function, which is also asymmetrical and sometimes used to fit experimental biological data. It differs from the other distribution in a fundamental way that becomes clear when considering the all-important central limit theorem (CLT). All these asymmetric distributions are qualitatively similar but quantitatively different. Thus, careful testing is necessary to decide which of these distributions better fits the empirical data sets. One way to do the testing is by calculating the Kolmogorov–Smirnov (K-S) distance between two distributions. I briefly discuss the K-S metric in this chapter. In several cases that we have studied, in particular autism spectrum disorder (ASD), we found that the Gamma distribution is the one that best fits the data (Figure 10.1). The Gamma distribution provides statistical inferences that help us interpret the data and discuss possible physiological consequences in ASD. These are discussed in more detail in other chapters in this volume (e.g., Chapters 1, 12, 13, and 14).

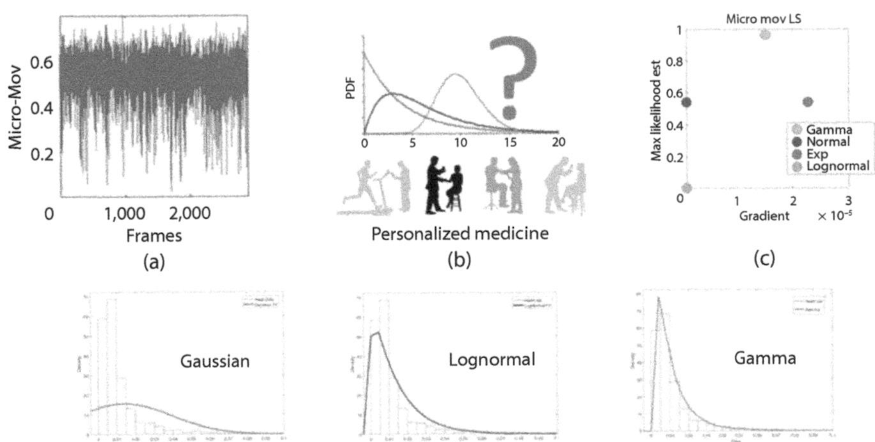

FIGURE 10.1 The continuous gamma family of probability distributions has fit well the biophysical data harnessed from the nervous systems of individual human subjects. (a) Micromovements extracted from involuntary head motions as a person is in the resting state during functional magnetic resonance imaging (fMRI) testing. (b) Different probability density functions (PDFs) can be used to characterize the motion data of different people, yet data from one single person can change distributions throughout development. This calls for a personalized approach to longitudinal data. (c) Output of maximum likelihood estimation testing the fit of different probability distributions to the data in (a). The gamma PDF produces the best fit in relation to the Gaussian, LN, and exponential cases. The bottom panel shows the frequency histograms and fitting curves corresponding to (a). (Prepared by E.B. Torres using MATLAB functions.)

The present review tries to be introductory and understandable for a general audience. I briefly review the relevant mathematical results that may not be common knowledge for behavioral neuroscientists. There are many sources and books in probability theory and stochastic processes that treat the material discussed here, although perhaps there is not a single place that does it in the way I do it here, and none that has the same type of emphasis on the biorhythms from the human nervous systems. Thus, I give a few appropriate references that relate to the material discussed here. There is no claim of originality, except for the way the presentation and some of the derivations are done.

Gaussian Distribution

Laplace was among the first to begin to discuss probabilistic processes. His work has led to many advances and applications developed by several authors over several centuries. These developments have included a variety of extensions, going from the very empirical to the very mathematical formulaic approaches of probability and stochastic theory. It was Gauss who, in the nineteenth century, first introduced his normal or Gaussian distribution while he was trying to understand the measurement errors while determining asteroids' orbits. The distribution is defined by the expression

$$N(x,\mu,\sigma)=\frac{1}{\sigma\sqrt{2\pi}}e^{-\frac{1}{2}\left(\frac{x-\mu}{\sigma}\right)^2} \tag{10.1}$$

Here μ is the mean value and σ the variance or standard deviation. What makes this probability distribution important is that (1) it is a *symmetric distribution* and (2) it is completely defined by its first two moments, that is, the mean and the variance, with expressions

$$\mu=\frac{1}{\sigma\sqrt{2\pi}}\int_{-\infty}^{\infty} xe^{-\frac{1}{2}\left(\frac{x-\mu}{\sigma}\right)^2}dx \tag{10.2}$$

$$\sigma^2=\frac{1}{\sigma\sqrt{2\pi}}\int_{-\infty}^{\infty} (x-\mu)^2 e^{-\frac{1}{2}\left(\frac{x-\mu}{\sigma}\right)^2}dx \tag{10.3}$$

with expressions $\langle x\rangle=\mu$; $Var(x)=\sigma^2$.

Of significant importance for the Gaussian distribution is what appears in the asymptotic limit of a sum of identically distributed independent random variables defined by an *arbitrarily bounded* probability distribution based on the CLT. I review how those connections arise, along with the conditions that have to be fulfilled by the probability distributions to reach this limit, leading, asymptotically, to Gaussian distributions.

POISSON RANDOM PROCESS

A random process consists of the change or evolution of a variable that does not follow a deterministic well-defined rule. This means, for example, that if we know the value of a variable at one time, we will not be able to assess with 100% certainty the value of that variable at a future time. We will only know its future value in a probabilistic sense. Among the most important random processes in probability theory, and of relevance for this chapter, is the family of Poisson random process (PRP). The PRP is characterized by having random variables that change within a time interval such that their values at any given time are completely independent of their values at any arbitrary time in the past. One limit of a PRP is given by the exponential probability distribution, which is defined as

$$P(x,\lambda)=\lambda e^{-\lambda x} \tag{10.4}$$

with the rate parameter $\lambda > 0$, $x \geq 0$; $P(x) = 0$ for $x \leq 0$. The mean value is $< x > = 1/\lambda$, and the variance $<x^2> - <x>^2 = 1/\lambda^2$.

An important property of the exponential probability distribution is that it is *memoryless*. This means that any exponential random variable will occur independent of any previous value this variable took. For example, if the random process describing the tossing of a coin is exponential, it means that if we observe heads in the first tossing, that tells us nothing about what the next tossing will be—either heads or tails. If we toss the coin several times and do not observe heads again, we do not know if the next toss will be tails since each time we toss the coin, it is like starting the process all over again. The exponential distribution is the most random of distributions (Feller 1967).

We can build a general expression for the PRP after the following process. Consider a set of n-exponential identically distributed random variables (i.d.r.v.) $S = (X_1, X_2, X_3, \ldots, X_n)$. We propose that the probability distribution for the *sum* of these random variables $\sum = X_1 + X_2 + X_{3,} + \ldots + X_n$ will be given by the general expression for PRP:

$$P_n(x,\lambda) = \lambda \frac{(\lambda x)^{n-1}}{(n-1)!} e^{-\lambda x} \tag{10.5}$$

with $n! = (n-1)(n-2)(n-3)\ldots(2)(1)$. For $n = 1$, this result is just the exponential distribution. One way of proving the result given in Equation 10.2 for arbitrary n is by extending the convolution property of the unrenormalized exponential distribution $P_U(x, \lambda) = e^{-\lambda x}$,

$$P_U(x+y) = P_U(x) \cdot P_U(y) \tag{10.6}$$

To prove Equation 10.2, we can use the mathematical induction approach, which means that first we assume that the result is true for $n = 1$. Then assume that it is true for n, proving that it is also true for $n + 1$. The expression for $(n + 1)$, $P_{n+1}(x, \lambda)$ can be derived by using the convolution property recursion relation in terms of the two known distributions, $P_n(x)$ and $P_1(x)$:

$$P_{n+1}(x,\lambda) = \int_0^x P_n(x-t)P_1(t)dt \tag{10.7}$$

Replacing the expression for $P_n(x, \lambda)$ given in Equation 10.2 and solving the integral, we have

$$P_{n+1}(x,\lambda) = \lambda \frac{(\lambda)^{n-1}}{(n-1)!} e^{-\lambda x} \int_0^x t^{n-1} dt = \lambda \frac{(\lambda x)^n}{n!} e^{-\lambda x} \text{QED} \tag{10.8}$$

which is the PRP result we wanted to prove: this probability distribution, defined for discrete n, is equivalent to several asymmetric distributions, in particular to the Gamma distribution for the continuous n variable that we discuss next.

Gamma Additive Distribution Function

One characteristic of the PRP is that it is not symmetric about the origin as the Gaussian distribution, as well as being defined for integer values of n. One important case of the PRP is the gamma probability distribution defined by

$$G(x,a,b) = \frac{1}{\Gamma(a) b^a} x^{a-1} e^{-x/b} \tag{10.9}$$

Here, $\Gamma(a)$ is the gamma function defined as

$$\Gamma(a) = \int_0^\infty x^{a-1} e^{-x} dx \tag{10.10}$$

a and b are called the *shape* and *scale* parameters, respectively. a takes continuous values in the interval $a \in (0, \infty)$, while $b > 0$. For n, an integer $\Gamma(n) = (n - 1)!$ The mean and the variance of the Gamma distribution are given by

$$<x> = a/b; \quad <x^2> - <x>^2 = a/b^2 \tag{10.11}$$

The Gamma distribution has the exponential distribution limit with

$$G(x, a = 1, b = 1/\lambda) = \lambda e^{-\lambda x} \tag{10.12}$$

As the shape a grows, with the scale parameter fixed, the Gamma distribution gets closer and closer to the Gaussian distribution. How close? We will discuss this later within the context of the CLT.

Note that the Gamma distribution, as is the case for the PRP, also satisfies the convolution property:

$$G(x, a + a', 1/b) = G(x, a, 1/b) \cdot G(x, a', 1/b) \tag{10.13}$$

The proof of this identity follows from carrying out the integrals:

$$\frac{1}{\Gamma(a)\Gamma(a')b^a b^{a'}} e^{-x/b} \int_0^x (x-y)^{(a-1)} y^{a'-1} dy \tag{10.14}$$

With the change of variable $y = xt$, the above expression becomes

$$P_{n+1}(x, \lambda) = \lambda \frac{(\lambda)^{n-1}}{(n-1)!} e^{-\lambda x} \int_0^x t^{n-1} dt = \lambda \frac{(\lambda x)^n}{n!} e^{-\lambda x} \text{QED} \tag{10.15}$$

This, except for a numerical constant, proves the result.

Weibull Additive Distribution Function

Another asymmetric distribution that is sometimes used to analyze empirical data is the Weibull distribution function, defined by

$$W(x, a, b) = \frac{a}{b^a} x^{a-1} e^{-(x/b)^a} \tag{10.16}$$

It is qualitatively similar to the Gamma distribution but not the same quantitatively. Here, $x \geq 0$; $a > 0$ is the *shape parameter* and $b > 0$ the *scale parameter*. The mean and the variance are

$$<x>_W = b\Gamma(1 + \frac{1}{a}); \quad \text{var}(x)_W = b^2[\Gamma(1 + \frac{2}{a}) - \Gamma^2(1 + \frac{1}{a})] \tag{10.17}$$

Just plotting the Gamma distribution, the Weibull distribution, or the LN distribution, as discussed later, for different values of the scale and shape parameters may not allow us to visually differentiate between the best of them to fit the empirical data. More quantitative modeling and testing is necessary to make sure which distribution is the one that more accurately represents the empirical data. Of significant importance is to have a large amount of data so that the differentiation can be done conclusively. But this is not always the case.

General Additive Probability Distribution Function

A more general version of probability distribution function that can be symmetric or asymmetric, including as particular limits for the Gaussian, gamma, or Weibull distribution, which is useful for generally testing the CLT, is defined as (Aitchison and Brown 1957; Firth 1988; Silva and Lisboa 2007)

$$R(x,a,b,\gamma,\mu)=\frac{\gamma(x-\mu)^{(a-1)}}{\Gamma(\frac{a}{\gamma})b^{a/\gamma}}e^{-(x-\mu)^{\gamma}/b} \tag{10.18}$$

Here $x > \mu$, and a, b, $\gamma > 0$. Setting $\mu = 0$, $\gamma = 1$, $a = 1$, we recover the exponential distribution. Taking $\mu = 0$, $\gamma = 1$ becomes the Gamma distribution, while setting $\gamma = 1/a = k$, $\mu = 0$, and choosing $\gamma = 1/a = k$, $\mu = 0$, $b = \lambda^{1/a}$, brings us back to the Weibull distribution. Notice that if we chose $\gamma = 2$; $\mu = 0$; $a = 1$; $\gamma = 1$, R becomes a Gaussian distribution function with the structure of the Maxwell–Boltzmann distribution of significant importance in statistical mechanics.

Lognormal Multiplicative Distribution Function

There are other distributions that are asymmetric and that could also be considered when trying to fit empirical data. One that differs in some ways from the ones given above, but which has been used extensively to fit biological empirical data, is the LN distribution. It is defined as

$$LN(x,\mu,\sigma)=\frac{1}{\sqrt{2\pi}\sigma x}\exp\left[-\frac{[\ln x-\mu]^2}{2\sigma^2}\right] \tag{10.19}$$

The parameter μ takes values in the reals, while $\sigma\varepsilon(0,\infty)$. e^{μ} is the scale parameter, while σ is the shape parameter, with $x\varepsilon(0,\infty)$. The LN's mean and variance are given by

$$<x>_{LN}=\exp(\mu+\frac{1}{2}\sigma^2);\quad Var<x>_{LN}=\exp[2(\mu+\sigma^2)]-\exp[2\mu+\sigma^2] \tag{10.20}$$

Although it looks like a normal distribution for ln x, the LN distribution *is not* symmetric or fully determined only by its first two moments, as is the case for the Gaussian distribution. For instance, the third and fourth moments defining the skewness and kurtosis are explicitly given by

$$Skew(x)_{LN}=(e^{\sigma^2}+2)\sqrt{e^{\sigma^2}-1};\quad Kurt<x>_{LN}=e^{4\sigma^2}+2e^{2\sigma^2}+3e^{2\sigma^2}-3 \tag{10.21}$$

In the Gaussian distribution, all moments can be related to its first and second moments. An important difference between the Gaussian and asymmetric probability distribution functions discussed before is that in the LN distribution the asymptotic limit of a multiplication of i.i.d.r.v. LN random variables leads to a Gaussian distribution, while in the previous cases, that happens when considering the sum of i.i.d.r.v. I will discuss this later within the CLT context.

Kolmogorov–Smirnov Test

One way of differentiating between two distributions is to *measure* how far apart they are from each other. One measure that is often used to determine the distance between two probability distribution function separations is the K–S distance between them, say, $R(x)$ and $T(x)$. The K–S is defined as

$$K-S=\sup_x|R(x)-T(x)| \tag{10.22}$$

Here “sup” is the supreme value between the separations of the two distributions at x. If the K–S distance is not small, it will be easy, as a function of the data size, to determine which one best fits the data. However, if the K–S distance is small, then only by increasing the data set size significantly can a clear determination of which one is the best distribution be made. Of course, if the separation distance is small and a phase parameter can be built from the *scale* and *shape* parameters, either distribution may work. This assumes a parameter set for the shape and scale parameters in the distributions. A similar equation as the one for the K–S distance above, can be used for the distance between the Gamma function and Weibull or LN distributions. This is not what we found in the ASD case. There we found that the distribution that best fit the empirical data was the Gamma distribution.

LAW OF LARGE NUMBERS AND THE CENTRAL LIMIT THEOREM

Two very important results in probability theory are the *law of large numbers* (LLN) and, as mentioned before, the CLT. These are two of most important theorems that make statistical theory work. Let me describe the essence of these two results and how the CLT connects to the distribution functions discussed above. Let us first consider the LLN. It pertains to doing a large number of identical measurements of the same quantity, and then asking about the relationship between the value of the asymptotic *geometric mean* and the *mean* calculated with the probability distribution function assumed to describe the random process.

Consider the set of n independent identically distributed random variables (i.i.d.r.v.) $\Omega_n = (X_1, X_2, X_3, \ldots, X_n)$, with n being an integer. Each one of these random variables is determined by the same probability distribution function $P(X_n)$, each having a mean μ and variance σ^2. The variance can take values in the interval $\sigma^2 \varepsilon(0, \infty)$.

Consider now the sum of random variables:

$$S_n = \sum_{i}^{n} X_i \tag{10.23}$$

with n being an integer.

The set $\vec{T} = (S_0, S_1, S_2, S_{3,} \ldots)$ represents a random sample determined from the probability distribution $P(X_n)$. Here we assume $S_0 = 0$. Next consider the geometric average

$$R_n = \frac{S_n}{n} = \frac{1}{n}\sum_{i=1}^{n} X_i \tag{10.24}$$

The LLN theorem states that

$$\lim_{n\to\infty} R_n \to \mu \tag{10.25}$$

Now let us briefly discuss the essence of the CLT: the theorem states that *the probability distribution function of the sum of a large set of i.i.d.r.v. will asymptotically become a Gaussian distribution*, regardless of the specific form of $P(X)$. The paramount importance of CLT in statistics is hard to overstate given that it is the reason why many statistical analyses work. Let us state the theorem more explicitly.

Note that the mean value is given by $<S_n> = n\mu$, for finite n, while the variance is $\text{var}(S_n) = <S_n{}^2> - <S_n{}^2> = n\sigma^2$, with σ^2 the variance of $P(X)$. The question then is, what is the asymptotic probability distribution for S_n in the $n \to \infty$ limit, given that the mean and variances diverge? To resolve that problem, we consider instead the alternative statistical variable:

$$Y_n = \frac{S_n - n\mu}{\sqrt{n}\sigma} \tag{10.26}$$

This expression has the advantage that the mean and variances are finite given that $<Y_n> = 0$, $\text{var}(Y_n) = 1$. The proof of the CLT states that the asymptotic distribution function for Y_n, in the limit that $n \rightarrow \infty$, is Gaussian. More explicitly,

$$\lim_{n \to \infty} D(Y_n) \rightarrow N(Y_\infty, 0, 1)\text{QED} \tag{10.27}$$

What this means is that regardless of the specific properties of $P(X)$, provided it is bounded and *well behaved statistically*, meaning that it is has bounded moments, the probability distribution of the sum of X_i values will asymptotically converge to a Gaussian distribution.

Let us now see how this would apply to the Gamma distribution defined in Equation 10.9. Let us consider first the exponential distribution, which means taking the scale parameter $1/\lambda$ and shape parameter equal to one. The corresponding Y_n random variable in this case is

$$Y_n = \frac{S_n - n/\lambda}{\sqrt{n}/\lambda} \tag{10.28}$$

In the $n \rightarrow \infty$, the distribution for the sum of exponentially distributed independent random variables asymptotically approaches a normal distribution. Similarly, we can define the Y_n variables for the full Gamma distribution, the Weibull distribution, or the Poisson distribution for integer n. The same applies in the case of the lognormal distribution; however, in this case, instead of the sum we define the alternative product or multiplicative random variable

$$\tilde{S}_n = \prod_i^n X_i \tag{10.29}$$

where the X_i values are chosen from the LN distribution function: the Y_n variable in this case is just given as before by replacing the mean value and the variance from Equations 10.2 and 10.3 into Equation 10.19, leading to a corresponding normal distribution with the corresponding multiplicative variables.

The basic difference then between LN distribution and the other asymmetric probability distributions we considered before is that the random processes in the LN case are multiplicative in nature and not additive, as in the other cases. This can lead to important quantitative consequences.

CONCLUSIONS

The goal of this chapter was to emphasize the importance of dealing with the overwhelming amounts of behavioral data being produced now from a large number of measurements or trials done in single individuals, in particular within the context of personalized medicine. We need to have completely open eyes of not making any a priori assumptions or prior hypotheses about the nature of the data that may not agree with the intrinsic statistical properties of what is measured. Often, a standard implicit assumption when analyzing public health data is that it has an inherent normal or Gaussian distribution. It is indeed true, as reviewed in this chapter, that many possible well-behaved probability distributions will in the "asymptotic" limit get very close to a Gaussian distribution. However, we have shown that only when some of the distribution parameters or number of trials goes to infinity does the distribution gets close—but how close to the Gaussian distribution is an important question. How far from the actually relevant distribution for the classification and interpretation of physiologically relevant data is a question that has to be determined. Of importance is to always start with the raw data, which may indeed contain a number of superfluous components that need to be separated from the relevant physiological or behavioral components of the data. To do this, the stability of the separation between the signals from noise has to be done extremely carefully.

ACKNOWLEDGMENTS

The author thanks Di Wu for useful comments about a draft of this chapter.

REFERENCES

Aitchison, J., and J. A. C. Brown. 1957. *The Lognormal Distribution, with Special Reference to Its Uses in Economics*, University of Cambridge Department of Applied Economics Monographs. Cambridge: Cambridge University Press.

American Psychiatric Association. 2013. *Diagnostic and Statistical Manual of Mental Disorders*. 5th ed. Washington, DC: American Psychiatric Association.

Eklund, A., T. E. Nichols, and H. Knutsson. 2016. Cluster failure: Why fMRI inferences for spatial extent have inflated false-positive rates. *Proc Natl Acad Sci USA* 113 (28):7900–5. doi: 10.1073/pnas.1602413113.

Feller, W. 1967. *An Introduction to Probability Theory and Its Applications*. 3rd ed. Wiley Series in Probability and Mathematical Statistics. New York: Wiley.

Firth, D. 1988. Multiplicative errors: Log-normal or gamma? *J R Stat Soc Series B* (2):266–8.

Friston, K. J., K. E. Stephan, R. Montague, and R. J. Dolan. 2014. Computational psychiatry: The brain as a phantastic organ. *Lancet Psychiatry* 1 (2):148–58. doi: 10.1016/S2215-0366(14)70275-5.

Hebb, D. O. 1949. *The Organization of Behavior: A Neuropsychological Theory*. Wiley Book in Clinical Psychology. New York: Wiley.

Hodgkin, A. L., and A. F. Huxley. 1952. A quantitative description of membrane current and its application to conduction and excitation in nerve. *J Physiol* 117 (4):500–44.

Insel, T. R. 2014. The NIMH Research Domain Criteria (RDoC) Project: Precision medicine for psychiatry. *Am J Psychiatry* 171 (4):395–7. doi: 10.1176/appi.ajp.2014.14020138.

Limpert, E., and W. A. Stahel. 2011. Problems with using the normal distribution—and ways to improve quality and efficiency of data analysis. *PLoS One* 6 (7):e21403. doi: 10.1371/journal.pone.0021403.

Limpert, E., W. A. Stahel, and M. Abbt. 2001. Log-normal distributions across the sciences: Keys and clues. *Bioscience* 51 (5):341–52.

Silva, L. E., and P. Lisboa. 2007. Analysis of the characteristic features of the density functions for gamma, Weibull and log-normal distributions through RBF network pruning with QLP. Presented at the Proceedings of the 6th WSEAS International Conference on Artificial Intelligence, Knowledge Engineering and Data Bases, Corfu Island, Greece, February 16–19.

Torres, E. B. 2011. Two classes of movements in motor control. *Exp Brain Res* 215 (3–4):269–83. doi: 10.1007/s00221-011-2892-8.

Torres, E. B. 2012. Atypical signatures of motor variability found in an individual with ASD. *Neurocase* 1:1–16 doi: 10.1080/13554794.2011.654224.

Torres, E. B., M. Brincker, R. W. Isenhower, P. Yanovich, K. A. Stigler, J. I. Nurnberger, D. N. Metaxas, and J. V. Jose. 2013. Autism: The micro-movement perspective. *Front Integr Neurosci* 7:32. doi: 10.3389/fnint.2013.00032.

Torres, E. B., R. W. Isenhower, J. Nguyen, C. Whyatt, J. I. Nurnberger, J. V. Jose, S. M. Silverstein, T. V. Papathomas, J. Sage, and J. Cole. 2016. Toward precision psychiatry: Statistical platform for the personalized characterization of natural behaviors. *Front Neurol* 7:8. doi: 10.3389/fneur.2016.00008.

Wang, X. J., and J. H. Krystal. 2014. Computational psychiatry. *Neuron* 84 (3):638–54. doi: 10.1016/j.neuron.2014.10.018.

11 Excess Success for a Study on Visual Search and Autism

Motivation to Change How Scientists Analyze Data

Gregory Francis

CONTENTS

Excess Success in Gliga et al. (2015) 165
Trust Your Data, But Not Too Much 168
An Alternative Approach 171
References 175

This chapter discusses how scientists use empirical results and statistical analyses to develop theoretical conclusions. Although such activities are an integral part of science, it is surprisingly difficult to relate theory to data, and it is often demonstrably done incorrectly. To keep the chapter relevant to the book, I discuss these issues in relation to a recent high-profile publication on autism that concluded that measurements on a visual search task among infants could predict emerging autism symptoms that appeared months later (Gliga et al. 2015). As shown in the chapter, a statistical analysis suggests that readers should be skeptical of the theoretical claims in Gliga et al. (2015). The reasons for this skepticism highlight general statistical issues that apply to investigations of autism and many other scientific topics.

EXCESS SUCCESS IN GLIGA ET AL. (2015)

At 9, 15, and 24 months (2 years) of age, Gliga et al. (2015) measured the ability of infants to (spontaneously) find an unusual target among a set of distractors. For the same infants at the same ages, they also assessed emerging autism symptoms using age-appropriate measures (Autism Observation Scale for Infants [AOSI] or Autism Diagnostic Observation Schedule [ADOS]). With three related analyses, they then explored relationships between visual search performance and emerging autism symptoms. The main theoretical claims were based on the presence or absence of significant correlations (described as regression weights) between different measurements. For example, a key finding was that 9-month visual search scores were significantly related to both 15-month AOSI scores ($p = 0.03$) and to 2-year ADOS scores ($p = 0.02$).

This primary result was then investigated in more detail with several follow-up analyses. One such follow-up analysis reported that the same relationships were present for the subset of infants classified as "high risk" for autism (due to having an older brother or sister diagnosed with the condition). Given the nature of infant recruitment for the study, around 85% of the infants were classified as high risk. Just as for the full data set, 9-month visual search scores were related to both 15-month AOSI scores ($p = 0.049$) and 2-year ADOS scores ($p = 0.02$).

A second follow-up analysis argued that the primary effects were due to a developmental pathway whereby visual search performance contributes to autism symptom measures, rather than the other way around. The argument involves considering the partial correlations that remain after taking into account other variables that differ in time. For example, the 9-month visual search scores were correlated with the 15-month AOSI scores, even when factoring out the contribution of 9-month AOSI scores ($p = 0.046$). However, the relationship between the 9-month visual search scores was not significantly correlated with the 2-year ADOS scores when factoring out the contribution of the 9-month and 15-month AOSI scores ($p = 0.13$). Gliga et al. (2015) argued that the presence and then absence of a significant correlation reflects the developmental progress of autism symptoms. This conclusion was bolstered by additional tests. Notably, the correlation was nonsignificant ($p = 0.44$) for 9-month visual search scores and 9-month AOSI scores (indicating development had not progressed enough to show a relationship). Along similar lines, it was noted that 9-month and 15-month visual search scores were significantly correlated ($p = 0.02$), but that the 15-month and 2-year visual search scores were not significantly correlated with the autism measures (p-values not given). This pattern of results was interpreted as indicating the importance of the early development of atypical perception.

Finally, significant correlations were found between the various autism measures taken at different ages. This is not a surprising outcome, given that the measures were designed for this purpose, but the absence of significant relationships among these measures would have undermined the other conclusions of the study.

An apparent strength of the findings in Gliga et al. (2015) is that the data precisely match the theoretical conclusions. The primary relationship between 9-month visual search scores and 15-month AOSI and 2-year ADOS holds for the full data set, a theoretically interesting subset of infants (the high-risk infants), and when factoring out other relevant measures. The other tests indicate, in a variety of ways, the early development of visual search data characteristics that are able to predict subsequent autism symptoms. Given how well the empirical data match these theoretical conclusions, it is not surprising that the findings were published in a prominent journal and mentioned in the popular press.

But there is something odd about the pattern of results in Gliga et al. (2015). The outcome of each statistical test matches the theoretical expectations (e.g., to be significant or not), but often only just below (or above) the significance criterion. Table 11.1 lists the different hypothesis tests and the associated statistics and p-values. The novel significant findings (not including the relationships between the various autism measures) have p-values of 0.02, 0.03, 0.02, 0.049, 0.02, and 0.046. It is strange that so many p-values should be between 0.02 and 0.05 (Cumming 2008; Simonsohn et al. 2014; van Assen et al. 2015). If the variables' relationships were as robust as is seemingly indicated by the consistency of the statistical tests (they are all successful), then one would commonly expect much smaller p-values than 0.02. Another way to say this is that if the combination of effects and sample sizes often produces p-values just below 0.05, then (due to random sampling) one would also expect to find p-values larger than 0.05 for some tests that are relevant to the theoretical claims (Francis 2012c; Ioannidis and Trikalinos 2007; Schimmack 2012). Gliga et al. (2015) do report nonsignificant results just above 0.05 (e.g., $p = 0.13$ for the partial correlation of 9-month visual search and 2-year ADOS), but the nonsignificant status of these tests were interpreted as support for the developmental properties of the theoretical claims, rather than as a failure to find a theoretically predicted outcome.

To rephrase the situation again, if the experiment is a proper test of the theoretical claims, then it is rather surprising that data with the level of noise that must be present (due to random sampling) should produce hypothesis test outcomes that are uniformly consistent with the theory. To estimate just how unusual such perfection should be, I generated a computer simulation in the R programming environment (R Core Team 2014) that defined normally distributed populations having the correlational structure of the data reported by Gliga et al. (2015). (The R source code for these simulations, and all other simulations described in this chapter, is available on the Open Science Framework at https://osf.io/q92sc/). When nonsignificant correlation values were unavailable, the simulation assigned zero to the population correlation, which maximizes the probability of producing a nonsignificant outcome. From these populations, random samples of size 100 were drawn and tested for the comparisons listed in Table 11.1. This process was repeated 100,000 times, and the final column of

TABLE 11.1
Hypothesis Tests Used by Gliga et al. (2015) to Support Their Theoretical Claims

Comparison	Correlation/Regression Weight	p	Probability of Success
9-month VS and 15-month VS	0.24	0.02	0.676
9-month VS and 9-month AOSI	0.08	0.44*	0.877
9-month VS and 15-month AOSI	0.22	0.03	0.602
9-month VS and 2-year ADOS	0.24	0.02	0.679
15-month VS and 15-month AOSI	NA	>0.05*	0.950
15-month VS and 2-year ADOS	NA	>0.05*	0.949
2-year VS and 2-year ADOS	NA	>0.05*	0.949
9-month AOSI and 15-month AOSI	0.34	0.0007	0.940
9-month AOSI and 2-year ADOS	0.31	0.002	0.888
15-month AOSI and 2-year ADOS	0.50	<0.0001	≈1.00
	High-risk Infants Only		
9-month VS and 15-month AOSI	0.223	0.049	0.454
9-month VS and 2-year ADOS	0.27	0.02	0.524
	Partial correlations		
9-month VS and 15-month AOSI, factoring out 9-month AOSI	0.182	0.046	0.546
9-month VS and 2-year ADOS, factoring out 9-month AOSI and 15-month AOSI	0.13	0.13*	0.655
All tests			0.052

Note: VS, visual search.
* The nonsignificant outcome was interpreted as consistent with the theoretical claims.

Table 11.1 reports the proportion of samples that produced the same outcome as reported by Gliga et al. (2015).

It should not be surprising that nearly all the estimated success probability values are above one-half. The estimated population correlations are based on the reported effects, which were all successful. Thus, random samples of the same size as the initial study from a population having these values should, most of the time, produce sample statistics that are successful (significant or nonsignificant, as appropriate). There is one exception; for the high-risk infants, a statistically significant correlation was found for the 9-month visual search scores and the 15-month AOSI scores. In the simulation experiments, the correlations and variances for the high-risk and control infants were assumed to be the same. The simulated test for high-risk infants simply used the first 70 scores in the sample (the actual number of high-risk infants that completed these conditions is not described in Gliga et al. [2015]). Consistent with this approach, the correlation for the full sample ($r = 0.22$) is nearly identical to that for the high-risk infants ($r = 0.223$). Nevertheless, the numbers reported in Gliga et al. (2015) for the test of the high-risk infants may contain an error. Using the reported beta, standard error, and a degrees of freedom of 68 gives $t = 2.027$ and $p = 0.0466$, which is smaller than the 0.049 reported in Gliga et al. (2015) and might suggest that the reported correlation is a bit too high (a correlation of 0.22, the same as for the full set, would give $p = 0.0495$). Whatever the source of the discrepancy, the effect on the estimated success probability is fairly small and does not substantively alter the conclusions given below.

In some cases, such as for the relationship between 15-month AOSI and 2-year ADOS scores, the probability of a significant result is very high. However, in more than half of the tests, the success probability is only around two-thirds, or lower. The final row of Table 11.1 shows the proportion of simulated experiments where all the tests produced a successful outcome (just as for the initial study).

This low value, 0.052, reflects the fact that when so many constraints are put on a data set, it is unlikely that a random sample of data will simultaneously satisfy them all.

If the effects are as estimated by the findings reported in Gliga et al. (2015), then 0.052 is the estimated probability that a replication experiment with the same sample size would reproduce the entire set of outcomes that support the theoretical conclusions. Thus, even if the theory is correct and the effects are real, the pattern of results used to support the theory is quite unlikely in a replication study. This prediction reflects the inherent uncertainty in measurements due to random sampling.

Given the rarity of uniform success for an experiment like the one reported by Gliga et al. (2015), readers should wonder how the original study happened to achieve such perfection. Recent investigations and analyses in psychology have revealed that many standard practices in psychological research tend to produce the kind of excess success that seems present in the findings of Gliga et al. (2015). These practices include publication bias, selective reporting of data and analyses, improper sampling methods, trying out various analyses to get $p < 0.05$, and hypothesizing after the results are known (HARKing) (Francis 2012a, 2012b; John et al. 2012; Kerr 1998; Schimmack 2012; Simmons et al. 2011). These practices are sometimes called "questionable research practices," "researcher degrees of freedom," and "*p*-hacking." From the available information, we cannot know which, if any, of these practices contributed to the excess success reported by Gliga et al. (2015). Indeed, following standard practice within psychological research, it is likely that the original authors do not have sufficient records to indicate whether they used some questionable research practices.

Regardless of the reasons for the apparent excess success in Gliga et al. (2015), readers should be skeptical about the accuracy of the reported data and/or the theory. Questionable research practices tend to inflate effect sizes (for significant outcomes) and increase Type I error rates. The impact of publication bias, improper sampling, and various forms of *p*-hacking have been well documented in previous studies (Francis 2012a, 2012b; Simmons et al. 2011). In the remainder of this chapter, I further explore the impact of what Kerr (1998) called HARKing.

TRUST YOUR DATA, BUT NOT TOO MUCH

Psychology is fundamentally an empirical science, where psychological scientists gather data and thereby draw theoretical conclusions. Such activities are a fundamental characteristic of every science, but due to random sampling, it is dangerous for a theory to follow too closely to experimental data. Fully trusting the data tends to generate overly complex models (with interactions and moderators) that track noise in the given sample and thereby perform poorly when used to predict future data.

A serious concern about HARKing is that it sometimes involves a misrepresentation of post hoc hypotheses as if they were prior hypotheses. In an extreme case, researchers explore their data set for various patterns and then generate hypotheses that are consistent with those patterns. If those hypotheses are subsequently reported as "predicting" the data, then researchers are lying about an important detail of their scientific investigation.

Importantly, the text of Gliga et al. (2015) does not suggest a misrepresentation of their hypotheses; rather, the text seems to indicate that their theory was intentionally designed to match their experimental findings. Had their data turned out differently, the authors would have reached different theoretical conclusions. It is understandable why Gliga et al. (2015) would behave this way; after all, scientists should change their theories when new data appears. Nevertheless, as shown below, staying too close to the experimental data creates implausible theories that will not appear valid on retesting.

Essentially every data set in psychological research contains noise, if for no other reason than the process of selecting a random sample from a population. Ideally, a theory ignores the noise and focuses on meaningful signals, but it is difficult to satisfy this ideal. Hypothesis testing uses statistical significance to determine whether a data set contains a signal (along with noise) or just noise. The standard $p < 0.05$ criterion reflects an effort to, over the long term, limit the probability of concluding the presence of a signal when there is only noise (make a Type I error). Of course, any criterion for deciding the presence of a signal also includes a risk of not detecting the signal (along with noise) when it really does exist (making a Type II error).

Researchers sometimes use statistical significance as a criterion for constructing a theoretical model. In this model construction process, significance is used to determine whether or not to include a factor, or level within a factor, as part of a theoretical model or explanation of an effect. For example, if there is a significant main effect of sex on the dependent variable, then sex becomes a relevant factor for the theoretical explanation of the effect. Likewise, if there is not a significant main effect of age on the dependent variable, then age is excluded from the theoretical explanation of the effect. If there is a significant interaction of age and sex, then researchers include the interaction in the model and often pursue various contrasts to determine the nature of the interaction and include these details as part of the theoretical explanation of the data. For some investigations, this kind of model construction process seems to be the whole point of testing for significance.

Unfortunately, model construction based on statistical significance is often a poor way to build theoretical models. The resulting models tend to become either unjustifiably complicated or unjustifiably simple. For example, when analyzing data from a 2 × 2 between-subjects analysis of variance (ANOVA), researchers may build their theoretical model by following the significant outcomes in the ANOVA: including or excluding terms as determined by statistical significance. But suppose the researcher then tested the resulting model by gathering a new set of data from the same population with the same sample sizes. What is the success probability of producing the same pattern of significant and nonsignificant outcomes?

The success probability depends on the details of the population, and can be explored with simulated data for a large number of 2 × 2 between-subjects designs. Figure 11.1 schematizes the structure of the simulations. On each run, the simulation first randomly selected four values from a normal distribution having a mean of zero and a standard deviation of SDp. These values were then set as population means for a simulated experiment. When SDp was small (e.g., 0.1), the four values tended to be close to each other, relative to the population standard deviation, which was set to the value 1. When SDp was large (e.g., 3), the four values tended to be quite different from each other.

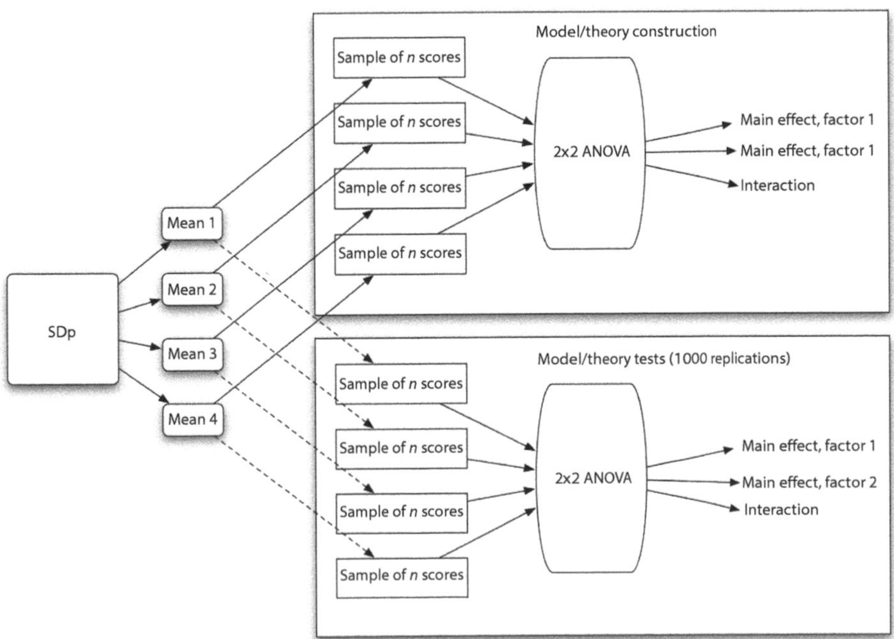

FIGURE 11.1 Schematic of simulations to examine the effects of HARKing on replication success.

With the population means defined, random samples of size n were then drawn from each population (assuming a normal distribution with a standard deviation of 1.0) and submitted to a 2 × 2 between-subjects ANOVA. The theoretical model was then defined by the pattern of significant and nonsignificant outcomes of the ANOVA. (In many cases, researchers would probably further specify the model by looking at various contrasts to explore the details of a significant interaction, and including contrasts in the model construction process would only amplify the problems described below.) This model construction process is a simulated version of HARKing.

To test the constructed theoretical model, 1000 replication experiments with the same sample size were randomly drawn from the same populations and analyzed in the very same way as the initial data set. To estimate success probability, the simulation calculated the proportion of replication experiments that produced the same pattern of significant and nonsignificant outcomes as the initial data set. This model construction and testing procedure was repeated 100 times with different population means, and Figure 11.2 plots the median proportion of replication experiments that matched the constructed model against the SDp value that was used to define the population means. The different curves are for different sample sizes, n.

To understand Figure 11.2, first look at the height of the curve on the far left when SDp = 0. In this case, the population means equal each other, so the null hypothesis is true. Most of the models (correctly) conclude that there is no difference between the means, but Type I errors will result in approximately 14% of the data sets producing at least one significant main effect or interaction. Regardless of the validity of the model, the replication studies agree with the created model about 85% of the time, and this property is largely unaffected by the sample size.

Now consider the right side of the curve, where the SDp value is large, and population means tend to be quite different relative to the standard deviation of the populations. Here the large-sample initial studies tend to find many significant results (main effects and an interaction) because such effects actually exist in the simulated populations. Because the effects are so strong, the large sample tests have high experimental power, so the replication studies also tend to reproduce the same pattern of significant and (some) nonsignificant outcomes. For smaller sample sizes, the replication studies are less successful, and that is to be expected because with lower experimental power, replication studies will often not produce the same outcomes as the initial sample, simply due to random sampling.

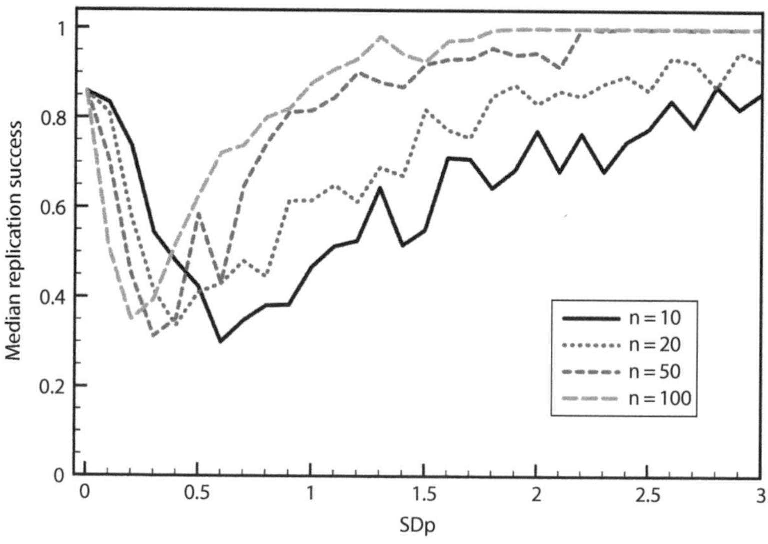

FIGURE 11.2 Replication success rate for experiments analyzed with a HARKing model creation method. Replicability is low when SDp is around 0.5 because the means tend to be modestly different from each other and the hypothesis tests are sensitive to random noise.

The really curious finding is for the relatively small values of SDp. Many of the values between 0 and 1 lead to poor reproducibility (as low as 30%) of the findings in the original data set, and this dip is present regardless of sample size. The frequent failure to replicate occurs because the population means created for these SDp values tend to be different enough to produce experiments with moderate power for one or more of the tests. Which tests have moderate power varies with the sample size. For example, if the original data set with $n = 10$ generates a significant main effect, there is a decent chance that a replication study will not produce the same significant main effect. At the same time, an initial data set with such a small sample is unlikely to produce a significant interaction effect (the power is lower), and replication studies will likewise usually produce the same nonsignificant outcome. In contrast, for a larger sample size, the power for the test of a main effect is high, and both the original and replication studies are likely to show it. However, power for an interaction is lower, and if the original data set happens to generate a nonsignificant interaction, there is a decent chance that a replication study will produce a significant interaction, and vice versa.

A researcher further exploring an interaction with various contrasts, or checking if significant effects also hold for a subset of the data, continues this exploration of tests with lower power. Thus, even if the power to find some effects is fairly strong, the researcher inadvertently undermines the replicability of the results by generating additional model characteristics (based on the outcome of additional tests) that inevitably reduce the probability of replication success. If scientists use a significant finding as incentive to pursue ever more model complexity until they are faced with nonsignificant outcomes, then they will interpret their data in a way that often fails to replicate in future studies.

I suspect that something similar to this model construction approach is what underlies, at least in part, the low predicted replicability of the findings in Gliga et al. (2015). If this interpretation is correct, then they analyzed the data to create a theoretical model with what seemed to be maximum accountability for the observed pattern of significant and nonsignificant outcomes. Unfortunately, such a model is unlikely to lead to successful replications. As a result, readers should doubt the validity of the model proposed by Gliga et al. (2015). The impression of the article would perhaps be worse if the apparent excess success in Gliga et al. (2015) is due to publication bias or improper sampling. In that case, the data itself might be called into question.

AN ALTERNATIVE APPROACH

The primary problem with model construction by statistical significance is that the resulting theoretical models fit both signal and noise and thereby do not generalize well when used to predict future data. There are alternative inferential analysis frameworks that try to control for model noise fitting (sometimes called "overfitting" the data) by balancing the goodness of the model's fit to the data against the model's complexity (Pitt and Myung 2002). A more complex model will generally do a better job matching a given data set, but the flexibility of a complex model also allows it to match noise in the data set. Since the noise will change for a new data sample, a complex model that fits noise will generally not perform well when used to predict future data. In terms of predicting future data, a simple model might perform better than a complex model, even though the simple model may not match the original data set as well as the complex model.

One approach for choosing among candidate models uses the Akaike information criterion (AIC) (Akaike 1974). For a given set of data and a given model, it combines a measure of how well the model fits the data and a measure of the model's complexity. The basic format is

$$\text{AIC} = 2\text{m} - 2\ln(L)$$

where m is the number of independent parameters in the model, L is the likelihood of the data given the best possible parameter values, and ln( ) refers to the natural logarithm. Larger values of L correspond to a better fit of the model to the data. The fit measure is subtracted from the number of parameters, so smaller values of AIC (perhaps being negative) indicate better support for the model. To understand the calculations, first consider the simplest (null) model for the 2×2 between-subjects design discussed above, where all the cells have a common mean value, μ, and a common standard deviation, σ. These ($m = 2$) parameter values can be estimated from the data using standard calculations for population parameters (these are maximum likelihood estimations). Designate these estimates as $\hat{\mu}$ and $\hat{\sigma}$. If the model assumes the population distribution follows a normal distribution, then the log likelihood for the null model is

$$\ln(L) = -\frac{N}{2}\ln(2\pi\hat{\sigma}^2) - \frac{1}{2\hat{\sigma}^2}\sum_{i=1}^{N}(X_i - \hat{\mu})^2$$

which is derived by multiplying the normal distribution probability density, using the estimated mean and standard deviation, that corresponds to each of the N points in the data set. This product is the likelihood of the entire data set, given this model. When taking the logarithm of the likelihood, the product becomes a sum.

By itself, a value of AIC does not mean very much. Its usefulness is in allowing comparison between models. For example, consider a slightly more complex ($m = 3$) model that supposes different means for the rows of the 2 × 2 between-subjects design, μ_1 and μ_2, along with a common standard deviation, σ. For this model, the calculation of log likelihood would be

$$\ln(L) = \left[-\frac{N_1}{2}\ln(2\pi\hat{\sigma}^2) - \frac{1}{2\hat{\sigma}^2}\sum_{i=1}^{N_1}(X_{i1} - \hat{\mu}_1)^2\right] + \left[-\frac{N_2}{2}\ln(2\pi\hat{\sigma}^2) - \frac{1}{2\hat{\sigma}^2}\sum_{i=1}^{N_2}(X_{i2} - \hat{\mu}_2)^2\right]$$

where $N_1 + N_2 = N$ reflects the sample sizes for the different rows of the design, X_{i1} indicates the data points from the first row, and X_{i2} indicates the data points from the second row. The null model is a special case of the row model (where the two means are equal), which means the row model will always produce a log-likelihood value at least as large as the null model, and it will typically produce a larger log-likelihood value than the null model. However, the AIC calculation includes the number of independent parameters ($m = 2$ for the null model and $m = 3$ for the row model). Smaller AIC values provide better support for a given model, and the question is whether the increase in the log likelihood of going from the null to the row model (better fit to the data) more than compensates for the increase in the number of parameters (higher complexity). To compare the two models, subtract their AIC values:

$$\Delta AIC = AIC(\text{null}) - AIC(\text{row})$$

Since smaller AIC values indicate more support for a model, if $\Delta AIC > 0$, then the data support the row model. If $\Delta AIC < 0$, then the data support the null model. Unlike the $p < 0.05$ rule that is popular in hypothesis testing, the ΔAIC criterion is not arbitrary. The "support" derived from the data reflects (estimated) performance of the selected model for predicting future data. We do not have to accept (or believe) that either the null or the row model is a very good model, but if $\Delta AIC > 0$, then the row model is expected to do a better job predicting future data than the null model. This property holds for large samples; for small samples, model selection based on ΔAIC tends to favor complex models over simple models. An extra penalty on the number of parameters for small samples corrects the AIC calculation (Hurvich and Tsai 1989):

$$AICc = AIC + \frac{2m(m+1)}{N-m-1}$$

For large sample sizes, the extra correction term goes to zero, so AIC and AICc become equivalent. The analysis is not limited to comparing just two models. It is easy to compute an AICc value for a "column" model ($m = 3$), for a model that considers effects of both the row and column structure of

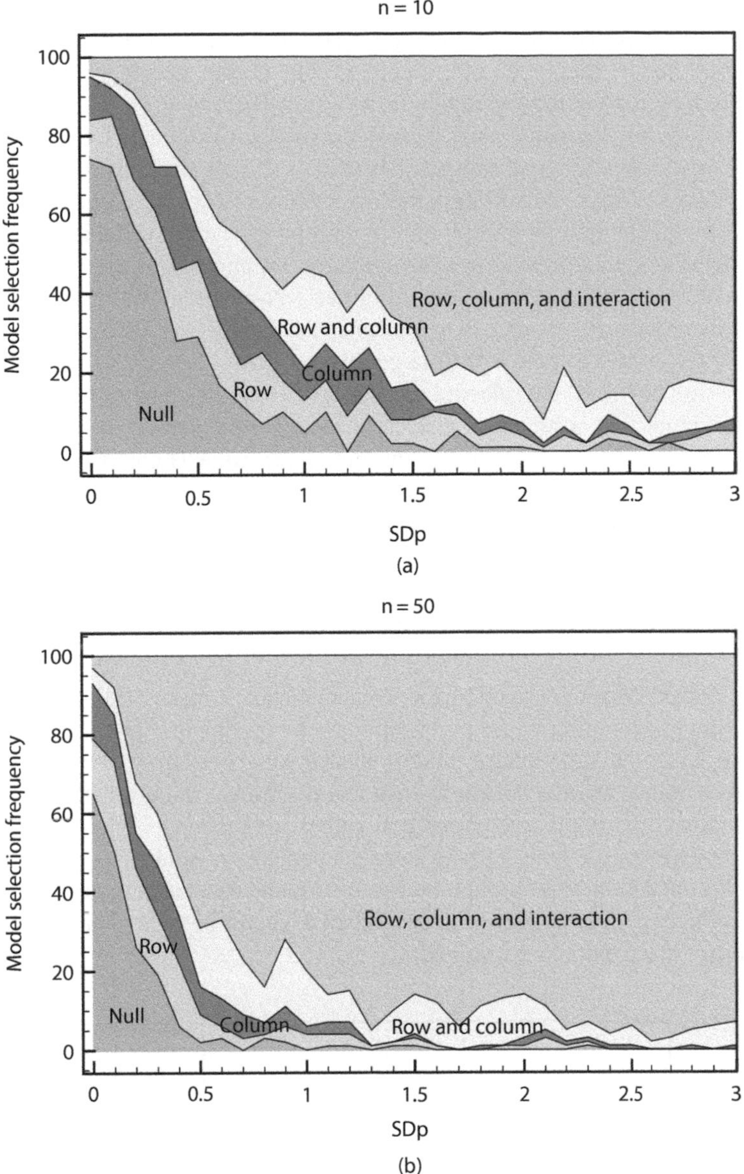

FIGURE 11.3 The frequencies of selecting different model types as a function of SDp. Larger values of SDp generally produce more variability among the population means. The null model is most commonly selected for SDp = 0, but as the population means become more variable, the most complicated model is usually selected. (a) Sample sizes of 10 for each of four cells. (b) Sample sizes of 50 for each of four.

the 2 × 2 design but does not consider an interaction ($m = 4$), and for a model that considers effects of the row, column, and interaction ($m = 5$). As before, the question is whether the increase in likelihood compensates for the increase in complexity. In terms of predicting future data, the best model is the one with the smallest AICc value.

Figure 11.3 shows how often different model types are selected as a function of the SDp parameter used to define the means of the 2 × 2 between-subjects design. In Figure 12.3a, the sample size for each cell is $n = 10$, and in Figure 12.3b, the sample size is $n = 50$. First, focus on the far left of each graph, where SDp = 0 and the null hypothesis is true (all population means are equal).

For data generated from such populations, the model selection process usually selects the null model, especially for the small sample size. Unlike hypothesis testing, inferences based on model selection do not directly try to control the Type I error rate, and with a larger sample size, the null model is less commonly selected, even when the population is truly null. The loss of Type I error control may seem like a big price to pay, but the gain is that the selected model is estimated to best predict future data (and one never knows when a hypothesis test has made a Type I error anyhow).

For nonzero values of SDp, the null hypothesis is almost always false (the population means are chosen randomly). As SDp increases, the sample means become more variable, so it is not surprising that the null model is less often selected and that the most complicated model (row, column, and interaction) is more often selected. A comparison of Figure 11.3a and b indicates that the switch in model selection preference occurs for smaller SDp values as the sample size increases, which is similar to how a hypothesis test increases power with larger sample sizes.

Figure 11.4 shows how well the selected models predict the outcome of replication experiments. To investigate the predictive accuracy of a selected model, 1000 simulated replication experiments (same sample size and population means as the initial experiment) compared new sample values with predicted values from the selected model. The performance of the model for a replication experiment was measured as mean squared error (MSE):

$$MSE = \frac{\sum_{i=1}^{N} (X_i - \hat{y}_i)^2}{N}$$

where $\hat{y}_i$ is the predicted value as derived by the selected model. A mean MSE value was computed for each selected model by averaging across every replication experiment. Figure 11.4 shows the average mean MSE value across the 100 selected models at each value of SDp. As is to be expected, MSE is larger for models based on smaller samples. With larger samples, the estimated means and standard deviation are usually closer to the true population values and the model produces better predictions. Prediction accuracy never goes below 1.0 because the population variance equals 1.0, and this variability cannot be accounted for by a model based on means and the standard deviation. That is, even if the true model (with the population means and standard deviation) were available, there would still be sampling variability that cannot be explained.

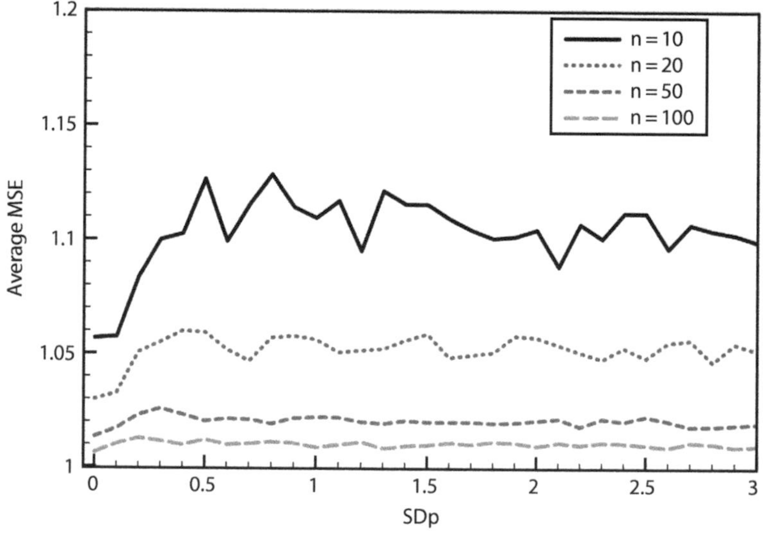

FIGURE 11.4 Average MSE for 1000 replication experiments as a function of SDp for models selected by the AICc analysis.

It might seem curious that average MSE is generally smallest for SDp = 0, but this makes sense because here the null model tends to be the most commonly selected model. When this model is selected, the single mean value is estimated by pooling data across all four cells of the 2 × 2 design. Thus, even for the smallest sample size ($n = 10$), 40 data points are used to estimate the mean, which generally produces a good estimate. In contrast, for larger SDp values, the most complicated model tends to be selected, but then each mean is estimated from only 10 data points. As a result, these relatively poor-quality estimates lead to poor predictions and higher MSE.

Importantly, the overfitting problems that plague hypothesis testing, as indicated in Figure 11.2, are addressed by the AIC type of analysis. In particular, the analysis does not enable researchers to develop ever more complex models that (eventually) fit noise in the data set. A researcher can consider more complicated models (e.g., with various contrasts between conditions), but at some point, the gain in terms of model fit is outweighed by the cost of using more parameters.

The reported findings and theoretical conclusions presented by Gliga et al. (2015) seem too good to be true. Given the sample sizes, estimated correlations, and experimental design, full success for the relevant hypothesis tests is rather unlikely. As such, readers should be skeptical about the validity of the data and/or the conclusions in Gliga et al. (2015). One possible explanation for such excess success is that the theoretical conclusions were derived directly from the outcomes of the hypothesis tests (HARKing). Such an explanation is plausible because it seems to be a common approach to theory development in psychological science. Unfortunately, further analysis indicates that models built with a HARKing approach are unreliable in the sense that their predicted outcomes are unlikely to fully replicate.

An alternative analysis approach to model development avoids HARKing by pitting a model's fit to empirical data against the model's complexity. These computations help researchers select a model that best predicts future data and thereby protect against selecting overly complex models that fit noise in a given sample. The AIC types of selection methods described in this chapter can be applied to many other situations (Burnham and Anderson 2003), and conceptually similar approaches using Bayesian analysis methods can take advantage of informative prior information (Gelman et al. 2014; Kruschke 2010; Lee and Wagenmakers 2014). Once starting these kinds of investigations, it often becomes apparent that model selection is not the only relevant inference that matters to researchers, and prediction through model averaging and related techniques is also sometimes valuable (e.g., Burnham and Anderson 2004).

The excess success that appears in Gliga et al. (2015) is arguably a reflection of standard theory construction methods in psychological science. Readers should recognize the dangers of this standard practice, and researchers should explore alternative theory construction methods that better satisfy their scientific goals.

REFERENCES

Akaike, H. 1974. A new look at the statistical model identification. *IEEE Trans Automat Contr* 19 (6):716–23.

Burnham, K. P., and D. R. Anderson. 2003. *Model Selection and Multimodel Inference: A Practical Information-Theoretic Approach*. Berlin: Springer Science & Business Media.

Burnham, K. P., and D. R. Anderson. 2004. Multimodel inference understanding AIC and BIC in model selection. *Sociol Methods Res* 33 (2):261–304.

Cumming, G. 2008. Replication and p intervals: p values predict the future only vaguely, but confidence intervals do much better. *Perspect Psychol Sci* 3 (4):286–300.

Francis, G. 2012a. The psychology of replication and replication in psychology. *Perspect Psychol Sci* 7 (6): 585–94.

Francis, G. 2012b. Publication bias and the failure of replication in experimental psychology. *Psychon Bull Rev* 19 (6):975–91.

Francis, G. 2012c. Too good to be true: Publication bias in two prominent studies from experimental psychology. *Psychon Bull Rev* 19 (2):151–6.

Gelman, A., J. B. Carlin, H. S. Stern, and D. B. Rubin. 2014. *Bayesian Data Analysis*. Vol. 2. Boca Raton, FL: CRC Press/Chapman & Hall.

Gliga, T., R. Bedford, T. Charman, M. H. Johnson, and BASIS Team. 2015. Enhanced visual search in infancy predicts emerging autism symptoms. *Curr Biol* 25 (13):1727–30.

Hurvich, C. M., and C.-L. Tsai. 1989. Regression and time series model selection in small samples. *Biometrika* 76:297–307.

Ioannidis, J. P. A., and T. A. Trikalinos. 2007. An exploratory test for an excess of significant findings. *Clin Trials* 4 (3):245–53.

John, L. K., G. Loewenstein, and D. Prelec. 2012. Measuring the prevalence of questionable research practices with incentives for truth telling. *Psychol Sci* 23 (5):524–32.

Kerr, N. L. 1998. HARKing: Hypothesizing after the results are known. *Pers Soc Psychol Rev* 2 (3):196–217.

Kruschke, J. K. 2010. *Doing Bayesian Data Analysis: A Tutorial with R and BUGS*. London: Academic Press.

Lee, M. D., and E.-J. Wagenmakers. 2014. *Bayesian Cognitive Modeling: A Practical Course*. Cambridge: Cambridge University Press.

Pitt, M. A., and I. J. Myung. 2002. When a good fit can be bad. *Trends Cogn Sci* 6 (10):421–5.

R Core Team. 2014. R: A language and environment for statistical computing. Vienna: R Foundation for Statistical Computing.

Schimmack, U. 2012. The ironic effect of significant results on the credibility of multiple-study articles. *Psychol Methods* 17 (4):551.

Simmons, J. P., L. D. Nelson, and U. Simonsohn. 2011. False-positive psychology: Undisclosed flexibility in data collection and analysis allows presenting anything as significant. *Psychol Sci* 22 (11):1359–66.

Simonsohn, U., L. D. Nelson, and J. P. Simmons. 2014. P-curve: A key to the file-drawer. *J Exp Psychol Gen* 143 (2):534.

van Assen, M. A. L. M., R. van Aert, and J. M. Wicherts. 2015. Meta-analysis using effect size distributions of only statistically significant studies. *Psychol Methods* 20 (3):293.

12 Contemporary Problems with Methods in Basic Brain Science Impede Progress in ASD Research and Treatments

Elizabeth B. Torres

CONTENTS

Introduction 178
Problem 1: Linear, Static Models Imposed on Neurodevelopmental Data That Are Inherently Nonlinear and have Complex Dynamics 179
Why Is This Important to Consider in ASD? 181
Problem 2: Imposition of Normality in Data That Are Not Normally Distributed 182
Why Is This Important to Consider in ASD? 184
Problem 3: Activity Required for Spontaneously Self-Supervised and Self-Corrective Internal Models 186
Why Is This Important to Consider in ASD? 188
From Neuromotor Control to Predictive Social Behavior 189
Orderly Development of Control Levels in the Infant's Nervous System 190
Problem 4: Lack of a Proper Taxonomy of Control Levels in Motor Research 191
Why Is This Important to Consider in ASD? 192
Problem 5: Lack of Models to Assess and Track Social Interactions in a Disorder Defined as a Social Communication Deficit 192
Conclusions and Take-Home Message 193
References 194

This chapter identifies and discusses five central problems concerning the basic scientific approaches for data gathering, analyses, and interpretation in the subfield of behavioral neuroscience. We illustrate these issues using empirical data where current assumption of linearity and normality in data that are inherently otherwise has masked important clinical phenomena and obstructed the path to Precision Medicine. Within the subfields of basic scientific research and clinical practices, we posit that these problems are preventing us from unveiling first principles of brain functioning, including those related to the question of how deliberate autonomy and intelligence may emerge in a nascent, developing nervous system. The chapter provides examples from several timelines of the human life span. These include neurodevelopment, childhood, youth, and adulthood. The hope is to provide enough evidence to convince our readership that we already have the proper tools to transform contemporary research and clinical practices toward personalized targeted treatments for precision psychiatry. All we need is not to impose any a priori assumptions on our data, and rather let their inherent variabilities guide our statistical inquiry.

INTRODUCTION

We are entering a new transformative era in the medical field—an era of precision medicine. With the advent of new technological advances and approaches to basic science, we are poised for an accelerated rate of change in our ability to generate, gather, integrate, analyze, and interpret data from the human brain and body in an attempt to deliver individualized target treatments. Amidst this transformation in the medical field are the scientific disciplines related to the studies of the nervous systems and their pathologies. Among the many disciplines addressing neuropsychiatric and neurological disorders of the nervous systems are those that for assessment and diagnoses of nervous system disorders primarily employ the bottom layers of the knowledge network of the precision medicine platform (shown in Figure 12.1). More specifically, these layers feed from participant-contributed data and ordinal data obtainable from subjective clinical tests. These tests rely on the observation of behaviors. In principle, subsequent layers under the realm of "behaviors" could connect the ordinal data from clinical inventories to the data from the top layers—those including genetic-related information. Nevertheless, now this is not possible because of the rather incomplete contemporary methods that psychiatry and psychology use to analyze behaviors.

The psychiatric and psychological constructs that have guided basic brain and health research in the medical fields related to mental health do not have a proper infrastructure in place to gather, analyze, and interpret physiological data underlying the types of ordinal data derived from observation and subjective interpretation of behavior. In this sense, the motor output generated by the nervous systems producing those behaviors provides a window into the brain functioning as it pertains to motor control, adaptive behavior, and plasticity in general. These physiological data could help bridge the ordinal scores from observation and interpretation of behaviors to the somatic motor physiology. If science really wanted to benefit from the new tenets of this revolutionary era of precision medicine (Figure 12.1) and build an interconnected knowledge network, the fields related to mental health may necessarily have to transform their methods to include analytics that can handle continuous output from the nervous systems. This output comes in the form of biorhythms, that is, time series of parameters harnessed from different levels of control, spanning from the autonomic to the involuntary to the voluntary layers of the peripheral nervous system (PNS) and central nervous system (CNS).

In this chapter, we identify five central problems concerning the basic scientific approaches for data gathering, analyses, and interpretation in the subfield of behavioral neuroscience. The lack of a proper analytical framework in this important subfield and several of its current approaches to

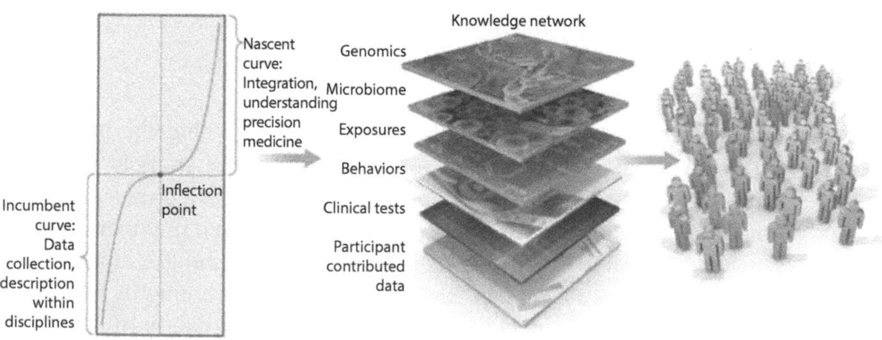

FIGURE 12.1 Toward true personalized medicine in new behavioral sciences. "An inflection point marks an opportunity or moment of dramatic change between the first, or incumbent curve, marking steady progress, and a second, or nascent, curve, indicating transformation and accelerated progress. In biomedical research, health, and health care, we are at an inflection point, poised for precision medicine". This chapter addresses some of the pitfalls and fundamental flaws in the conceptualization and analyses of the layer of behaviors currently obstructing the proper integration between the lower and upper layers of the knowledge network. (Reproduced with permission from Hawgood et al. *Sci Transl Med* 7(300):300ps17, 2015.)

attempt to connect clinical scores and electrophysiology may be preventing the field of autism from unveiling first principles of brain functioning, including those related to the question of how deliberate autonomy and intelligence may emerge in a nervous system.

More specifically, throughout this chapter we expose a subset of problems at the level of *behaviors* in the knowledge network of Figure 12.1. We argue that so long as these problems remain unaddressed, the bottom layers of the knowledge network concerning clinical data will remain disconnected from the higher layers concerning genomics—the latter are critical not only to develop target drugs for personalized treatments of disease, but also to identify and longitudinally track off-target side effects. Indeed, since observing behaviors is the main method to catalogue disorders of the nervous systems, these subjective means lead to highly heterogeneous disorders. Further, the observational methods in use to track disease progression and/or intervention effectiveness are not appropriate. They miss the physiological evolution of a coping biological system suffering from such disorders. Several classes of psychotropic drugs, originally developed for other purposes in an adult system, are now commonly prescribed under the *Diagnostic and Statistical Manual of Mental Disorders* (DSM) criteria (American Psychiatric Association 2013) to treat observable symptoms of *neurodevelopmental* disorders like autism spectrum disorder (ASD) and attention deficit hyperactivity disorder (ADHD). As mentioned in the concluding remarks of Section I of the book, the accelerated rates of change of physical growth and neurodevelopment in the young nervous systems stand in marked contrast to the steady-state rate of change of the adult nervous systems. As such, it is dangerous to use psychotropic drugs in infants and children without proper monitoring treatment outcomes. Psychotropic drugs by definition alter the nervous systems' functioning and have unknown long-term consequences for neurodevelopment.

We argue in favor of the use of new data types and new personalized statistical approaches to analyze natural behaviors as a transformative means to help accelerate the discovery of targeted treatments and dynamically track both changes in targeted symptoms and off-target side effects in each child.

PROBLEM 1: LINEAR, STATIC MODELS IMPOSED ON NEURODEVELOPMENTAL DATA THAT ARE INHERENTLY NONLINEAR AND HAVE COMPLEX DYNAMICS

One of the top priorities in current ASD research is to identify biomarkers that could flag risk of potential stunting in neurodevelopment at an early age—to facilitate early intervention. The methods used to measure progress in physical development, however, are doing so under the implicit assumption that the processes governing neurodevelopment are linear in nature. As such, researchers and clinicians primarily use parametric, linear methods to chart and track physical growth despite their extremely accelerated rate of change (Figure 12.2). Take, for instance, the population growth charts used by pediatricians today to measure physical parameters, such as infant body length, body weight, and head circumference.

The standardized population growth charts have been created and produced by both the Centers for Disease Control and Prevention (CDC) (Kuczmarski et al. 2000) and the World Health Organization (WHO) (Grummer-Strawn et al. 2010), with recommendations to use the CDC-WHO charts due to discrepancies and variation in data collection and thus chart formulation (de Onis and Onyango 2003). These growth charts reflect adjustments for breast-feeding, race, sex, and other important parameters that the WHO has considered (de Onis and Onyango 2003; Zorlu and de Onis 2011). Since 2006, the standard charts have been adopted by more than 140 nations, including the United States. They remain the gold standard to assess mortality indexes and determine milestones of physical growth. The growth charts are not a diagnostic tool. Nonetheless, pediatricians often use them to infer general aspects of neurodevelopmental progress. The charts conform to statistical rigor (Flegal and Cole 2013; Kuczmarski et al. 2002) and use incremental (velocity-dependent) values to capture the rates of physical change of the infant. Pediatricians may also combine their use with a handful of motor milestones to track early developmental progress. Yet, these charts alone may not necessarily

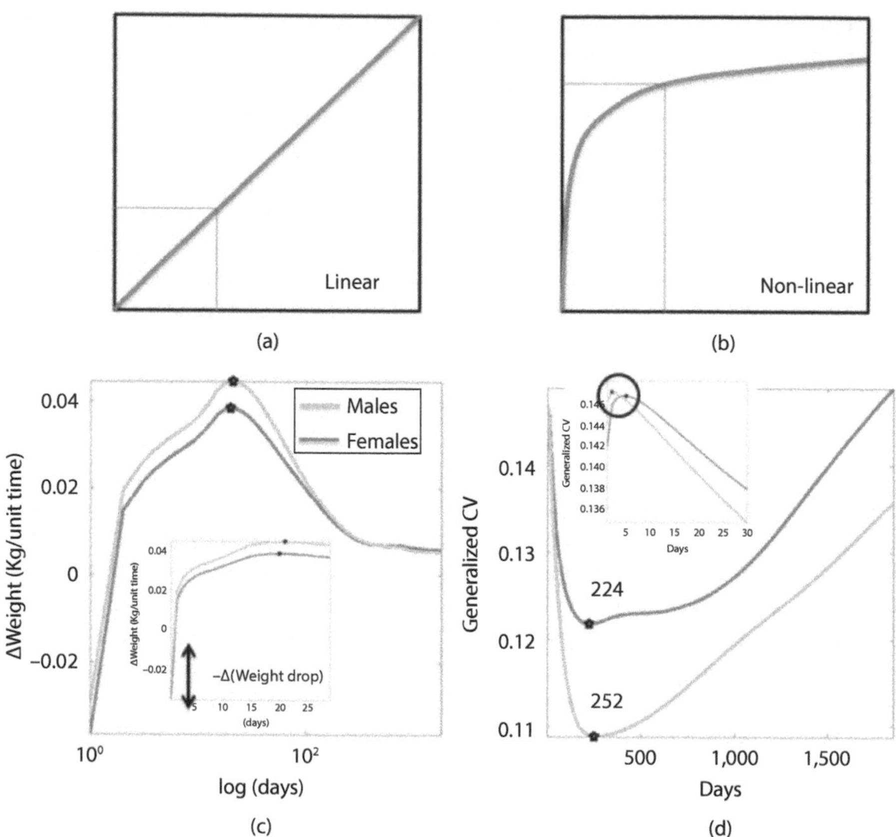

FIGURE 12.2 Nonlinear nature of physical growth reflected in the rate of change of weight of the newborn expressed in kilograms per day. (a, b) Linear vs. nonlinear changes presented in schematic form. (c) Curves representing longitudinal changes in body weight (kg/day) collected from 2 years of age and then switched to cross-sectional data up to 5 years of age (log day units). Each data point is from the day-to-day change in the median value of the weight, taken across 26,985 babies per summary point (13,623 females and 13,362 males). Note the accelerated rate of change in the initial month (as in the nonlinear curve in (b)), whereby the inset graph zooms in and shows the highly variable patterns, i.e., the initial drop in weight the typical newborn experiences followed by accelerated increase. Note as well the early separation between the female and male typical baby already visible in (d), where an inflexion point of the generalized coefficient of variation (CV) indicates marked differences in weight variations. Females lead by almost a month in attaining that inflexion point, marking the switch from steady increase to a drop in the rate of change appreciated in (c). The inset zooms in the first month, where by the first week the males reach a peak in generalized CV before the females do. Under the linear umbrella currently used by pediatricians to assess babies (using absolute values visit by visit), such important changes will be missed. (Reproduced with permission from Torres et al., *Front. Pediatr.*, 4:121, 2016.)

capture the true nature of early neurodevelopment—particularly those aspects of neurodevelopment pertaining to the type of neural control of movements reached by 4–5 years of age—the limiting age of the growth charts.

The methods to develop the charts are openly available (along with the data used to derive the growth parameters) (de Onis and Onyango 2003; Kuczmarski et al. 2002). We made use of such data to help illustrate our point on the nonlinear nature of infant growth (Figure 12.2). In Figure 12.2, we illustrate the results of reexamining these publicly available data under a different lens to track the longitudinal incremental progression of the weight change, day by day, in male and female newborn babies. To that end, we used the median weight drawn from 26,985 babies per summary point (13,623 females and 13,362 males). The data reflect the longitudinal tracking of these babies for the first 2 years of life, upon which the tracking switches to cross-sectional data until 5 years of age is reached. The nonlinear, accelerated rate of change of all physical parameters (head circumference, body length, and body weight) hints at the need to use nonlinear mathematical frameworks for analyses of infant data in general.

Why Is This Important to Consider in ASD?

Rapid changes in the functioning of the nervous systems embedded in the physical body of the developing infant accompany the accelerated rates of change of that physical body during the first years of life. Indeed, when such changes stunt and their effects on socialization become evident, clinicians may confer a diagnosis of an ASD. This typically takes place around 3 years of age, when some degree of uncertainty about the diagnosis still prevails. As the child grows and does not develop language or other social and/or communicative skills, the initial diagnosis acquires more certainty. Evidently, the first 3 years of life are critical in the formation of synapses and self-organization of neural networks of the (peripheral) somatic motor systems and their projections to the cerebrocortical (central) systems. Through the sensing of the physical rhythms that the baby's system itself causes, the brain can learn to self-regulate and self-track self-generated actions. In turn, attaining a balance between the rates of physical change and the rates of neuromotor control seems critical to learn to adapt, self-correct, self-predict, and self-control the bodily motions that the brain gradually learns to own.

Our study of the newborn baby revealed that early neuromotor control typically develops at rates comparable to those of physical body growth (Torres et al. 2016c). In babies that undergo stunting in neuromotor development, it is possible to detect the slowdown or the altogether halting of typical rates in motor control acquisition within the first 4–5 months. We believe that it may be possible to detect the problem even earlier to immediately intervene.

The growth of motor and sensory neuronal nerves embedded in the body and head accompanies their nonlinear growth. To develop autonomous control, the nervous systems must develop proper myelination, form synapses, and build circuits to communicate neural information to and from the CNS and PNS. The emergence of the self as a percept, the development of self-supervised control, and eventually self-supervised corrections must be critical to attain the overall development of agency and volition. Scientists in the fields of development and pediatrics may need to adopt proper mathematical tools and data types that enable the continuous longitudinal measurements of such processes in the very early stages of life. Because they initially unfold so fast, if we wait 3 months to start quantifying them in the newborn, we will surely miss a critical period to scaffold the development of the nervous systems and their acquisition of autonomy.

The individualized treatment of the problem of stunting in neuromotor control or in the rate of physical growth is important because when developmental stagnation occurs, the nervous systems of the neonate will develop compensatory coping strategies specific to each individual. In this sense, the "one-size-fits-all" model of traditional behavioral analysis and population growth charts will obscure information required to enable early detection of risk for stunting. A personalized analytical approach would also follow the tenets of precision medicine in Figure 12.1.

We need to build dynamic and individualized growth charts. Owing to the accelerated rate of physical growth of the neonate, we need to update the chart on a daily basis. This would not be difficult to do today if we were to combine daily physical measurements of body growth with daily tracking of neuromotor control using wearable sensing technology. Indeed, one model to follow may be the use of a simple home-based application (app) coupling commercially available smartphones to other smart sensing devices located on the baby's body (e.g., Figure 12.3). If the rates of change in neuromotor control are not congruent with those in physical growth, a potential problem should be flagged and an intervention recommended within the first months of life (Torres et al. 2016c).

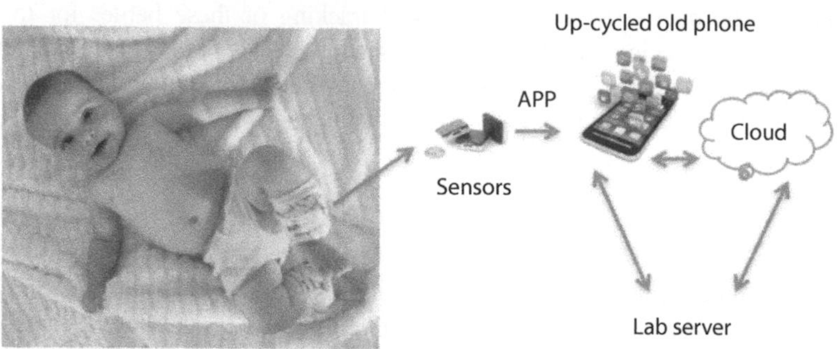

FIGURE 12.3 Toward a new path of early detection and early intervention combining concepts and methods from mobile-health, big data analytics and the tenets of personalized precision medicine.

PROBLEM 2: IMPOSITION OF NORMALITY IN DATA THAT ARE NOT NORMALLY DISTRIBUTED

The data employed to construct the WHO-CDC growth charts also revealed the non-Gaussian nature of the variability in physical growth across the population. The variable skewness of the probability distributions characterizing individual development and those characterizing the trends across the population were captured by tracking the Box–Cox L transformation parameter. This is used in a power transformation reported in the "Methods" paper (Kuczmarski et al. 2002) to enforce symmetry in skewed probability distributions (Flegal and Cole 2013). Quoting from the original "Methods" paper (emphasis added by the author),

> The distributions of some anthropometric data used in the growth charts are skewed. To remove skewness, a power transformation can be used to stretch one tail of the distribution while the other tail is shrunk. A Box-Cox transformation can make the distribution nearly normal (Box and Cox 1964). *The assumption is that, after the appropriate power transformation, the data are closely approximated by a normal distribution* (Cole 1990). The transformation does not adjust for kurtosis, which is a less important contributor to non-normality than skewness (Cole and Green 1992).
>
> In the LMS* technique, three parameters are estimated: the median (M), the generalized coefficient of variation (S), and the power in the Box-Cox transformation (L). The L reflects the degree of skewness. The LMS transformation equation is:
>
> $$X = M\,(1 + LSZ)^{1/L} \quad L \neq 0$$
>
> $$X = M\,e^{(SZ)} \quad L = 0$$
>
> where X is the physical measurement and Z is the z-score that corresponds to the percentile.
>
> The key task of the transformation was to estimate parameters L, M, and S.
>
> With estimates of L, M, and S, values of X are connected to the values of Z through the above equation. The percentile is obtained from a *normal distribution table* where the z-score corresponds to the percentile of interest. For example, a z-score of 0.2019 corresponds to the 58th percentile. In the case of growth charts, with the L, M, and S parameters, it is possible to evaluate any single measure in a population as an exact z-score or percentile.

It is rather unfortunate that the methods enforced normality on the skewed distributions underlying the anthropometric parameters used to build the population growth charts (e.g., see incremental weight [kg/day] distribution in Figure 12.4a). In this regard, it is not clear how to interpret the reported

* LMS stands for lambda, mu, sigma, the transformation parameters defined on page 6 of the "Methods" section of the 2000 CDC Growth Charts for the United States: Methods and Development, Department of Health and Human Services, Centers for Disease Control and Prevention, National Center for Health Statistics Series 11, Number 246, May 2002.

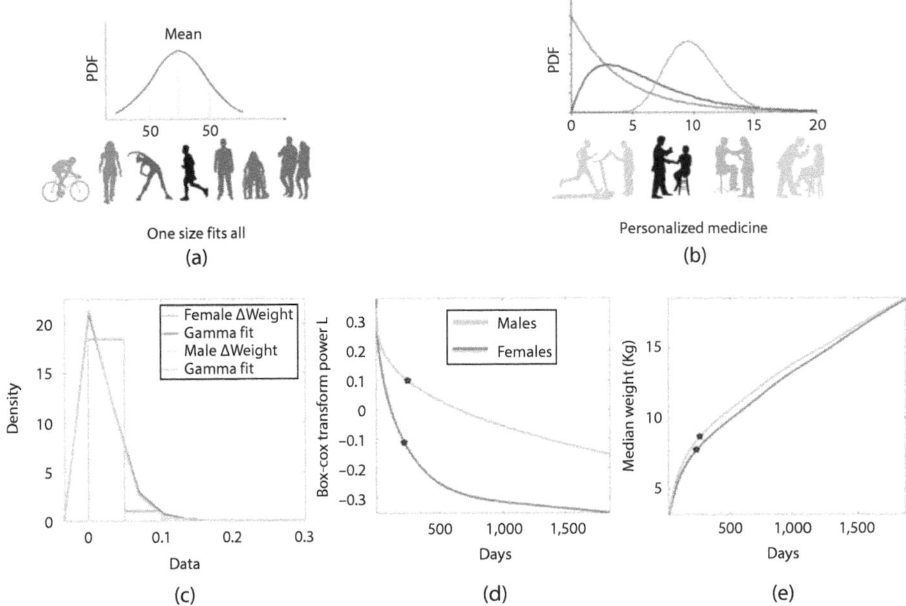

FIGURE 12.4 Non-Gaussian nature of the velocity-based (incremental) anthropomorphic neurodevelopmental data in Figure 12.2. (a) vs. (b) contrasts two statistical approaches to assess developmental data. In (a), the one-size-fits-all model currently dominating basic science leaves out individual nuances of neurodevelopment and applies an assumed normal distribution to all human behavioral data. Researchers harness these data from nervous systems that evolve over time with different rates of change, but throw away as noise inherent features of the data. (b) The personalized approach proposed by our group does not assume anything about the underlying statistical signatures of the developmental data. It rather estimates the statistical parameters of the individual as he or she evolves over time subject to varying degrees of maturation and adaptation rates. As a result, a family of probability distributions characterizes the person's biorhythms. This approach stands in contrast to the researcher's enforced assumption of the normal distribution across the population. (c) Sample skewed distributions of the change in weight (kg/day) of female and male babies taken across the first 5 years of development. (d) Curves of the reported Box–Cox transformation power quantity L indicating the nonnormal distribution. (e) Median weight changes over time (note the nonlinear curve, particularly in the first year of life). (Reproduced with permission from Torres et al., *Front. Pediatr.*, 4:121, 2016.)

generalized coefficient of variation S, derived from the skewed-to-normal transformed data, or even understand how S was obtained in the first place, given the different options for additive and multiplicative cases (Forkman 2009; Koopmans et al. 1964; Singh et al. 2004). This information is critical to obtain an estimate of the growth parameters and their summary statistics. For example, we can gain some sense of the evolution of skewness by profiling the L parameter in Figure 12.4b, but we do not know how the kurtosis of the underlying probability distributions may change with age and development. This is the case where the above-mentioned power transformation to enforce normality on the data does not adjust for kurtosis.

It is pertinent to mention that we have studied the evolution of skewness and kurtosis of distributions related to the linear speed of pointing movements in cross-sectional data from 176 participants. In typical controls, their ages ranged from 3 to 77 years old. There we found that these empirically estimated moments change over time with typical aging (Torres et al. 2016a and see Figure 12.5). As such, it may be important to track their evolution during early neurodevelopment.

Owing to those recent results, we know today that the non-Gaussian nature of these distributions calls for a systematic study of both the skewness and kurtosis of the empirical distributions of growth parameters obtained in early neurodevelopment, that is, prior to 3 years of age, before the child receives an observational diagnosis of ASD. Likewise, the inherent variability of the original growth

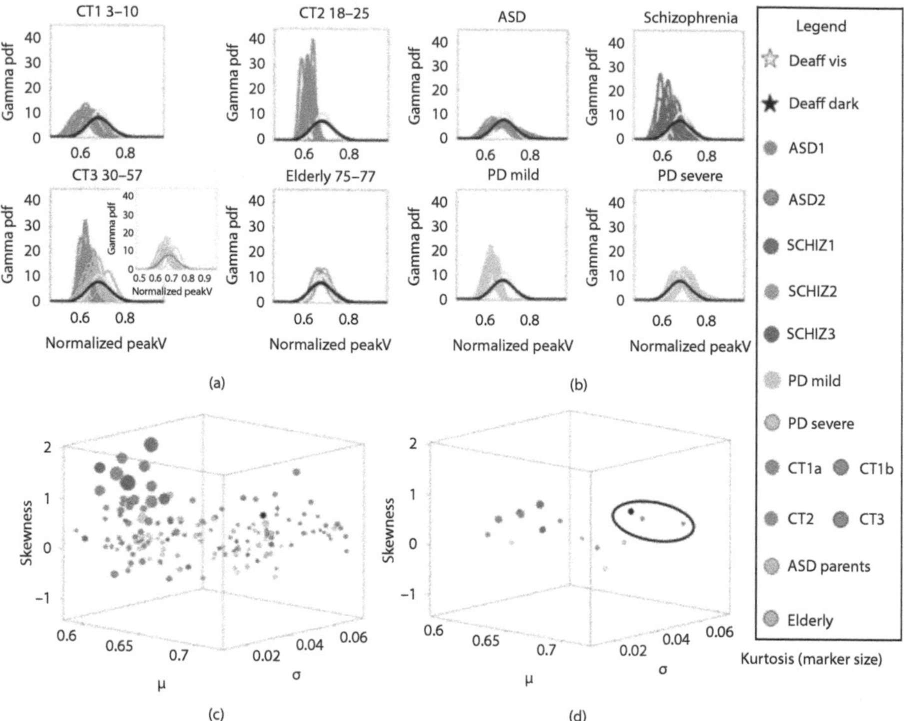

FIGURE 12.5 Evolution of probability distribution functions (PDFs) characterizing biophysical rhythms of target-directed reaches in typically aging individuals and in individuals aging with pathology of the nervous systems. (a) Typical aging from 3 to 77 years old shows changes in the empirically estimated PDFs whereby the shape and dispersion of the distributions shift values. Specifically, early in infancy, the children's goal-directed motions manifest higher dispersion and more skewness. During college years (18–25 years old) the noise-to-signal ratio (NSR) decreases and the shape of the distribution turns more symmetric. Typical aging after midlife reveals distributions with higher dispersion and skewness. Green curves correspond to young parents of children with ASD (below 40 years old) who manifest atypically higher dispersion and skewness than other participants of comparable age and same sex. Black and yellow PDFs are from deafferented subject Ian Waterman, who lost sensory (kinesthetic reafference) feedback from movement, pressure, and touch at the age of 19 due to a viral infection. His stochastic signatures are different from those of controls. (b) PDFs empirically estimated from different pathologies, including ASD. Note that Waterman has stochastic signatures closer to those of ASD participants (from 3 to 25 years old) and to those of patients with Parkinson's disease (PD) of high severity (according to the Unified Parkinson's Disease Rating Scale). (c) Summary statistics of the estimated PDFs, including estimated mean, variance, skewness, and kurtosis, reveal a map of the different pathologies of the nervous systems in relation to controls. (d) The centroids of the clusters in (c) highlight Waterman's signatures as he moves in complete darkness in relation to the ASD centroids. (Reproduced with permission from Torres et al., *Front. Neurol.* 7:8, 2016.)

data, lost when applying such transformations, may hold important cues to intervene. In other words, the tails of those skewed distributions may contain the important information we seek. Current analytics often throw away such information as noise by averaging the data under the enforced assumption of normality. One must keep in mind that these population charts are the gold standard to track neurodevelopment in the infant population worldwide. As such, they should be exhaustive and empirically driven.

Why Is This Important to Consider in ASD?

Autism is the by-product of a developmental process gone awry. Framing the condition in this way, one can conceive the nervous systems that evolve to receive this diagnosis as coping systems that adapt to change along different developmental pathways than typical. In this sense, it is not that the statistical methods used to track development are flawed, for example, those used to build the population growth charts. They are sound *under the statistical assumptions made*. The problem rather lies in the assumptions made, as they are not empirically justified by the inherent neurodevelopmental process linked to accelerated, nonlinear physical growth. The linear parametric assumptions imposed on the original data go entirely orthogonal to the true nature of the empirical data at hand. As such, the analytical approaches in use erase the very information that we need in order to detect and flag risk for neurodevelopmental stunting in the very early stages of life.

The information we are searching for is right in front of our eyes, but we are looking at it through the wrong lens. Pediatricians are not aware of these statistical nuances. They measure the baby every visit and compare those absolute measurements with the measurements of previous visits in order to attain some sense of change, rather than to assess its rate. The comparison also involves considering growth relative to the population growth chart for the "typical" values. Yet given the empirical finding, that growth bears a nonlinear, non-Gaussian signature, and given that physicians rely on charts that are forcedly defining linear, Gaussian processes, this methodology obscures the true underlying potential risk. This is particularly the case when such risk is present early (according to the accelerated rate of change in physical growth within the first month, as reflected in the inset of Figure 12.2c). It is not surprising then that by 3 years of age, the clinicians detect ASD with a degree of certainty that increases as the child further ages. The clinician misses a critical window to intervene as precious time goes by during those early months of life.

I note here another complication related to the growth charts. Once we learned in my lab the details of the methods employed to build the growth charts, we called various pediatricians to ask them how they used the WHO CDC charts to track development. When asking about population growth charts, we would invariably hear, "Ah! The Nestle chart!" or "Yes! The Johnson & Johnson chart!" These formula-based charts from major food companies are readily available to pediatricians, but they are not the breast-feeding-based charts recommended by the WHO-CDC. We do not know the differences between formula-feeding- and breast-feeding-based charts, or the impact that recommending formula may have on a neonate with stunted neuromotor control that the pediatrician has no way of detecting by eye. Consider, for instance, accelerating the rate of physical growth when the rate of development in networking capacity of the underlying nerves is somehow compromised (e.g., issues with myelination, excess synaptic noise from lacking scaffolding proteins at the postsynaptic terminals, etc.). In such cases, the body may grow, but neurodevelopment may fall behind because reentrant feedback from the periphery is not properly contributing to the brain's development (e.g., somatic motor maps, synapses, and circuits and systems at the cortical, subcortical, and spinal cord levels).

Another important aspect of the growth chart data refers to the differences between female and male neonates. Notice in Figure 12.4d that the time course of the required transformation power L is different for male and female babies, denoting different families of probability distributions underlying the variability in physical growth related to weight. Although not shown here, body length and head circumference follow similar trends, so overall physical growth rates are congruent to rates of neuromotor control when the baby develops normally (Torres et al. 2016c), but this linear relationship (shown in Figure 12.6b for the weight parameter) breaks down as development becomes stagnant.

The early sex differences in physical development are relevant to ASD because there is a large diagnosis disparity between males and females—approximately 5.5:1 boys to girls (Mandy et al. 2012; Newschaffer et al. 2007; Volkmar et al. 1993). Current observational diagnostics also impose a priori the Gaussian distribution to cast and analyze their subjective hand-coded data. These methods applied to ordinal data drawn from observation obscure differences between males and females that are nonetheless quantifiable very early on in the physical development of the newborn baby.

Infant development is indeed a process that when looked at through the appropriate lens, already reveals fundamental differences in the physical development of the two sexes linked to differences in the development and maintenance of neuromotor control (Torres et al. 2013b, 2016b). As the baby develops and early childhood gives way to adolescence and then college, the signatures of motor

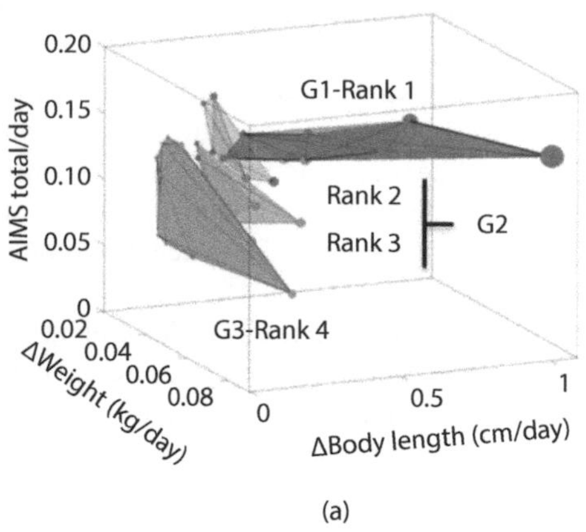

(a)

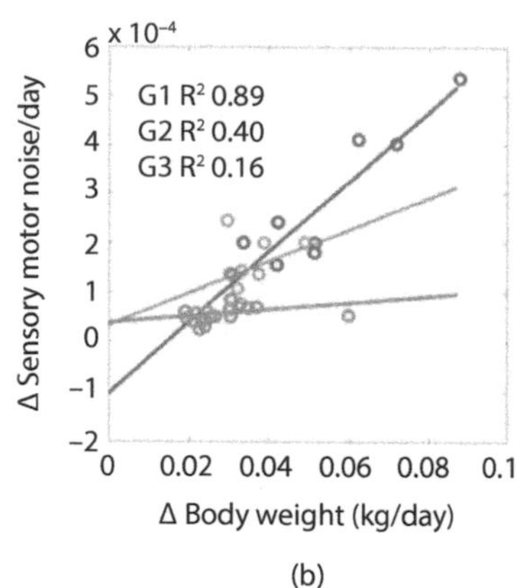

(b)

FIGURE 12.6 Stunting in neurodevelopment captured by objective physical metrics. (a) In a group of 36 neonates with 24 at risk from complications at birth (some preterm) and 12 typically born (full-term) with no complications, we were able to blindly separate babies at risk in Groups 2 and 3 based on the emerging longitudinal relationship between physical growth and neuromotor control. Specifically, the growth measurements across 6 months automatically clustered babies based on the median ranking of their measurements and plotted in a three-dimensional surface using Delaunay triangulation. The babies growing at the fastest daily rate across all three parameters made up Group G1 of typical physical development (head circumference represented by the size of the circle). They came from the original group of 12 babies born without complications, but also contained two babies from the group at risk. These babies underwent intensive physical and occupational therapy. (b) The tracking of leg motions using wearable inertial measurement units revealed the transition of fluctuations in the amplitude of self-generated acceleration from spontaneous random noise to well-structured signal from visit to visit. These transitions markedly registered in Group G1 comprised the highest-ranked babies in (a). To a lesser extent, the data showed such transitions in Group G2 comprised by Rank 2 and Rank 3 babies. However, Group G3 of Rank 4 babies showed stunting in the transitions denoting neuromotor control (flat slope). From visit to visit, their somatic motor patterns did not evolve. As such, the linear relation uncovered between the nonlinear rate of physical growth and the nonlinear, stochastic motor parameters failed to appear for this group at risk of neurodevelopmental derail. Panel (b) focuses on weight, but the stunting manifested as well in head circumference and body length (not shown). Note in (a) that the Alberta Infant Motor Scale (AIMS) score on the z-axis is a scoring system of readiness to walk. Higher scores were found in the babies with the highest ranking in the rates of physical growth. (Reproduced with permission from Torres et al., *Front. Pediatr.*, 4:121, 2016.)

variability shift values (Figure 12.5), but in ASD, they remain stagnant throughout the human life span across the population at large (Torres et al. 2013a). As mentioned above, and further illustrating this point in data from newborn infants, Figure 12.6 shows an example of a data-driven approach from our lab that readily detects stunting of neuromotor development and flags risk within the first 6 months of life. The methods employed to compute such biometrics are amenable to embed in baby-ready Fitbits, an approach that would enable the monitoring of the rates of growth and the rates of neurodevelopment on a daily basis.

Why wait until 3 years of age to detect problems with social exchange when by 2–3 months problems with stunting in neuromotor control are already detectable?

Social interactions require, by necessity, neuromotor control because we are always in a constant state of motion—even when seemingly standing still.

PROBLEM 3: ACTIVITY REQUIRED FOR SPONTANEOUSLY SELF-SUPERVISED AND SELF-CORRECTIVE INTERNAL MODELS

Behavioral neuroscience employs subjective hand-coding methods for data gathering. Since these methods draw the ordinal data from observation, they rely primarily on the limited capacity of conscious vision. Furthermore, the analyses and interpretation of the subjective data are naturally biased by experiments that constrain the experimental task design a priori by rather elaborate hand-crafted hypotheses that rarely leave room for spontaneous findings. Under the current significant hypothesis testing paradigm, there is a sort of "self-fulfilling prophesy" circularity to the scientific method that is employed by the brain health disciplines. This "evidence-based science" has limited the field, while constraining the methodological approaches. The consequences in the translation of these approaches to the clinical realm lead to problematic diagnosis, treatment, and behavioral interventions of ASD. They have not contributed to improvements in quality of life of the affected person and the affected family.

One of the problems we face in the analyses of behavior is a lack of grounding in the neuroanatomy and neurophysiology of the systems underlying the planning, execution, adaptation, and correction of actions making up behaviors. Indeed, the curricula of fields like psychology and psychiatry often lack a study of the computational models and electrophysiology of sensory and motor control.

Many clinicians that diagnose, treat, and track ASD (and other neurodevelopmental disorders) have a limited understanding and awareness of the anatomical structures of sensory and motor nerves and/or their functional physiology. Rarely mentioned or measured in any way are the functioning of afferent-sensory channels conducting information on movement, pressure, and touch versus those conducting information on pain and temperature. Yet many of these neurological supporting facets of motor control and affect (respectively) are malfunctioning in a large number of people with ASD (Damasio and Maurer 1978). For instance, our lab has documented a number of cases of children that report not feeling their body properly (as further illustrated in the parental chapters in Section V of the book). As illustrated in the case of Daniel (Chapter 24), some children have excess tolerance to pain, while others may demonstrate temperature dysregulation. These anecdotal accounts by parents, and pediatricians, described in Chapters 21 through 25, add to our own scientific observations. Such qualitative reports—a body of information that may be considered scientific in other fields—raise the question, *why are we ignoring these parental accounts?* The lack of or the atypical bodily and facial sensations in ASD ought to be quantified in light of different ganglia innervating the face and body and different phylogenetic orders of maturation for the above-mentioned systems (Figure 12.7). These underlie many aspects of the social and communication axes.

For instance, this sense of touch that we tend to take for granted is of utmost importance in the formation of somatic bodily maps and their projections to the brain.

How does our brain discover the physical body that it needs to own and control, when those maps and the PNS-CNS connections fail to form?

The very notion of the self, spontaneously emerging from self-supervision and prospective self-corrective error codes, is indispensable to form a stable percept of the world around us. It is also important to develop deliberate autonomy over one's own physical body in motion.

The systems' acquired ability to differentiate between the efferent flow caused by the CNS and the returning streams of sensory (reafference) feedback must be difficult to attain if sensory neurons are not properly transducing a form of energy into action potentials. They may also fail to appear if the transmission channels of the transduced neural signal are somehow impeded by poor myelination, or if pre- and postsynaptic sites lack proper scaffolding to communicate, or if in general the returning afferent signals are such that it is difficult to discern endo- from exoafferent influences (among others).

Under such conditions, likely co-occurring in ASD, how are the nervous systems then going to own self-generated actions and deliberately predict their control at will?

We know today that involuntary minute fluctuations in bodily and head rhythms (Torres et al. 2013a; Torres and Denisova 2016) pollute the signals harnessed from the nervous systems with a diagnosis of ASD across ages, sex, and developmental stages. This feature is detectable in deliberate and spontaneous aspects of goal-directed actions (Torres et al. 2013a, 2016a), in automated actions without a goal (Torres et al. 2016b), and during the resting state while the person attempts to remain still (Torres and Denisova 2016). They are present across the body, including the head, trunk, and upper and lower limbs. Under such conditions, it must be very difficult for a nervous system trying

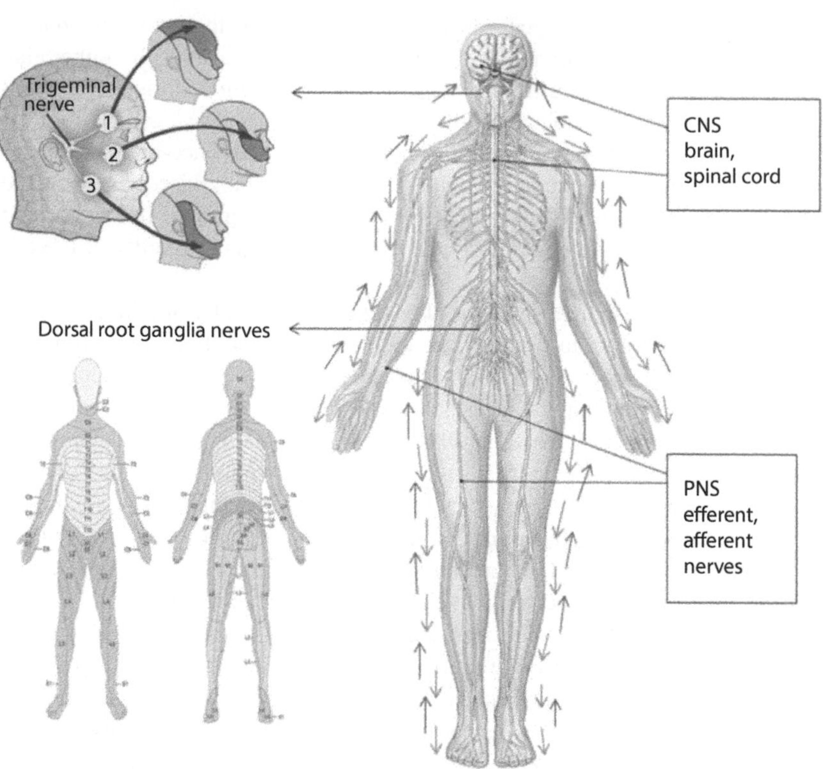

FIGURE 12.7 Distinct maps for the face and body sensory-motor nerves conduct neural impulses and enable communication between the CNS and PNS. These somatic maps in the periphery project to central cerebrocortical structures and require proper maturation to eventually contribute to the neuromotor control required in all social behaviors. These structures build prenatally from nerve cell differentiation and, upon birth, follow a phylogenetically guided maturation order, whereby the emergence of cortical circuits and neural systems depends on the intactness and proper maturation of peripheral circuits and neural systems. (Reproduced with permission from Torres et al., *Front. Integr. Neurosci.* 10:22, 2016.)

to self-monitor its self-generated actions to separate internally caused rhythms from extraneous rhythms to understand sensory consequences and eventually correctly predict them ahead of time.

Why Is This Important to Consider in ASD?

The intactness of somatic peripheral information from the start of life, even prenatally, seems critical to form proper cerebrocortical connections, circuits, neural systems, and maps of changes in physical rhythms. These are important elements to facilitate central control of the internal dynamics of self-generated physical actions.

In ASD, we need to begin the path of better understanding the important roles of the PNSs on the development of self-supervision and autonomy. We need to better understand the relationships between the enteric system, where autonomy exists in its own right (Gershon 1998), and the immune system, where self-supervision must exist from the conception of life, if the organism is to survive the dramatic switch of environments at birth. These two primordial systems already contain two critical ingredients that the CNS will need to autonomously control, regulate, and supervise self-generated actions at will, to build an abstract model of the dynamic self in motion and be able to create dynamically modifiable forward and inverse maps of the motions of others in the social scene. Under those conditions, mental navigation and timely dynamic interactions in the social medium are possible.

Otherwise, such processes would not take place. The following is a proposed plausible scenario in early neurodevelopment: as the newborn spontaneously moves at random, and sensory and motor noise systematically transition into well-structured signals, deliberate trial and error may begin to separate from spontaneous activity. Under such conditions, the uncertainty of the outcomes from predicting sensory consequences of self-generated actions (e.g., arm flailing) may reduce. At some point, then, self-regulation may emerge as the infant learns body ownership and prospective control. It is possible that around the time of reaching such milestones, the social medium begins to make sense to the nascent nervous systems. Consequently, agency and the need for interaction with others in that medium may naturally follow.

In marked contrast, the newborn infant that never reaches the stage of internally and autonomously generated self-supervision may never attain a model of the self. This infant will have difficulties communicating socially. If this pattern persists after 3 years of age, visible signs differing from the expected typical developmental social trajectory may lead to the observational diagnosis of ASD. Yet, those differences readily detectable after 3 years of age are likely the by-product of a process that may have started even before birth. *Why delay measuring the evolutions of the sensory and somatic motor activities from birth?* After all, the biorhythms directly output by the nervous systems of the newborn infant are accessible through noninvasive means, including wearable sensing technologies of various kinds. New analytics and data types derived from such waveforms continuously harnessed from the nervous systems are also available today.

If we want to understand ASD origins, we need to move away from superficial observations and delve deep into the elements that ultimately give rise to the levels of body ownership, self-control, and autonomy required for social behavior. The one-size-fits-all, linear, static, deterministic approach to ASD research, driven primarily by subjective clinical criteria, will continue to keep the bottom layers of the knowledge network disconnected from the top layers (in Figure 12.1). In this sense, the implementation of the tenets of precision medicine and their specific application to the fields of psychiatry and pediatrics will continue to remain obstructed if we do not change or expand the methods to gather and analyze nervous systems data.

From Neuromotor Control to Predictive Social Behavior

We posit that predictive behavior is the by-product of interactions between bottom-up and top-down processes that develop since birth (see Figure 2 in the closing remarks of Section I). Predictive behavior is an emergent property of the system guided by neurodevelopmental processes that involve, from an early age, the self-sensing of the dynamic changes in the physical rhythms caused by the nervous system itself. Such a recursive schema of self-supervision and self-correction must lead to the transition from passive stimulus–response associations and built-in reflexes to active prospective behavior, guided by successful outcomes from predicting the actions' sensory consequences. The successful emergence of anticipatory behavior must then depend on the balance between subconscious and conscious levels of control presumably mediated by different structures within the nervous systems. Subconscious processes mediated by subcortical structures (brainstem, limbic system, basal ganglia, cerebellum, spinal cord, and peripheral nerves) provide support and fast, automatic, and autonomous processing to support and maintain conscious processes. The latter, presumably mediated by neocortical networks, are conceivably slower and dependent on the continuous sensory feedback from the subconscious systems to compensate for the sensory transduction and transmission delays, thus enabling timely and successful decisions mediated by timely actions producing behavior.

Based on empirical results, we have previously proposed that the balance between these conscious and unconscious systems is critical to link mental intent and autonomous physical volition. In this sense, we have found that patients with PD have lost this balance and overcompensate with excess deliberateness in their motions (Torres et al. 2011). In contrast, patients with schizophrenia (SCHIZ) manifest avolition and motor delusions characterized by marked inversion between the roles of deliberate and spontaneous segments of their pointing motions, to the extent that it is not possible to distinguish between intentional and extemporaneous aspects of their movements (Nguyen et al. 2016).

The autistic conditions manifest both of these cases, but the general feature all individuals report that remains congruent with our objective quantification and statistical characterization of their motions is the disconnect between the intention to move and their agency over the execution of their motions. In the words of the ASD participants, it is as though the body has acquired a mind of its own or the intended plan "kicks in" too late. Interestingly, the timeline of these manifestations differs across these conditions. In ASD, they manifest very early in neurodevelopment, around 3 years of age. In SCHIZ, they become more evident during puberty, when the transition toward youth occurs, around 19–21 years old. In PD, they are obvious after 40–50 years of age, when neurodegeneration begins the slow yet visible decline of the nervous systems. In each case, sensory feedback emerging from kinesthetic input plays an important role to maintain performance. However, its role has different weight on the timely formation of action maps and the updating of maps reflecting the actions' sensory consequences.

When there is persistent corrupted (random and noisy) feedback tied to the sensing of the body in motion, it is very likely that the development of prospective self-correction codes stalls and the system somehow lives in the "here and now" (see Chapter 1). In this regard, a developing nervous system ought to be able to sense its own self-generated rhythms in the first place. Sensory organs, sensory transducers, and transmission channels must be working properly throughout the nervous systems, from the gut to the heart to the brain. The questions are then, once reafference is adequately flowing, how do the nervous systems attain self-supervision and self-corrective codes? Moreover, how does the organism discover the limiting values of those self-corrections? Are those self-corrections stored as part of a general code that perpetuates self-regulation across different systems? Where does that ability for self-discovery and self-control of such rhythms come from in the first place? Is it a by-product of the genetic code itself, or is it a self-emergent property of the organism, unveiled through a combination of spontaneous activity and deliberate trial and error during early life? One must wonder if such mechanisms are inherited and already exist, for example, built into the immune systems, or if the autonomic nervous systems in their own right create and keep them to hand them down to the systems in charge of voluntary control.

As we have stated, the accelerated rates of change in physical growth and neuromotor development are important to consider during the early stages of the neonate's existence. Their unfolding may enhance our understanding of key ingredients leading to the proper development of intelligent (predictive) behavior. If there are complications at birth, there will be a major insult to the nervous systems development, and very likely, the expected temporal trajectory of such processes will stunt or derail. As such, monitoring the systems' evolution with adequate instruments and analytical frameworks becomes very important.

At the neonatal intensive care unit (NICU), one can see the baby transitioning from the womb's environment to the regular environment we live in. At that stage, amidst tubes, cables, humidifiers, and temperature probes, life emerges in a rather miraculous way, while following some seemingly required order. Once the heartbeat is in place, developing autonomous respiration patterns seems fundamental to survival. Even after the autonomous respiration patterns are in place, the gut and digestive systems' autonomy will need to stabilize, to enable survival. Indeed, gastrointestinal complications in premature babies are largely responsible for fatal outcomes (e.g., from a condition called necrotizing enterocolitis [NEC]) (Denning et al. 2017; Sisk et al. 2016). The achievement of autonomy and stability seems to be a key precursor to the start of successful nervous systems' development (neurodevelopment).

Orderly Development of Control Levels in the Infant's Nervous System

The phylogeny and ontogeny of the proposed taxonomy of neuromotor control and somatosensation (Torres 2011) with regard to autonomous biophysical rhythms generated by the nervous systems may also help us understand the projection of adaptable body maps onto brain regions. These maps that begin to develop since conception are later in life expressed as diverse topographic representations of sensory and motor cortical and subcortical structures of the developing brain (Purves 2012). Indeed, many such critical structures seem altered in postmortem studies of brains from individuals who had a diagnosis of ASD (Broek et al. 2014; Edmonson et al. 2014; Purcell et al. 2001). These have included the frontal, parietal, and cerebellar cortices (Fatemi et al. 2002; Laurence and Fatemi 2005), as well as brainstem areas important for multisensory integration and the proper development and maintenance of neuromotor control (see Chapter 8 for a review).

The development of such maps ought to require in the first place the ability to sense the brain's self-caused rhythms and separate endo- from exoafference along the continuous reafferent flow (kinesthetic or otherwise). These steps seem critical to scaffold different aspects of the formation, maintenance, and updating of internal models of the dynamically changing self. Such internal models are required to update abstract mental existence in general, but in particular, they are required for the types of abstract mental navigation that emerge during neurodevelopment as a fundamental component of intelligent or predictive behavior required and expected in a highly dynamic social scene. The latter aspect is particularly relevant to the theme of this book since most conditions categorized as mental illnesses affect the person's ability to relate to the social medium. The social medium also fails to embrace the affected individual. The social scene seems to be operating at different frequencies and timescales than those of the nervous systems of the affected individual. In light of neurodevelopment, without the type of deliberate control of autonomy that the newborn baby develops early on, it is hard to create a "perceptual bubble" inclusive of the frequencies attuned to both the social medium and those of the person affected by nervous systems' disorders that necessarily affect bodily agency and willful prospective control.

Part of the ASD conundrum is how to relate somatomotor aspects of behaviors and social communication exchange. Social interactions require the solution of many difficult computational problems, most of which involve controlling facial and bodily rhythms caused and self-supervised by the brain itself. The self-production and emergent self-control of such rhythms since birth necessarily lead to neurodevelopmental processes that are inherently dynamic, nonlinear, and variable (stochastic). The very nature of the internal space that the physical body generates (spanning more than 200 degrees of freedom [DoF] [Zatsiorsky et al. 2000]), the broad range of frequencies and timescales that define external sensory stimuli (Purves 2012), and the very problem of integrating these signals through the parietal, vestibular, and other structures in the spinal cord make the problem of developing proper motor control rather challenging. To make sense of the self in the world and the world in the self, the nervous systems of the newborn infant must operate under principles that agree with the very nature of the signals it must produce, sense, simulate, and process.

Why, therefore, does brain science tend to a priori impose rather linear, static, deterministic approaches on the neurodevelopmental phenomena at hand?

PROBLEM 4: LACK OF A PROPER TAXONOMY OF CONTROL LEVELS IN MOTOR RESEARCH

The field of neuromotor control could help define biometrics based on sensory and motor processes. Yet, the paucity of models that consider appropriate levels of control has made it difficult to translate them into actual clinical applications. Most of the basic research in neuromotor control remains disconnected from social and cognitive aspects of naturalistic behaviors. The experimental paradigms in human motor psychophysics remain much too constrained to allow for the study of freely moving bodies performing actions in activities of daily life. The advent of wearables with high sampling resolution and the introduction of a new taxonomy of neuromotor control (Torres 2011), that maps different ranges of variability in biophysical rhythms from the nervous systems to different levels of control, are starting to enable the translation of biometrics developed in the laboratory settings to more naturalistic environments (Kalampratsidou and Torres 2016). Under this new approach, we can track the signatures of variability of a person's daily routines, from exercising and walking around during the day, to sleeping cycles at night. Movement classes spanning different control levels, ranging from those spontaneously occurring to those performed rather deliberately, bring a new vision to the study of motor control (Nguyen et al. 2016; Torres 2011; Torres et al. 2011) with direct applications to ASD movement research (Torres et al. 2013a).

Why Is This Important to Consider in ASD?

The recent above-mentioned developments are very relevant to the clinical arena. They enable habilitation and rehabilitation of self-bodily awareness. At present, we are poised to explore new avenues to enhance neuromotor control and (consequently) improve volition in ASD (Torres 2016; Torres et al. 2013c). This path of intervention will be crucial to connect in each individual with ASD the mental intent to act with the physical realization of the desired act. Developing body ownership and agency is a first step toward being able to interact socially and ultimately regain the basic freedom that many on the spectrum have been (perhaps unintentionally) robbed of by interventions that force the person to conform to expected social appropriateness. They enforce such behaviors while discounting coping mechanisms and accommodations that nervous systems naturally create to survive. Such interventions indeed disregard the constraints of a coping developing nervous system. They do not leave room for spontaneous exploration conducive of the type of self-discovery a baby naturally experiences.

PROBLEM 5: LACK OF MODELS TO ASSESS AND TRACK SOCIAL INTERACTIONS IN A DISORDER DEFINED AS A SOCIAL COMMUNICATION DEFICIT

The criteria for both research and clinical diagnosis of ASD involve very elaborate social interactions between the person who administers the test and the person under examination. At present, there are no models to simulate and measure such dyadic exchange. No one scores the examiner administering the test to the child. We do not know, for example, what influences the examiner may have on the child when he or she prompts the social presses in search for spontaneous "overtures" from the child. How spontaneous a response may be will depend in great part on the nature of the prompt to initiate the ensuing reaction. If the examiner is having a bad day, this may be indirectly reflected in the prompting and consequently affect the response of the child. If the child does not like the examiner from the start, this may also affect the outcome and skew the scores in ways that do not reflect the child's best capabilities. We can think of many different reasons to avoid having such a one-sided test for a scoring system that will directly affect the life of the child without any scientific examination of dyadic social exchange. Indeed, the paucity of models of dyadic exchange that can handle the two interacting bodies in motion with rapidly changing dynamics prevents us from better characterizing ASD in an unbiased, reliable way. In recent years, our lab has deployed a platform to study dyadic social exchange within the Autism Diagnostic Observation Schedule 2 (ADOS-2) settings (Whyatt et al. 2015). We have also extended the use of these new methods to therapeutic settings in pediatric occupational therapy specifically focused on sensory-motor integration. We hope that the new platform technology helps advance basic science in ASD. We also hope to generate outcome measures needed to provide insurance companies with the evidence needed to cover such therapies. We refer the reader to Chapter 7 of examining physiological somatic motor measures of dyadic social exchange in the context of the ADOS administration.

As of today, coverage of sensory-motor-oriented therapies in ASD is not possible. This lacking impedes the type of diversification in therapies needed to tackle the disorder's heterogeneity and implementation of personalized approaches to address problems in each child. In this regard, we hope that the proposed neuromotor control taxonomy (Torres 2011) helps define different subtypes of ASD.

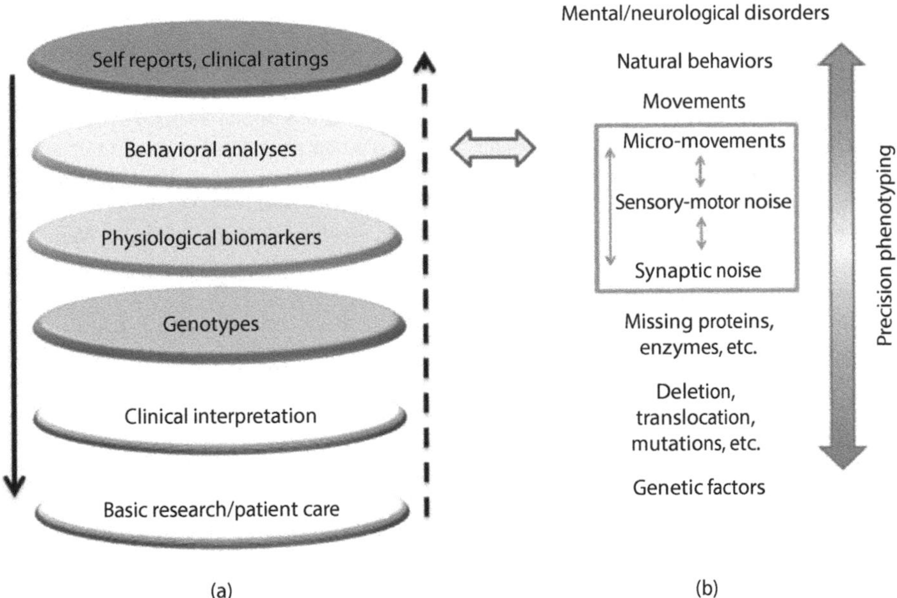

FIGURE 12.8 Toward precision psychiatry. (a) Transforming behavioral analyses to attain objective biometrics and help connect the various layers of the knowledge network. (b) Precision phenotyping can be achieved by mapping sensory-motor noise signatures to synaptic noise signatures of known etiology. Instead of correlating discrete clinical scores of the top layer with genotypic information, we propose mapping objective biometric results from natural behaviors to genetic information. (Reproduced with permission from Torres, E.B., et al., *Front. Integr. Neurosci.*, 10, 22, 2016.)

This taxonomy also maps different levels of phylogenetically appearing control with different levels of somatic motor variability. Under such scheme, it may be possible to provide a classification system evaluating the functioning of different nerve groups (e.g., efferent-motor vs. afferent-sensory), and within those subgroups further separate facial versus bodily maps (as in Figure 12.7). An important component in this regard is the level of deliberate autonomy of the brain over the body. When paired with genetics, such taxonomy would also be amenable to map different types of synaptic noise (Figure 12.8) with corresponding signatures of somatic motor noise along the facial and bodily maps (in Figure 12.7). If the autonomic nervous systems, or the level of involuntary motions, overpower deliberate autonomy of the brain over the body, we may be able to classify autism based on the quantification of such interference with volitional control and agency of the brain over the physical body.

CONCLUSIONS AND TAKE-HOME MESSAGE

The implementation of precision medicine is currently underway in disciplines like cancer research and medical practices. The recent success in targeted treatments of different cancer types strongly points at the high potential of the integrative and individualized approach to medical practices. We need to disrupt the present models of the psychological and socioeconomic construct of ASD, shift gears into a more holistic brain–body approach to this set of conditions, and begin the path of precision psychiatry. New approaches to handle nonlinear dynamic and stochastic data with the appropriate mathematical machinery will enable the implementation of precision psychiatry in mental health. Such approaches will not impose a priori overly simplifying assumptions, which currently obstruct the path of spontaneous scientific discovery.

REFERENCES

American Psychiatric Association. 2013. *Diagnostic and Statistical Manual of Mental Disorders*. 5th ed. Washington, DC: American Psychiatric Association.

Box, G. E., and D. R. Cox. 1964. An analysis of transformations. *J R Stat Soc Series B* 26:211–52.

Broek, J. A., P. C. Guest, H. Rahmoune, and S. Bahn. 2014. Proteomic analysis of post mortem brain tissue from autism patients: Evidence for opposite changes in prefrontal cortex and cerebellum in synaptic connectivity-related proteins. *Mol Autism* 5:41. doi: 10.1186/2040–2392–5-41.

Cole, T. J. 1990. The LMS method for constructing normalized growth standards. *Eur J Clin Nutr* 44 (1):45–60.

Cole, T. J., and P. J. Green. 1992. Smoothing reference centile curves: The LMS method and penalized likelihood. *Stat Med* 11 (10):1305–19.

Damasio, A. R., and R. G. Maurer. 1978. A neurological model for childhood autism. *Arch Neurol* 35 (12):777–86.

Denning, T. L., A. M. Bhatia, A. F. Kane, R. M. Patel, and P. L. Denning. 2017. Pathogenesis of NEC: Role of the innate and adaptive immune response. *Semin Perinatol* 41 (1):15–28.

de Onis, M., and A. W. Onyango. 2003. The Centers for Disease Control and Prevention 2000 growth charts and the growth of breastfed infants. *Acta Paediatr* 92 (4):413–9.

Edmonson, C., M. N. Ziats, and O. M. Rennert. 2014. Altered glial marker expression in autistic post-mortem prefrontal cortex and cerebellum. *Mol Autism* 5 (1):3. doi: 10.1186/2040–2392–5-3.

Fatemi, S. H., A. R. Halt, J. M. Stary, R. Kanodia, S. C. Schulz, and G. R. Realmuto. 2002. Glutamic acid decarboxylase 65 and 67 kDa proteins are reduced in autistic parietal and cerebellar cortices. *Biol Psychiatry* 52 (8):805–10.

Flegal, K. M., and T. J. Cole. 2013. Construction of LMS parameters for the Centers for Disease Control and Prevention 2000 growth charts. *Natl Health Stat Report* (63):1–3.

Forkman, J. 2009. Estimator and tests for common coefficients of variation in normal distributions. *Commun Stat Theory Methods* 38 (2):233–51.

Gershon, M. D. 1998. *The Second Brain: The Scientific Basis of Gut Instinct and a Groundbreaking New Understanding of Nervous Disorders of the Stomach and Intestine*. 1st ed. New York: HarperCollins Publishers.

Grummer-Strawn, L. M., C. Reinold, N. F. Krebs, Centers for Disease Control and Prevention. 2010. Use of World Health Organization and CDC growth charts for children aged 0–59 months in the United States. *MMWR Recomm Rep* 59 (RR-9):1–15.

Hawgood, S., I. G. Hook-Barnard, T. C. O'Brien, and K. R. Yamamoto. 2015. Precision medicine: Beyond the inflection point. *Sci Transl Med* 7 (300):300ps17. doi: 10.1126/scitranslmed.aaa9970.

Kalampratsidou, V., and E. B. Torres. 2016. Outcome measures of deliberate and spontaneous motions. Presented at the Third International Symposium on Movement and Computing, MOCO'16, Thessaloniki, Greece, July 5–6, 2016.

Koopmans, L. H., D. B. Owen, and J. I. Rosenblatt. 1964. Confidence intervals for the coefficient of variation for the normal and log normal distributions. *Biometrika* 51:25–32.

Kuczmarski, R. J., C. L. Ogden, L. M. Grummer-Strawn, K. M. Flegal, S. S. Guo, R. Wei, Z. Mei, L. R. Curtin, A. F. Roche, and C. L. Johnson. 2000. CDC growth charts: United States. *Adv Data* (314):1–27.

Kuczmarski, R. J., C. L. Ogden, S. S. Guo, L. M. Grummer-Strawn, K. M. Flegal, Z. Mei, R. Wei, L. R. Curtin, A. F. Roche, and C. L. Johnson. 2002. 2000 CDC growth charts for the United States: Methods and development. *Vital Health Stat 11* (246):1–190.

Laurence, J. A., and S. H. Fatemi. 2005. Glial fibrillary acidic protein is elevated in superior frontal, parietal and cerebellar cortices of autistic subjects. *Cerebellum* 4 (3):206–10. doi: 10.1080/14734220500208846.

Mandy, W., R. Chilvers, U. Chowdhury, G. Salter, A. Seigal, and D. Skuse. 2012. Sex differences in autism spectrum disorder: Evidence from a large sample of children and adolescents. *J Autism Dev Disord* 42 (7):1304–13. doi: 10.1007/s10803–011–1356–0.

Newschaffer, C. J., L. A. Croen, J. Daniels, et al. 2007. The epidemiology of autism spectrum disorders. *Annu Rev Public Health* 28:235–58. doi: 10.1146/annurev.publhealth.28.021406.144007.

Nguyen, J., U. Majmudar, T. V. Papathomas, S. M. Silverstein, and E. B. Torres. 2016. Schizophrenia: The micro-movements perspective. *Neuropsychologia* 85:310–26. doi: 10.1016/j.neuropsychologia.2016.03.003.

Purcell, A. E., O. H. Jeon, A. W. Zimmerman, M. E. Blue, and J. Pevsner. 2001. Postmortem brain abnormalities of the glutamate neurotransmitter system in autism. *Neurology* 57 (9):1618–28.

Purves, D. 2012. *Neuroscience*. 5th ed. Sunderland, MA: Sinauer Associates.

Singh, A. C., M. Westlake, and M. Feder. 2004. A generalization of the coefficient of variation with application to suppression of imprecise estimates. *Am Stat* 4359–4365.

Sisk, P. M., T. M. Lambeth, M. A. Rojas, T. Lightbourne, M. Barahona, E. Anthony, and S. T. Auringer. 2016. Necrotizing enterocolitis and growth in preterm infants fed predominantly maternal milk, pasteurized donor milk, or preterm formula: A retrospective study. *Am J Perinatol*. doi: 10.1055/s-0036-1597326.

Torres, E. B. 2011. Two classes of movements in motor control. *Exp Brain Res* 215 (3–4):269–83. doi: 10.1007/s00221–011–2892–8.

Torres, E. B. 2016. Rethinking the study of volition for clinical use. In *Progress in Motor Control: Theories and Translations*, ed. J. Lazcko and M. Latash. New York: Springer.

Torres, E. B., M. Brincker, R. W. Isenhower, P. Yanovich, K. A. Stigler, J. I. Nurnberger, D. N. Metaxas, and J.V. Jose. 2013a. Autism: The micro-movement perspective. *Front Integr Neurosci* 7:32. doi: 10.3389/fnint.2013.00032.

Torres, E. B., and K. Denisova. 2016. Motor noise is rich signal in autism research and pharmacological treatments. *Sci Rep* 6:37422. doi: 10.1038/srep37422.

Torres, E. B., K. M. Heilman, and H. Poizner. 2011. Impaired endogenously evoked automated reaching in Parkinson's disease. *J Neurosci* 31 (49):17848–63. doi: 31/49/17848 [pii] 10.1523/JNEUROSCI.1150–11.2011.

Torres, E. B., R. W. Isenhower, J. Nguyen, C. Whyatt, J. I. Nurnberger, J. V. Jose, S. M. Silverstein, T. V. Papathomas, J. Sage, and J. Cole. 2016a. Toward precision psychiatry: Statistical platform for the personalized characterization of natural behaviors. *Front Neurol* 7:8. doi: 10.3389/fneur.2016.00008.

Torres, E. B., R. W. Isenhower, P. Yanovich, G. Rehrig, K. Stigler, J. Nurnberger, and J. V. Jose. 2013b. Strategies to develop putative biomarkers to characterize the female phenotype with autism spectrum disorders. *J Neurophysiol* 110 (7):1646–62. doi: 10.1152/jn.00059.2013.

Torres, E. B., J. Nguyen, S. Mistry, C. Whyatt, V. Kalampratsidou, and A. Kolevzon. 2016b. Characterization of the statistical signatures of micro-movements underlying natural gait patterns in children with Phelan McDermid syndrome: Towards precision-phenotyping of behavior in ASD. *Front Integr Neurosci* 10:22. doi: 10.3389/fnint.2016.00022.

Torres, E. B., B. Smith, S. Mistry, M. Brincker, and C. Whyatt. 2016c. Neonatal diagnostics: Toward dynamic growth charts of neuromotor control. *Front Pediatr* 4 (121):1–15.

Torres, E. B., P. Yanovich, and D. N. Metaxas. 2013c. Give spontaneity and self-discovery a chance in ASD: Spontaneous peripheral limb variability as a proxy to evoke centrally driven intentional acts. *Front Integr Neurosci* 7:46:1–7. doi: 10.3389/fnint.2013.00046.

Volkmar, F. R., P. Szatmari, and S. S. Sparrow. 1993. Sex differences in pervasive developmental disorders. *J Autism Dev Disord* 23 (4):579–91.

Whyatt, C., A. Mars, E. DiCicco-Bloom, and E. B. Torres. 2015. Objective characterization of sensory-motor physiology underlying dyadic interactions during the Autism Diagnostic Observation Schedule-2: Implications for research and clinical diagnosis. Presented at the Annual Meeting of the Society for Neuroscience, Chicago, October 17–21.

Zatsiorsky, V. M., IOC Medical Commission, and International Federation of Sports Medicine. 2000. *Biomechanics in Sport: Performance Enhancement and Injury Prevention, Encyclopaedia of Sports Medicine*. Oxford: Blackwell Science.

Zorlu, G., and M. de Onis. 2011. New WHO child growth standards catch on. In *Bull World Health Organ* 89: 250–1.

13 Inherent Noise Hidden in Nervous Systems' Rhythms Leads to New Strategies for Detection and Treatments of Core Motor Sensing Traits in ASD

Elizabeth B. Torres

CONTENTS

Introduction 197
Background on Motor Dysfunction Assessment in ASD 198
Why Choose Pointing and Gait in Our Examples? 200
New Data Type: From Discrete Segments to Continuous, Naturalistic Behaviors 202
Noise in the Periphery 203
Deafferented Subject IAN Waterman 205
Can We Shift from Random and Noisy Motor Patterns in ASD to Predictable Motor Signals? 206
Take-Home Lesson: Disconnected Brain Science Needs to Bridge the Mind–Body Dichotomy in ASD Definition, Research, and Treatments 209
References 210

This chapter provides examples of new data types to use with the statistical platform for individualized behavioral analysis so as to both simulate important aspects of inherent variations in natural behaviors and test predictions about signal-to-noise ratios and randomness in empirical data. Through several statistical lenses, we "zoom in and out" of deliberate and spontaneous biorhythms generated by the nervous systems during pointing and walking. We study the stochastic properties of these biorhythms with subsecond time precision. We analyze these data with an eye for corrective feedback information of use to the autism spectrum disorder researchers and clinicians alike. The chapter presents new experimental paradigms and methods that, for the first time, begin the challenging path of attempting to connect sociomotor cognition and neuromotor control. These attempts are grounded in the study of self-sensing and self-supervision or corrections of the motions derived from the continuous rhythms caused by the nervous systems.

INTRODUCTION

There is a long history of movement deficits and neurological conditions in disorders that are otherwise described as mental (Rogers 1992). In autism spectrum disorders (ASDs), accounts of motor deficits have largely originated from first- and secondhand testimonies given by self-advocates, parents, and caregivers (Donnellan and Leary 1995, 2012; Donnellan et al. 2012; Robledo et al. 2012) and beautifully describe a neurological construct (Damasio and Maurer 1978). Yet, for the most part, basic science and contemporary psychological and psychiatric approaches have not seriously considered such accounts or proposed models to study this constellation of disorders. This is self-evident in the current clinical criteria for diagnosis employed by the fifth edition of the *Diagnostic and Statistical Manual of Mental Disorders* (DSM-5) in psychiatry (American Psychiatric Association 2013) and by tools such as the Autism Diagnostic Observation Schedule (ADOS) in psychology (Lord et al. 2000). Such highly subjective criteria also currently dominate our scientific inquiry in basic science.

The insistence by these clinical fields that sensory and somatic motor dysfunctions are not core issues of ASD has been partially reinforced by the paucity of methods to extract patterns in the movements that make up natural behaviors. This chapter shows examples of new data types and analytics that challenge the current clinical criteria. The new approaches can provide information hidden in fluctuations of the nervous systems' rhythms that are much too fast or occurring at frequencies undetectable by the naked eye of the clinician. The aim is to provide scientists, from a broad range of disciplines, with new analytical means to examine natural behaviors through difference lenses and across multiple layers of the nervous systems. This is analogous to "zooming in" and "zooming out" of the data we observe and record. In other words, we would examine the movements that make up observable and unobservable aspects of behaviors using different temporal and frequency scales. The new methods and analytics would permit descriptions ranging from years, days, and hours to millisecond or submillisecond precision according to our instruments' capabilities. This is in stark contrast to limiting our inquiry exclusively by conscious observational capabilities restricted to ordinal data from discrete behavioral observations. Importantly, the data we proposed to use come from wearable sensors "listening" to the neural signals from peripheral nerves. Such flowing signals are amplified by the muscles (Kuiken et al. 2009; Schultz et al. 2009). They carry information about neuromotor control exerted by the central nervous system (CNS) on the periphery. As such, they provide a proxy for non-invasive evaluation of centrally generated volitional control.

The methods presented in this chapter contrast with current state-of-the-art machine learning techniques that use signals extracted from remote sensing cameras. In such cases, a layer of image processing is required to isolate potentially physiologically relevant behavioral modules (Wiltschko et al. 2015). As such, those approaches may experience difficulties when isolating a path to "deconvolve" the contributions from different layers of the efferent and afferent nerves throughout the periphery, from those inherent to the instrument. Likewise, they may be constrained by a priori chosen criteria denoting discrete behavioral segments rendered to be the relevant ones, at the expense of missing other segments, for example, those spontaneously occurring largely beneath awareness. Indeed, physiological signal extraction is an important future goal of research, as it enables the further development of methods with the potential to close the sensory-motor feedback loops in the face of excess noise and randomness. In autism research, these features of noise and randomness have been a hallmark of the motor output data directly obtainable from sensors that continuously listen to the self-generated motor activity through the skin (Torres et al. 2013a and 2013b).

Discrete behavioral module identification has been rather common in behavioral research and clinical practices that are based on observation. These methods are also used in the descriptions of animal models of neurodevelopmental disorders (Harony-Nicolas et al. 2015), a field that shall benefit from new emerging technological advances in motion capture (Wiltschko et al. 2015). Nonetheless, as noted earlier, we may miss important patterns in these data when segmenting behavioral epochs a priori during data preprocessing. Perhaps by complementing such methods with those from computational neuroscience, we may obtain a more complete individualized profile of the nervous system we study.

BACKGROUND ON MOTOR DYSFUNCTION ASSESSMENT IN ASD

The scientific community interested in ASD motor phenomena has accumulated mounting evidence quantifying movement differences in various action types (Green et al. 2009; Jansiewicz et al. 2006;

Ming et al. 2007). Along those lines, examples abound concerning deficits, such as excess repetitive motions (Bodfish et al. 2000), impairments in handwriting (Fuentes et al. 2009), dyspraxia (Dowell et al. 2009; Dziuk et al. 2007), problems with feed-forward and feedback mechanisms during force production control (Mosconi et al. 2015; Mosconi and Sweeney 2015), and problems in posture stability (Molloy et al. 2003), among many others (Deitz et al. 2007; Haswell et al. 2009; Marko et al. 2015; Torres and Donnellan 2015; Whyatt and Craig 2012). These types of neuromotor dysfunction have also been associated with cerebellar issues (D'Mello et al. 2015; Kaufmann et al. 2003; Mostofsky et al. 2009), as well as with cortical (Mahajan et al. 2016; Nebel et al. 2014) and subcortical (Qiu et al. 2010) areas critical for sensory-motor function.

This recent body of work has started to gain momentum, thus inviting the clinical community to reconsider motor deficits and quantify movement disorders of various kinds as core symptoms of ASD (Whyatt and Craig 2012, 2013). Throughout this book, we argue that despite the compilation of abundant evidence for neuromotor dysfunction across different cross sections of the population with a diagnosis of ASD, there has been a paucity of models with the potential to eventually connect neuromotor dysfunction with deficits in sensory processing, sensory transduction, and sensory transmission. An ability to augment these fields is particularly relevant, as impairments at these levels could prevent sensory-motor integration and transformation processes required for the neurodevelopment of sensory and motor maps.

The development of sensory and somatic motor maps is vital for the development of coordination and volitional motor control over the developing body, a body with abundant degrees of freedom (DoF) (Bernshteĭn 1967) that rapidly grows during early development. The nervous systems embedded in the rapidly changing body will need to adapt fast in order to move timely and smoothly to communicate intentions in the social scene. Understanding such issues will help with understanding the emergence of prospective planning. In turn, quantifying how the nervous system of a child gradually starts predicting the sensory consequences of (impending) self-generated actions (Feĭgenberg and Linkova 2014) may help us begin to connect key elements of neuromotor control development with different levels of sociomotor decisions. The characterization of motor physiology in relation to such social and cognitive issues may help us pave the way to understand impairments in key ingredients necessary to generally scaffold sociomotor behavior.

A key ingredient to the development of sensory and motor maps that is explicitly explored in this book is the use of movement as a form of reafferent sensory input, that is, flowing from the peripheral nervous system (PNS) to the CNS (Torres et al. 2013, 2016a). However, the conceptualization of the motor problem as a movement sensing issue will require the development of new data types and new analytics to tackle major motor control dysfunctions that are poorly understood today, even within the typical population.

How can we begin to quantify possible deficits in motor output that potentially impede the sensing of actively self-produced movements as a form of sensory feedback?

In this chapter, we introduce pointing- and gait-related behaviors to provide examples of new data types and new analytical techniques that are amenable to characterize different levels of neuromotor control, ranging from a descriptive level bounded by our limits in conscious perception, to a more implicit level capturing details at millisecond temporal scales escaping the naked eye. In the first part of the chapter, we illustrate "open-loop" approaches to the study of simple goal-directed or automatic behaviors, such as pointing to a target or walking. These approaches merely record and characterize the statistics of biophysical rhythms caused by the nervous systems during the implementation of such actions. There is no intervention on our part to attempt to close the PNS-CNS loops by providing feedback driven by the features extracted from their own outcomes. In the second part of the chapter, we shift to "closed-loop" approaches whereby the stochastic signatures of the biorhythms of the nervous systems are used as a form of continuous feedback to change and guide the nervous systems' performance. We use a form of sensory augmentation to implement noise dampening or noise cancellation in the kinesthetic reafferent signals from self-generated actions. In this closed-loop case, we explain the potential benefits of using such an approach to influence and steer movement sensing and bodily awareness in ASD.

WHY CHOOSE POINTING AND GAIT IN OUR EXAMPLES?

Pointing develops as a precursor of communication in early stages of life when the infant begins to gesture in order to identify objects or people of interest in the social scene (Konczak and Dichgans 1997; Konczak et al. 1995; Scorolli et al. 2016; Spencer et al. 2006; Thelen et al. 1996, 2001). Effective pointing to communicate needs, desires, and decisions requires coordination and coarticulation across multiple joints of the body, along with timely synergies of the underlying muscles. A large body of research has investigated these issues in the typical population, including children (Corbetta and Thelen 1995; Konczak et al. 1995; Thelen et al. 1993) and adults (Domkin et al. 2002; Gottlieb et al. 1996; Torres and Zipser 2004; Tseng et al. 2003; Verrel et al. 2012), but very little work has been done within the field of ASD to separate different manifestations of deficits in sensory-motor control in relation to other features defining the phenotype.

One common phenotypic feature of ASD is the lack of spoken language, or the difficulties and delays to articulate speech. Further, a number of studies have illustrated a reduction in the use of gestures, including communicative pointing actions to indicate a cognitive decision (Torres et al. 2013) in children with ASD—with recent work indicating such children may even have difficulties perceiving these acts (Swettenham et al. 2013). This could be due to nervous system developmental delay, as when an individual has a genetic disorder that results in lengthy maturation of upper-body nerve circuitry. In such cases, the onset of proper eye–hand coordination necessary for accurate visuomotor control may be challenged for both perception and action. The question then is, *could there be a hidden relation between spoken language and pointing movements buried in the motor code that we could automatically extract?*

Indeed, both pointing and talking require a lengthy maturation period. They require the mastering of timely synergies and prospective coarticulation (Hardcastle and Hewlett 1999; Menard et al. 2013; Ryalls et al. 1993; Smith 2006), but developing these abilities requires continuous sensory feedback, particularly as the returning stream of self-generated movements is sensed back through afferent nerves of the periphery and autonomously supervised by the nervous systems. This continuous flow must be further integrated with other sensory inputs from external sources. If the processing of any of these components is impeded during neurodevelopment, proper map and sensory-motor transformation will also be affected.

In the absence of proper self-supervision, instructing a child with pronounced developmental differences how to perform an experimental task could be taxing to both the child and the experimenter. Indeed, the latter may misread the child's responses and interpret the results inappropriately, while the affected child may not deliver the outcome expected by the experimenter. Why not design simple tasks that evoke a natural response by the child, one the child spontaneously would have? Much as when playing at home or simply performing activities of daily living, experiments can be fun and natural to the child. When this is the case, experiments involving gait or pointing may be more feasible to assess the stochastic properties of the biophysical rhythms generated by the nervous systems. Figure 13.1 provides examples of tasks involving naturalistic pointing and walking patterns to assess these stochastic properties in children with neurodevelopmental issues who may not yet gesture or talk fluently.

Walking and its embedded gait patterns requiring high levels of balance and turning control start to develop early in life (Jensen et al. 1994; Smith and Thelen 2003; Thelen and Ulrich 1991; Vereijken and Thelen 1997), although as with pointing, full maturation is not typically attained until several years later (Cowgill et al. 2010; Dierick et al. 2004; Ivanenko et al. 2004; Menkveld et al. 1988; Rose-Jacobs 1983; Stolze et al. 1997). Indeed, the literature on pointing reports that by 4–5 years of age, the nervous system of the typically developing child transitions into mature patterns of pointing kinematics resembling those of young adulthood (Konczak and Dichgans 1997; Thelen and Smith 1994; Torres et al. 2013; Von Hofsten 2009). In contrast, full gait maturation typically manifests later, after 6 years of age (Bisi and Stagni 2016; Belmonti et al. 2013; Menkveld et al. 1988; Sutherland et al. 1980). As such, impairments in the natural development of these multijointed motions may

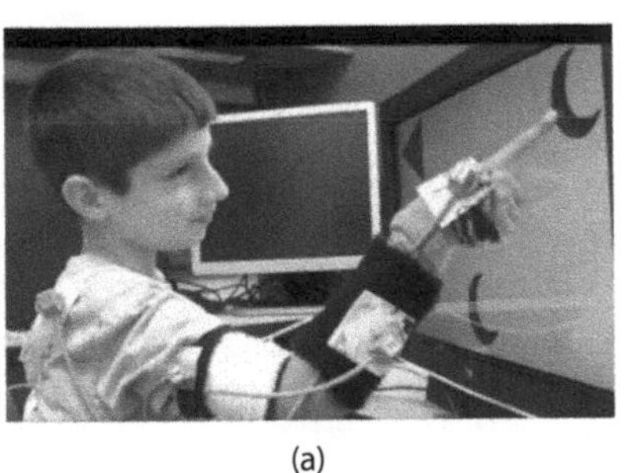

(a)

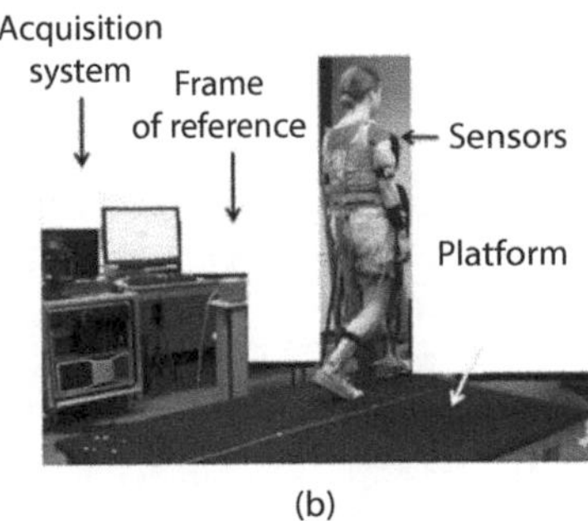

(b)

FIGURE 13.1 Pointing and gait as experimental paradigms to study natural behaviors continuously unfolding different layers of movement classes and cognitive decisions, ranging from deliberate to spontaneous and highly automated. (a) Complex pointing convolved with decision making in a match-to-sample task where the child is asked to decide which figure (out of two choices displayed on the upper left and right corners of the screen) matches the sample in the lower center location. This task is performed by the child, at the child's own pace. He determines the flow of the experiment as the touch of the screen evokes the display of the figures to be matched. He has enough time to decide and then point through self-generated actions. However, the instructions may be challenging, thus calling for a simpler pointing task to be used instead. (b) When pointing is too taxing for the child, natural walking involving gait patterns can be used as a proxy to probe neuromotor control. (Reproduced with permission from Torres et al., *Front. Integr. Neurosci.* 10:22. 2016.)

manifest around the typical transitional ages and help foretell a potential problem with overall maturation in sensory-motor systems. Several of these milestones may be necessary precursors to effectively execute and control intentional acts at will (i.e., needed for the development of volitional control).

A rich body of literature has investigated gait during development (Berger et al. 1984; Menkveld et al. 1988) and helped us gain important insights into issues like "toe walking" (Weber 1978) and other gait disturbances in comorbid conditions like ASD (Calhoun et al. 2011; Kindregan et al. 2015; Vernazza-Martin et al. 2005; Vilensky et al. 1981) and attention deficit hyperactivity disorder (ADHD) (Buderath et al. 2009; Papadopoulos et al. 2014). Some of these studies forecast language impairments from gait disturbances like toe walking (Accardo and Whitman 1989) that are common in ASD and other related disorders. How can we begin a new path of data-driven research connecting the emergence of cognitive disturbances with early manifestations of bodily driven sensory-motor disturbances?

To do so, we need to create new data types, analytical techniques and visualization methods (e.g., see Figures 13.2 and 13.3) enabling the continuous (dynamic) assessment of the nervous systems of the child to create the opportunity to intervene, while being well informed of the moment-by-moment corrective reactions of the child's nervous system to the intervention. We need frameworks for statistical analyses that agree with the nonlinear dynamic nature of neurodevelopment (Thelen and Smith 1994) and with the stochastic features of naturally variable actions (Brincker and Torres 2013; Torres et al. 2013). The new platform for data gathering and analyses should also be amenable to capture longitudinal changes and characterize their rates over time. Further, an important component of this new platform should be features that allow near-real-time use of statistical estimation to close feedback loops corrupted by noise via sensory substitution and sensory augmentation techniques. Lastly, big data rapidly accumulate when using high-grade wearable sensors to continuously track motions over days and months. As such, the new methods should be able to handle large amounts of data rapidly accumulated from wearable sensors, both off- and on-line, a contemporary problem of mobile health for personalized (precision) medicine. In the next sections, we examine some of these issues and provide examples of how they can be addressed in the context of ASD.

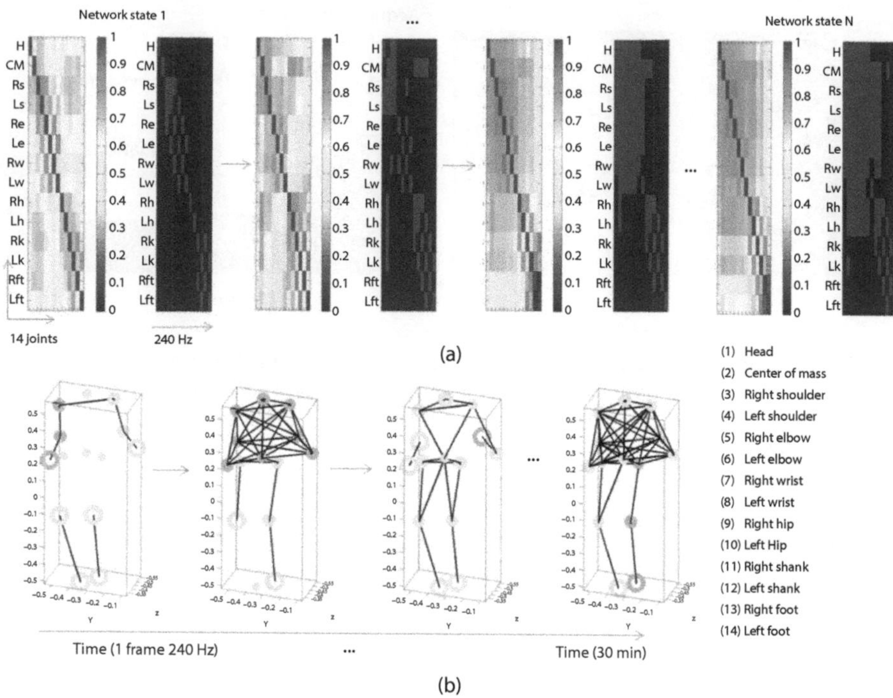

FIGURE 13.2 Visualization of peripheral network of joints as the states of the network dynamically evolve in time (Torres et al. 2016b). Network measures of connectivity and modularity can be automatically tracked as the child walks. (a) Phase-locking value matrices show patterns of synchronicity across the body with corresponding binary matrices obtained by thresholding for high values (Phase Locking Value (PLV) index of 0 means no synchronicity, whereas values close to 1 mean synchronous patterns). (b) Evolution of the network across the body during a 30-minute experimental session. Circle sizes denote clustering coefficient values (higher values of the clustering coefficient represented by larger circles). The gray shades represents the modules that emerge and dissolve during the session. (Reproduced with permission from Torres et al., *Front. Integr. Neurosci.* 10:22, 2016.)

New Data Type: From Discrete Segments to Continuous, Naturalistic Behaviors

The extent to which we can continuously measure a signal from the nervous systems and feed it back in some parameterized form (e.g., to steer the nervous systems' performance) greatly depends on the sampling rate of our instrumentation, the way in which we instruct the individual to move, and the specific data parameters that we choose to extract for analysis.

Let us begin with the latter point. Most pointing, reaching, and grasping experiments in motor control often use targets to study this family of movements as a form of goal-directed behavior. Such studies often segment the motion trajectories into epochs spanning from the onset of the movement to its ending at the target. When the end effector reaches the target or the hand stops, the error between the desired position of the end effector and the position of the target is quantified using some norm. With a few recent exceptions (Torres 2011; Torres et al. 2010, 2011), the retracting segment of the reach is discarded and often treated as a nuisance. However, by doing so, we risk losing information about interconnecting segments of movement, for example, movements away from the target, spontaneously performed, largely beneath awareness. Indeed, such segments do not seem to have a useful purpose in motor control research (Shadmehr and Wise 2005). They are ambiguous, highly variable, and more sensitive to changes in the motion dynamics than the movement segments directed to the goal (Torres et al. 2013).

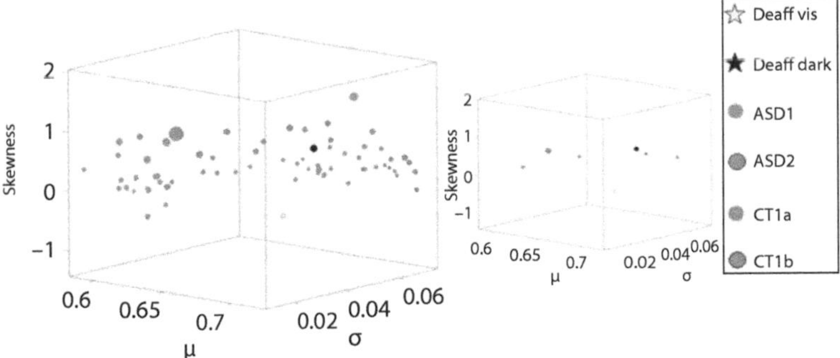

FIGURE 13.3 Signatures of motor output as kinesthetic reafferent input in ASD, controls, and deafferented subject IW. Cross-sectional map of the population contrasting two self-emerging clusters of controls (CT) of various ages (CT1a are older, college-aged students, and CT2 are young children from 3 to 16 years old) and age-matching participants with ASD (ASD1 are young children from 3 to 16 years of age, and ASD2 are young ASD adults from 17 to 25 years of age). IW is represented by a black circle when in complete darkness he points relying on motor imagery, and a yellow circle when he explicitly uses continuous vision of the visual target. Inset shows the centers of the clusters. Note the location of IW signatures centered at the ASD group, and in particular, the inset shows the proximity of the older children to IW's location. The cluster is made up by the estimated moments of the gamma process, estimated with 95% confidence using maximum likelihood estimation (Reproduced with permission from Torres et al., *Front. Neurol.* 7:8, 2016.)

To our surprise however, we found that the "ambiguous" spontaneously performed movement segments that do not seem to follow a specific goal do carry important information about the person's adaptive capabilities (Torres 2011); the degree of motor learning, for example, in sports (Torres 2012); and the ability to predict impending speed in future trials from acceleration and speed in prior trials (Torres 2013). They can also serve as indicators of a lack of balanced control between deliberate and automatic motions in patients with Parkinson's disease (Torres et al. 2011), or reveal adequate strategies to guide the injured nervous systems of some stroke patients (Torres et al. 2010).

It is not always straightforward to characterize continuous behaviors. Instrumentation and sensors sample discrete measurements per unit time. A time series of such discrete occurrences must then be converted to a continuous signal representing a continuous random point process (Clamann 1969; Fee et al. 1996; Salcido et al. 2012) before being able to analyze it with appropriate statistical methods. Once a proper analytical platform is in place to handle real-time estimation and continuous longitudinal tracking of neurodevelopment, we can characterize the noise-to-signal ratios of various parameters extracted from biophysical rhythms output by the various parts of the nervous systems. In this sense, the waveform variability in amplitude and timing will be critical to attain such empirical characterization and determine parameter ranges across multiple layers of control.

NOISE IN THE PERIPHERY

Since motor variability and its sensation may be at the core of a necessary foundation to scaffold cognition at various levels (see Chapter 1 and Brincker and Torres 2013), it becomes crucial to identify critical ingredients in the kinematics data to help better characterize the motor output in great detail.

An important aspect of neurodevelopment may emerge by mapping the signal-to-noise ratios at the motor output onto the various levels of control the nervous systems have. Determining the ranges of proper levels of signal-to-noise ratios may help us design therapies aimed at attaining prospective control of actions and decision (Torres et al. 2016a). These could include (among others) the ability of the newborn to autonomously control the respiration rhythms during food intake, to avoid choking—a skill developed early during infancy that could provide clues to help us unveil their mechanisms (Craig et al. 1999, 2000; Craig and Lee 1999). This form of autonomous neuromotor control must precede other abilities to coarticulate muscles in the orofacial structures and produce timely sounds (Barlow and Estep 2006). It remains to be seen if such abilities also precede or help scaffold language. We believe that structures suffering from persistent noisy output, and thus noisy reafference, will certainly have difficulties developing prospective motor control.

In the presence of excess noise and randomness, how would these structures continuously sense back vibrations from sound production and build an error correction code possibly operating a step ahead to compensate for motor sensing transductions and transmission delays?

Today, we lack knowledge about the typical levels of proprioception across facial structures involved in neuromotor control. Yet we know that bodily sensations partly depend on perceiving the self in motion. Indeed, proprioception and kinesthetic reafference are important to build and to continuously update internal models for action control (Kawato and Wolpert 1998). Even when the motor apparatus is intact to facilitate the contraction and relaxation of bodily muscles and produce forces, continuous movement production and control are impossible if continuous kinesthetic sensing is impeded (Balslev 2007a, 2007b; Cole 1995; Ingram et al. 2000; Miall and Cole 2007; Miall et al. 1995, 2000). These models and views motivate us to search for signatures of kinesthetic sensing that differ from typical ones; that is, unveiling the typical ranges and building normative data to that end should be our priority. What sort of impairments could emerge from a persistent noisy kinesthetic code in autism?

It is worthwhile to point out that the extant methods in the autism literature used to interpret results from motor control studies, such as those implying that individuals with ASD lack or have intact proprioception, have yielded inconclusive outcomes. For example, impaired proprioception in ASD has been suggested as a source of problems with one-leg balancing with eyes closed (Weimer et al. 2001). Yet, studies of reaching or decision-making behavior have claimed that no proprioceptive deficits have been identified (Fuentes et al. 2011; Sharer et al. 2016), particularly during force adaptation studies (Gidley Larson et al. 2008). Part of the reasons for such contradictory interpretations may lie in the methods and paradigms employed. A large majority of motor assessment is performed through clinical inventories and self-reports that do not actually measure the underlying physiology of the motor outputs. More recent developments in our lab are moving toward a more objective approach to the study of neurodevelopment (e.g., the visualization and quantification of gait patterns in Figure 13.2).

Other experimental paradigms in psychology assess reaction times in behavioral responses using mouse-clicks, where movement is restrained and not measured at all. Furthermore, studies that employ analyses of continuously evolving kinematics parameters tend to smooth out minute fluctuations in motor performance as noise and measure only discrete epochs of the continuous motions. This smoothing process is completed under the assumption of Gaussian processes and theoretical Gaussian mean and variance parameters (see Chapter 11). We have, however, found that parameters of the kinematics do not distribute normally (Torres 2011, 2012; Torres et al. 2013a). In autism, the variability of such motion parameters is atypical, and the minute changes in amplitude and timing of kinematics events that are traditionally averaged out as noise contain large amounts of information illuminating more than one area of inquiry in this condition of the nervous systems. It is indeed worthwhile to explore these variations with new methods that do not a priori assume anything about the random processes under examination.

As explained above, we have recently characterized the fluctuations in amplitude and timing of parameters using a gamma process under the assumption that events are independent and identically distributed (iid). To that end, we have used maximum likelihood estimation to fit the gamma family of probability distributions to empirical data and estimate the shape and dispersion parameters of the probability distributions of each individual in a group. The moments of the estimated distributions are subsequently computed to uncover normative ranges of these stochastic parameters. Then we can compare those ranges with empirically estimated ranges found in individuals with a diagnosis of ASD (Torres et al. 2016a). Figure 13.3 shows the self-emerging clusters separating individuals in the spectrum from typical controls. Note how prominent this separation is, with much higher variability in ASD and slower motions on average than neurotypical controls.

DEAFFERENTED SUBJECT IAN WATERMAN

In addition to typical controls, we included in our studies of movement in autism a participant named Ian Waterman (IW). IW is an individual who has been physically deafferented from C3 down since the age of 19 years old (aged 42 at the time of data collection). It is worthwhile to explain why this was a critical step in our inquiry.

IW is the only documented case of an individual with physical deafferentation that can walk and move in a highly controlled manner (Cole 1995). He has attained this major accomplishment by teaching himself a form of sensory substitution. Specifically, IW has learned to replace continuous kinesthetic reafference with continuous visual reafference and motor imagery to deliberately plan every aspect of his motions. After many years of use, he has created a large repertoire of cognitive maps of all his bodily movements. He uses those maps on demand and is capable of adapting and readapting them on-line. Indeed, we were able to witness this ability firsthand when IW visited our lab for experiments. In particular, we used the aforementioned pointing (forward and back) paradigm to ask if there were any similarities between the stochastic signatures of speed peak modulations in amplitude for IW and those of the individuals with ASD. To that end, we examined the global speed peaks of the forward and back, point-to-point ballistic segments and extracted their micromovements to characterize them using a gamma process.

Why would this question be of any relevance in light of the type of data we analyze and the analyses we perform? The data that we analyze are continuously read out from the nervous systems at the motor output level. They are a spike train of fluctuations in the signals' amplitude and timing. Yet this efferent output signal is convolved with sensory input from afferent channels that continuously update internally sensed kinesthetic information and externally sensed sensory inputs from the environment. In the words of Von Holst and Mittelstaedt (1950), we need to separate exoafference from reafference in the efferent motor signal that we track. Clearly, electrodes inserted in the sensory and motor nerves would give us a better waveform to work with to that end, but we would lose the non-invasive feature of the wearable sensors, and would then be constrained to lab work, or to work in clinics with such facilities. Yet, ASD is a worldwide condition, with a number of families with an affected child struggling to afford the luxury of health care or direct access to basic scientific research. In this sense, we aim to design methods that can work with a signal that we can harness using off-the-shelf technology, readily and massively available to many in the world population at large.

The case of IW without afferent signals from the self-generated movements that his brain causes served as a control subject to help us better understand and interpret the potential meaning of the noise patterns we found in ASD. We reasoned that if the signatures of the individuals with ASD clustered near or around IW's signatures, it was likely that their movement-based sensing was impeded. To test this question, we used two conditions for IW. One was with explicit and continuous visual feedback of the target. The other was in complete darkness. In the former, he continuously and deliberately updates the ongoing pointing path based on the visual information that changes the distance between his moving hand and the fixed target. In the second case, the information IW uses for updating his hand path comes from motor imagery. He imagines the movement explicitly, and the hand–target distance reduction occurs internally in his mind.

The work with IW provided a valuable insight into the possible interpretation of the random and noisy patterns that we found in ASD using the new statistical platform for the personalized analyses of continuous kinematics data. It alerted us of the possibility that persistent noisy and random motion patterns continuously fed back to the CNS as reafferent kinesthetic sensory input may give rise to a form of virtual deafferentation. While IW is physically deafferented and the signatures of his motions are due to this physical cutoff of information between the CNS and the PNS, we do not know the extent to which the afferent nerves of the ASD individual may be impaired (e.g., poor myelination and pre- and/or post-synaptic issues). Further, IW's brain developed in typical fashion and formed maps to scaffold pointing behavior from an early age. His physical deafferentation took place as a young adult at 19 years old. In ASD, the neurodevelopment of the brain circuitry and cortical and subcortical structures supporting the planning and execution of pointing motions has been reportedly atypical since birth (D'Mello et al. 2015; Kaufmann et al. 2003; Mahajan et al. 2016; Mostofsky et al. 2009; Nebel et al. 2014; Qiu et al. 2010). As such, the source of the problem could be not only in the faulty sensory feedback that continuous self-produced motions provide, but also in the implementation of the output itself. Indeed, many children with ASD suffer from hypotonia (muscle weakness) at birth and beyond. This condition could in principle impede the transmission of the signal from central structures. In this data set, however, the motor implementation of the pointing motion was possible, and although slower on average and more variable than that of the age-matched controls (Figure 13.3), it was comparable in speed and variability to that of IW. IW has no visible problem outputting and implementing the motor command. His signatures and those of the ASD match in statistical features. As such, it is likely that the level of noise that we find in the motor output patterns of individuals with ASD contributes to corrupted reafferent feedback. These results provide evidence to suggest that sensory feedback from actively produced movements may be impeded in ASD.

CAN WE SHIFT FROM RANDOM AND NOISY MOTOR PATTERNS IN ASD TO PREDICTABLE MOTOR SIGNALS?

One of the advantages of the types of methods presented in this chapter is the ability to update, in near real time, the estimates of the stochastic signatures from moment to moment. This possibility enables us to close the feedback loops and provide the end user of computer-based interfaces with well-informed somatic motor feedback along appropriately working sensory channels. Such an approach opens new avenues to employ sensory substitution techniques to design personalized treatments. Having the ability to identify appropriate sensory channels for therapy is crucial, as we may help improve the internal states of the physiology of the child. In the adult system, it has been possible to identify sources of sensory guidance that improve the system toward typical ranges. The adequacy of the sensory input for guidance is different across populations of patients. For example, appropriate sensory guidance for a stroke patient with a lesion in the left posterior parietal cortex comes from external sources, such as continuous visual feedback from the target (Torres et al. 2010). In contrast, patients with Parkinson's disease benefit from continuous visual feedback of their moving finger as they point to a memorized target (Torres 2011).

Therapies that are designed without consideration of somatic motor issues in ASD may induce stress in excess. In turn, such therapies may prove ineffective because the pace of learning and adaptive sensory-motor control may be negatively impacted by excess stress. As such, tailoring the feedback that the therapist or clinician provides to the child to abide by the inherent sensory-motor processing capabilities of that child is important. Some relevant questions in this regard may then be, what sensory channel or combination of sensory channels may be more effective to deliver stimulus and influence the behavior effectively? How often shall we reassess the child's behavioral output during a session to estimate the trends we see with the therapy on any given day? And how often shall we do so across months of therapy?

These questions are important because at present, there is no coverage in the United States for many therapies that are reportedly effective in ASD (e.g., developmental, individual difference, relationship-based [DIR] or floor time [Greenspan and Wieder 2006], sensory-motor-based occupational therapy [Miller and Fuller 2006], and American hippotherapy [Engel and MacKinnon 2007]). The forms of therapeutic interventions proposed here could rely on objective outcome measures and provide updates to insurance companies in the United States on their effectiveness to justify coverage.

Further, all therapies involving a dyadic interaction between the child and the clinician could benefit from the tracking of synergistic relations between the two. In turn, improvements in dyadic synergistic relations in real time can translate into improvements in sociomotor behavior. The latter are ultimately required in social dynamics of the social scene at large. The methods presented here can help the tracking of individual patterns in synthetic scenarios where the dyad is formed between an end user and an avatar (Figure 13.4) or in real dyadic interactions between a clinician and a child (e.g., see ADOS interactions in Chapter 7).

Along the lines of individual tracking of motor sensing signatures, we have also developed ways to engage the individual child with interactive media and tailor the media to the child's sensory and somatic-motoric preferences. This has been done by continuously reassessing (through the motor output signal) the outcome of such interactions, while determining within the session which media brings the motion patterns away from noisy and random (according to the outcome measurements we have described above) and toward less noisy and more predictable regimes. Importantly, a distinct feature of our application was that we did not explicitly prompt the child in these experimental interventions (Torres et al. 2013). Instead, we evoked the exchange between the child motions and the media by using the real-time output from the wearable sensors affixed to the child's hand, arm, and trunk.

To that end, we created a scenario whereby the child's real-time movement patterns were tracked as a gamma process. Moment by moment, we estimated the shape and scale of the gamma probability distribution function best fitting the frequency histogram of the micromovements embedded in the

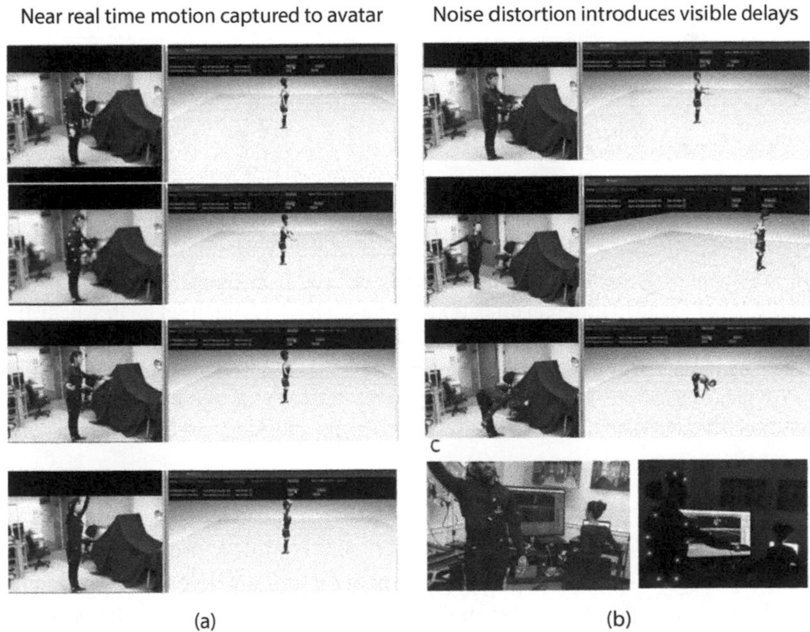

FIGURE 13.4 Synthetic dyadic exchange between a human user and a computer avatar where the present methods are used to provide mirrored and distorted versions of the near-real-time motions as output by high-speed cameras (the phase space). (a) The avatar projected on a large screen within the unity environment that renders the three-dimensional images is endowed with the veridical motions directly harnessed with the active light-emitting diodes (LEDs) located on the person. (b) The present methods are then used to estimate the moment-by-moment gamma process of the motions and feed back to the person via the avatar distorted versions of the ongoing movements. By introducing well-informed delays, parameterizing the motions in different ways, we can build a computational platform to simulate and explore effective, as well as ineffective, scenarios in motion-based feedback during interventions. (Courtesy of Rutgers University Sensory Motor Integration Lab, New Brunswick, NJ, work by Vilelmini Kalampratsiduo.)

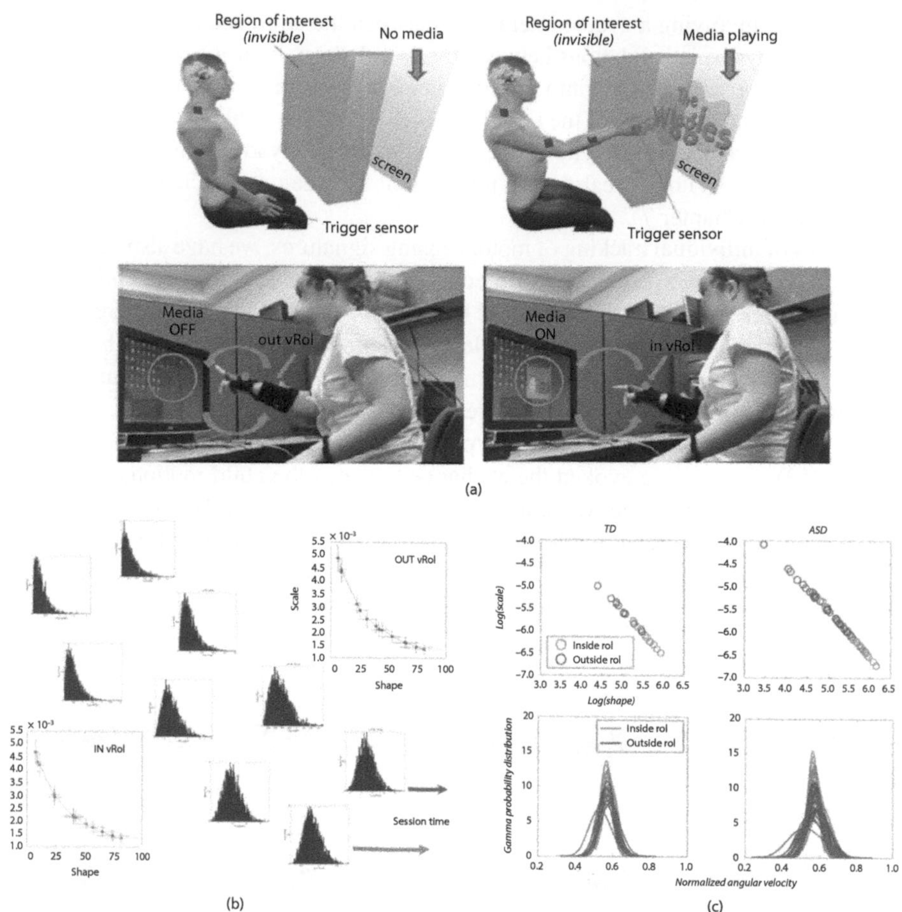

FIGURE 13.5 Spontaneously evoking changes in behavior in ASD using parameterized motor output–based feedback and audiovisual media in near real time. (a) Experimental intervention set up in schematic form and real implementation. (b) Evolution of gamma process within one session for intentional seeking vRoI (light gray) vs. spontaneously leaving it (dark gray). (c) Transitioning from excess noise and randomness (dark gray) in the ASD motor signal to typical signatures (light gray) comparable to those of age-matched neurotypical controls. (Reproduced with permission from Torres, E. B., Yanovich, P., and Metaxas, D. N. *Front. Integr. Neurosci.* 7:46, 2013.)

angular (or linear) velocities of the hand as the hand entered or left a virtual region of interest (vRoI) that we defined. This region spanned a preprogrammable volume whereby we could change the size of the volume (shrink it or expand it) and shift the location of its center across the personal space comfortably reachable by the hand without having to stretch out (the peripersonal workspace). While the child comfortably sat (Figure 13.5a), we let the child spontaneously explore the peripersonal workspace. As the hand entered the vRoI, the media output was triggered in front of the child. This established a loop of cause and effect that in the initial stages was not obvious. To the child, the event initially looked as a random occurrence. Yet, as any curious child would, the children with ASD (each one of 25 with no fluent spoken language in this experiment) explored the peripersonal workspace in search for that "magic spot" that caused the media to play. Since we were quantifying the changes in the gamma process from moment to moment, we could see which media was most effectively shifting the hand angular (and/or linear) speed patterns from random and noisy to predictively periodic. We could also assess the emergence of high signal-to-noise ratios.

We varied the media stimuli, identifying the child's preferred stimulus. For instance, the child's self-image was displayed from the real-time video of the session (captured from a video camera facing the child), whereas other media included cartoon clips. We then examined which children preferred what stimulus in the precise sense of which stimulus was the most effective (i.e., shifting at the fastest rate) toward those of age-matched neurotypical controls. Notably, these shifts occurred in a matter of minutes. Most importantly, when we returned for a follow-up session 4–5 weeks later, all children had remembered the task and retained the exploratory abilities, along with the adaptive capacity to shift the signatures of motor output as a function of the media type.

This consistent change in behavioral signatures quantified in one session was retained when we returned weeks later (Figure 13.5b). This type of retention without training strongly suggests that something vital is spared in the autistic condition, that is, the ability to spontaneously, through trial and error, infer the goal of the task and solve it to attain a reward. In our case, unlike in other interventions, this reward was internally triggered, that is, self-motivated, once the children established cause and effect. Indeed, the children were not externally rewarded with food or tokens in this case. They were not explicitly prompted to complete the task either. They obtained their reward of self-controlling the projection of their preferred cartoon or their self-video image by *spontaneously* exploring the peripersonal workspace. Much as any newborn baby would do, the children with ASD in this study had the ability to self-discover basic causal relations in the world.

We just had to step back and watch the process unfold in front of our eyes. It was the most rewarding experience we ever had in our autism research. In some cases, a child who would only script or use echolalia uttered sounds and words that for the first time fit the occasion perfectly (i.e., "What's happening? … Happening now …"). As that child became in control of the situation, driving the flow of the interaction and not being told what to do, his or her nervous systems became self-regulated. Something really profound about human volition and its deliberate control revealed itself to our faces during those days of experimentation at the Rutgers Douglass Developmental Disability Center and at the Christian Sarkine Autism Treatment Center of Indianapolis.

TAKE-HOME LESSON: DISCONNECTED BRAIN SCIENCE NEEDS TO BRIDGE THE MIND–BODY DICHOTOMY IN ASD DEFINITION, RESEARCH, AND TREATMENTS

Perhaps owing to the disembodied approach prevalent in cognitive psychology, it has been challenging to connect motor deficits with the evident cognitive and social impairments that later appear during neurodevelopment and that, in many cases, give rise to the ASD phenotype. In recent years, embodied cognition has emerged as a new subfield of cognitive psychology to begin considering the possible influences of bodily maps on mental navigation (Clark 2006, 2007; Gallese 2007), affordances (Brincker 2014), and cognitive motor control (Garbarini and Adenzato 2004; Gallese 2007; Thelen et al. 2001), among other ingredients required to scaffold proper social dynamics.

This promising subfield known to many as embodied cognition has yet to make contact with clinical ASD, where a psychological-psychiatric construct prevails to describe disembodied social issues as mental illnesses. In contrast, the approaches described in this chapter are congruent with the views of embodied cognition (Lobel 2014; Shapiro 2011; Ziemke et al. 2007) and ecological psychology (Gibson 1979, 1983). They afford the types of closed-loop approaches used in the fields of brain–machine and body–machine interfaces and neural smart prosthetics that use sensory substitution and sensory augmentation techniques to guide and adapt the nervous systems' functioning in real time. These techniques that reparameterize the nervous systems' output and feed it back to the end user in near real time in a highly controlled manner hold tremendous promise in ASD interventions, as shown here by the related work from our lab (Torres et al. 2013).

We consider the types of social behaviors used to evaluate and detect an autistic condition as a continuous bundle of movements with variable degrees of voluntary control feeding information back to the brain through afferent nerves in the body, some occurring largely beneath awareness and some performed rather deliberately with a concrete goal or purpose. The types of top-down decision-making processes required during social exchange and ultimately executed by sensory-motor systems are not merely mental in our conceptualization of cognitive control. They emerge over time and are embodied in the early stages of development. As such, they require the early development of neuromotor control from the bottom up (see Chapter 3).

As discussed in Chapter 3, bridging such aspects of behavior with cognitive-social exchange that uses discrete inventories is impossible under the disembodied schema of cognitive psychology. Well-known theories of ASD, such as the theory of mind (ToM) (Baron-Cohen et al. 1985, 1995), the empathizing-systematizing theory (Baron-Cohen 2009), or the lack of central coherence theory (Briskman et al. 2001), rely on the description of observed phenomena through inventories and surveys. But self-reporting or reporting on the behaviors of others by observation alone misses much of the nuances and subtleties of behavior occurring at frequencies and timescales that escape conscious processing. These aspects of behavior do not enter in the clinical inventories used to validate such theories (e.g., the autism quotient [Baron-Cohen et al. 2001] and the ADOS-2 [Lord et al. 2000]). And much of the related ongoing kinematics research involving eye motions or pointing behavior during ToM experiments tends to average motion trajectories and discard as noise important fluctuations in subtle aspects of social exchange that high-grade instrumentation could detect. Because of these methodological issues, a critical need exists today for (1) paradigms that encourage continuously flowing natural behaviors with the potential to generate new data types in embodied-cognitive approaches to brain research, (2) proper analytics to quantify motor phenomena as they naturally occur in unconstrained behaviors that are inevitably embedded in the social scene, and (3) analytics that permit corrective feedback to the user provided in near real time and derived from statistically well-informed patterns along sensory channels that the person's nervous system may naturally prefer. If we follow these fundamental steps, there is a chance to connect mind and body and build a bridge between the intent to act and the (deliberate) volitional control of the actions caused by that intent. The methods presented in this chapter provide a unifying framework to implement research programs centered on the preferences of the person and, above all, presuming the person's competence for communication and social exchange.

REFERENCES

Accardo, P., and B. Whitman. 1989. Toe walking. A marker for language disorders in the developmentally disabled. *Clin Pediatr (Phila)* 28 (8):347–50.

American Psychiatric Association. 2013. *Diagnostic and Statistical Manual of Mental Disorders*. 5th ed. Washington, DC: American Psychiatric Association

Balslev, D., J. Cole, and R. C. Miall. 2007a. Proprioception contributes to the sense of agency during visual observation of hand movements: Evidence from temporal judgments of action. *J Cogn Neurosci* 19 (9): 1535–41. doi: 10.1162/jocn.2007.19.9.1535.

Balslev, D., R. C. Miall, and J. Cole. 2007b. Proprioceptive deafferentation slows down the processing of visual hand feedback. *J Vis* 7 (5):12 1–7. doi: 10.1167/7.5.127/5/12 [pii].

Barlow, S. M., and M. Estep. 2006. Central pattern generation and the motor infrastructure for suck, respiration, and speech. *J Commun Disord* 39 (5):366–80. doi: 10.1016/j.jcomdis.2006.06.011.

Baron-Cohen, S. 2009. Autism: The empathizing-systemizing (E-S) theory. *Ann NY Acad Sci* 1156:68–80. doi: 10.1111/j.1749-6632.2009.04467.x.

Baron-Cohen, S., A. M. Leslie, and U. Frith. 1985. Does the autistic child have a "theory of mind"? *Cognition* 21 (1):37–46. doi: 0010-0277(85)90022-8 [pii].

Baron-Cohen, S., L. Cosmides, and J. Toobv. 1995. *Mindblindness: An Essay on Autism and Theory of Mind*. Cambridge, MA: MIT Press.

Baron-Cohen, S., S. Wheelwright, R. Skinner, J. Martin, and E. Clubley. 2001. The autism-spectrum quotient (AQ): Evidence from Asperger syndrome/high-functioning autism, males and females, scientists and mathematicians. *J Autism Dev Disord* 31 (1):5–17.

Belmonti, V., G. Cioni, and A. Berthoz. 2013. Development of anticipatory orienting strategies and trajectory formation in goal-oriented locomotion. *Exp Brain Res* 227 (1):131–47. doi: 10.1007/s00221-013-3495-3.

Berger, W., E. Altenmueller, and V. Dietz. 1984. Normal and impaired development of children's gait. *Hum Neurobiol* 3 (3):163–70.

Bernshteĭn, N. A. 1967. *The Co-ordination and Regulation of Movements.* 1st English ed. Oxford: Pergamon Press.

Bisi, M. C., and R. Stagni. 2016. Development of gait motor control: What happens after a sudden increase in height during adolescence? *Biomed Eng Online* 15 (1):47. doi: 10.1186/s12938-016-0159-0.

Bodfish, J. W., F. J. Symons, D. E. Parker, and M. H. Lewis. 2000. Varieties of repetitive behavior in autism: Comparisons to mental retardation. *J Autism Dev Disord* 30 (3):237–43.

Brincker, M. 2014. Navigating beyond "here & now" affordances—On sensorimotor maturation and "false belief" performance. *Front Psychol* 5:1433. doi: 10.3389/fpsyg.2014.01433.

Brincker, M., and E. B. Torres. 2013. Noise from the periphery in autism. *Front Integr Neurosci* 7:34. doi: 10.3389/fnint.2013.00034.

Briskman, J., F. Happe, and U. Frith. 2001. Exploring the cognitive phenotype of autism: Weak "central coherence" in parents and siblings of children with autism. II. Real-life skills and preferences. *J Child Psychol Psychiatry* 42 (3):309–16.

Buderath, P., K. Gartner, M. Frings, H. Christiansen, B. Schoch, J. Konczak, E. R. Gizewski, J. Hebebrand, and D. Timmann. 2009. Postural and gait performance in children with attention deficit/hyperactivity disorder. *Gait Posture* 29 (2):249–54. doi: 10.1016/j.gaitpost.2008.08.016.

Calhoun, M., M. Longworth, and V. L. Chester. 2011. Gait patterns in children with autism. *Clin Biomech (Bristol, Avon)* 26 (2):200–6. doi: 10.1016/j.clinbiomech.2010.09.013.

Clamann, H. P. 1969. Statistical analysis of motor unit firing patterns in a human skeletal muscle. *Biophys J* 9 (10):1233–51. doi: 10.1016/S0006-3495(69)86448-9.

Clark, A. 2006. Language, embodiment, and the cognitive niche. *Trends Cogn Sci* 10 (8):370–4. doi: 10.1016/j.tics.2006.06.012.

Clark, A. 2007. Re-inventing ourselves: The plasticity of embodiment, sensing, and mind. *J Med Philos* 32 (3): 263–82. doi: 780168855 [pii].10.1080/03605310701397024..

Cole, J. 1995. *Pride and a Daily Marathon.* 1st MIT Press ed. Cambridge, MA: MIT Press.

Corbetta, D., and E. Thelen. 1995. A method for identifying the initiation of reaching movements in natural prehension. *J Mot Behav* 28 (3):285–93.

Cowgill, L. W., A. Warrener, H. Pontzer, and C. Ocobock. 2010. Waddling and toddling: The biomechanical effects of an immature gait. *Am J Phys Anthropol* 143 (1):52–61. doi: 10.1002/ajpa.21289.

Craig, C. M., and D. N. Lee. 1999. Neonatal control of nutritive sucking pressure: Evidence for an intrinsic tau-guide. *Exp Brain Res* 124 (3):371–82.

Craig, C. M., D. N. Lee, Y. N. Freer, and I. A. Laing. 1999. Modulations in breathing patterns during intermittent feeding in term infants and preterm infants with bronchopulmonary dysplasia. *Dev Med Child Neurol* 41 (9):616–24.

Craig, C. M., M. A. Grealy, and D. N. Lee. 2000. Detecting motor abnormalities in preterm infants. *Exp Brain Res* 131 (3):359–65.

Damasio, A. R., and R. G. Maurer. 1978. A neurological model for childhood autism. *Arch Neurol* 35 (12): 777–86.

Deitz, J. C., D. Kartin, and K. Kopp. 2007. Review of the Bruininks-Oseretsky test of motor proficiency, (BOT-2). *Phys Occup Ther Pediatr* 27 (4):87–102.

Dierick, F., C. Lefebvre, A. van den Hecke, and C. Detrembleur. 2004. Development of displacement of centre of mass during independent walking in children. *Dev Med Child Neurol* 46 (8):533–9.

D'Mello, A. M., D. Crocetti, S. H. Mostofsky, and C. J. Stoodley. 2015. Cerebellar gray matter and lobular volumes correlate with core autism symptoms. *Neuroimage Clin* 7:631–9.

Domkin, D., J. Laczko, S. Jaric, H. Johansson, and M. L. Latash. 2002. Structure of joint variability in bimanual pointing tasks. *Exp Brain Res* 143 (1):11–23. doi: 10.1007/s00221-001-0944-1.

Donnellan, A. M., and M. R. Leary. 1995. *Movement Differences and Diversity in Autism/Mental Retardation: Appreciating and Accommodating People with Communication and Behavior Challenges.* Movin on Series. Madison, WI: DRI Press.

Donnellan, A. M., and M. R. Leary. 2012. *Autism: Sensory-Movement Differences and Diversity*. 1st ed. Cambridge, WI: Cambridge Book Review Press.

Donnellan, A. M., D. A. Hill, and M. R. Leary. 2012. Rethinking autism: Implications of sensory and movement differences for understanding and support. *Front Integr Neurosci* 6:124 doi: 10.3389/fnint.2012.00124.

Dowell, L. R., E. M. Mahone, and S. H. Mostofsky. 2009. Associations of postural knowledge and basic motor skill with dyspraxia in autism: Implication for abnormalities in distributed connectivity and motor learning. *Neuropsychology* 23 (5):563–70. doi: 10.1037/a0015640.

Dziuk, M. A., J. C. Gidley Larson, A. Apostu, E. M. Mahone, M. B. Denckla, and S. H. Mostofsky. 2007. Dyspraxia in autism: Association with motor, social, and communicative deficits. *Dev Med Child Neurol* 49 (10):734–9. doi: 10.1111/j.1469-8749.2007.00734.x.

Engel, B. T., and J. R. MacKinnon. 2007. *Enhancing Human Occupation through Hippotherapy: A Guide for Occupational Therapy*. Bethesda, MD: AOTA Press.

Fee, M. S., P. P. Mitra, and D. Kleinfeld. 1996. Variability of extracellular spike waveforms of cortical neurons. *J Neurophysiol* 76 (6):3823–33.

Feĭgenberg, I. M., and J. Linkova. 2014. *Nikolai Bernstein: From Reflex to the Model of the Future, Studien zur Geschichte des Sports*. Zurich: Lit Verlag.

Fuentes, C. T., S. H. Mostofsky, and A. J. Bastian. 2009. Children with autism show specific handwriting impairments. *Neurology* 73 (19):1532–7.

Fuentes, C. T., S. H. Mostofsky, and A. J. Bastian. 2011. No proprioceptive deficits in autism despite movement-related sensory and execution impairments. *J Autism Dev Disord* 41 (10):1352–61.

Gallese, V. 2007. Before and below 'theory of mind': Embodied simulation and the neural correlates of social cognition. *Philos Trans R Soc Lond B Biol Sci* 362 (1480):659–69. doi: 10.1098/rstb.2006.2002.

Garbarini, F., and M. Adenzato. 2004. At the root of embodied cognition: Cognitive science meets neurophysiology. *Brain Cogn* 56 (1):100–6. doi: 10.1016/j.bandc.2004.06.003.

Gibson, J. J. 1979. *The Ecological Approach to Visual Perception*. Boston: Houghton Mifflin.

Gibson, J. J. 1983. *The Senses Considered as Perceptual Systems*. Westport, CT: Greenwood Press.

Gidley Larson, J. C., A. J. Bastian, O. Donchin, R. Shadmehr, and S. H. Mostofsky. 2008. Acquisition of internal models of motor tasks in children with autism. *Brain* 131 (11):2894–903.

Gottlieb, G. L., Q. Song, D. A. Hong, and D. M. Corcos. 1996. Coordinating two degrees of freedom during human arm movement: Load and speed invariance of relative joint torques. *J Neurophysiol* 76 (5):3196–206.

Green, D., T. Charman, A. Pickles, S. Chandler, T. Loucas, E. Simonoff, and G. Baird. 2009. Impairment in movement skills of children with autistic spectrum disorders. *Dev Med Child Neurol* 51 (4):311–6.

Greenspan, S. I., and S. Wieder. 2006. *Infant and Early Childhood Mental Health: A Comprehensive, Developmental Approach to Assessment and Intervention*. 1st ed. Washington, DC: American Psychiatric Association.

Hardcastle, W. J., and N. Hewlett. 1999. *Coarticulation: Theory, Data, and Techniques*. Cambridge: Cambridge University Press.

Harony-Nicolas, H., S. De Rubeis, A. Kolevzon, and J. D. Buxbaum. 2015. Phelan McDermid syndrome: From genetic discoveries to animal models and treatment. *J Child Neurol* 30 (14):1861–70. doi: 10.1177/0883073815600872.

Haswell, C. C., J. Izawa, L. R. Dowell, S. H. Mostofsky, and R. Shadmehr. 2009. Representation of internal models of action in the autistic brain. *Nat Neurosci* 12 (8):970–2. doi: 10.1038/nn.2356.

Ingram, H. A., P. van Donkelaar, J. Cole, J. L. Vercher, G. M. Gauthier, and R. C. Miall. 2000. The role of proprioception and attention in a visuomotor adaptation task. *Exp Brain Res* 132 (1):114–26.

Ivanenko, A., V. M. Crabtree, and D. Gozal. 2004. Sleep in children with psychiatric disorders. *Pediatr Clin North Am* 51 (1):51–68.

Jansiewicz, E. M., M. C. Goldberg, C. J. Newschaffer, M. B. Denckla, R. Landa, and S. H. Mostofsky. 2006. Motor signs distinguish children with high functioning autism and Asperger's syndrome from controls. *J Autism Dev Disord* 36 (5):613–21. doi: 10.1007/s10803-006-0109-y.

Jensen, J. L., K. Schneider, B. D. Ulrich, R. F. Zernicke, and E. Thelen. 1994. Adaptive dynamics of the leg movement patterns of human infants. *I. The effects of posture on spontaneous kicking. J Mot Behav* 26 (4):303–12. doi: 10.1080/00222895.1994.9941686.

Kaufmann, W. E., K. L. Cooper, S. H. Mostofsky, G. T. Capone, W. R. Kates, C. J. Newschaffer, I. Bukelis, M. H. Stump, A. E. Jann, and D. C. Lanham. 2003. Specificity of cerebellar vermian abnormalities in autism: A quantitative magnetic resonance imaging study. *J Child Neurol* 18 (7):463–70.

Kawato, M., and D. Wolpert. 1998. Internal models for motor control. *Novartis Found Symp* 218:291–304; discussion 304–7.

Kindregan, D., L. Gallagher, and J. Gormley. 2015. Gait deviations in children with autism spectrum disorders: A review. *Autism Res Treat* 2015:741480. doi: 10.1155/2015/741480.

Konczak, J., and J. Dichgans. 1997. The development toward stereotypic arm kinematics during reaching in the first 3 years of life. *Exp Brain Res* 117 (2):346–54.

Konczak, J., M. Borutta, H. Topka, and J. Dichgans. 1995. The development of goal-directed reaching in infants: Hand trajectory formation and joint torque control. *Exp Brain Res* 106 (1):156–68.

Kuiken, T. A., G. Li, B. A. Lock, R. D. Lipschutz, L. A. Miller, K. A. Stubblefield, and K. B. Englehart. 2009. Targeted muscle reinnervation for real-time myoelectric control of multifunction artificial arms. *JAMA* 301 (6):619–28. doi: 10.1001/jama.2009.116.

Lobel, T. 2014. *Sensation: The New Science of Physical Intelligence*. 1st Atria Books hardcover ed. New York: Atria Books.

Lord, C., S. Risi, L. Lambrecht, E. H. Cook Jr., B. L. Leventhal, P. C. DiLavore, A. Pickles, and M. Rutter. 2000. The Autism Diagnostic Observation Schedule-Generic: A standard measure of social and communication deficits associated with the spectrum of autism. *J Autism Dev Disord* 30 (3):205–23.

Mahajan, R., B. Dirlikov, D. Crocetti, and S. H. Mostofsky. 2016. Motor circuit anatomy in children with autism spectrum disorder with or without attention deficit hyperactivity disorder. *Autism Res* 9 (1):67–81. doi: 10.1002/aur.1497.

Marko, M. K., D. Crocetti, T. Hulst, O. Donchin, R. Shadmehr, and S. H. Mostofsky. 2015. Behavioural and neural basis of anomalous motor learning in children with autism. *Brain* 138 (Pt 3):784–97. doi: 10.1093/brain/awu394.

Menard, L., M. A. Cathiard, S. Dupont, and M. Tiede. 2013. Anticipatory lip gestures: A validation of the movement expansion model in congenitally blind speakers. *J Acoust Soc Am* 133 (4):EL249–55. doi: 10.1121/1.4793436.

Menkveld, S. R., E. A. Knipstein, and J. R. Quinn. 1988. Analysis of gait patterns in normal school-aged children. *J Pediatr Orthop* 8 (3):263–7.

Miall, R. C., and J. Cole. 2007. Evidence for stronger visuo-motor than visuo-proprioceptive conflict during mirror drawing performed by a deafferented subject and control subjects. *Exp Brain Res* 176 (3):432–9. doi: 10.1007/s00221-006-0626-0.

Miall, R. C., H. A. Ingram, J. D. Cole, and G. M. Gauthier. 2000. Weight estimation in a "deafferented" man and in control subjects: Are judgements influenced by peripheral or central signals? *Exp Brain Res* 133 (4): 491–500.

Miall, R. C., P. N. Haggard, and J. D. Cole. 1995. Evidence of a limited visuo-motor memory used in programming wrist movements. *Exp Brain Res* 107 (2):267–80.

Miller, L. J., and D. A. Fuller. 2006. *Sensational Kids: Hope and Help for Children with Sensory Processing Disorder (SPD)*. New York: G. P. Putnam's Sons.

Ming, X., M. Brimacombe, and G. C. Wagner. 2007. Prevalence of motor impairment in autism spectrum disorders. *Brain Dev* 29 (9):565–70.

Molloy, C. A., K. N. Dietrich, and A. Bhattacharya. 2003. Postural stability in children with autism spectrum disorder. *J Autism Dev Disord* 33 (6):643–52.

Mosconi, M. W., and J. A. Sweeney. 2015. Sensorimotor dysfunctions as primary features of autism spectrum disorders. *Sci China Life Sci* 58 (10):1016–23. doi: 10.1007/s11427-015-4894-4.

Mosconi, M. W., S. Mohanty, R. K. Greene, E. H. Cook, D. E. Vaillancourt, and J. A. Sweeney. 2015. Feedforward and feedback motor control abnormalities implicate cerebellar dysfunctions in autism spectrum disorder. *J Neurosci* 35 (5):2015–25. doi: 10.1523/JNEUROSCI.2731-14.2015.

Mostofsky, S. H., S. K. Powell, D. J. Simmonds, M. C. Goldberg, B. Caffo, and J. J. Pekar. 2009. Decreased connectivity and cerebellar activity in autism during motor task performance. *Brain* 132 (Pt 9):2413–25. doi: 10.1093/brain/awp088.

Nebel, M. B., S. E. Joel, J. Muschelli, A. D. Barber, B. S. Caffo, J. J. Pekar, and S. H. Mostofsky. 2014. Disruption of functional organization within the primary motor cortex in children with autism. *Hum Brain Mapp* 35 (2):567–80. doi: 10.1002/hbm.22188.

Papadopoulos, N., J. L. McGinley, J. L. Bradshaw, and N. J. Rinehart. 2014. An investigation of gait in children with attention deficit hyperactivity disorder: A case controlled study. *Psychiatry Res* 218 (3):319–23. doi: 10.1016/j.psychres.2014.04.037.

Qiu, A., M. Adler, D. Crocetti, M. I. Miller, and S. H. Mostofsky. 2010. Basal ganglia shapes predict social, communication, and motor dysfunctions in boys with autism spectrum disorder. *J Am Acad Child Adolesc Psychiatry* 49 (6):539–51, 551.e1–4. doi: 10.1016/j.jaac.2010.02.012.

Robledo, J., A. M. Donnellan, and K. Strandt-Conroy. 2012. An exploration of sensory and movement differences from the perspective of individuals with autism. *Front Integr Neurosci* 6:107. doi: 10.3389/fnint.2012.00107.

Rogers, D. M. 1992. *Motor Disorder in Psychiatry: Towards a Neurological Psychiatry*. Chichester: John Wiley & Sons.

Rose-Jacobs, R. 1983. Development of gait at slow, free, and fast speeds in 3- and 5-year-old children. *Phys Ther* 63 (8):1251–9.

Ryalls, J., S. Baum, R. Samuel, A. Larouche, N. Lacoursiere, and J. Garceau. 1993. Anticipatory co-articulation in the speech of young normal and hearing-impaired French Canadians. *Eur J Disord Commun* 28 (1):87–101.

Salcido, D. D., Y. M. Kim, L. D. Sherman, G. Housler, X. Teng, E. S. Logue, and J. J. Menegazzi. 2012. Quantitative waveform measures of the electrocardiogram as continuous physiologic feedback during resuscitation with cardiopulmonary bypass. *Resuscitation* 83 (4):505–10. doi: 10.1016/j.resuscitation.2011.09.018.

Schultz, A. E., P. D. Marasco, and T. A. Kuiken. 2009. Vibrotactile detection thresholds for chest skin of amputees following targeted reinnervation surgery. *Brain Res* 1251:121–9. doi: 10.1016/j.brainres.2008.11.039.

Scorolli, C., E. Daprati, D. Nico, and A. M. Borghi. 2016. Reaching for objects or asking for them: Distance estimation in 7- to 15-year-old children. *J Mot Behav* 48 (2):183–91. doi: 10.1080/00222895.2015.1070787.

Shadmehr, R., and S. P. Wise. 2005. *The Computational Neurobiology of Reaching and Pointing: A Foundation for Motor Learning, Computational Neuroscience*. Cambridge, MA: MIT Press.

Shapiro, L. A. 2011. *Embodied Cognition, New Problems of Philosophy*. New York: Routledge.

Sharer, E. A., S. H. Mostofsky, A. Pascual-Leone, and L. M. Oberman. 2016. Isolating visual and proprioceptive components of motor sequence learning in ASD. *Autism Res* 9 (5):563–9. doi: 10.1002/aur.1537.

Smith, A. 2006. Speech motor development: Integrating muscles, movements, and linguistic units. *J Commun Disord* 39 (5):331–49. doi: 10.1016/j.jcomdis.2006.06.017.

Smith, L. B., and E. Thelen. 2003. Development as a dynamic system. *Trends Cogn Sci* 7 (8):343–8.

Spencer, J. P., M. Clearfield, D. Corbetta, B. Ulrich, P. Buchanan, and G. Schoner. 2006. Moving toward a grand theory of development: In memory of Esther Thelen. *Child Dev* 77 (6):1521–38. doi: 10.1111/j.1467-8624.2006.00955.x.

Stolze, H., J. P. Kuhtz-Buschbeck, C. Mondwurf, A. Boczek-Funcke, K. Johnk, G. Deuschl, and M. Illert. 1997. Gait analysis during treadmill and overground locomotion in children and adults. *Electroencephalogr Clin Neurophysiol* 105 (6):490–7.

Sutherland, D. H., R. Olshen, L. Cooper, and S. L. Woo. 1980. The development of mature gait. *J Bone Joint Surg Am* 62 (3):336–53.

Swettenham, J., A. Remington, K. Laing, R. Fletcher, M. Coleman, and J. C. Gomez. 2013. Perception of pointing from biological motion point-light displays in typically developing children and children with autism spectrum disorder. *J Autism Dev Disord* 43 (6):1437–46. doi: 10.1007/s10803-012-1699-1.

Thelen, E., and B. D. Ulrich. 1991. Hidden skills: A dynamic systems analysis of treadmill stepping during the first year. *Monogr Soc Res Child Dev* 56 (1):1–98; discussion 99–104.

Thelen, E., and L. B. Smith. 1994. *A Dynamic Systems Approach to the Development of Cognition and Action*. MIT Press/Bradford Books Series in Cognitive Psychology. Cambridge, MA: MIT Press.

Thelen, E., D. Corbetta, and J. P. Spencer. 1996. Development of reaching during the first year: Role of movement speed. *J Exp Psychol Hum Percept Perform* 22 (5):1059–76.

Thelen, E., D. Corbetta, K. Kamm, J. P. Spencer, K. Schneider, and R. F. Zernicke. 1993. The transition to reaching: Mapping intention and intrinsic dynamics. *Child Dev* 64 (4):1058–98.

Thelen, E., G. Schoner, C. Scheier, and L. B. Smith. 2001. The dynamics of embodiment: A field theory of infant perseverative reaching. *Behav Brain Sci* 24 (1):1–34; discussion 34–86.

Torres, E. B. 2011. Two classes of movements in motor control. *Exp Brain Res* 215 (3–4):269–83. doi: 10.1007/s00221-011-2892-8.

Torres, E. B. 2012. Atypical signatures of motor variability found in an individual with ASD. *Neurocase* 1:1–16. doi: 10.1080/13554794.2011.654224.

Torres, E. B. 2013. Signatures of movement variability anticipate hand speed according to levels of intent. *Behav Brain Funct* 9:10.

Torres, E. B., A. Raymer, L. J. Gonzalez Rothi, K. M. Heilman, and H. Poizner. 2010. Sensory-spatial transformations in the left posterior parietal cortex may contribute to reach timing. *J Neurophysiol* 104 (5):2375–88. doi: 10.1152/jn.00089.2010.

Torres, E. B., and A. M. Donnellan. 2015. Editorial for research topic "Autism: The movement perspective." *Front Integr Neurosci* 9:12. doi: 10.3389/fnint.2015.00012.

Torres, E. B., and D. Zipser. 2004. Simultaneous control of hand displacements and rotations in orientation-matching experiments. *J Appl Physiol (1985)* 96 (5):1978–87. doi: 10.1152/japplphysiol.00872.2003.

Torres, E. B., J. Nguyen, S. Mistry, C. Whyatt, V. Kalampratsidou, and A. Kolevzon. 2016b. Characterization of the statistical signatures of micro-movements underlying natural gait patterns in children with Phelan McDermid syndrome: Towards precision-phenotyping of behavior in ASD. *Front Integr Neurosci* 10: 22. doi: 10.3389/fnint.2016.00022.

Torres, E. B., K. M. Heilman, and H. Poizner. 2011. Impaired endogenously evoked automated reaching in Parkinson's disease. *J Neurosci* 31 (49):17848–63. doi: 10.1523/JNEUROSCI.1150-11.2011.

Torres, E. B., M. Brincker, R. W. Isenhower, P. Yanovich, K. A. Stigler, J. I. Nurnberger, D. N. Metaxas, and J. V. Jose. 2013a. Autism: The micro-movement perspective. *Front Integr Neurosci* 7:32. doi: 10.3389/fnint.2013.00032.

Torres, E. B., P. Yanovich, and D. N. Metaxas. 2013b. Give spontaneity and self-discovery a chance in ASD: Spontaneous peripheral limb variability as a proxy to evoke centrally driven intentional acts. *Front Integr Neurosci* 7:46. doi: 10.3389/fnint.2013.00046.

Torres, E. B., R. W. Isenhower, J. Nguyen, C. Whyatt, J. I. Nurnberger, J. V. Jose, S. M. Silverstein, T. V. Papathomas, J. Sage, and J. Cole. 2016a. Toward precision psychiatry: Statistical platform for the personalized characterization of natural behaviors. *Front Neurol* 7:8. doi: 10.3389/fneur.2016.00008.

Tseng, Y. W., J. P. Scholz, G. Schoner, and L. Hotchkiss. 2003. Effect of accuracy constraint on joint coordination during pointing movements. *Exp Brain Res* 149 (3):276–88. doi: 10.1007/s00221-002-1357-5.

Vereijken, B., and E. Thelen. 1997. Training infant treadmill stepping: The role of individual pattern stability. *Dev Psychobiol* 30 (2):89–102.

Vernazza-Martin, S., N. Martin, A. Vernazza, A. Lepellec-Muller, M. Rufo, J. Massion, and C. Assaiante. 2005. Goal directed locomotion and balance control in autistic children. *J Autism Dev Disord* 35 (1):91–102.

Verrel, J., M. Lovden, and U. Lindenberger. 2012. Normal aging reduces motor synergies in manual pointing. *Neurobiol Aging* 33 (1):200.e1–10. doi: 10.1016/j.neurobiolaging.2010.07.006..

Vilensky, J. A., A. R. Damasio, and R. G. Maurer. 1981. Gait disturbances in patients with autistic behavior: A preliminary study. *Arch Neurol* 38 (10):646–9.

Von Hofsten, C. 2009. Action, the foundation for cognitive development. *Scand J Psychol* 50 (6):617–23. doi: 10.1111/j.1467-9450.2009.00780.x.

Von Holst, E., and H. Mittelstaedt. 1950. The principle of reafference: Interactions between the central nervous system and the peripheral organs. In *Perceptual Processing: Stimulus Equivalence and Pattern Recognition*, ed. P. C. Dodwell, 41–72. New York: Appleton-Century-Crofts.

Weber, D. 1978. "Toe-walking" in children with early childhood autism. *Acta Paedopsychiatr* 43 (2–3):73–83.

Weimer, A. K., A. M. Schatz, A. Lincoln, A. O. Ballantyne, and D. A. Trauner. 2001. "Motor" impairment in Asperger syndrome: Evidence for a deficit in proprioception. *J Dev Behav Pediatr* 22 (2):92–101.

Whyatt, C., and C. Craig. 2013. Sensory-motor problems in autism. *Front Integr Neurosci* 7:51. doi: 10.3389/fnint.2013.00051.

Whyatt, C. P., and C. M. Craig. 2012. Motor skills in children aged 7–10 years, diagnosed with autism spectrum disorder. *J Autism Dev Disord* 42 (9):1799–809. doi: 10.1007/s10803-011-1421-8.

Wiltschko, A. B., M. J. Johnson, G. Iurilli, R. E. Peterson, J. M. Katon, S. L. Pashkovski, V. E. Abraira, R. P. Adams, and S. R. Datta. 2015. Mapping sub-second structure in mouse behavior. *Neuron* 88 (6): 1121–35 doi: 10.1016/j.neuron.2015.11.031.

Ziemke, T., J. Zlatev, and R. M. Frank. 2007. *Body, Language, and Mind, Cognitive Linguistics Research*. Berlin: Mouton de Gruyter.

14 Micromovements
The s-Spikes as a Way to "Zoom In" the Motor Trajectories of Natural Goal-Directed Behaviors

Di Wu, Elizabeth B. Torres, and Jorge V. José

CONTENTS

Introduction 217
From Continuous Signals to "Spiking" Information 219
Simulating Patterns and Empirically Verifying Them 220
Random versus Periodic Behavior of Motor Output Fluctuations 220
Conclusions and Take-Home Message 222
References 223

Computer simulations of spike trains generated by brain neurons have been a useful tool to generate questions in the field of computational neuroscience. There is, however, a paucity of such methods in the study of complex behaviors, including analyses of kinematics parameters from movement trajectories embedded in natural purposeful behaviors. This chapter explores new data types and computational techniques leading to the simulation of patterns present in actual empirical data, along with synthetic patterns generated by computational models. We discuss their utility in setting normative bounds to compare modeled data with actual data obtained from individuals with the pathology of the developing nervous systems leading to a diagnosis of autism spectrum disorder (ASD).

INTRODUCTION

In this new era of wearable sensors and mobile-health concepts, it will be very useful to have methods that exploit various layers of variability in biophysical signals. Indeed, transitioning from instrumentation output to interpretable signal readout from the nervous systems is challenging. For example, if we seek to understand the timely synchronization in repeated pointing behaviors (e.g. in Figure 14.1) to begin to relate movement and gestural language in autism, we may want to preserve the original temporal dynamics of the raw data we acquire. To do so, we may want to select smoothing techniques to convert the discretely acquired signal into a continuous waveform representing a continuous random process. Then we can examine the stochastic properties of such a waveform and assess the levels of noise and signal that the nervous systems of the person are most likely accessing from moment to moment.

What types of filtering and smoothing may be most appropriate to attain our goals of capturing signals with the potential to be physiologically informative? And what types of data could we derive from such filtering with the potential to help us automatically classify heterogeneous phenomena in autism? Figure 14.1 invites some thoughts on these questions and shows some sample data types that we can extract from noninvasive wearable sensors.

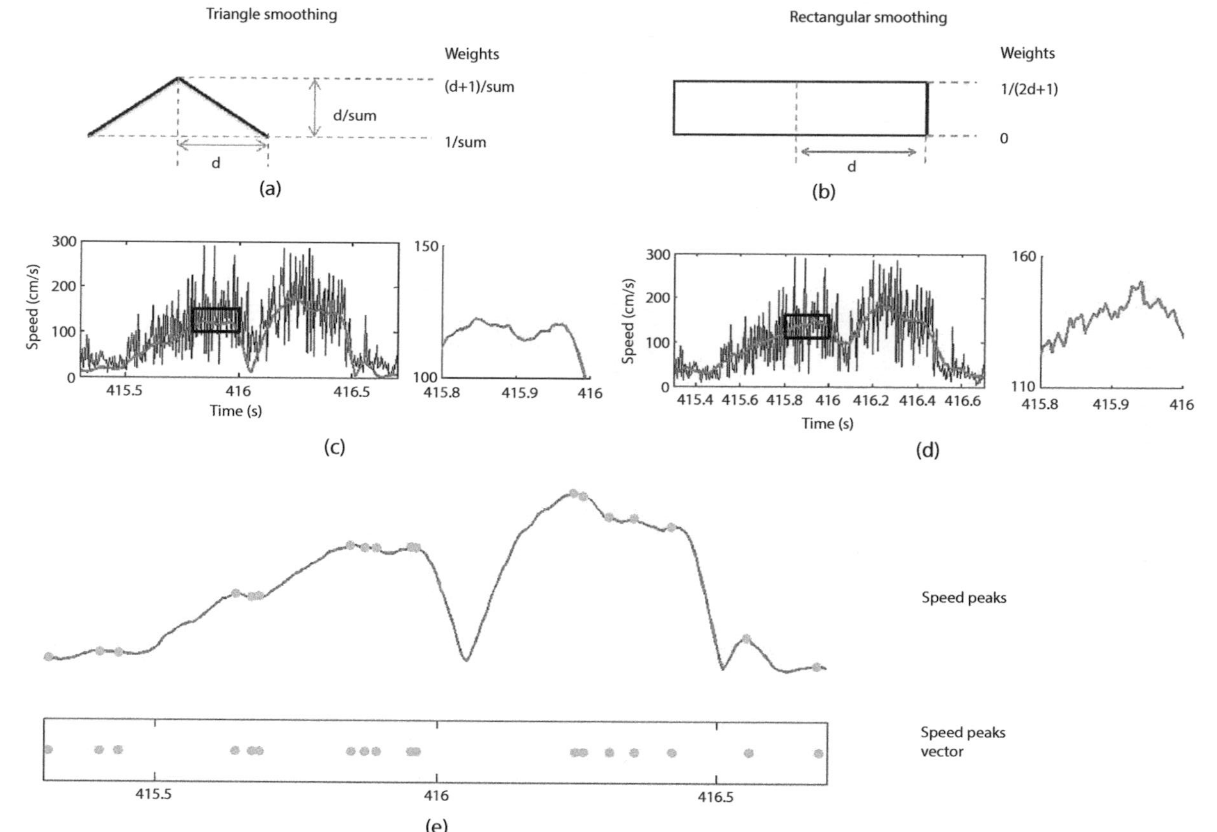

FIGURE 14.1 Filtering and smoothing process preserving the original raw data temporal dynamics while extracting new data types. Illustration of the triangular (a) and rectangular (b) smoothing algorithms. (c) The triangular smoothing algorithm preserves the internal fluctuation timings, removing the high-frequency external noise. (d) The rectangular smoothing algorithm fails to eliminate high-frequency noise, smearing the internal fluctuations. (e) New data type quantifying motor noise noninvasively at the millisecond range: identifying s-Peaks along the time profiles building up the s-Peaks' vector containing the temporal peaks' information.

An appropriate filtering algorithm should remove the unwanted nonphysiological external noise while retaining the internal motion fluctuations. Inherent motion fluctuations usually appear in the speed profile in the form of extra peaks sporadically appearing along the profile. To preserve the information possibly contained in these peaks, like their occurring rates and patterns, we selected a triangular smoothing algorithm. This algorithm was implemented by using a moving triangular window (Figure 14.1a), which replaces each point in the profile with the average of the data points in that window (the data points are weighted accordingly, as shown in Figure 14.1a). In comparison, traditional smoothing algorithms usually use rectangular filtering windows to calculate the average of the data points inside the window with the same weights (Figure 14.1b). Figure 14.1c and d plots and compares the results from applying the triangular and rectangular smoothing algorithms (having the same window size, 25 frames) on the same raw data. The zooming in of the profiles (right panels) clearly shows that the triangular smoothing algorithm works better at getting rid of the high-frequency external noise, while maintaining the curve's shape. In this chapter, the smoothing parameter was carefully selected to extract most of the information discussed below. The robustness of the parameter selection was also tested.

From Continuous Signals to "Spiking" Information

The minute fluctuations here and there along the speed profile can now be studied because their temporal dynamics were preserved. As such, Figure 14.1e shows how, after implementing the smoothing algorithm, those minute fluctuations in the speed profiles become evident. We identified the local peaks appearing along the speed profile (green dots in the plot) and named them speed peaks (s-Peaks). Temporal information about the s-Peaks (time when the s-Peaks appear) was extracted in the form of an s-Peak vector (bottom plot): when there is an s-Peak, the vector element is assigned a 1; otherwise, it is assigned a 0. In analogy to the widely used neuron action potential spike raster-gram in computational neuroscience, we then built up an s-Peak matrix with the s-Peaks' temporal information across cycles.

This new data type resembling spike trains commonly studied in the cortical neurons invites us to now think about possible peripheral activity transmitted by the peripheral nerves. Since the moment-by-moment events that these s-Peaks illustrate accumulate probabilistic information over time, it is possible to import several of the techniques already developed in the field of computational neuroscience and adapt them to understand the statistical signatures that the new data type provides.

The advantages and critical features that distinguish our approach from others in kinematics analyses within the ASD community studying motor dysfunction are that under this new platform of work, it is possible to:

1. Build analytical simulations
2. Test the predictions in the empirical arena

Further, new empirical questions can be designed to explore theoretical model-driven predictions not yet found in the empirical data. This ability to explore and empirically test artificial behaviors that can be evaluated against actual empirical data is an advantage of computational neuroscience that sets this approach apart from the traditional experimental paradigms often employed in ASD research—often constrained to the fields of psychology and psychiatry. Such fields are somehow often forced into hypothesis testing, with little to no scope for the discovery of novel or unexpected outcomes. Indeed, in our approach we use analytical techniques that later permit derivations of patterns in normative data for comparison with patterns in real experimental data obtainable from persons with pathologies of the nervous systems.

This interchange between analytical simulations and data-driven analyses is amenable to uncover self-emerging patterns and provide easier ways to interpret their possible meanings in light of the stochastic signatures they reveal. For example, we can focus on two features of the motor output data: their randomness and noise-to-signal ratio (NSR). Examining their presence and evolution over time in large cross sections of the autistic population can be rather illuminating, particularly when we do so in the context of other neurological and/or neuropsychiatric disorders. In this sense, the inherent variability in the continuously recorded data, as captured by critical points of change and temporal dynamics fluctuations, will no longer be treated as "noise." As we will see, noise can be a signal to the nervous systems.

SIMULATING PATTERNS AND EMPIRICALLY VERIFYING THEM

Random versus Periodic Behavior of Motor Output Fluctuations

Figure 14.2a presents the results of simulations that help us generate indexes distinguishing between random and periodic patterns across trials of s-Peaks. More specifically, we simulated the s-Peaks' matrix for two processes: one as a homogenous Poisson process, representing a motion process with high randomness, and the other for a partially synchronized process, representing a motion process with more control and higher periodicity.

We further introduced two tests to characterize the differences between these two processes. The first test was to measure synchronicity among cycles by calculating the cross-correlation function as a function of the binning width (Figure 14.2b). A somewhat related approach was used by Wang and Buzsaki (1996) for neuronal cortical spikes. The second test consisted of calculating the statistics of the temporal intervals between adjacent s-Peaks. This is analogous to the interspike interval (ISI) analyses done in computational neuroscience (Figure 14.2c).

When examining the actual empirical data in search of patterns of randomness and periodicity (synchronicity) in the s-Peaks, we found that in ASD the former is more common, while in typical development the latter prevails. Representative results are shown in Figure 14.3. They characterize the s-Peaks of pointing motions from children with ASD and varying degrees of spoken language capacity at the time of the experiments. Their more random s-Peak patterns contrast to the well-structured periodic ones of a neurotypical control child of similar age.

Note that the more random the patterns were, the lesser was the ability to articulate language. We posit that this type of randomness, which we also found in such motions when "zooming out" and examining the global peak speed of each forward and backward segment trajectory discussed in Chapter 7 (also see; Torres et al. 2013), may be a systemic issue in ASD. That is, these random patterns may also be found in motions executed by the orofacial structures involved in language. These structures are responsible for the control and feedback of the sensory motor apparatus responsible for the sound production, sound reception, and anticipatory synergies necessary to timely coarticulate modules of continuous speech.

The neuroanatomical structures of the face and body invite some thoughts on their functional interrelations and/or degree of independence, particularly those between the trigeminal ganglia innervating facial structures and the dorsal root ganglia underlying the structures involved in arm movements, upper-body control, and control of upright locomotion. These relations must be understood in light of the important roles of the information exchange of the peripheral nervous system (PNS) to the central nervous system (CNS) and the CNS to the PNS via efferent and afferent nerves. The above results are a first step in beginning to connect gestural and spoken language to underlying motion patterns. This connection is proposed under a unifying statistical framework that for the first time unveils potential avenues to link communication and neuromotor-sensing-based control.

In this sense, the maps in the periphery must develop properly to send proper feedback and help scaffold their corresponding projections across cortical and subcortical structures of the CNS. We posit that systems with impeded (random and noisy) peripheral feedback will have difficulties with the continuous correction and prediction of sensory motor delays. The moment-by-moment persistent randomness will most likely force the person to live in the "here and now" (Brincker and Torres 2013), relying on the current sensory information, but having difficulties anticipating the

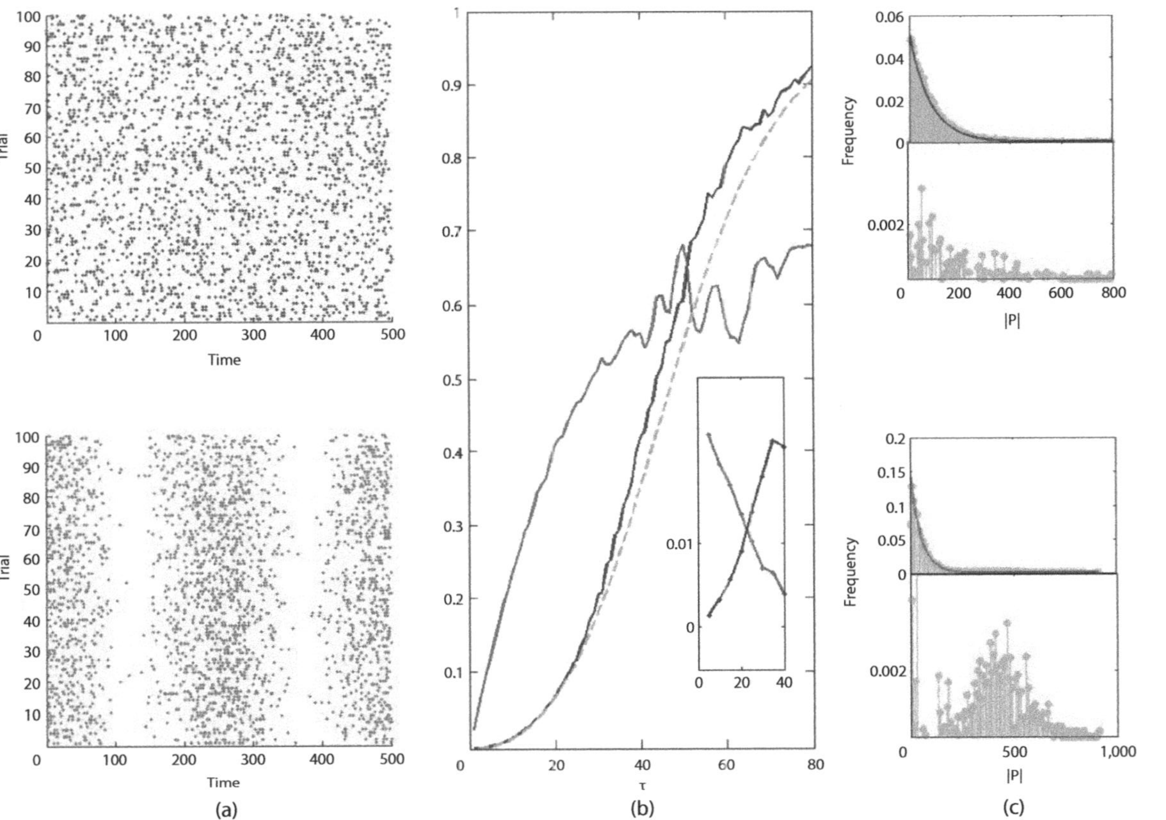

FIGURE 14.2 Simulation patterns and feature characterizations. (a) Raster-gram-like s-Peak matrices for simulated homogeneous Poisson peak train (upper) and simulated partially synchronized peak trains (bottom). (b) Population cross-correlation function, C, as a function of binning window size, τ, for (a and b). Green dashed line denotes the analytically calculated curve for random Poisson train peaks. Blue curve shows the simulated Poisson random train peaks, and the red curve the simulated partially synchronized peaks' train. Inset shows the corresponding slopes of the $C(\tau)$ curves. (c) Histogram of temporal intervals between nearest-neighbor s-Peaks in two simulated cases. Solid lines indicate the exponential fit (for values lower than 50). Bottom panels plot the histograms of the intervals outside of the exponential fit region, which distinguish these two cases.

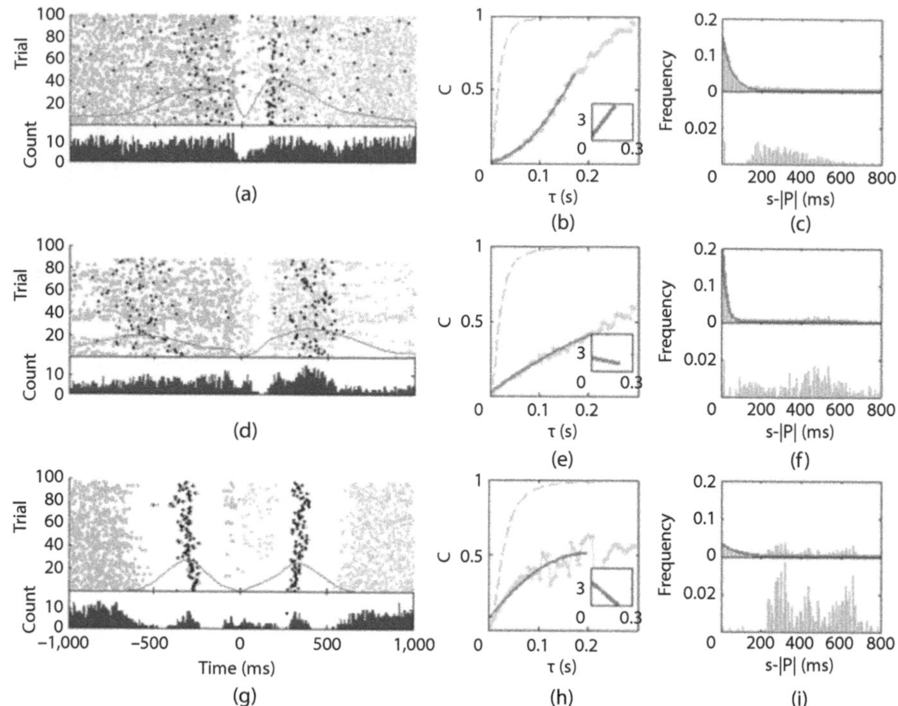

FIGURE 14.3 Sample data sets from three representative children and patterns similar to those found from the simulations in Figure 13.1. (a) Child with ASD and no spoken language. Black dots mark the global peak of the segment, while green dots are local s-Peaks forward and orange dots are s-Peaks backward. (b) Excess randomness predicted by analytical simulations and present in the actual data. (c) Inter-s-Peak times fit by the exponential and residual distributions in the tail highlighted in the bottom panel. (d) A child with ASD able to express some phrases shows a more periodic structure than the child in (a). (e, f) As before, mark differences in the periodicity and inter-s-Peak interval distributions. Specifically the s-Peaks that do not fit the exponential distribution (i.e., longer-range intervals between s-Peaks) are more noticeable than those in (a). (g) Well-structured (periodic) patterns in the neurotypical control. (h) Distinct patterns captured by a biometric developed analytically with the simulations. (i) Very distinct patterns for the inter-s-Peak interval distributions away from the exponential fit.

future sensory consequences of actions from the past sensory events that those actions themselves caused. In the face of such challenge and the disparate temporal and frequency scales of multimodal sensory transduction, how can the organism sense and perceive the world simultaneously? Clearly, if in addition to the excess randomness there is excess motor noise, the problem of neuromotor prospective control will be even harder.

CONCLUSIONS AND TAKE-HOME MESSAGE

This chapter underscores the importance of examining and modeling more than one layer of precision in data harnessed from the nervous systems. By taking seemingly smooth overt movement trajectories of the hand toward targets and obtaining variations in micromovements, we have identified a new type of spike train with the potential to facilitate detection and systematic quantification of excess noise and randomness in developing nervous systems. Such information, considered a nuisance and treated as noise under traditional averaging techniques, proves to contain signals with great utility to detect and track atypical neurodevelopment of motor control. Such involuntary micromotions possibly affect timely feedback and consequently impede the ability to properly articulate language. This work paves the way to quantify and possibly bridge elements of motor control with elements of cognition and communication at subsecond timescales.

REFERENCES

Brincker, M., and E. B. Torres. 2013. Noise from the periphery in autism. *Front Integr Neurosci* 7:34. doi: 10.3389/fnint.2013.00034.

Torres, E. B., M. Brincker, R. W. Isenhower, P. Yanovich, K. A. Stigler, J. I. Nurnberger, D. N. Metaxas, and J. V. Jose. 2013. Autism: The micro-movement perspective. *Front Integr Neurosci* 7:32. doi: 10.3389/fnint.2013.00032.

Wang, X. J., and G. Buzsaki. 1996. Gamma oscillation by synaptic inhibition in a hippocampal interneuronal network model. *J Neurosci* 16 (20):6402–13.

Section IV

The Therapeutic Model

Movement as a Percept to Awaken the Mind

Preface to Section IV

Elizabeth B. Torres

In the United States, the availability of therapeutic interventions to remediate autism spectrum disorder (ASD) is subject to insurance coverage (Wang et al. 2013) and deeply entangled with the public educational system. The child that receives a diagnosis of ASD before school age has access to an early intervention program (EIP) (Zwaigenbaum et al. 2015), while children of school age who receive the diagnosis generally gain access to the programs at the school (Corsello 2005).

Interventions may include a mixture of different philosophies, ranging from behavioral modification methods (e.g., applied behavioral analysis [ABA]) (Simmons et al. 1966; Lovaas et al. 1974) to developmental interventions (DIR or floor time) (Wieder and Greenspan 2003) to some form of occupational therapy (OT) (Schaaf and Miller 2005).

All approaches aim at changing the child's behavior into more socially appropriate manifestations. As such, they have many overlapping features with differences in how the ultimate goal is achieved. Despite availability of some of these therapies through the public school systems or in-home programs, there is a paucity of research on their true individualized effectiveness. More precisely, there is a lack of data on longitudinal outcome measures using objective means. Consequently, we do not know what therapies may work best for a given child versus which therapies may work best in another child. Furthermore, there is a lack of sensory-motor-oriented therapies that would consider the accelerated rates of growth of the infant alongside with the stochastic nature of neurodevelopment. The lack of proper outcome measures also restricts the diversification of therapies for any given child. Out-of-pocket expenses in the United States are much too high for many middle-class families to afford, let alone low-income families who may not even have access to diagnosis. The lack of research on interventions, combined with the scarce coverage of the few interventions available today, makes the therapeutic arena of ASD rather uncertain in the years to come.

In this section, we consider some alternative forms of accommodations and interventions that are gaining some popularity in mainstream circles. We open this section with a chapter on neurological music therapy and its visible benefits to the nonverbal child with ASD. Chapter 16 provides an example of finding accommodations to support the child's learning path and, using very simple means, facilitate various aspects of his or her education in the classroom and in the home environment.

To contrast the U.S. approach to intervention and those in use in other countries, we bring some examples of interventions in other cultures. Notably, we provide examples from Argentina, where a mixture of different forms of interventions guided by different philosophies is made available to the family. Collaboration between the family and a multidisciplinary team of clinicians and physicians provides an example of alternative approaches that converge faster to improvements of the child's social life than any one therapy in isolation (Chapter 17). Chapter 18 delves into the physical education approach, exploiting movements and their sensations to gradually build a sense of self and others, and to help the child learn the intricacies of social interactions using well-structured, team-oriented sports. The programs in Chapters 17 and 18 offer integrative approaches to therapy in ASD amenable for such heterogeneous conditions. Chapter 19 returns to the school setting and examines the problem of intervention and education through the eyes of a U.S. teacher.

REFERENCES

Corsello, C. M. 2005. Early intervention in autism. *Infants Young Children* 18 (2):74–85.

Lovaas, O. I., L. Schreibman, and R. L. Koegel. 1974. A behavior modification approach to the treatment of autistic children. *J Autism Child Schizophr* 4 (2):111–29.

Schaaf, R. C., and L. J. Miller. 2005. Occupational therapy using a sensory integrative approach for children with developmental disabilities. *Ment Retard Dev Disabil Res Rev* 11 (2):143–8.

Simmons, J. Q., 3rd, S. J. Leiken, O. I. Lovaas, B. Schaeffer, and B. Perloff. 1966. Modification of autistic behavior with LSD-25. *Am J Psychiatry* 122 (11):1201–11.

Wang, L., D. S. Mandell, L. Lawer, Z. Cidav, and D. L. Leslie. 2013. Healthcare service use and costs for autism spectrum disorder: A comparison between Medicaid and private insurance. *J Autism Dev Disord* 43 (5): 1057–64.

Wieder, S., and S. I. Greenspan. 2003. Climbing the symbolic ladder in the DIR model through floor time/ interactive play. *Autism* 7 (4):425–35.

Zwaigenbaum, L., M. L. Bauman, R. Choueiri, et al. 2015. Early identification and interventions for autism spectrum disorder: Executive summary. *Pediatrics* 136 (Suppl 1):S1–9.

15 Rhythm and Movement for Autism Spectrum Disorder

A Neurodevelopmental Perspective

Blythe LaGasse, Michelle Welde Hardy, Jenna Anderson, and Paige Rabon

CONTENTS

Introduction 230
Rhythm for Motor Movement 230
Music and Cortical Plasticity 231
Music Therapy for Autism Spectrum Disorder 232
Clinical Case Vignettes 234
Gross Motor 234
  Example of Naturally Evoking Sustained Motor Output through Music 234
  Example of Improving Initiation of Motor Output 234
  Example of Treating Issues with Motor Inhibition 235
Speech 235
  Example of the Use of Music Therapy to Help with Functional Speech Communication 235
  Example of the Use of Music Therapy to Help with Phoneme Production 236
  Example of the Use of Music Therapy to Help with Speech Pacing 236
Cognition/Attention 237
  Example of the Use of Music Therapy to Help with Switching Attention 237
  Example of the Use of Music Therapy to Help with Impulse Control 237
  Example of the Use of Music Therapy to Help with Working Memory 237
Conclusion 238
References 238

The biorhythms of the nervous systems spontaneously entrain with external vibrations in the environment. Such external input can come from musical instruments outputting signals that we can control from the outside. By controlling those signals externally, we can steer the biorhythms of the somatic motor systems of another person and help that person self-regulate his or her self-generated motions. This chapter explores neurological music therapy as a new important avenue to help the person with autism spectrum disorder (ASD) habilitate and rehabilitate his or her self-produced biorhythms. We review the extant literature on music therapy and neurological music therapy in light of concrete examples and vignettes from our clinical practice and our basic scientific lab experiments. We provide evidence of the benefits of pairing music and movement in ASD to effortlessly retrain the tempo and rhythms of the body in motion and improve many aspects of sociomotor control.

INTRODUCTION

Autism spectrum disorder (ASD) is characterized by deficits in social interaction, and restricted and repetitive patterns of behaviors, interests, and activities (American Psychiatric Association 2013). According to the fifth edition of the *Diagnostic and Statistical Manual of Mental Disorders* (DSM-5), the criterion of restricted and repetitive behaviors includes stereotyped or repetitive motor movements (American Psychiatric Association 2013). Researchers have expanded on the movement aspect of autism, demonstrating that movement differences exist in individuals on the autism spectrum (Bhat et al. 2011; Torres 2012; Torres et al. 2013a, 2016). As coordination and regulation of sensory and movement information is required for social communication (Donnellan et al. 2012), movement differences have the potential to be observed within social and communicative differences. There are few research studies focused on accommodations or treatments to improve movement in children with ASD. One accommodation that has some emerging evidence is the use of rhythmic cueing to improve sensorimotor functioning in ASD.

Recent systematic reviews have established that auditory rhythmic cueing is an effective tool for gross motor rehabilitation in populations including stroke (Bradt et al. 2010) and Parkinson's disease (de Dreu et al. 2012). Success observed with these populations has been attributed to the ability for neurons to quickly synchronize to an auditory stimulus, despite neurological disease or disorder. Furthermore, rhythmic cueing is proposed to prime the motor system, allowing individuals with movement differences increased success in performing movement sequences (Rossignol and Jones 1976; Thaut 2008). More recently several researchers have proposed that rhythm may also be used in the treatment of movement differences in individuals with ASD (Hardy and LaGasse 2013; Srinivasan et al. 2014). The purpose of this chapter is to illustrate the use of music therapy for sensorimotor regulation in persons with ASD. We will also provide examples of how changes in movement can impact cognitive and social functioning.

RHYTHM FOR MOTOR MOVEMENT

The neurological basis of music in the brain, especially rhythm in the brain, has become more understood by researchers over the past two decades. Music processing and production have been shown to activate areas throughout the brain, including the cortex, subcortex, and cerebellum (Peretz and Zatorre 2005; Thaut et al. 2014). Interestingly, music engages areas of the brain that are commonly recruited for nonmusical tasks, including speech, motor movement, and attention networks (Schwartze et al. 2011; Thaut 2005; Thaut et al. 2005). These activations include areas beyond the typical area recruited for a particular nonmusical task, which has been attributed to the preservation of musical functions despite the loss of a related nonmusical function. For example, persons with nonfluent aphasia have lost the ability to speak, yet retain the ability to sing—distributed cortical activations are seen in singing but not speech (Forgeard et al. 2008; Ozdemir et al. 2006; Schlaug et al. 2009). Research findings in musical neuroscience have been used in music therapy, where trained clinicians use aspects of music to facilitate cortical plasticity.

Rhythm is the organizing factor in all music, serving as a timekeeper in the therapeutic application of music for motor rehabilitation goals. Rhythmic cueing is provided with a reoccurring stimulus that maintains a fixed interstimulus interval. This type of external cueing has been shown to activate motor areas of the brain, including the premotor cortex, supplementary motor areas, presupplementary motor area, and lateral cerebellum (Bengtsson et al. 2009). Furthermore, rhythmic cueing can be used to achieve rapid motor synchronization in persons with and without neurological disability (Thaut et al. 1999). The use of external rhythmic cueing has been studied extensively in the rehabilitation sciences, where auditory rhythmic cueing has been utilized as an effective treatment in motor rehabilitation for more than a decade (LaGasse and Knight 2011).

External auditory cuing has been well established as a therapeutic intervention in the rehabilitation of motor movement. Of particular interest to this chapter is clear evidence that external rhythmic cueing can improve freezing of gait and increase stride length in persons with basal ganglia and cerebellar disorders, including Parkinson's disease (Arias et al. 2009; Chouza et al. 2011; Howe et al. 2003; McIntosh et al. 1997; Rochester et al. 2009; Thaut et al. 1996) and cerebellar ataxia (Abiru et al. 2008). Rhythmic cueing for upper-body volitional movement has been used in individuals with hemiparesis, including decreased movement variability and a decrease of compensatory trunk movements (Malcolm et al. 2009). Recent work provides a comprehensive review of rhythm in motor movement research with a focus on autism (Hardy and LaGasse 2013; LaGasse and Knight 2011).

Motor planning deficits and adaptation difficulties have been demonstrated in individuals with cerebellar disorder (Block and Bastian 2012; Fisher et al. 2006); however, these individuals are relatively unimpaired in sensory adaptation (Block and Bastian 2012). Therefore, the intact sensory adaptation ability may be utilized to facilitate development of motor networks. Although studies on rhythmic entrainment in individuals with cerebellar impairments are limited (Molinari et al. 2003), research has demonstrated that this population displays unimpaired motor synchronization to an external auditory cue. For instance, Provasi et al. (2014) found that children with tumors in the cerebellum demonstrated an ability to synchronize finger tapping to an external auditory rhythm, in contrast to excess variability during an uncued self-paced task. Taken together, this initial research suggests that external rhythmic auditory cueing and motor coupling may facilitate rehabilitation or habilitation of motor patterns in individuals with movement disorders.

MUSIC AND CORTICAL PLASTICITY

Engaging in music experiences has been shown to change the brain. For example, adult musicians have cortical differences in sensorimotor areas, auditory areas, and areas involved in multisensory integration (Bermudez and Zatorre 2005; Gaser and Schlaug 2003a, 2003b; Imfeld et al. 2009; Luo et al. 2012; Oechslin et al. 2009). Shorter-term musical training has also been shown to change the brain. Indeed, as illustrated by Hyde et al. (2009), 15 months of musical training can result in changes within the motor, auditory, frontal, and occipital regions of children. Moreover, Pascual-Leone (2001) demonstrated increased connectivity in motor brain areas after only a few weeks of training on the piano, while motor regions of the brain have been shown to increase in activations following a 6-week bilateral arm training program (Luft et al. 2004; Whitall et al. 2011). Since therapeutic interventions may not be feasible for long periods of time, evidence of cortical changes after short-term interventions may be most interesting for therapeutic application. In another study, music-supported therapy (playing drums and keyboard) for individuals with chronic stroke was shown to improve connectivity in auditory-motor regions of the brain, supporting the notion that engagement in a musical task can lead to changes in the cortex after insult or injury (Ripolles et al. 2015; Rodriguez-Fornells et al. 2012).

Prior chapters in this text have established that there is an underlying motor difference in persons on the autism spectrum. In this sense, the book treats motor as output but also as sensory input to the brain. Indeed, one of the critical theoretical constructs to link movement research and autism in recent years (Torres and Donnellan 2012) has been the principle of reafference connecting the peripheral to the central nervous systems (Von Holst and Mittelstaedt 1950). The sensing of motor variability at different levels of control (Torres 2011) can be paired with the habilitation and enhancement of volition (Torres et al. 2010) in individuals with autism (Torres et al. 2013b). In the context of music therapy, motor output can be guided by auditory stimuli as a modified reafferent stream that combines exoafferent information from the external world with endoafferent information internally generated by physiological processes, including self-produced movements. This principle and its tenet speak directly to the relations among systems in charge of body autonomy and self-control as they interact with the higher-level control centers of the brain, that is, the centers in the brain in charge of executive function, motor decision making, forward planning, and anticipatory control. Music therapy may serve to bridge top-down with bottom-up functions, including those from subcortical regions, central pattern generators, and various layers of the peripheral autonomic nervous systems that in autism somehow seem to have "a mind of their own." Indeed, across the broad spectrum of autism, individuals often express their frustration with trying to control their bodies at will (Robledo et al. 2012).

Music and its rich elements seem to serve as a "glue" that brings balance to all these systems and, in this way, explicitly help volitional control of movement. The therapist first guides these movements, but then the individual gradually sees spontaneous movements emerge with therapeutic support. Through intervention, the individual learns to control movements that are self-generated and at will, without having to think about it or be prompted to do so. Music seems to enable the communication between body and brain, coordinating automatic physical and cognitive exchange.

One of the important ingredients to support the potential of music therapy as a tool to intervene in neurodevelopmental disorders such as autism is the very early ability of the nervous system to entrain its internal rhythms with those of the external environment. For example, newborn babies spontaneously synchronize the rhythms of their body to those of their mom's speech (Condon and Sander 1974). Other findings in patients with cerebellar lesions suggest that rhythmic synchronization of behavior remains intact (Arias and Cudeiro 2010; Howe et al. 2003; McIntosh et al. 1997; Miller et al. 1996; Molinari et al. 2005; Prassas et al. 1997; Rochester et al. 2009). Thus, despite evidence that motor network abnormalities may be present in autism, the findings concerning rhythmic behavior in babies and cerebellar patients suggest the possibility that rhythm could be utilized to treat motor differences in ASD. Rhythmic auditory cues may facilitate activations in these affected areas to elicit shared networks for motor performance, bypassing the damaged areas, reorganizing the networks, or providing perhaps compensatory accommodations to recruit other areas. See Hardy and LaGasse (2013) for a more complete review of music and cortical plasticity.

MUSIC THERAPY FOR AUTISM SPECTRUM DISORDER

Areas of particular interest in this chapter include how music therapy can be used to improve functioning of children on the autism spectrum, specifically how rhythmic stimuli can provide a foundation for acquisition or demonstration of motor, speech, and cognitive skills. Music therapy is the therapeutic application of music to improve motor, cognition, and communication in children with neurodevelopmental disorders. Traditionally, music therapy has been utilized to address social, communicative, and cognitive needs of children with ASD (Kern et al. 2013). However, we would like to propose the use of a neurodevelopmental music therapy approach with persons on the autism spectrum. Current evidence in music therapy has indicated that rhythmic cueing may provide a template for organizing and executing motor movement in persons with autism (Hardy and LaGasse 2013). However, this evidence must be combined with current knowledge of neural and musical development in childhood, with a particular emphasis on how music can impact the developing brain.

In addition to neural and musical development, nonmusical development must also be considered when using music therapy in the treatment of children on the spectrum. Assessing the child's developmental level in motor, communication, and cognitive skills is essential, but must be completed with consideration of how motor output and movement sensing difficulties could be impacting these skills. Movement is present in many of the core deficits in persons with autism. Examples of this include the timing involved in speech production, responses to social cues through speech or movement, and the ability to execute a motor plan to complete a task, such as hugging a family member. Motor regulation is essential for many elements of daily living, including interaction, expression, and communication—all areas of impairment for individuals with ASD (Robledo et al. 2012). Therefore, the use of auditory rhythms may promote social, communication, and cognitive skills by providing a foundation for which these skills may be attained or demonstrated.

The predictability of musical stimuli may improve motor planning; however, the ability of a child on the spectrum to use this rhythmic accommodation would be dependent on factors such as age and perceptual motor processing abilities. Although there is an overall lack of research on synchronization abilities in children, the available research indicates that children can entrain to external tactile stimuli in infancy, demonstrated in oral motor entrainment and respiratory entrainment studies (Barlow and Estep 2006; Barlow et al. 2008; Ingersoll and Thoman 1994), as well as social studies concerning language acquisition abilities in the neonate (Condon and Sander 1974).

The ability to synchronize appears to improve in children as they age, with 7-year-old children performing at 77% accuracy in a finger-tapping synchronization task and 11-year-olds performing at 98% accuracy for the same task (Volman and Geuze 2000). Children between the ages of 6 and 9 have been shown to perform rhythmic synchronization tasks better at a faster pace than at a slower pace (Mastrokalou and Hatziharistos 2007). The finding that children better synchronize motor movement to a faster tempo has been supported in the extant literature (Kumai and Sugai 1997; Rao et al. 2001). Differences in synchronization abilities in infants and errors seen in developing children are most likely due to the ongoing maturational process that takes place at that time of perceptual motor development (Smith and Thelen 2003; Torres et al. 2013a). In infancy, these tasks are affecting central pattern–generated behavior without a need for cognitive thought. In childhood, the child is asked to perform a task in a certain manner. His or her processing time, motor response time for a volitional movement, and cortical disorganization or noise may impact his or her ability to complete the task. However, the ability to synchronize with near-adult levels appears to emerge in early adolescence (Hardy and LaGasse 2013; Volman and Geuze 2000).

In the clinical setting, children are observed to complete synchronization tasks in and out of phase with an external stimulus. This observation is supported by research indicating that although children can respond to a beat, this response is seldom accurately timed (Schaefer and Overy 2015); in fact, children may synchronize better to the "offbeat" than the instance of the stimulus (Volman and Geuze 2000). This is not to indicate that children will not be able to synchronize or predict rhythmic cues, but rather that continuous synchronization is evolving as they develop a more mature motor percept with high predictive power. The child would be more likely to perform a synchronization task in and out of phase, with corrections being more rapidly made as he or she ages. In music therapy, however, continuous synchronization is not a goal; rather, the anticipatory nature of rhythmic structure is used to help with motor planning. For example, if the child is working on reaching for an item, rhythm is used to support the planning and execution of reaching, rather than his or her ability to continuously maintain a steady beat while reaching. Similar to how music is used in individuals with stroke, the underlying principle of rhythmic synchronization and anticipation is used to facilitate precise motor movement in children on the autism spectrum.

This notion may be supported by the many music therapy intervention studies that have shown improvements in social (Brownell 2002; Finnigan and Starr 2010; Kern and Aldridge 2006; Kern et al. 2007; Kim et al. 2008, 2009; LaGasse 2014) and communication skills (Lim 2010; Wan et al. 2011) and attention regulation (Pasiali et al. 2014). Improvements seen in these studies may be, in part, due to improved motor regulation of motions with an underlying rhythmic structure. Because rhythms are present throughout many motions making up our activities of daily living, it is very likely that their improvements in autism would have a positive impact on their daily routines. These improvements would also most likely transfer to social-cognitive aspects of behaviors, as many of the sociomotor axes require synchronization across several rhythmic layers of the system, including automatic entrainment of bodily rhythms in conversations and joint attention from synchronous eye rhythms in dyadic interactions. We would like to illustrate how music therapy interventions with a strong rhythmic structure can promote functions, including motor, speech, and cognition. Here we present several clinical case vignettes where rhythm and music are used to promote skills. We start by safely assuming that motor differences in these children impact their ability to acquire certain skills, yet through the evoked self-organization of bodily rhythms, aided by music, and the use of this newly self-organized motor output as reafferent feedback, we induce marked improvements in their overall behavior.

CLINICAL CASE VIGNETTES

The following case vignettes highlight how rhythm and music can be used to facilitate functional outcomes in children on the autism spectrum. All the examples provided involve one-on-one interaction with the person during individual therapy. This form of interaction provides an opportunity to directly address that person's needs, and observe and record the immediate outcome of the therapy during a session. The music therapist typically begins sessions by first addressing motor regulation, as this can directly impact the ability to produce spontaneous speech utterances that help demonstrate cognitive abilities. Rhythm is then used as a foundation in all exercises in order to assist in motor production, anticipation of responses, and overall self-organization. Singing is used for directives, as initial evidence supports that individuals on the spectrum may process singing differently than speech (Lai et al., 2012; Paul et al., 2015). Furthermore, singing provides for additional anticipatory cueing through the harmonic and melodic structure.

GROSS MOTOR

Example of Naturally Evoking Sustained Motor Output through Music

Dylan is a 14-year-old boy with autism who displays difficulty walking consistently to a desired destination (i.e., walking to the car in the parking lot or walking to the restroom at school). He frequently stops or hesitates and often becomes distracted by objects or people in the environment. The music therapist instructs Dylan to hold a medium-sized frame drum while she plays a steady beat that corresponds to his pace of walking. During the exercise, the therapist sings lyrics that provide functional information to Dylan: (1) where they are walking and (2) the desired goal—to keep his body moving. This facilitates Dylan's continuous walk from one destination to another without stopping, and the functional goal of the exercise. Upon success in goal completion, the therapist is then able to add layers of difficulty that will aid the client in self-regulation. These include variations along the walking path with respect to direction (forward to backward to forward again) and variations in speed, evoked by changing the tempo as a natural cue to speed up or slow down. The therapist gradually fades the musical and vibrotactile support of the drum as Dylan walks independently to a desired location.

Example of Improving Initiation of Motor Output

Jason is a 6-year-old boy diagnosed with autism who displays difficulty using his left arm and often does not participate in bilateral and crossing midline exercises. When asked to reach up with his left arm, he will often scream and stop participating. When engaged in crossing midline exercises, he keeps his left arm close to his side and will only reach across with his right arm. Jason has been assessed by physical and occupational therapists, and there are no documented physical impairments to explain his limited use of the left arm.

Jason prefers the guitar and often brings one from home to the therapy session. A song is selected and a metronome is set to keep the rhythmic structure. The therapist holds the guitar, plays the chord progression, and sings while Jason strums the guitar with his stronger, dominant right hand to facilitate his success and motivate him to the task. The therapist only sings when Jason strums, encouraging him to continue strumming to keep the songs going. After the first verse, the therapist moves to a position that allows for Jason to play with his left hand to address the goal of utilizing his left side. The therapist uses the structure of the song to frame the expectation of playing with his right hand for the verse, and then playing with his left hand for the chorus. Gradually, the therapist moves the guitar up to encourage Jason to stretch his left arm while he plays to increase his range of motion and his awareness of his body in space. The rhythm supports the motor system to sustain the motor output, while the preferred instrument and song choice reduce anxiety while doing a nonpreferred task. After the song is finished, the therapist reaches up for a high five from Jason with his left hand.

Example of Treating Issues with Motor Inhibition

Cole is a 10-year-old boy with autism who has a hard time regulating his motor output, specifically inhibiting his gross motor movement. He often "elopes" from his behavioral aide at school and has a particularly difficult time transitioning from one task to the next. To work on increasing Cole's motor control during transitions, the music therapist initially structures two exercises: (1) sitting on a t-stool while crossing the midline to play drums one hand at a time and (2) bouncing on a ball while playing the xylophone with both hands simultaneously. Each exercise was selected to provide varied sensory information to his body during active engagement (the t-stool promotes body control through balance, and the ball promotes body awareness through active proprioception). The metronome is initially set based on Cole's speed of bouncing, matching his cadence at first and then modulating the tempo to reflect a functional speed for his output. This functional tempo is maintained throughout the entire experience. The therapist first gave clear parameters for each task. Cole is asked to play 10 times on the drums, alternating left to right, with a preparatory beat provided prior to the expectation to play, until the count of 10. Upon completion of this task, a melodic transitional line is sung by the therapist to indicate movement to the next task (i.e., "and now I can walk to play the xylophone"). This recognizable melodic line paired with the rhythmic template provides Cole with the cueing he needs, as well as a time frame, to move directly to the other task. As Cole demonstrates success within transitions, more tasks are added so that by the end of treatment, he is able to transition to up to five different tasks within one session without eloping. This repetitive melody gradually turns into a more recognizable melodic line to the extent that it could then be used by his behavioral aide when he needs it to transition Cole between tasks in the school environment. To this end, the aide used lyrics at first, but then was able to fade that into just humming the melody so as to facilitate a continuous flow of the activity without eloping.

Variations of this strategy with respect to time length and frequency prevented rote memorization or buildup of anticipation, which in this context would be detrimental to the overall goal of maximally inhibiting the eloping in the middle of the task. Indeed, Cole could not predict when the specific task prior to the transition would occur. Counting down to indicate the number of times remaining for each task was initially the most effective accommodation to assist with Cole's motor control. Within this context, the length of time changed within each task, but eventually, the therapist used songs as the structure within which the verse, chorus, and bridge represented a different task and the transitions were built between them. In this sense, transitioning between tasks became spontaneous, natural events—events that did not have to be deliberately prompted, but rather were evoked beneath Cole's awareness.

SPEECH

Example of the Use of Music Therapy to Help with Functional Speech Communication

Joshua is a 6-year-old boy with autism that displays limited speech; however, the output can be echolalic (i.e., repeating words) or rote in nature. He responds well and appears to be motivated by instrument play during his music therapy session. The therapist facilitates a vocal output exercise with a song structured to provide an engagement section, a speech response section, and a validation section. In the engagement portion, Joshua plays an instrument with rhythmic cues for initiation and inhibition. Once he demonstrates gross motor regulation, the therapist transitions to the response section. In this section, the therapist rhythmically presents a phrase that Joshua completes based on choices presented prior to the experience: "Now I want to play __________ (fast, slow, loud, soft)." This is followed by a validation section where the therapist plays the way he described.

Visual accommodations may be added if needed (i.e., word choices and choice board). This strong predictable musical structure allows Joshua to be successful in producing functional communication rather than echolalia.

Example of the Use of Music Therapy to Help with Phoneme Production

Becky is a 4-year-old girl with autism that presents with no functional verbal speech. She uses an augmented aid communication device with picture word icons to communicate her wants and needs independently and is now being encouraged to pair the initial phoneme with her communication request, like "bathroom." She demonstrates low arousal most of the time and struggles to initiate and sustain body movements. She also displays low muscle tone that impacts her posture.

The music therapist places Becky on a therapy ball (appropriate for her height and weight) and rhythmically facilitates her to bounce to the music. The bouncing and sensory input give appropriate feedback for Becky to now maintain an upright posture and overall improved arousal state. The therapist transitions Becky into phoneme exercises paired with the current rhythm and bounce of her movements. The therapist sings a repetitive song structure that provides opportunities to practice the targeted phoneme within a functional phrase. For example, "I can /b/ (bounce), on the /b/ (ball)." The therapist fades her voice and allows Becky to use her voice independently. Other phonemes are also targeted based on her needs.

Example of the Use of Music Therapy to Help with Speech Pacing

William is a 7-year-old boy diagnosed with autism and apraxia who exhibits cluttering of speech, where the syllables of the words are spoken rapidly with irregular rhythm. This makes him difficult to understand, and his words and phrases tend to jumble together in a disorganized fashion. He becomes frustrated when he is not understood, as evidenced by his increasing his volume and intensity to make his point, which only makes him less intelligible.

To help William, his speech therapist has a specific language program tailored to his immediate and most pressing needs. This program consists of repetition and production of sentences consisting of words in his working memory capacity. It also includes sentences emphasizing pronouns and past and present tenses that he frequently confuses. During the implementation of the program, the therapist notes that when William repeats the requested phrases, he often "clutters" words within the sentence, decreasing intelligibility. The immediate goal is to try to slow his rate of speech to decrease the mispronunciations and slurring of speech sounds, and allow for greater functionality and intelligibility.

William appears to enjoy music and often chooses to sing in music therapy. When singing familiar songs, William's articulation is much clearer and his pacing is slower and more controlled within the musical structure. The therapist identifies a functional tempo (slower than his speech output) and uses the metronome to facilitate a functional rhythm for his speech exercises so as to try to transfer to the speech production the intrinsic ability that William has during his singing, which allows him greater organization, planning, and intelligibility within the song.

The language program phrases are then sung within a melodic, rhythmic structure, and William is able to articulate and pace each phrase in a way that is clearly understood. Within the context of the song, the predictable cueing of the metronome primes the speech motor apparatus, thus evoking a sort of continuity in the speech that supersedes the appearance of cluttering words. In turn, this new flow allows for improved intelligibility. The melody is then faded and the phrase is spoken to the rhythm of the metronome. Over time, the metronome is also faded and William is encouraged to pace his speech output by thinking about a song in his head and slowing down his speech.

COGNITION/ATTENTION

Example of the Use of Music Therapy to Help with Switching Attention

Megan is a 10-year-old girl with autism that presents with difficulties switching her attention to her teacher at school and her classmates when engaged in a group project or social activity. The music therapist sets up an exercise to help Megan practice switching her attention to two different stimuli. With a metronome set at a steady beat in the background, the therapist introduces two dramatically different musical cues that correspond to two different ways for Megan to move (i.e., bear crawl and jumping). Our assumption is that the movement flow under these different postural requirements helps Megan maintain her arousal level and gives her the sensorimotor information she needs to successfully sustain and switch her attention in the exercise. The use of the metronome in the background provides a rhythmic foundation for the entire exercise with the ability to distinguish between postural modes. This extrinsic timing from the metronome can be naturally superimposed on the intrinsic timing of the self-produced movements without the need for explicit prompting. In this sense, the transition into more fluid behaviors can be gradually achieved, whereby the external stimuli gradually become internally driving stimuli to affect the motor system. In other words, the stimuli become naturally congruent with the very system producing them as output and receiving them in a metronome-transformed way as input. When Megan's body demonstrates greater awareness to the two varying stimuli, and this awareness reaches her cognition of them, then the exercise difficulty can be gradually increased by making the differences in cues more subtle. In this way, a gradual transition from discrete sets to continuous sets of stimuli can be used to evoke (rather than to explicitly prompt) fluidity in her behavior. As in other examples provided, the aim is to bridge autonomic motor with automatic motor output so as to impact voluntary motor output and ultimately achieve volition and intent: the hallmarks of cognitive control.

Example of the Use of Music Therapy to Help with Impulse Control

Sarah is an 8-year-old girl diagnosed with autism who demonstrates difficulty with impulse control in the classroom setting. She often gets up and runs to different areas of the classroom. To help with this, the therapist sets up a variety of hand percussion instruments around the room, whereby all the instruments are visible from where Sarah is sitting against one wall, but are at least 5 or more feet away. The therapist creates a lyric structure with directions in which an instrument is named, she is asked to wait, and then go play. The musical structure of the song utilizes a steady rhythm to prime the sensorimotor system, and a descending chord progression is used to allow for anticipation and then resolve to the tonic when it is time to move and play. To generalize this skill, the music and instruments can be removed and the teacher can utilize the same space in the classroom to provide directions and wait time before moving to and participating in the next classroom task.

Example of the Use of Music Therapy to Help with Working Memory

Kyle is a 14-year-old boy with autism. His assessment indicates a working memory difficulty, as he is not retaining information that is presented to him and requires constant prompting. The therapist sets the metronome to a tempo based on previous motor exercises to prime Kyle's system and prepare him for this cognitive task. Eight different-colored bells are placed on the desk in front of Kyle, and a sequence of four colors are verbalized rhythmically for him to play, but he has to hear the order of all the bells before he is allowed to play. For example, the therapist says, "Red, yellow, purple, blue; now play," and he has to retain the information in his working memory and play the sequence requested. As he demonstrates the ability to remember the four units in the sequence, the therapist increases the challenge by adding more units and also delaying the directive to play (green, blue, orange, red … pause … pause … pause … now play).

CONCLUSION

Music is a form of sensory input that is naturally predictable and organized. Because primitive subcortical brain areas are involved in the processing and decoding of musical stimuli, researchers have proposed that auditory-motor coupling drives motor control. This coupling may help with the development of autonomy and organization in natural behaviors. We combine this tenet in our basic scientific research and our therapeutic practices to help the sensory-motor systems of individuals with autism find a way to intrinsically and spontaneously learn volition. The evidence from our practice and research invites further exploration into music therapy and the various potential applications of it to help individuals with autism gain automatic control of their bodies in motion.

Music experiences are fun and create an emotionally harmonious social (dyadic) environment between the person and the therapist (or the researcher). This context can also be motivating, thus providing opportunities for individuals to practice skills that can then be generalized into their everyday routines. We recommend a neurodevelopmental approach to music therapy treatment, where neurological factors of autism are considered alongside the individual's development. By integrating developmental and neurological knowledge, as well as current research findings, the music therapist can provide an optimal environment for skills acquisition and the development and maintenance of motor control conducive of action ownership, self-agency, and ultimately, independent, autonomous control.

REFERENCES

Abiru, M., Y. Kikuchi, K. Tokita, Y. Mihara, M. Fujimoto, and B. Mihara. 2008. The effects of neurologic music therapy on gait disturbance in a cerebellar ataxia: A case study. *Gunma Med J* 87:213–8.

American Psychiatric Association. 2013. *Diagnostic and Statistical Manual of Mental Disorders*. 5th ed. Washington, DC: American Psychiatric Association.

Arias, P., and J. Cudeiro. 2010. Effect of rhythmic auditory stimulation on gait in Parkinsonian patients with and without freezing of gait. *PLoS One* 5 (3):e9675.

Arias, P., M. Chouza, J. Vivas, and J. Cudeiro. 2009. Effect of whole body vibration in Parkinson's disease: A controlled study. *Mov Disord* 24 (6):891–8.

Barlow, S. M., and M. Estep. 2006. Central pattern generation and the motor infrastructure for suck, respiration, and speech. *J Commun Disord* 39 (5):366–80.

Barlow, S. M., D. S. Finan, J. Lee, and S. Chu. 2008. Synthetic orocutaneous stimulation entrains preterm infants with feeding difficulties to suck. *J Perinatol* 28 (8):541–8.

Bengtsson, S. L., F. Ullen, H. H. Ehrsson, T. Hashimoto, T. Kito, E. Naito, H. Forssberg, and N. Sadato. 2009. Listening to rhythms activates motor and premotor cortices. *Cortex* 45 (1):62–71.

Bermudez, P., and R. J. Zatorre. 2005. Differences in gray matter between musicians and nonmusicians. *Ann NY Acad Sci* 1060:395–9.

Bhat, A. N., R. J. Landa, and J. C. Galloway. 2011. Current perspectives on motor functioning in infants, children, and adults with autism spectrum disorders. *Phys Ther* 91 (7):1116–29.

Block, H. J., and A. J. Bastian. 2012. Cerebellar involvement in motor but not sensory adaptation. *Neuropsychologia* 50 (8):1766–75.

Bradt, J., W. L. Magee, C. Dileo, B. L. Wheeler, and E. McGilloway. 2010. Music therapy for acquired brain injury. *Cochrane Database Syst Rev* (7):CD006787.

Brownell, M. D. 2002. Musically adapted social stories to modify behaviors in students with autism: Four case studies. *J Music Ther* 39 (2):117–44.

Chouza, M., P. Arias, S. Vinas, and J. Cudeiro. 2011. Acute effects of whole-body vibration at 3, 6, and 9 Hz on balance and gait in patients with Parkinson's disease. *Mov Disord* 26 (5):920–1.

Condon, W. S., and L. W. Sander. 1974. Neonate movement is synchronized with adult speech: Interactional participation and language acquisition. *Science* 183 (4120):99–101.

de Dreu, M. J., A. S. van der Wilk, E. Poppe, G. Kwakkel, and E. E. van Wegen. 2012. Rehabilitation, exercise therapy and music in patients with Parkinson's disease: A meta-analysis of the effects of music-based movement therapy on walking ability, balance and quality of life. *Parkinsonism Relat Disord* 18 (Suppl 1):S114–9.

Donnellan, A. M., D. A. Hill, and M. R. Leary. 2012. Rethinking autism: Implications of sensory and movement differences for understanding and support. *Front Integr Neurosci* 6:124.

Finnigan, E., and E. Starr. 2010. Increasing social responsiveness in a child with autism. A comparison of music and non-music interventions. *Autism* 14 (4):321–48.

Fisher, B. E., L. Boyd, and C. J. Winstein. 2006. Contralateral cerebellar damage impairs imperative planning but not updating of aimed arm movements in humans. *Exp Brain Res* 174 (3):453–66.

Forgeard, M., E. Winner, A. Norton, and G. Schlaug. 2008. Practicing a musical instrument in childhood is associated with enhanced verbal ability and nonverbal reasoning. *PLoS One* 3 (10):e3566.

Gaser, C., and G. Schlaug. 2003a. Brain structures differ between musicians and non-musicians. *J Neurosci* 23 (27):9240–5.

Gaser, C., and G. Schlaug. 2003b. Gray matter differences between musicians and nonmusicians. *Ann NY Acad Sci* 999:514–7.

Hardy, M. W., and B. LaGasse. 2013. Rhythm, movement, and autism: Using rhythmic rehabilitation research as a model for autism. *Front Integr Neurosci* 7 (19):1–9.

Howe, T. E., B. Lovgreen, F. W. Cody, V. J. Ashton, and J. A. Oldham. 2003. Auditory cues can modify the gait of persons with early-stage Parkinson's disease: A method for enhancing parkinsonian walking performance? *Clin Rehabil* 17 (4):363–7.

Hyde, K. L., J. Lerch, A. Norton, M. Forgeard, E. Winner, A. C. Evans, and G. Schlaug. 2009. Musical training shapes structural brain development. *J Neurosci* 29 (10):3019–25.

Imfeld, A., M. S. Oechslin, M. Meyer, T. Loenneker, and L. Jancke. 2009. White matter plasticity in the corticospinal tract of musicians: A diffusion tensor imaging study. *Neuroimage* 46 (3):600–7.

Ingersoll, E. W., and E. B. Thoman. 1994. The breathing bear: Effects on respiration in premature infants. *Physiol Behav* 56 (5):855–9.

Kern, P., and D. Aldridge. 2006. Using embedded music therapy interventions to support outdoor play of young children with autism in an inclusive community-based child care program. *J Music Ther* 43 (4):270–94.

Kern, P., M. Wolery, and D. Aldridge. 2007. Use of songs to promote independence in morning greeting routines for young children with autism. *J Autism Dev Disord* 37 (7):1264–71.

Kern, P., N. R. Rivera, A. Chandler, and M. Humpal. 2013. Music therapy services for individuals with autism spectrum disorder: A survey of clinical practices and training needs. *J Music Ther* 50 (4):274–303.

Kim, J., T. Wigram, and C. Gold. 2008. The effects of improvisational music therapy on joint attention behaviors in autistic children: A randomized controlled study. *J Autism Dev Disord* 38 (9):1758–66.

Kim, J., T. Wigram, and C. Gold. 2009. Emotional, motivational and interpersonal responsiveness of children with autism in improvisational music therapy. *Autism* 13 (4):389–409.

Kumai, M., and K. Sugai. 1997. Relation between synchronized and self-paced response in preschoolers' rhythmic movement. *Percept Mot Skills* 85 (3 Pt 2):1327–37.

LaGasse, A. B. 2014. Effects of a music therapy group intervention on enhancing social skills in children with autism. *J Music Ther* 51 (3):250–75.

LaGasse, A. B., and A. Knight. 2011. Rhythm and music in rehabilitation: A critical review of current research. *Crit Rev Phys Rehabil Med* 23 (1–4):49–67.

Lim, H. A. 2010. Effect of "developmental speech and language training through music" on speech production in children with autism spectrum disorders. *J Music Ther* 47 (1):2–26.

Luft, A. R., S. McCombe-Waller, J. Whitall, L. W. Forrester, R. Macko, J. D. Sorkin, J. B. Schulz, A. P. Goldberg, and D. F. Hanley. 2004. Repetitive bilateral arm training and motor cortex activation in chronic stroke: A randomized controlled trial. *JAMA* 292 (15):1853–61.

Luo, C., Z. W. Guo, Y. X. Lai, W. Liao, Q. Liu, K. M. Kendrick, D. Z. Yao, and H. Li. 2012. Musical training induces functional plasticity in perceptual and motor networks: Insights from resting-state FMRI. *PLoS One* 7 (5):e36568.

Malcolm, M. P., C. Massie, and M. Thaut. 2009. Rhythmic auditory-motor entrainment improves hemiparetic arm kinematics during reaching movements: A pilot study. *Top Stroke Rehabil* 16:69–79.

Mastrokalou, N., and D. Hatziharistos. 2007. Rhythmic ability in children and the effects of age, sex, and tempo. *Percept Mot Skills* 104 (3 Pt 1):901–12.

McIntosh, G. C., S. H. Brown, R. R. Rice, and M. H. Thaut. 1997. Rhythmic auditory-motor facilitation of gait patterns in patients with Parkinson's disease. *J Neurol Neurosurg Psychiatry* 62 (1):22–6.

Miller, R. A., M. H. Thaut, G. C. McIntosh, and R. R. Rice. 1996. Components of EMG symmetry and variability in parkinsonian and healthy elderly gait. *Electroencephalogr Clin Neurophysiol* 101 (1):1–7.

Molinari, M., M. G. Leggio, M. De Martin, A. Cerasa, and M. Thaut. 2003. Neurobiology of rhythmic motor entrainment. *Ann NY Acad Sci* 999:313–21.

Molinari, M., M. G. Leggio, V. Filippini, M. C. Gioia, A. Cerasa, and M. H. Thaut. 2005. Sensorimotor transduction of time information is preserved in subjects with cerebellar damage. *Brain Res Bull* 67 (6):448–58.

Oechslin, M. S., A. Imfeld, T. Loenneker, M. Meyer, and L. Jancke. 2009. The plasticity of the superior longitudinal fasciculus as a function of musical expertise: A diffusion tensor imaging study. *Front Hum Neurosci* 3:76.

Ozdemir, E., A. Norton, and G. Schlaug. 2006. Shared and distinct neural correlates of singing and speaking. *Neuroimage* 33 (2):628–35.

Pascual-Leone, A. 2001. The brain that plays music and is changed by it. *Ann NY Acad Sci* 930:315–29.

Pasiali, V., A. B. LaGasse, and S. L. Penn. 2014. The effect of musical attention control training (MACT) on attention skills of adolescents with neurodevelopmental delays: A pilot study. *J Music Ther* 51 (4): 333–54.

Peretz, I., and R. J. Zatorre. 2005. Brain organization for music processing. *Annu Rev Psychol* 56:89–114.

Prassas, S. G., M. H. Thaut, G. C. McIntosh, and R. R. Rice. 1997. Effect of auditory rhythmic cuing on gait kinematic parameters in stroke patients. *Gait Posture* 6:218–23.

Provasi, J., V. Doyere, P. S. Zelanti, V. Kieffer, H. Perdry, N. El Massioui, B. L. Brown, G. Dellatolas, J. Grill, and S. Droit-Volet. 2014. Disrupted sensorimotor synchronization, but intact rhythm discrimination, in children treated for a cerebellar medulloblastoma. *Res Dev Disabil* 35 (9):2053–68.

Rao, S. M., A. R. Mayer, and D. L. Harrington. 2001. The evolution of brain activation during temporal processing. *Nat Neurosci* 4 (3):317–23.

Ripolles, P., N. Rojo, J. Grau-Sanchez, et al. 2015. Music supported therapy promotes motor plasticity in individuals with chronic stroke. *Brain Imaging Behav* 10 (4):1289–1307.

Robledo, J., A. M. Donnellan, and K. Strandt-Conroy. 2012. An exploration of sensory and movement differences from the perspective of individuals with autism. *Front Integr Neurosci* 6:107.

Rochester, L., D. J. Burn, G. Woods, J. Godwin, and A. Nieuwboer. 2009. Does auditory rhythmical cueing improve gait in people with Parkinson's disease and cognitive impairment? A feasibility study. *Mov Disord* 24 (6):839–45.

Rodriguez-Fornells, A., N. Rojo, J. L. Amengual, P. Ripolles, E. Altenmuller, and T. F. Munte. 2012. The involvement of audio-motor coupling in the music-supported therapy applied to stroke patients. *Ann NY Acad Sci* 1252:282–93.

Rossignol, S., and G. M. Jones. 1976. Audiospinal influences in man studied by the h-reflex and its possible role in rhythmic movement synchronized to sound. *Electroencephal Clin Neurophysiol* 41:203–8.

Schaefer, R. S., and K. Overy. 2015. Motor responses to a steady beat. *Ann NY Acad Sci* 1337:40–4.

Schlaug, G., M. Forgeard, L. Zhu, A. Norton, A. Norton, and E. Winner. 2009. Training-induced neuroplasticity in young children. *Ann NY Acad Sci* 1169:205–8.

Schwartze, M., P. E. Keller, A. D. Patel, and S. A. Kotz. 2011. The impact of basal ganglia lesions on sensorimotor synchronization, spontaneous motor tempo, and the detection of tempo changes. *Behav Brain Res* 216 (2):685–91.

Smith, L. B., and E. Thelen. 2003. Development as a dynamic system. *Trends Cogn Sci* 7 (8):343–8.

Srinivasan, S. M., L. S. Pescatello, and A. N. Bhat. 2014. Current perspectives on physical activity and exercise recommendations for children and adolescents with autism spectrum disorders. *Phys Ther* 94 (6):875–89.

Thaut, M. 2008. *Rhythm, Music, and the Brain: Scientific Foundations and Clinical Applications*. 1st paperback ed. Studies on New Music Research. New York: Routledge.

Thaut, M. H. 2005. The future of music in therapy and medicine. *Ann NY Acad Sci* 1060:303–8.

Thaut, M. H., D. A. Peterson, and G. C. McIntosh. 2005. Temporal entrainment of cognitive functions: Musical mnemonics induce brain plasticity and oscillatory synchrony in neural networks underlying memory. *Ann NY Acad Sci* 1060:243–54.

Thaut, M. H., G. C. McIntosh, R. R. Rice, R. A. Miller, J. Rathbun, and J. M. Brault. 1996. Rhythmic auditory stimulation in gait training for Parkinson's disease patients. *Mov Disord* 11 (2):193–200.

Thaut, M. H., G. P. Kenyon, M. L. Schauer, and G. C. McIntosh. 1999. The connection between rhythmicity and brain function. *IEEE Eng Med Biol Mag* 18 (2):101–8.

Thaut, M. H., P. D. Trimarchi, and L. M. Parsons. 2014. Human brain basis of musical rhythm perception: Common and distinct neural substrates for meter, tempo, and pattern. *Brain Sci* 4 (2):428–52.

Torres, E. B. 2011. Two classes of movements in motor control. *Exp Brain Res* 215 (3–4):269–83.

Torres, E. B. 2012. Atypical signatures of motor variability found in an individual with ASD. *Neurocase* 1:1–16.

Torres, E. B., A. Raymer, L. J. Gonzalez Rothi, K. M. Heilman, and H. Poizner. 2010. Sensory-spatial transformations in the left posterior parietal cortex may contribute to reach timing. *J Neurophysiol* 104 (5): 2375–88.

Torres, E. B. and A. M. Donnellan. 2012. Autism: The movement perspective, *Frontiers in Integrative Neuroscience*. p. 1–374.

Torres, E. B., M. Brincker, R. W. Isenhower, P. Yanovich, K. A. Stigler, J. I. Nurnberger, D. N. Metaxas, and J. V. Jose. 2013a. Autism: The micro-movement perspective. *Front Integr Neurosci* 7:32.

Torres, E. B., P. Yanovich, and D. N. Metaxas. 2013b. Give spontaneity and self-discovery a chance in ASD: Spontaneous peripheral limb variability as a proxy to evoke centrally driven intentional acts. *Front Integr Neurosci* 7:46.

Torres, E. B., R. W. Isenhower, J. Nguyen, C. Whyatt, J. I. Nurnberger, J. V. Jose, S. M. Silverstein, T. V. Papathomas, J. Sage, and J. Cole. 2016. Toward precision psychiatry: Statistical platform for the personalized characterization of natural behaviors. *Front Neurol* 7:8.

Volman, M. J., and R. H. Geuze. 2000. Temporal stability of rhythmic tapping "on" and "off the beat": A developmental study. *Psychol Res* 63 (1):62–9.

Von Holst, E., and H. Mittelstaedt. 1950. The principle of reafference: Interactions between the central nervous system and the peripheral organs. In *Perceptual Processing: Stimulus Equivalence and Pattern Recognition*, ed. P. C. Dodwell, 41–72. New York: Appleton-Century-Crofts.

Wan, C. Y., L. Bazen, R. Baars, A. Libenson, L. Zipse, J. Zuk, A. Norton, and G. Schlaug. 2011. Auditory-motor mapping training as an intervention to facilitate speech output in non-verbal children with autism: A proof of concept study. *PLoS One* 6 (9):e25505.

Whitall, J., S. M. Waller, J. D. Sorkin, L. W. Forrester, R. F. Macko, D. F. Hanley, A. P. Goldberg, and A. Luft. 2011. Bilateral and unilateral arm training improve motor function through differing neuroplastic mechanisms: A single-blinded randomized controlled trial. *Neurorehabil Neural Repair* 25 (2):118–29.

16 Use of Video Technology to Support Persons Affected with Sensory-Movement Differences and Diversity

Sharon Hammer, Lisa Ladson, Max McKeough, Kate McGinnity, and Sam Rogers

CONTENTS

Introduction 243
Monty 245
Sam 247
David 247
Max 248
Dakota 249
Conclusion 250
Referenccs 250

This chapter illustrates a simple and yet powerful accommodation to help individuals with movement differences in the spectrum of autism. Through the use of widely available video technology designed by the authors and supported by the anecdotal contribution of several self-advocate individuals in the spectrum, we can learn to appreciate the importance of flexibly adapting external dynamics present in video images with variable degrees of speed and highly variable self-generated bodily rhythms used to control the flow of the image presentation. The positive outcome of the intervention underscores once again the importance of taking into consideration the person's physical needs and neurological predispositions. Guiding the person from the bottom up, rather than merely imposing the guidance from the top down through prompting or other unilateral means, helps the person respond better to adaptable visuomotor support.

INTRODUCTION

Donnellan and Leary (2012) remind us of the access difficulties experienced by many individuals who are affected by movement and sensory differences and diversity. Donnellan and Leary (1995) examine the notion that people might "behave in unusual ways due to the way their body is organized," especially as related to sensory and movement. These sensory-movement differences and diversity can, in fact, affect and even block a person's access to their skills and knowledge (Donnellan et al. 2012). It is our premise that collaborating with the individual to create video technology supports can increase consistency of access to current skills and knowledge, as well as create an easier path to learning new skills.

Video technology supports seem uniquely designed to create more movement fluidity for individuals who experience access issues and think in pictures. Dr. Temple Grandin was one of the first individuals affected with autism to explain her neurological difference of "thinking in pictures" (Grandin 1995, 19):

> I think in pictures. Words are like a second language to me. I translate both spoken and written words into full-color movies, complete with sound, which run like a VCR tape in my head.

To paraphrase a more recent description from Dr. Grandin, when she hears a spoken word, images "pop" into her head that display different pictorial representations of that word, which she likens to "Google Images."* The visual processing strength and style that is often reported by individuals with autism and captured in brain imaging research (Samson et al. 2012) suggests that video technology is not only compatible with the neurology of autism but, in fact, may be speaking what is considered by Judy Endow to be her "first language" (Endow 2013). Further, Judy Endow reminds us that "if a picture speaks a thousand words, how many words does a video speak?"

For those who process information more easily when it is presented visually (i.e., instead of verbally), teaching through pictures may be more "friendly" to that individual's neurological style. In particular, the dynamics of frame-by-frame pictures in video may be more amenable to map onto bodily rhythms and motion patterns that the person naturally and inherently already possesses. In this sense, to provide a more flexible, more adaptable, and broader picture-display dynamics, our definition of *video technology* is "any visual image that moves and has an electronic display" (McGinnity et al. 2013). Some current examples of media we would consider as video technology include videos, either homemade, purchased, or accessed through YouTube, TeacherTube, or other public video posting sites; computer software; PowerPoint or Keynote presentations on the computer or iPad or tablet; video games; and applications for computers, tablets, or handheld devices.

The critical point here is that the speed of the flow inherent in the pictures being presented to the person must be adaptable to accommodate the person's own bodily dynamics, that is, the rate of change of his or her internally generated bodily rhythms. Following this adaptable rate, the externally presented video technology has the potential to coherently entrain the flow of the videos with the flow of the body. Since the entrainment of these two rhythms can increase the likelihood of better integrating them, it then may be possible to latch onto the external one and guide the internal one to become "unstuck," for example, as when freezing of the body occurs. The notion of closing in this way the sensory (visual) motor loops and augmenting externally sensed dynamic-visual input (from the ongoing video technology) with internally sensed kinesthetic input (from the self-generated ongoing bodily motion dynamics) can be a very powerful ally of the person with autism (see Chapter 1 and Torres et al. 2013). The notion can also help caregivers provide proper support to the affected person because of the broad availability of such video technology today.

For individuals with autism, the use of video technology as a means to support has been groundbreaking. Max McKeough, a teenager with autism spectrum disorder (ASD) (previously, Asperger's syndrome), who was introduced to video technology several years ago, sums up his exposure to its use in this way: "I expect that I will continue to be aided in my future activities by a technology that has so vastly improved my life thus far." An increasing number of professionals, friends, and family members who collaborate with and support individuals with autism recognize that video technology has dramatically changed the way that they provide assistance. Using technology-based supports has opened up a range of diverse uses; limits to their use seem confined only by the imagination. The authors would like to briefly examine why these supports are so successful for individuals affected with autism.

There are several factors that make video technology compatible with autistic neurology. Unlike the constantly moving and changing pictures that the world provides, video technology allows access to these images in a way that gives the individual more control: "The individual watching the video

---

* T. Grandin, keynote address presented at the Autism Society of America Conference, Orlando, Florida, 2011.

has control over the speed, repetition, and volume of the viewing" (McGinnity et al. 2013). It is possible for the same content to be reviewed again and again. Within the use of this type of support, the viewer will not be "surprised" by unexpected social demands or expectations. As one author put it, "Video technology allows us to teach without the 'distraction of human interaction'" (Neumann 2004). The technology may also help to limit the distractions of the rest of the world. Every screen upon which an individual might access a video support has a built-in border:

> The edges of a TV screen, a computer monitor, or an iPod Touch offer a crystal clear border of where to start and where to stop attending. Unlike real life, there is no ambiguity as to where the attention is to be. (McGinnity et al. 2013)

Unlike other often-used supports, these technology-based supports seem to assist individuals affected with autism in the process of generalization.* In a formal study (Charlop-Christy et al. 2000), video modeling was shown to be more effective than in-vivo (i.e., live) modeling; the subjects that used video modeling had faster rates of acquisition of new skills than their control group that had access to live models. Further, the video modeling was more effective in promoting generalization of the newly learned skills. In the authors' use of video technology to support affected individuals, it seems we acknowledge the processing strengths and outsmart some of the challenges that are inherent in ASDs. Because every affected person experiences the world uniquely, it is vital to collaborate to better understand and respect the individual's experience when creating supports. As Ralph Waldo Emerson reminds us, "The secret of education lies in respecting the pupil" (Sealts 1982, 180–190).

In recent years, McGinnity et al. (2013) have discussed a variety of ways to use video technology to support people affected with movement differences and diversity: to teach new skills, to train staff, to support more consistent access to skills and knowledge, to enhance life and support competence, and to support new behaviors. In this chapter, we provide some examples of using video technology to try new things, to transition, to support staff understanding of sensory-movement differences and diversity, to support access of verbal language, to access inclusive environments, and to support more fluid movement of thoughts.

Carl Jung (1931) was one of the first individuals to identify the phenomenon of "stuck thoughts." Jung wrote, "I only know one thing: when my conscious mind no longer sees any possible road ahead and consequently gets stuck, my unconscious psyche will react to the unbearable standstill." More recently, this phenomenon of "stuckness" has been described by researchers, as well as individuals affected with autism to describe their experiences. Stuck thoughts, emotions, movements, or words† (Endow 2009; McGinnity et al. 2013; Vitikos 2009); brain freeze and freezing or stopping of movements and thoughts (Damasio and Maurer 1978; Maurer and Damasio 1982); and "brain jam"‡ or "access denied," as one adolescent put it, have been widely reported in first-person accounts and our personal communication with individuals affected by movement diversity and differences.

MONTY

Monty was an 11-year-old boy affected with autism. He was in the sixth grade and attended general education classes at the public middle school. Every one of Monty's teachers agreed that he was very bright. The district's standardized tests revealed the same to be true. Monty was a smart, cooperative, motivated, interested student, yet he was struggling in the majority of his classes.

A time was set up to meet with Monty to discuss what was happening for him. During this meeting, Monty described that he was able to focus for the first few minutes of each class. Then, at some point during some classes, the teacher would say something that would trigger a "tornado video" to start in

---

* T. Buggey, presented at the Autism Society of America Conference, Orlando, Florida, 2007.

† Retrieved from judyendow.com (2015).

‡ Retrieved from www.autismmind.com (2015).

his head. Upon further investigation, Monty was able to explain that the teacher did not actually have to say the word *tornado* or even talk about weather. One example that Monty shared was when a teacher was talking about some materials she left at her house. Because the materials were missing, and he had no picture of what they looked like, in his mind, an image of a tornado came up swirling around a generic house (again, because he did not have a specific picture of his teacher's house). In the tornado, there were random pieces of paper flying about (the materials the teacher forgot).

Monty said that thinking so much about tornadoes was upsetting to him. It was not something that he wanted to keep doing. Once a tornado video started "playing" in his brain, Monty did not know how to stop it. When the video was playing, he was not able to focus on the teacher or process what was happening in class. He reported wanting to pay attention in class and wanting to do well, but he just could not move the stuck thoughts in his brain.

Monty was able to clearly explain what was going on for him. In setting up a support for him, it was vital to incorporate the way he was talking about and thinking about what was happening in his thought process. With Monty's input, a PowerPoint presentation was created to support him with his self-described stuck thoughts of tornadoes.

The PowerPoint presentation comprised 10 slides (Figure 16.1). The slides consisted of some still pictures and pictures with animation added. Monty helped in deciding what pictures to use, the correct terms to use, and the size of the pictures (at one point in the process of creating a PowerPoint slide, he said, "No, it is way bigger than that in my head"). The animation function was used on some of the slides to represent the movement of information in his head. This animation allows the "schoolwork" in one slide to slowly fade away and the tornado video to come in quickly and in a more "solid" way. The support was meant to recreate, as closely as possible, what Monty was experiencing in his processing. Then, we used Monty's words to come up with a solution. Using animation, a finger is shown pressing the "pause" button on the tornado video. On the next slide, we inserted a breathing exercise that Monty had been practicing to help him to relax. Originally, we thought that this was going to be enough to help Monty stop the movie from playing in his head.

Upon trying it for a few weeks, Monty reported that the images within the tornado videos were just "too strong" and kept coming back after he was done breathing. So, with Monty's direction, we added a slide giving Monty time to watch "another, happier video" in his head before getting back to focus on his schoolwork. Monty gave us some ideas for what this happier video could be (McGinnity et al. 2013).*

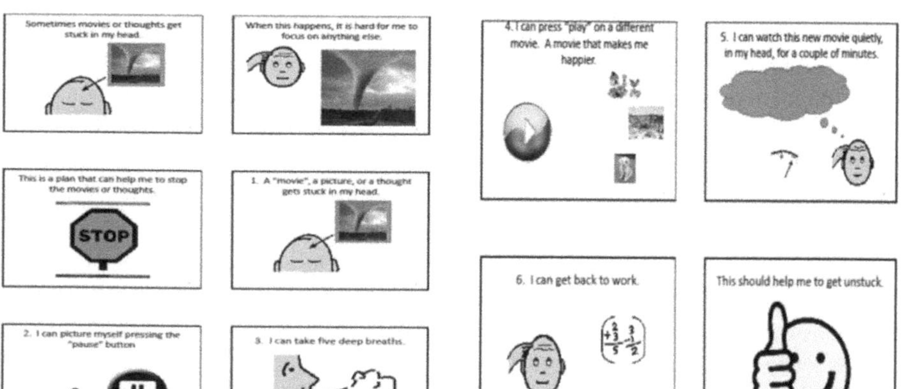

FIGURE 16.1 Monty's Stuck Thoughts PowerPoint

* Images used with permission from Boardmarker. www.boardmarker.com.

This final version of the support was introduced to Monty as a way to help him stop the tornado video from playing in his head. He watched the PowerPoint every day before going to any classes. Monty clicked through the slides independently. He had control over the speed in which he viewed the presentation. He did this for 3 weeks. At the end of this 3-week period, Monty told his teacher that he no longer needed to watch the PowerPoint support. He now knew how to "stop the tornado videos from playing in my mind." Monty's teachers corroborated Monty's reported success. When asked, each of them said that Monty was more focused in class, participated more actively in classroom discussions, and seemed happier in general.

The development of this PowerPoint for Monty resulted in a template that can be adapted for others who are affected with an internal (i.e., neurological) stuckness around ideas, thoughts, or pictures. It has been adapted for one young child with autism who had a fear of squirrels and had trouble stopping himself from thinking about a squirrel once he saw one. A similar support was developed for a high school student with ASD whose thinking could get stuck on violent images and websites, which resulted in his expulsion from public school and his being banned from using computers at home or school. While such measures by the school district may have kept the high school student and those around him safe, they did not provide the support he needed to shift his thinking when it became stuck on violent images.

In both of these cases, personalizing Monty's template to each individual's situation resulted in less stress and stuckness, and the ability to shift out of the stuck idea or picture. For the high school student, once he was able to shift out of the violent images, he was again able to use computers in a safe and meaningful manner, which was a great boon to his overall education and quality of life.

SAM

I am 31 years old. I live in a house in the country with a roommate and staff supporting us. I have two sisters and I am an uncle twice! My history: I attended early childhood special education from the ages of 3–5, and then I was fully included into a general education 5-year-old kindergarten, and I learned in a classroom with my same-aged, general education peers through all of elementary and most of middle school. In late middle school and high school, I attended a combination of general education classes and special education classes. My family moved from Lodi, Wisconsin, to Poynette, Wisconsin, when I was 10 years old. I graduated from Poynette High School in Poynette, Wisconsin.

I use video for myself to help my neurology—that means my brain—to understand and process information. I also make videos for my staff to tell them how my supports work and to teach them how I want to be supported as an adult male. Like many other people with autism, I think in pictures. Also, like many other people with autism, I depend on consistency in the way I am supported, to maximize access to my skills, feelings, and life! The way I make the videos is this:

1. My autism consultant and I write a script when I have a session with her. The script describes how the visual support works and what I want my staff to do to support me to use the visual.
2. I take the script home, and my staff and I transcribe the script onto big cue cards.
3. Then, my staff tapes me saying the script into a video camera.

The videos I make to train my staff help them support me in a consistent way and make my life a lot better!

DAVID

David, an early childhood student with autism, was having difficulty participating in the morning circle time. He would often move about the classroom and stop intermittently in various areas. An adult consistently prompted David, both verbally and visually, to come back to his spot on the carpet. He would comply with the request, but was unable to sustain the attention for more than a few seconds. An observer in the classroom used an iPad to videotape the activity in order to consult with the teacher at a later time.

During the observation, David showed an interest in the iPad and sat near the observer and watched the teacher and other students through the iPad. This lasted for the entire activity. The behavior was curious to both the teacher and the observer. After a lengthy discussion, it was hypothesized that "in real time," the activity, with all of its movement and engagement, was overstimulating for David. It was further hypothesized that the iPad may have given David clues as to where to attend and what was the salient activity in which he was expected to engage. The border around the iPad seemed to provide the perfect structure and boundary to highlight where David's attention needed to be focused. The next day, the teacher set up an iPad on a tripod and encouraged David to participate by "watching" circle time through the iPad. David sat behind the iPad and over time consistently engaged in the 20-minute activity for its entirety. Ultimately, the iPad was faded from circle time, having apparently "taught" David where and how to focus his attention. David no longer needs the iPad to engage in the 20 minutes of circle time on a regular basis. However, he occasionally requests the iPad at circle time via the Picture Exchange Communication System (Frost 2002).

The use of video technology with David was expanded to include preteaching of lessons. David watched a video of the lesson being taught, after which he was able to focus on the teacher during that lesson. Currently, David is learning play schemes through the use of video technology in the same way, first viewing activities through video and then engaging with a peer. His frequency and success with play behaviors have increased as a result.

MAX

I am currently in my second year of attendance at the University of Illinois, Chicago (UIC) studying bioengineering. I hope to explain how video technology played a role in my ability to try something completely new, and to describe some of the other ways video technology has improved ease and access in my life.

My family enjoys downhill skiing, and I was interested in trying it. Some of the reasons that I wanted to try skiing are:

- I wanted to try something new.
- I did not want to feel like I was missing out on something the whole family was doing.
- It looked like others were having fun.

The chair lift was an experience that could be visually engaged in from afar. At first glance, I was very intimidated. I watched for nearly an hour but could not muster the courage to try it. I had several family members do reconnaissance for me on the aspects of skiing that I could not see (e.g., my sister and others checked it all out and came back with a verbal report). I still had serious doubts that I would ever ride it. Additional verbal assurance (that was available in copious amounts) was *not* helping and was, in fact, more damaging to my ability to process.

Several family members made videos for me in hopes that if I could *see* the entire sequence of skiing, I might feel more comfortable trying it. Each aspect of the skiing experience was caught on video from various perspectives (e.g., from the perspective of the skier and from the perspective of a person ahead of the skier looking back). Not all points of view were helpful. I learned that the types of videos that are most useful to me are those that are filmed from *my* perspective—whatever I will be seeing as I execute the task.

These are the ways that the videos helped me:

- Confidence: Removed the element of surprise and the wild things that my imagination could conjure up.
- Video made the challenge seem very doable; it looked like I could handle what I saw.
- Video also established an idea of set terms of the event: speed, motion, and so forth, because of the perspective the video was filmed from.
- Final thoughts about skiing: I am glad that I conquered this.
- The video was the push that I needed.

I returned to the slopes annually; however, I no longer ski. I tried skiing one more time and decided it was not for me. This is by choice, not by fear. I may return or not, my choice. Once I realized that video could help me try something new, I sought out other uses of it in my life. Some of the doors that video technology has opened in my life include:

1. I had an opportunity to present publicly at an autism institute for educators. Once I realized how much video had helped me in skiing, I asked that I be videotaped in each presentation I have done since. Viewing the video let me see what I was doing on stage and helped me to understand what I could do to improve, but also what I could do each time on stage progressively. I could see how the audience reacted to certain tones of mine on stage, so I could continue to use them or dispense with them in future presentations. My increasing confidence on the stage led to my willingness to successfully audition to be the commencement speaker at my high school graduation of my class of 327 students and their families and friends.
2. I watched video footage of myself giving speeches as a way to support my thinking so that I could write a paper on it. The video helped me put my experience into context. That context was pivotal to the success of the paper, my senior writing project.
3. I continue to utilize video technology in numerous aspects of my life, the most recent of which has been to acclimate myself to campus life at the UIC. I made myself a video following my class schedule. Watching it helped me prepare myself not only for the timing involved, but also so I could get a sense of where I was on campus. Initially, the video helped me memorize my class route. Now that I am more familiar with the campus, the video assists me in knowing where I am in relation to other familiar locations on campus.

I expect that I will continue to be aided in my future activities by a technology that has so vastly improved my life thus far. I hope that sharing my experiences helps others to try new things.

DAKOTA

Dakota, a 17-year-old young man with autism, had never had a reliable communication system. He communicated through gestures, leading his parents and school support staff to items that he wanted and/or would get items himself. This method had its limitations. If the item was not in view or unknown to Dakota, he was unsuccessful at meeting his wants and needs. Many attempts at using assistive technology devices, teaching sign language, and using the Picture Exchange Communication System (Frost 2002) were ineffective in teaching Dakota to independently utilize a communication system.

When initial attempts to use a video model to teach skills to Dakota were made, he would push away the iPad. It was hypothesized that the movement of information on the screen was too much for Dakota to process. School personnel went back to traditional visual supports but added in short video model clips to engage Dakota. Through a slow process, Dakota began to engage with the video models, and ultimately, he was able to utilize an assistive technology device through the use of a series of video models. The video models consisted of teacher demonstrations on how to use the assistive technology device. Dakota began using the device with support and then independently. At 18, Dakota finally had a way to communicate his wants and needs consistently.

CONCLUSION

Throughout these case studies, the use of video technology seems to scaffold firm grounding to reduce unexpected stimuli—providing a predictive platform to extrapolate salient information and better integrate (moment by moment) that extraneous information into the internally self-generated bodily rhythms. This aversion to unexpected stimuli, a characteristic often reported by individuals with ASD, is specifically implicated in the high uncertainty the stimuli generate in the ensuing natural actions. In particular, as illustrated throughout the preceding chapters, individuals with ASD display difficulty finding a stable pattern of predictable actions. This can be statistically quantified within the variability patterns of fluctuations inherently present in their motions, indicative of high noise and randomness leading to high uncertainty in action planning and dynamic execution (see Chapters 1 and 14). Through principles of kinesthetic reafference, such actions provide a foundation to habilitate and rehabilitate internal maps of bodily rhythms and schema of the external environment—to translate and transform external information into purposeful action (see Chapter 1). It may be that such underlying latent sensory-motor difficulties preventing the establishment of a predictable pattern to "translate" external information may further underpin these higher-level issues with unexpected, unpredictable information. However, we hope these examples inspire readers to consider using readily available video technology to support themselves and others affected with sensory-movement differences and disorders. Do not give up on technology. Be creative in its use, brainstorm alternatives, and be consistent. Success can be right around the corner.

REFERENCES

Charlop-Christy, M. H., L. Le, and K. A. Freeman. 2000. A comparison of video modeling with in vivo modeling for teaching children with autism. *J Autism Dev Disord* 30 (6):537–52.

Damasio, A. R., and R. G. Maurer. 1978. A neurological model for childhood autism. *Arch Neurol* 35 (12): 777–86.

Donnellan, A. M., and M. R. Leary. 1995. *Movement Differences and Diversity in Autism/Mental Retardation: Appreciating and Accommodating People with Communication and Behavior Challenges*. Madison, WI: DRI Press.

Donnellan, A. M., and M. R. Leary. 2012. *Autism: Sensory-Movement Differences and Diversity*. 1st ed. Cambridge, WI: Cambridge Book Review Press.

Donnellan, A. M., D. A. Hill, and M. R. Leary. 2012. Rethinking autism: Implications of sensory and movement differences for understanding and support. *Front Integr Neurosci* 6:124. doi:10.3389/fnint.2012.00124.

Endow, J. 2009. *Paper Words: Discovering and Living with My Autism*. Shawnee, KS: AAPC Publishing.

Endow, J. 2013. *Painted Words: Aspects of Autism Translated*. 1st ed. Cambridge, WI: Cambridge Book Review Press.

Frost, L. 2002. *The Picture Exchange Communication System Training Manual*. 2nd ed. Newark, DE: Pyramid Educational Products.

Grandin, T. 1995. *Thinking in Pictures: And Other Reports from My Life with Autism*. 1st ed. New York: Doubleday.

Jung, C. A. 1931. *The Aims of Psychotherapy*. Princeton, NJ: Princeton University Press.

Maurer, R. G., and A. R. Damasio. 1982. Childhood autism from the point of view of behavioral neurology. *J Autism Dev Disord* 12 (2):195–205.

McGinnity, K., S. Hammer, and L. Ladson. 2013. *Lights! Camera! Autism! 2: Using Video Technology to Support New Behavior*. Cambridge, WI: Cambridge Book Review Press.

Neumann, L. 2004. *Video Modeling: A Visual Teaching Method for Children with Autism*. Croton, MD: Willerik Publishing.

Samson, F., L. Mottron, I. Soulieres, and T. A. Zeffiro. 2012. Enhanced visual functioning in autism: An ALE meta-analysis. *Hum Brain Mapp* 33 (7):1553–81. doi:10.1002/hbm.21307.

Sealts, M. M., Jr. 1982. Emerson as teacher. In *Emerson Centenary Essays*, ed. J. Myerson, 180–190. Carbondale: Southern Illinois University Press.

Torres, E. B., P. Yanovich, and D. N. Metaxas. 2013. Give spontaneity and self-discovery a chance in ASD: Spontaneous peripheral limb variability as a proxy to evoke centrally driven intentional acts. *Front Integr Neurosci* 7:46. doi:10.3389/fnint.2013.00046.

Vitikos, T. 2009. Counseling people with autism using FC. *Communicator* 18 (3):9–10.

17 Argentinian Ambulatory Integral Model to Treat Autism Spectrum Disorders

Silvia Baetti[*]

CONTENTS

Introduction 254
Cognitive and Academic Program 256
Communication Skills Program 258
Social Skills Program 259
Program of Musical Therapy for Sensory Modulation 260
Motor Skills Program 262
Program for Self-Reliance and Sensory Regulation 264
Strategies 264
Parent Support Program 265
Conclusion 265
References 265

This chapter describes a therapeutic model designed and implemented at the Pediatric Mental Health Division of the Hospital Italiano de Buenos Aires, Argentina. The services offered by this division adopt a holistic brain–body approach that integrates elements from several disciplines spanning from psychiatry and psychology to physical education. The approach combines techniques designed in our private practices with the existing methods of Treatment and Education of Autistic and Communication related handicapped CHildren (TEACCH); the developmental, individual difference, relationship-based (DIR) model or floor time; the Picture Exchange Communication System (PECS), and applied behavioral analysis (ABA), along with physical movement–based training to develop social interactive skills. This interdisciplinary concept emerged from the lack of treatments for autism spectrum disorder that would help children transition from the home to the classroom environment—a problem that was identified in special education and mainstream schools. Besides the development of integrated interventions of various types, the model works with the parents of the child and the school personnel to extend the interventions at the clinic to the home and school environments. To that end, the coordination among parents, educators, and clinicians permits the identification of the main needs, strengths, and weaknesses of each individual child with the purpose of tailoring the treatments and home or school environment of the child.

[*] Translated from Spanish by E. B. Torres.

INTRODUCTION

Autism spectrum disorder (ASDs) is a highly heterogeneous complex and systemic set of conditions. As we have seen in previous chapters, ASD affords more than one level of description, but at present, the main focus is on problems with social communications and restricted interests—which are also manifested in some repetitive (ritualistic or stereotypical) motions. As personnel with medical training working at a hospital, our team places an emphasis not only on the psychological and psychiatric aspects of the condition, but also on the physiological components of the nervous system disorders. In the face of such complexity, our best bet is to bring together a highly interdisciplinary team and integrate into our intervention several aspects of the human behavior that can be conducive to better social interactions.

The schematic in Figure 17.1 depicts the interdisciplinary nature of the program we have designed for ASD and lists the six main areas of focus. However, the order in the figure is not the order in which the child receives the interventions. Since the objectives of each program are interdependent and individualized according to the areas of strength of the child, there is no particular order to follow. The starting point is the strongest area the child may have. As such, one of the first steps in the treatment is the identification of that area of potential capability, predisposition, or preference that parents often know well. Using the child's strengths helps the child with build self-esteem and opens up new possibilities for the team members to gain access to other weaker areas, or other areas that may be more challenging, to help the team accomplish the ultimate goal of successful social exchange. For example, a child that may have a predisposition toward music therapy is encouraged in that area with the purpose of discovering psychological and cognitive components that could benefit from that strength. Likewise, the presence of motion in every aspect of behavior permits the simultaneous use of motor control to permeate all aspects of other therapies through the actions that the child is prompted to perform and/or from the actions the child spontaneously performs.

In tandem with the therapies depicted in Figure 17.1, other interventions are also used. These include biochemical treatment (prescription drugs as needed); neurosensory treatment (treatment

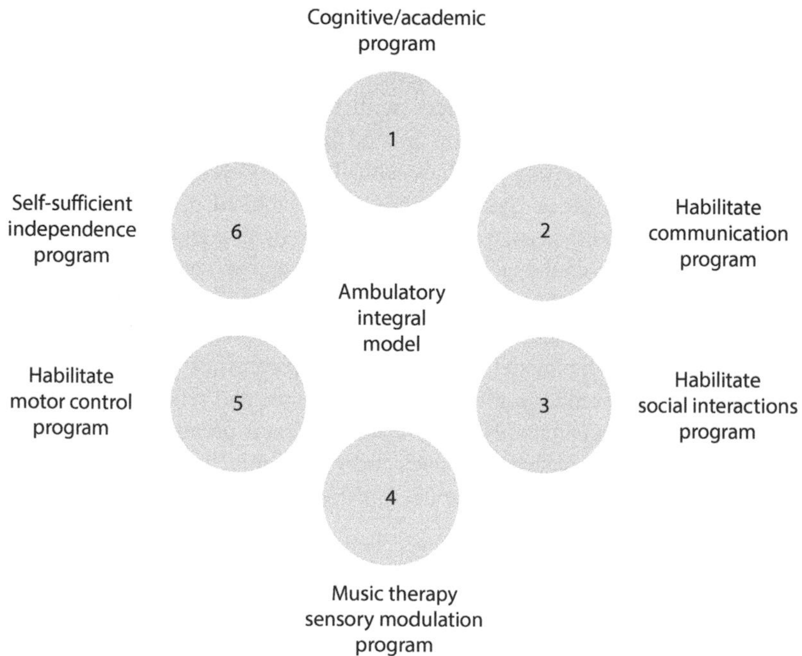

FIGURE 17.1 Ambulatory integral model to treat ASDs.

of sensory regulation by auditory training and communicational rehabilitation); behavioral model treatment using applied behavioral analysis (ABA); the educational model using the Treatment and Education of Autistic and Communication related handicapped CHildren (TEACCH) model; the developmental, individual difference, relationship-based (DIR) or floor-time model; and the Picture Exchange Communication System (PECS). The integration model does not place emphasis on one separate area at a time, but rather combines all areas in a balanced manner defined by all therapists. As such, the cohesive nature of the team is the most important component of the model. Coordinating all activities and communicating all outcomes as the child receives the individual sessions promotes an integrated approach that one could not possibly get using a single approach or applying a "one-size-fits all-model" to all children that come to the clinic.

Similar to most therapies for ASD, our program aims to focus on behaviors associated with this diagnosis. We aim to enhance positive behaviors that ultimately increase quality of life. However, unlike many other programs, we do not define behavior as a negative manifestation of the child's symptomatology. Indeed, within many fields related to ASD, the term *behavior* has a bad connotation—used to denote challenging or inappropriate manifestations of the child toward the self or others (self-injurious acts or acts to injure others). We argue that these behaviors are a manifestation of an underlying sensory and nervous system trying to find consistency or dampen uncertainty within the world. These unintentional behaviors are thus beyond the individual's control, and may be a by-product of intense fear and/or a signal of a nervous system that cannot regulate itself.

The program we have developed aims to look at behaviors as possible forms of adaptation of a coping system that lives immersed in a random, seemingly chaotic, stream of sensory information intensifying the uncertainty of the child's perceptual experience (Markram et al. 2007). Indeed, in recent years a form of high uncertainty has been quantified in the readout of the child's body, illustrating excess noise and randomness across the rhythms generated by the nervous systems (Brincker and Torres 2013), during both voluntary (Torres et al. 2013) and involuntary (Torres and Denisova 2016) motions. Our program provides various forms of support to try to help reduce this uncertainty. We provide social and communication cues in advance (feed-forward mode) to help the child figure out the situation he or she is in, or what may be needed (in the social sense) to open a communication channel and succeed in getting a response from the interlocutor. We aim at improving the adaptive skills of the person to induce the spontaneous self-discovery of possible objectives in a given conversation or situation taking place in the social domain. Presenting the child, ahead of time, with possible scenarios and evoking responses (rather than directly prompting him or her or telling him or her what to do) seems to help the child gain self-esteem and self-motivation. Above all, we search for improvement in the child's quality of life. To that end, we promote relevant dimensions in the domain of affect and aim at enhancing interpersonal relations, emotional growth, physical well-being, self-determination, and ultimately, social inclusion and social rights.

The program is rather intensive and highly interactive with two other critical elements in the life of the child: the parents or caregivers and the school teachers. Many elements of the program are inspired by basic scientific research and are updated according to the scientific advances in the various fields they draw from. Among the works we have used are those of Peter Hobson (2004), Theo Peeters (1997); Peeters and Gillberg (1999), Hilde Le Clercq (1985), and Ami Klin (2003; Klin et al. 2003; Volkmar et al. 2005). Our team is composed of psychologists, educational psychologists, physical education teachers, therapists, a social worker, a speech therapist, and medical doctors. Each patient attends treatment two, three, or four times a week and receives two or three treatment sessions per day. Each session is 40 minutes. The overarching program consists of a range of main areas (Figure 17.1), including a cognitive and academic program, a communication skills program (including social skills), a music therapy program for sensory modulation, and a motor skills program. Each of these individual programs aims to work on an axis of development within each child, and draws on multiple therapists and therapeutic programs to achieve useful gains for the individual. Each of these programs and the core focus are presented in turn.

COGNITIVE AND ACADEMIC PROGRAM

One of the focuses of the cognitive program is the issue of imitation. From the start of life, imitation is an important component of social interactions. Typically, many aspects of imitation seem overtly innate, for example, when a baby naturally and automatically imitates several of the mom's facial gestures and entrains with her sounds (Condon 1996; Condon and Sander 1974). There is inconsistent evidence on whether the child with ASD has a similar ability to imitate or if overt imitation is also impeded (Hobson 2004). Some authors argue that imitation is impeded in ASD (Gopnik et al. 1999; Meltzoff et al. 2012; Rogers et al. 1996), while others argue that some aspects of imitation are relatively intact (Charman et al. 1997; Morgan et al. 1989). On the basis of the results obtained by Peter Hobson, Melissa Moore, and Allyson Ann Lee (Ledbetter-Cho et al. 2015, 2016; Lee et al. 2015; Ninci et al. 2013), one may hypothesize that children with ASD are able to perceive and copy the actions of others, but are unable to do so in the same way as typically developing children do.

Perhaps the problem is more subtle. Children with ASD appear to have preferences for objects as they are less ambiguous; that is, their dynamics are more predictable than those of humans. Indeed, we know from researchers using point-light displays during motion perception studies that children with ASD seem to prefer to recognize objects' motions over the motions of others (Klin et al. 2009, 2015). As such, children with ASD may be more inclined to imitate the dynamics of the objects located on those who they are supposed to imitate. That is, the children move with the objects on people and seemingly imitate the person, but in reality, they are just following the dynamics of objects these persons wear or carry. This gives us something to work with during therapies that involve imitation, as we would try to encourage a holistic approach to motion from objects and people's bodies in our program by, for example, getting the child acquainted with learning to sense his or her own body dynamics in the first place. This is why our program has a section devoted to the step-by-step development of motor control through physical education (explained in detail in Chapter 18). However, the ability to identify the extent to which the child was actually able to capture the essence of the person's dynamics and map those onto his or her own dynamics is unknown. This is an important to further disentangle that question because in the social scene, adopting others' dynamics is part of entraining and reciprocating to show agreement (Richardson et al. 2015; Varlet et al. 2016). The fact that some of the implicit aspects of the imitation process—precisely those that seem to make imitation a success in the social scene—occur largely beneath awareness constitutes a great challenge for therapists trying to teach the child how to imitate successfully.

Imitation of action can also serve as the means to learn about, and guide, other aspects of the holistic approach to ASD. Several elements of intentionality in action are present during imitation that require the therapist to enhance attentional skills (e.g., joint attention) and nurture the emotional relations of the child. In this regard, the program is mindful of the needs of each child during the imitation sessions. The strong Argentinean training tradition in psychodynamics in the areas of psychiatry and psychology has been our best ally in this regard. The novelty of our approach rests on the comprehensive and cohesive nature of the team. There are some core aspects of ASD that this interdisciplinary team are fully aware of and draw on. These are:

- The autistic brain seems to process sensory information differently and, as such, seems to arrive at different percepts of the self and others.
- The autistic nervous system seems to have a different set of rules that impede the reduction of information in ways similar to those of neurotypical nervous systems.
- The autistic child seems to rely more on direct sensory information than on the representational concepts derived from it.
- The autistic child has limited ability to interpret gestures in the same way as neurotypical individuals.
- All the above differences manifest in the lack of the type of imaginative, representational, or abstract thought process we observe in typical developing children.

Importantly, successful imitation relies on different types of gestures, including:

- Instrumental gestures: They have great iconic meaning in that there is a visible connection between the image and its meaning.
- Expressive gestures: They are subtle, their effect is not as direct, and they are used to convey complex emotions and the overall states of mind.
- The difficulty adding representation or abstract meaning to perception results in the "different cognitive style" associated with communication, social interaction, stereotyped behavior, and restricted interests affecting individuals with ASD.

Through the therapy program, we also attempt to address the following problems with imagination:

- Failing to understand the "whole" at the expense of focusing on the details of the parts, with fragmented actions lacking the fluidity of typical motions
- Responding to the stimulus but not processing it to perceive it in the abstract
- A form of "inflexible" thinking leading to illogical "fears"
- Constant search for consistency
- Excessive reactions (too much or too little) to visual, auditory, and tactile stimuli

Using the above information, we have outlined a range of guidelines for the development of an educational or schooling program that integrates these core elements to promote cognitive development in children with ASD. The core guidelines include:

- Prevent factors that trigger behavior.
- Use stereotypic behavior as a reward.
- Enforce predictability in the daily routine, for example, consistent duration of activities.
- Use tasks that are guided by visual feedback.
- When changing the routine or the environment, introduce changes gradually.
- Reach agreements with the child so he or she participates in the decision-making process.
- Stop activity (with visual aids) and start another activity.
- Use stereotyped interests constructively.
- Promote school readiness.

As part of the overarching program of cognitive skills, we therefore have designed a methodology for acquisition of key educational skills, such as literacy. However, as we initiate and maintain that program, the child receives toilet training, food intake (diet) training, and sleep assessment, while we treat fears and phobias to decrease tantrums, self-injurious behaviors, and aggressiveness. There are some key points we keep in mind when addressing psychoeducational programs for ASD. These include:

- What to teach? Every therapist must know the psychology of typical child development in all aspects and sociocommunication interactions.
- How do you teach? Use structuring and systematizing units. Education is a basic priority for the student with ASD, but it needs to be guided without an emphasis on the errors the child makes, but rather with gentle emotional support promoting affect.
- Why teach? To encourage maximum personal development to attain the highest possible quality of life. One should always aim to improve the social knowledge of children with ASD and foster their communication skills.
- Aim at achieving a self-regulatory behavior adapted to the environment, and try to achieve functional generality of what is taught in natural environments.

COMMUNICATION SKILLS PROGRAM

Children with ASD tend to display fewer orienting behaviors when called by name at 12 months of age (Dawson et al. 2002; Osterling et al. 2002), although some other work also observed this type of difficulty for 8–10 months (Werner et al. 2005). In children that go on to develop ASD, certain characteristics are nonetheless unique; namely, the differences seem more strictly communicative, and they are observed at 24 months of age. Around that time, infants tend to focus on the use of proto-declarative language (Osterling and Dawson 1994; Osterling et al. 2002). Not only do these elements appear less, but also they are used in qualitatively different ways than typical, for example, without looking at the face of the speaker. In prospective studies, both verbal and nonverbal communication difficulties were found from 12 months of age in high-risk children who were later diagnosed with ASD; such investigations have found no previous markers (Landa and Garrett-Mayer 2006; Landa et al. 2007; Sullivan et al. 2007; Yirmiya et al. 2006; Yoder et al. 2009).

To describe the program involving communication intervention for people with ASD, we follow the principles that emerge from the most recent functional and evolutionary research. The acquisition of different skills that make language possible within a critical period depends on multiple neurocognitive mechanisms. Owing to their properties and characteristics, these mechanisms can be grouped into three systems (Tager-Flusberg 1999; Tager-Flusberg and Cooper 1999): computational, theory of mind, and general cognition. Under normal conditions, these three kinds of systems develop harmoniously and interact to facilitate language development during the critical period (Fuentes-Biggi et al. 2006; Golinkoff et al. 1996, 2002; Weisberg et al. 2013, 2014). However, in ASD certain developmental dissociations between conceptual and grammatical skills have been described. It is possible that certain functional autonomy may be selectively altered by neurobiological, cognitive, and/or very different socioemotional deficits (Campo et al. 2013, 2016; Fuentes-Biggi et al. 2006; Poch et al. 2015).

The classification of Riviére (2011) offers many advantages from practical and theoretical standpoints. The former is useful for diagnosing and designing intervention programs. The latter offers some plausible explanations with regards to language in ASD. It allows some comparison with stages of normal language developmental, and the development of functional hypotheses about the evolutionary processes that may be altered in people with an autistic disorder.

As noted, each overarching program is devised upon core foundational therapies. Some of those included with the communication program target the following:

- Training in understanding or receptive language
- Training in expressive language
- Methods that emphasize individualized intervention language (e.g., PECS)
- Improved nonverbal communication (signs, symbols, drawings, and objects)
- Use of computerized systems
- Use of rooms with minimal clutter and sound or noise to avoid overstimulation of other senses

The intervention is fine-tuned according to the intellectual and linguistic level of each child. The Derbyshire Language Scheme (Masidlover 1979) or pragmatic aspects of the first communication skills (Cocquyt et al. 2015) are used as a guide to improve conversational skills and language comprehension. Further, improving communication skills with others involves the help of the parents and the use of language appropriate for the child's level. More precisely, the program encourages effective communication through positive interactions.

It is important to note in this section that when a child comes to our program with a suspicion of ASD, even before the formal diagnosis, we begin intensive therapeutic intervention so as not to waste time. We are well aware of a popular myth in the face of language delays—"the child will eventually talk"—yet as time goes by, language does not appear. This early intervention focuses on all aspects of Figure 17.1, even when ASD has yet to be diagnosed. This program is tailored to neurodevelopment in general, so it is important that the autistic condition is only a specific mode of intervention that requires additional elements to aim for inclusion of the child in society at large. Our main goal, however, is to enhance quality of life throughout this process of intervention. In this regard, it is fundamental to train language specialists that treat autistic children to gain a more holistic view of the condition and to go beyond the nuances of language to help the child attain autonomy and self-control. More often than not in other programs, one specialist treats the child with ASD with an exclusive focus on his or her area, disregarding or not fully acknowledging the complexity of the ASD phenomena.

SOCIAL SKILLS PROGRAM

This part of the program targeting social skills considers five important steps: (1) identify the social skill deficit, (2) distinguish between skill acquisition and performance deficits, (3) select intervention strategies, (4) initiate the intervention, and (5) adapt and modify the intervention as needed. Although some specific targets for intervention may emerge during the initial stages, none of them become the exclusive focus. Instead, the integrated holistic approach is used. Some basic foundational strategies of the program are:

1. Teaching in the basic rules of conduct, for example, maintaining proper distance in an interaction
2. Teaching in social routines: Greetings, farewells, strategies for initiating contact, contact termination strategies, and so forth
3. Training in the socioemotional key: Through the use of video showing emotions, letters of emotional expressions, adaptation strategies of emotional expression context, and so forth
4. Strategies to respond to the unexpected: For example, teaching social "buzzwords" to "muddle through"
5. Training of social cooperation strategies: For example, in a construction game, provide half the pieces to each child and moderate their interactions with an emphasis for collaboration
6. Teaching games with simple rules so the child learns about the rules of social engagement and the importance of order
7. Encourage helping peers
8. Design tasks to help the child learn how to distinguish between concrete reality and fake reality: For example, someone with a costume that makes him "look fat" but he is actually "thin"
9. Teaching paths to knowledge: Designing tasks for teaching verbal routines on knowledge of the type "I know because I've seen" versus "I do not know because I have not seen"
10. Teach to adopt someone else's perspective: For example, guess what a partner may be watching even when the child is not directly watching it

Simple instrumental strategies (physical or social) are encouraged in patients with a lower development level. For example, the perception of contingencies or stimulus–response associations will be encouraged to build a map between their actions and reactions within a given environment. The social skills program seeks to increase interest in social situations by encouraging self-awareness and self-esteem. In turn, the program helps with the development of learning skills by creating a fun atmosphere where the therapist builds skills from very simple, basic blocks to more complex interactions. These procedures are embedded in all components of the program to increase the capacity of the individual to generate social initiative and learn to identify and follow social rules. The program is also mindful of age and developmental stages of other children within a social scene. The developmental disparities associated with ASD are kept in mind when gradually inserting the child with others in a play situation. The therapists encourage specific rules, including:

- Promote the use of gestures and nonverbal elements of communication
- Develop skills of self-knowledge
- Learn to correctly identify differences in self-mood and the mood of others
- Learn to team up, cooperate, show solidarity, and respect the rules of social engagement
- Learn to problem-solve in a dynamic social context
- Learn to wait for others, tolerate others, and share with others
- Learn to communicate desires and needs in a kind manner
- Manage negative thoughts that deteriorate self-esteem and social competence

The therapist also practices some physical exercises to help with social anxiety. These include muscle relaxation techniques and breathing techniques. Further, higher-level exercises are also in place, for example, turn taking and starting and finishing conversations with another person within a social context. By combining the physical exercises and the high-level instructions, the child can also learn to differentiate different contextual situations, such as the right time to initiate participation in a dialogue, and how to autoregulate behaviors that enhance positive interactions with a partner.

PROGRAM OF MUSICAL THERAPY FOR SENSORY MODULATION

The music therapy program provides core sensory modulation that has repercussions at all levels of the program, including cognitive development, social skills, and motor control. At its core, it consists of two parts. One is grounded on scientific findings (e.g., neurological music therapy tailored to neurological disorders or disorders of the nervous systems, including ASD [Thaut 2005, 2015; Thaut et al. 2014]). The other is more therapeutic in nature and guided by evidence from clinical practices.

The clinical practice is conceived as a discipline that uses music to achieve therapeutic goals, for example, the restoration, maintenance, and improvement of both the mental and physical health of the individual. The therapy facilitates changes in behavior, contributes to the understanding of self, and promotes better adaptation to society—which is expressed at both the individual and group level. The universal character of music contributes to the development and integration of physical, emotional, and mental balance across a group. Chapter 15 provides an example of such practices.

One of the most important aspects of music therapy according to Thayer Gaston (de L'Etoile 2000) is the habilitation and rehabilitation of interpersonal relationships. Indeed, music helps to establish desirable interpersonal relationships through group activities, whereby emphasis is naturally placed on social integration, recognition of others, and learning to respect and value others, as well as being respected and valued by others. The music therapy approach uses the unique and universal powers of rhythm to provide self-regulation and self-organization of the person's nervous systems. According to Rolando Benenzon (1981, 1997), music therapy integrates the following principles:

- *ISO principle:* This principle in music therapy refers to the sound identity. It implies respect for the other and knowledge of it before starting work. We all have a sound identity that distinguishes and characterizes us. It is a dynamic and not a static principle. As such, the sound identity may shift across different contexts and situations. The Benenzon method of music therapy (Schwabe 1976) distinguishes various types of ISO:
  - *ISO gestalt:* The characteristic of an individual.
  - *ISO complementary:* Small changes are cooperating each day or each music therapy session. Default environmental and dynamic circumstances.
  - *ISO group:* The ISO established in a group of therapeutics. They have to take into account the individual ISOs.

- *Cultural ISO:* Depends on the culture in which it was born.
- *Universal ISO:* Typical of the human species and distinguishes us as human beings.
- *Principle of object broker:* You can define music as a communication tool capable of acting on the patient therapeutically by building the relationship with the therapist, without triggering states of intense alarm (e.g., adopt a sound through which the patient communicates).
- *Principle of integrated object:* Refers to the capacity of music to integrate and unify others. Often, instruments of great impact are chosen by a person who leads the group.

In our program, we classify the techniques used in music therapy in two large blocks, expressive and receptive techniques, depending on the patient's response in relation to internal or external aspects of the therapy, respectively.

Some methods used in the program include the guided imagery and music (GIM) method, which engages the listener to achieve a relaxed state to suggest images, symbols, or emotions with a creative purpose, and as a basis for the therapeutic action method. The therapist helps the patient to explore his or her inner world, to search through the unknown states of consciousness, growth, and welfare.

Another method related to thc ISO principle (aka Nordoff–Robbins method [Nordoff and Robbins 1971]), or method of musical improvisation therapeutics. This method is based on improvisation at the piano by the therapist, who performs what the patient expresses through percussion instruments and piano. The method aims to encourage the patient to express his or her feelings through music. It is an individualized method, and is particularly aimed at children with problems: ASD, mental retardation, neurological problems, etc.

- *Behavioral method:* As with other behaviorist approaches, this one uses music to encourage "appropriate" social behaviors or to discourage "inappropriate" social behavior through rewards that help establish stimulus–response pairs.
- *Psychoanalytic method:* This method uses music therapy improvisation and musical dialogue to explore the subconscious by sound expression. It is used with psychiatric patients, troubled couples, social relations, and so forth. Psychoanalysis also uses reciprocal improvisation duets between the therapist and patient, in addition to verbal speech.
- *Benenzon method:* Creates a space between the therapist and patient that leads to the opening of communication channels through an intermediary object that mediates the patient–therapist interaction. It is applied in hospitals, mental health centers, and special education; with adults and children; and so forth (Benenzon 1997, 1981).

The music therapy program aims to:

- Increase group cohesion and social skills.
- Increase attention.
- Improve fine and gross motor coordination.
- Improve auditory, visual, and tactile perception.
- Redirect nonadaptive behavior.
- Stimulate cognitive functions: joint attention (the extent and quality), attention, working memory, anticipation, flexibility, the different types of memory, and executive functions. Sensory stimulation as music encompasses all but auditory stimulation, engaging other channels, such as visual, tactile, and kinesthetic.

MOTOR SKILLS PROGRAM

The portion of the program devoted to motor control is run by professionals in the areas of physical education, sports, psychology, and alternative communication systems. These professionals have received special training to become acquainted with the unique features of the children in the spectrum so as to develop programs tailored to their social needs.

Although many in the clinical field admit that visible clumsiness and lack of bodily coordination are characteristics of the movements performed by children in the spectrum, very little emphasis has been placed on movements and their sensations as specific parts of intervention programs in ASD. Occupational therapy with an emphasis on sensory-motor integration is an example of programs in the United States (Miller and Fuller 2006) that have placed some emphasis on functional goals in activities of daily living that are impacted by sensory-motor issues in ASD. However, the lack of scientific literature on their methods and reliable outcome measures to track progress during interventions forced us to develop our own programs in our hospital settings with homologue programs in homes and school environments.

One of the first signs of motor problems that Tony Attwood (2008) refers to in his guide for professionals in the field is the delay children with ASD experience in reaching walking milestones. In young children, there may be additional limitations on the ability to play ball games, difficulty learning to tie shoelaces, and a strange way of walking or running. During school years, other motor difficulties surface, as the teacher soon becomes aware of poor handwriting and lack of aptitude for school sports. In adolescence, a small minority develop facial tics, for example, involuntary spasms of the muscles of the face, or rapid blinking and occasional grimaces (Donnellan and Leary 1995). Corina and Christopher Gillberg (Gillberg et al. 1994) have included motor clumsiness as one of six diagnostic criteria. Conversely, Peter Szatmari and his colleagues follow the American Psychiatric Association (APA) criteria in that they do not make a direct reference to motor coordination. Moreover, the APA has a list of features associated with Asperger syndrome, including the presence of clumsiness in the preschool period and delayed motor milestones, but no specific criteria exist in the *Diagnostic and Statistical Manual of Mental Disorders* (DSM) to include motor issues as a core symptom of the condition. Such motor issues are not present only in the children with severe ASD. Some studies suggest that between 50% and 90% of children and adults with Asperger syndrome or high-functioning ASD may have motor coordination problems as well (Gowen and Miall 2005; Nayate et al. 2005, 2012; Rinehart et al. 2006a; Szatmari et al. 1990; Weimer et al. 2001).

While there is debate and confusion as to how to categorize and measure motor clumsiness, or whether to include it as part of the diagnostic criteria, there is no doubt that these issues, when present, have a devastating and pervasive influence in the social life of the child. Even that alone should be a reason for concern and treatment. Indeed, all these features are specific indicators of clumsiness and movement disorders that we consider essential to target when attempting to improve social interactions. Indeed, these external behavioral symptoms of ASD may increase an individual's chance of becoming a subject of bullying once he or she starts school (see Chapter 26), and so it becomes critical to help change the perception of ASD by others.

Research has begun to profile the prevalence of motor difficulties across the ASD spectrum using standardized tests of motor proficiency, such as the Griffiths, Bruninks–Oseretsky (Poulsen et al. 2011), and gross motor impairment (Manjiviona and Prior 1995; Ulrich 1985) tests. When used to test children in the spectrum, the results suggest that poor motor coordination affects a wide range of abilities involving gross and fine motor skills (e.g., Whyatt and Craig 2012, 2013). As researchers, parents, and self-advocates demonstrate in this book, the motor problems are indeed important in ASD.

Our program addresses some specific areas of motor control in the following sections.

Locomotion: The gait of children with ASD is different from that of typical peers (Chester and Calhoun 2012; Esposito et al. 2011; Lim et al. 2016; Rinehart et al. 2006a, 2006b; Torres et al. 2016). There seems to be lack of coordination between the upper and lower limbs (see also Chapter 14). This feature can be quite visible once the child reaches school age. At that point, other children might tease the affected child, thus inducing reluctance to participate in sports and physical education in school. The therapeutic program is designed to ensure that movements become well coordinated. It is our experience that in contrast to gait, swimming appears less affected in the children. The program encourages swimming, so the child has the opportunity to experience genuine competence and admiration about the movements in this sport.

Ball Skills: Basic skills to catch and throw accurately seem to be particularly affected (Whyatt and Craig 2012, 2013). When the autistic child grabs a ball with both hands, arm movements are often poorly coordinated and dysregulated; that is, hands may close in the correct position, but a split second later, thus missing the ball (Whyatt and Craig 2013). A study shows that children often cannot look in the direction of the target before launch (Manjiviona and Prior 1995). One of the consequences of failing to be good at ball games is the exclusion of children from some of the most popular social games in the Argentinean playground (football, or soccer). For instance, they may avoid some of the activities because they know their lack of competence, or they may be deliberately excluded by their peers, because they are a liability to the team's performance. From an early age, parents need to teach and practice skills with the ball, not to be exceptional athletes, but to ensure that the child has the basic tools to be included in the games at school. Further, since these sports require eye–hand coordination and vision may be also impaired, it is important to check eye vision and obtain prescription eyeglasses as needed.

Balance: There may be problems with balance in ASD. For example, if the child tries to stand up on one leg with eyes closed, the outcome may be a fall (Manjiviona and Prior 1995; Minshew et al. 2004; Molloy et al. 2003). Temple Grandin (Ratey et al. 1992) describes how she is unable to keep her balance when she puts one foot before the other to attempt walking on a straight line. This is common to many children we see in the clinic. It is problems like this that can affect a child's ability to use the recreational facilities and activities in the gym along with his or her peers (Riquelme et al. 2016; Thompson et al. 2017). The child may need practice and encouragement with activities that require balance, as this component of motor control is very important for early social exchange and inclusion.

Dexterity: This area of motor skills is very important in the performance of daily living activities that require coordination of both hands (Riquelme et al. 2016; Thompson et al. 2017), an area considered problematic in ASD (e.g., Manjiviona and Prior 1995; Whyatt and Craig 2012). They include, for example, learning to dress, tying the shoelaces, drinking from a bottle or glass, and eating with utensils. Dexterity includes foot and leg coordination as well. These are required during games and other activities that require social interactions. They are also necessary when learning to ride a bicycle or operate tools. Because of their importance, we place a special emphasis on tasks that require both manual and foot dexterity.

Dyspraxias: Tasks that require the use of tools are problematic in ASD (Dziuk et al. 2007; Miller et al. 2014; Schumacher et al. 2015; Steinman et al. 2010; Williams et al. 2004). The planning stages necessary to execute the actions that synergistically coordinate the body with external objects seem to be affected in ASD (Bodison 2015; McAuliffe et al. 2017; Miller et al. 2014; Mosconi and Sweeney 2015). As such, the child may need supervision and encouragement to work at an appropriate pace, and take time to correct mistakes. Sometimes, the child can be encouraged to reduce the rate having to count between actions and using a timer to indicate an appropriate pace (Russell et al. 2016).

Lax Joints or Hypermobility Syndrome in ASD: One of the features we examine during a diagnostic assessment is the presence of lax joints (Shetreat-Klein et al. 2014). The origins of this somewhat common feature in ASD are unknown: Is this a structural abnormality, or is it due to low muscle tone? The prevalence of this difficulty is also unknown, but it is present in children with ASD who also have SHANK3 deletion syndrome (Sarasua et al. 2014).

When problems such as lax joints or immature or unusual pressure occur, the child is included in a program with the occupational therapist (OT) to carry out therapeutic activities conducive of attaining functional goals. This is a priority in our program with young children, as many school activities require the use of a pen or pencil, scissors, and so forth, and those in turn recruit the fingers and hand–arm joints.

Rhythm: This feature of sound and motion has been described in autobiographical books by Temple Grandin (Grandin 1996; Grandin and Scariano 1986) as a different way to synchronize the bodily rhythms of the feet and hands with other people or within the self. When two people walk next to each other, they tend to automatically synchronize the movements of their extremities, such as when soldiers are marching on parade. Their movements spontaneously acquire the same rhythm. This also happens when two people hold a conversation and the entrainment their bodies undergo is entirely beneath their awareness (Funahashi et al. 2014; Gepner et al. 1995; Stins et al. 2015). In contrast, the person with ASD seems to walk to the beat of a different drum (see Chapter 20) and requires effortful and deliberate thoughts to keep up with the other person's rhythms. This problem can also affect the ability to interact with another person, or a group, or to play with, share, or use an instrument in a social group. Our program uses various strategies to improve the autistic child rhythms. These include integrating the music therapy and the physical education programs and coordinating the individual therapist plan in an integral manner.

PROGRAM FOR SELF-RELIANCE AND SENSORY REGULATION

Parents appreciate this part of the program as much as children do. The ability to dress independently, eat or drink independently, or simply use the toilet or shower independently is often taken for granted by typically developing fellows; yet it is a major challenge when the neurodevelopment of the child is compromised. Accomplishing these daily living tasks is an important milestone in our program. To that end, the OT works hand in hand with all other therapists, the parents, and the teachers of each child. The OT sessions are tailored to the child's needs so as to help with daily living activities across multiple environments.

STRATEGIES

One way to facilitate the training across different therapies is by building accommodations that help the child dampen the uncertainty of his or her surrounding environment. If we make the environment well structured and predictable, if we avoid overstimulation and are mindful of the child sensory processing issues, there is a chance that the child will respond better to the intervention and make visible progress. We aim for the program to be rewarding for each child in ways that increase the self-esteem and encourage the child to want to continue each activity. Activities that are easy and simple to control pose less of a challenge and also help the therapist reach the next milestone in the individualized program.

PARENT SUPPORT PROGRAM

The program meets with the parents on a monthly basis, setting up a group therapy that includes all relevant parties, that is, the child, the parents, the teacher (if the child is of school age), and the therapist.

The role of families in the therapeutic-educational intervention for people with ASD is of great significance, but is conditioned by several stages in the process of discovering the child is indeed affected by ASD:

- *The family may be in a passive stage:* This stage is when the parents may still be in a state of "shock," in dire need of developing coping mechanisms to overcome the initial paralysis and move forward to help the child. They will learn that the child will need very intense and specialized support for most of his or her life, although these are more evident in the early years of onset of the disorder. The team will help the family understand the child's needs and work closely with the therapists to achieve the goals and contribute to the child's progress in the program.
- *The family may already be in the active stage:* This is the stage where the family is actively seeking help and gathering information to better understand the disorder and appropriately intervene.

We provide guidelines for organizing the child's living conditions at home (and at school) in a manner consistent with the therapy that we tailor to the child's needs, but also to the predispositions and capabilities we identify in the child. We encourage parents to support the child and reassure him or her in his or her activities and cheer at every accomplishment the child has. Our model is to increase the child's self-esteem in the first place to guide him or her toward a better life.

Another aspect of the program is to encourage social exchange of the parents with other affected parents so as to empathize and learn from each other. This type of moral support helps the team, the parents, and the child. As such, we hold monthly meetings at the Pediatric Mental Health Section of the Hospital Italiano de Buenos Aires with all parents and talk about different relevant topics that we derive from our sessions and interactions with the families. The call is open to all parents and/or caregivers who receive treatment in the Treatment of ASD Service. The turnout is relatively low, but that open space is maintained to provide education for all families. Family discussions can help group members to better cast their own issues in relation to those of others, so as to gain a broader perspective of the autistic condition and its heterogeneous nature.

CONCLUSION

The comprehensive outpatient model provides an individual intervention plan for each patient with an educational program for parents and caregivers and teachers. This program has been successful in leading the child toward self-regulation and independence with a decrease in disruptive behaviors that are deleterious for social exchange. Through this holistic approach, the child, with the emotional support of the parents, the educators, and the therapists, can begin the path of inclusion in the social medium and, as such, increase his or her quality of life.

REFERENCES

Attwood, T. 2008. *The Complete Guide to Asperger's Syndrome*. London: Jessica Kingsley Publishers.

Benenzon, R. O. 1981. *Music Therapy Manual*. Springfield, IL: C. C. Thomas.

Benenzon, R. O. 1997. *Music Therapy Theory and Manual: Contributions to the Knowledge of Nonverbal Contexts*. 2nd ed. Springfield, IL: Charles C. Thomas.

Bodison, S. C. 2015. Developmental dyspraxia and the play skills of children with autism. *Am J Occup Ther* 69 (5):6905185060. doi: 10.5014/ajot.2015.017954.

Brincker, M., and E. B. Torres. 2013. Noise from the periphery in autism. *Front Integr Neurosci* 7:34. doi: 10.3389/fnint.2013.00034.

Campo, P., C. Poch, R. Toledano, J. M. Igoa, M. Belinchon, I. Garcia-Morales, and A. Gil-Nagel. 2013. Anterobasal temporal lobe lesions alter recurrent functional connectivity within the ventral pathway during naming. *J Neurosci* 33 (31):12679–88. doi: 10.1523/JNEUROSCI.0645-13.2013.

Campo, P., C. Poch, R. Toledano, J. M. Igoa, M. Belinchon, I. Garcia-Morales, and A. Gil-Nagel. 2016. Visual object naming in patients with small lesions centered at the left temporopolar region. *Brain Struct Funct* 221 (1):473–85. doi: 10.1007/s00429-014-0919-1.

Charman, T., J. Swettenham, S. Baron-Cohen, A. Cox, G. Baird, and A. Drew. 1997. Infants with autism: An investigation of empathy, pretend play, joint attention, and imitation. *Dev Psychol* 33 (5):781–9.

Chester, V. L., and M. Calhoun. 2012. Gait symmetry in children with autism. *Autism Res Treat* 2012:576478. doi: 10.1155/2012/576478.

Cocquyt, M., M. Y. Mommaerts, H. Dewart, and I. Zink. 2015. Measuring pragmatic skills: Early detection of infants at risk for communication problems. *Int J Lang Commun Disord* 50 (5):646–58. doi: 10.1111/1460-6984.12167.

Condon, W. S. 1996. Sound-film microanalysis: A means for correlating brain and behavior in persons with autism. Presented at Autism Society of America National Conference, Milwaukee, WI, July 19.

Condon, W. S., and L. S. Sander. 1974. Neonate movement is synchronized with adult speech: Interactional participation and language acquisition. *Science* 183 (4120):99–101. doi: 10.1126/science.183.4120.99.

Dawson, G., J. Munson, A. Estes, J. Osterling, J. McPartland, K. Toth, L. Carver, and R. Abbott. 2002. Neurocognitive function and joint attention ability in young children with autism spectrum disorder versus developmental delay. *Child Dev* 73 (2):345–58.

de L'Etoile, S. 2000. The history of the undergraduate curriculum in music therapy. *J Music Ther* 37 (1):51–71.

Donnellan, A. M., and M. R. Leary. 1995. *Movement Differences and Diversity in Autism/Mental Retardation: Appreciating and Accommodating People with Communication and Behavior Challenges.* Movin on Series. Madison, WI: DRI Press.

Dziuk, M. A., J. C. Gidley Larson, A. Apostu, E. M. Mahone, M. B. Denckla, and S. H. Mostofsky. 2007. Dyspraxia in autism: Association with motor, social, and communicative deficits. *Dev Med Child Neurol* 49 (10):734–9. doi: 10.1111/j.1469-8749.2007.00734.x.

Esposito, G., P. Venuti, F. Apicella, and F. Muratori. 2011. Analysis of unsupported gait in toddlers with autism. *Brain Dev* 33 (5):367–73. doi: 10.1016/j.braindev.2010.07.006.

Funahashi, Y., C. Karashima, and M. Hoshiyama. 2014. Compensatory postural sway while seated posture during tasks in children with autism spectrum disorder. *Occup Ther Int* 21 (4):166–75. doi: 10.1002/oti.1375.

Gepner, B., D. Mestre, G. Masson, and S. de Schonen. 1995. Postural effects of motion vision in young autistic children. *Neuroreport* 6 (8):1211–4.

Gillberg, I. C., C. Gillberg, and G. Ahlsen. 1994. Autistic behaviour and attention deficits in tuberous sclerosis: A population-based study. *Dev Med Child Neurol* 36 (1):50–6.

Golinkoff, R. M., H. L. Chung, K. Hirsh-Pasek, J. Liu, B. I. Bertenthal, R. Brand, M. J. Maguire, and E. Hennon. 2002. Young children can extend motion verbs to point-light displays. *Dev Psychol* 38 (4):604–14.

Golinkoff, R. M., R. C. Jacquet, K. Hirsh-Pasek, and R. Nandakumar. 1996. Lexical principles may underlie the learning of verbs. *Child Dev* 67 (6):3101–19.

Gopnik, A., A. N. Meltzoff, and P. K. Kuhl. 1999. *The Scientist in the Crib: Minds, Brains, and How Children Learn.* 1st ed. New York: William Morrow & Co.

Gowen, E., and R. C. Miall. 2005. Behavioural aspects of cerebellar function in adults with Asperger syndrome. *Cerebellum* 4 (4):279–89. doi: 10.1080/14734220500355332.

Grandin, T. 1996. *Thinking in Pictures: And Other Reports from My Life with Autism.* 1st ed. New York: Vintage Books.

Grandin, T., and M. Scariano. 1986. *Emergence, Labeled Autistic.* 1st ed. Novato, CA: Arena Press.

Hobson, R. P. 2004. *The Cradle of Thought: Exploring the Origins of Thinking.* Oxford: Oxford University Press.

Fuentes-Biggi, J., M. J. Ferrari-Arroyo, L. Boada-Muñoz, et al. 2006. Guía de buena práctica para el tratamiento de los trastornos del espectro autista. *Rev Neulog* 43:425–38.

Klin, A. 2003. Asperger syndrome: An update. *Rev Bras Psiquiatr* 25 (2):103–9.

Klin, A., D. J. Lin, P. Gorrindo, G. Ramsay, and W. Jones. 2009. Two-year-olds with autism orient to non-social contingencies rather than biological motion. *Nature* 459 (7244):257–61. doi: 10.1038/nature07868.

Klin, A., S. Shultz, and W. Jones. 2015. Social visual engagement in infants and toddlers with autism: Early developmental transitions and a model of pathogenesis. *Neurosci Biobehav Rev* 50:189–203. doi: 10.1016/j.neubiorev.2014.10.006.

Klin, A., W. Jones, R. Schultz, and F. Volkmar. 2003. The enactive mind, or from actions to cognition: Lessons from autism. *Philos Trans R Soc Lond B Biol Sci* 358 (1430):345–60. doi: 10.1098/rstb.2002.1202.

Landa, R., and E. Garrett-Mayer. 2006. Development in infants with autism spectrum disorders: A prospective study. *J Child Psychol Psychiatry* 47 (6):629–38. doi: 10.1111/j.1469-7610.2006.01531.x.

Landa, R. J., K. C. Holman, and E. Garrett-Mayer. 2007. Social and communication development in toddlers with early and later diagnosis of autism spectrum disorders. *Arch Gen Psychiatry* 64 (7):853–64. doi: 10.1001/archpsyc.64.7.853.

Le Clercq, H. 1985. *Autism from Within—A Handbook*. Belgium: Intermediate Books.

Ledbetter-Cho, K., R. Lang, K. Davenport, M. Moore, A. Lee, A. Howell, C. Drew, D. Dawson, M. H. Charlop, T. Falcomata, and M. O'Reilly. 2015. Effects of script training on the peer-to-peer communication of children with autism spectrum disorder. *J Appl Behav Anal* 48 (4):785–99. doi: 10.1002/jaba.240.

Ledbetter-Cho, K., R. Lang, K. Davenport, M. Moore, A. Lee, M. O'Reilly, L. Watkins, and T. Falcomata. 2016. Behavioral skills training to improve the abduction-prevention skills of children with autism. *Behav Anal Pract* 9 (3):266–70. doi: 10.1007/s40617-016-0128-x.

Lee, A., R. Lang, K. Davenport, M. Moore, M. Rispoli, L. van der Meer, A. Carnett, T. Raulston, A. Tostanoski, and C. Chung. 2015. Comparison of therapist implemented and iPad-assisted interventions for children with autism. *Dev Neurorehabil* 18 (2):97–103. doi: 10.3109/17518423.2013.830231.

Lim, B. O., D. O'Sullivan, B. G. Choi, and M. Y. Kim. 2016. Comparative gait analysis between children with autism and age-matched controls: Analysis with temporal-spatial and foot pressure variables. *J Phys Ther Sci* 28 (1):286–92. doi: 10.1589/jpts.28.286.

Manjiviona, J., and M. Prior. 1995. Comparison of Asperger syndrome and high-functioning autistic children on a test of motor impairment. *J Autism Dev Disord* 25 (1):23–39.

Markram, H., T. Rinaldi, and K. Markram. 2007. The intense world syndrome—An alternative hypothesis for autism. *Front Neurosci* 1 (1):77–96. doi: 10.3389/neuro.01.1.1.006.2007.

Masidlover, M. 1979. The Derbyshire language scheme: Remedial teaching for language delayed children. *Child Care Heath Dev* 5 (1):9–16. doi: 10.1111/j.1365-2214.1979.tb00105.x.

McAuliffe, D., A. S. Pillai, A. Tiedemann, S. H. Mostofsky, and J. B. Ewen. 2017. Dyspraxia in ASD: Impaired coordination of movement elements. *Autism Res.* 10 (4):648–52. doi: 10.1002/aur.1693.

Meltzoff, A. N., A. Waismeyer, and A. Gopnik. 2012. Learning about causes from people: Observational causal learning in 24-month-old infants. *Dev Psychol* 48 (5):1215–28. doi: 10.1037/a0027440.

Miller, L. J., and D. A. Fuller. 2006. *Sensational Kids: Hope and Help for Children with Sensory Processing Disorder (SPD)*. New York: G. P. Putnam's Sons.

Miller, M., L. Chukoskie, M. Zinni, J. Townsend, and D. Trauner. 2014. Dyspraxia, motor function and visual-motor integration in autism. *Behav Brain Res* 269:95–102. doi:10.1016/j.bbr.2014.04.011.

Minshew, N. J., K. Sung, B. L. Jones, and J. M. Furman. 2004. Underdevelopment of the postural control system in autism. *Neurology* 63 (11):2056–61.

Molloy, C. A., K. N. Dietrich, and A. Bhattacharya. 2003. Postural stability in children with autism spectrum disorder. *J Autism Dev Disord* 33 (6):643–52.

Morgan, S. B., P. S. Cutrer, J. W. Coplin, and J. R. Rodrigue. 1989. Do autistic children differ from retarded and normal children in Piagetian sensorimotor functioning? *J Child Psychol Psychiatry* 30 (6):857–64.

Mosconi, M. W., and J. A. Sweeney. 2015. Sensorimotor dysfunctions as primary features of autism spectrum disorders. *Sci China Life Sci* 58 (10):1016–23. doi: 10.1007/s11427-015-4894-4.

Nayate, A., B. J. Tonge, J. L. Bradshaw, J. L. McGinley, R. Iansek, and N. J. Rinehart. 2012. Differentiation of high-functioning autism and Asperger's disorder based on neuromotor behaviour. *J Autism Dev Disord* 42 (5):707–17. doi: 10.1007/s10803-011-1299-5.

Nayate, A., J. L. Bradshaw, and N. J. Rinehart. 2005. Autism and Asperger's disorder: Are they movement disorders involving the cerebellum and/or basal ganglia? *Brain Res Bull* 67 (4):327–34 doi: 10.1016/j.brainresbull.2005.07.011.

Ninci, J., R. Lang, K. Davenport, A. Lee, J. Garner, M. Moore, A. Boutot, M. Rispoli, and G. Lancioni. 2013. An analysis of the generalization and maintenance of eye contact taught during play. *Dev Neurorehabil* 16 (5): 301–7. doi: 10.3109/17518423.2012.730557.

Nordoff, P., and C. Robbins. 1971. *Therapy in Music for Handicapped Children*. New ed. London: Gollancz.

Osterling, J., and G. Dawson. 1994. Early recognition of children with autism: A study of first birthday home videotapes. *J Autism Dev Disord* 24 (3):247–57.

Osterling, J. A., G. Dawson, and J. A. Munson. 2002. Early recognition of 1-year-old infants with autism spectrum disorder versus mental retardation. *Dev Psychopathol* 14 (2):239–51.

Parish-Morris, J., E. A. Hennon, K. Hirsh-Pasek, R. M. Golinkoff, and H. Tager-Flusberg. 2007. Children with autism illuminate the role of social intention in word learning. *Child Dev* 78 (4):1265–87. doi: 10.1111/j.1467-8624.2007.01065.x.

Peeters, T. 1997. *Autism: From Theoretical Understanding to Educational Intervention*. San Diego: Singular Publishing Group.

Peeters, T., and C. Gillberg. 1999. *Autism: Medical and Educational Aspects*. 2nd ed. London: Whurr Publishers.

Poch, C., M. I. Garrido, J. M. Igoa, M. Belinchon, I. Garcia-Morales, and P. Campo. 2015. Time-varying effective connectivity during visual object naming as a function of semantic demands. *J Neurosci* 35 (23):8768–76. doi: 10.1523/JNEUROSCI.4888-14.2015.

Poulsen, A. A., L. Desha, J. Ziviani, L. Griffiths, A. Heaslop, A. Khan, and G. M. Leong. 2011. Fundamental movement skills and self-concept of children who are overweight. *Int J Pediatr Obes* 6 (2–2):e464–71. doi: 10.3109/17477166.2011.575143.

Ratey, J. J., T. Grandin, and A. Miller. 1992. Defense behavior and coping in an autistic savant: The story of Temple Grandin, PhD. *Psychiatry* 55 (4):382–91.

Richardson, M. J., S. J. Harrison, R. W. Kallen, A. Walton, B. A. Eiler, E. Saltzman, and R. C. Schmidt. 2015. Self-organized complementary joint action: Behavioral dynamics of an interpersonal collision-avoidance task. *J Exp Psychol Hum Percept Perform* 41 (3):665–79. doi: 10.1037/xhp0000041.

Rinehart, N. J., B. J. Tonge, J. L. Bradshaw, R. Iansek, P. G. Enticott, and J. McGinley. 2006a. Gait function in high-functioning autism and Asperger's disorder: Evidence for basal-ganglia and cerebellar involvement? *Eur Child Adolesc Psychiatry* 15 (5):256–64. doi: 10.1007/s00787-006-0530-y.

Rinehart, N. J., B. J. Tonge, R. Iansek, J. McGinley, A. V. Brereton, P. G. Enticott, and J. L. Bradshaw. 2006b. Gait function in newly diagnosed children with autism: Cerebellar and basal ganglia related motor disorder. *Dev Med Child Neurol* 48 (10):819–24. doi: 10.1017/S0012162206001769.

Riquelme, I., S. M. Hatem, and P. Montoya. 2016. Abnormal pressure pain, touch sensitivity, proprioception, and manual dexterity in children with autism spectrum disorders. *Neural Plast* 2016:1723401. doi: 10.1155/2016/1723401.

Riviére, A. 2011. A history of autism: Conversations with the pioneers. In *A History of Autism*, ed. A. Feinstein, 108. Hoboken, NJ: Wiley-Blackwell.

Rogers, S. J., L. Bennetto, R. McEvoy, and B. F. Pennington. 1996. Imitation and pantomime in high-functioning adolescents with autism spectrum disorders. *Child Dev* 67 (5):2060–73.

Russell, D. M., J. L. Haworth, and C. Martinez-Garza. 2016. Coordination dynamics of (a)symmetrically loaded gait. *Exp Brain Res* 234 (3):867–81. doi: 10.1007/s00221-015-4512-5.

Sarasua, S. M., L. Boccuto, J. L. Sharp, A. Dwivedi, C. F. Chen, J. D. Rollins, R. C. Rogers, K. Phelan, and B. R. DuPont. 2014. Clinical and genomic evaluation of 201 patients with Phelan-McDermid syndrome. *Hum Genet* 133 (7):847–59. doi: 10.1007/s00439-014-1423-7.

Schumacher, J., K. E. Strand, and M. Augustyn. 2015. Apraxia, autism, attention-deficit hyperactivity disorder: Do we have a new spectrum? *J Dev Behav Pediatr* 36 (2):124–6. doi: 10.1097/DBP.0000000000000132.

Schwabe, C. 1976. Theroretical and methodological aspects of music therapy in children with special reference to international developmental tendencies [in German]. *Psychiatr Neurol Med Psychol (Leipz)* 28 (5):290–7.

Shetreat-Klein, M., S. Shinnar, and I. Rapin. 2014. Abnormalities of joint mobility and gait in children with autism spectrum disorders. *Brain Dev* 36 (2):91–6. doi: 10.1016/j.braindev.2012.02.005.

Steinman, K. J., S. H. Mostofsky, and M. B. Denckla. 2010. Toward a narrower, more pragmatic view of developmental dyspraxia. *J Child Neurol* 25 (1):71–81. doi: 10.1177/0883073809342591.

Stins, J. F., C. Emck, E. M. de Vries, S. Doop, and P. J. Beek. 2015. Attentional and sensory contributions to postural sway in children with autism spectrum disorder. *Gait Posture* 42 (2):199–203. doi: 10.1016/j.gaitpost.2015.05.010.

Sullivan, M., J. Finelli, A. Marvin, E. Garrett-Mayer, M. Bauman, and R. Landa. 2007. Response to joint attention in toddlers at risk for autism spectrum disorder: A prospective study. *J Autism Dev Disord* 37 (1): 37–48. doi: 10.1007/s10803-006-0335-3.

Szatmari, P., L. Tuff, M. A. Finlayson, and G. Bartolucci. 1990. Asperger's syndrome and autism: Neurocognitive aspects. *J Am Acad Child Adolesc Psychiatry* 29 (1):130–6.

Tager-Flusberg, H. 1999. A psychological approach to understanding the social and language impairments in autism. *Int Rev Psychiatry* 11 (4):325–34. doi: 10.1080/09540269974203.

Tager-Flusberg, H., and J. Cooper. 1999. Present and future possibilities for defining a phenotype for specific language impairment. *J Speech Lang Hear Res* 42 (5):1275–8.

Thaut, M. H. 2005. The future of music in therapy and medicine. *Ann N Y Acad Sci* 1060:303–8. doi: 10.1196/annals.1360.023.

Thaut, M. H. 2015. The discovery of human auditory-motor entrainment and its role in the development of neurologic music therapy. *Prog Brain Res* 217:253–66. doi: 10.1016/bs.pbr.2014.11.030.

Thaut, M. H., G. C. McIntosh, and V. Hoemberg. 2014. Neurobiological foundations of neurologic music therapy: Rhythmic entrainment and the motor system. *Front Psychol* 5:1185. doi: 10.3389/fpsyg.2014.01185.

Thompson, A., D. Murphy, F. Dell'Acqua, C. Ecker, G. McAlonan, H. Howells, S. Baron-Cohen, M. C. Lai, M. V. Lombardo, MRC Aims Consortium, and C. Marco. 2017. Impaired communication between the motor and somatosensory homunculus is associated with poor manual dexterity in autism spectrum disorder. *Biol Psychiatry* 81 (3):211–9. doi: 10.1016/j.biopsych.2016.06.020.

Torres, E. B., J. Nguyen, S. Mistry, C. Whyatt, V. Kalampratsidou, and A. Kolevzon. 2016. Characterization of the statistical signatures of micro-movements underlying natural gait patterns in children with Phelan McDermid syndrome: Towards precision-phenotyping of behavior in ASD. *Front Integr Neurosci* 10: 22. doi: 10.3389/fnint.2016.00022.

Torres, E. B., and K. Denisova. 2016. Motor noise is rich signal in autism research and pharmacological treatments. *Sci Rep* 6:37422.

Torres, E. B., M. Brincker, R. W. Isenhower, P. Yanovich, K. A. Stigler, J. I. Nurnberger, D. N. Metaxas, and J. V. Jose. 2013. Autism: The micro-movement perspective. *Front Integr Neurosci* 7:32. doi: 10.3389/fnint.2013.00032.

Ulrich, D. A. 1985. Test of gross motor development. Austin, TX: PRO-ED.

Varlet, M., R. C. Schmidt, and M. J. Richardson. 2016. Influence of internal and external noise on spontaneous visuomotor synchronization. *J Mot Behav* 48 (2):122–31. doi: 10.1080/00222895.2015.1050548.

Volkmar, F., K. Chawarska, and A. Klin. 2005. Autism in infancy and early childhood. *Annu Rev Psychol* 56: 315–36. doi: 10.1146/annurev.psych.56.091103.070159.

Weimer, A. K., A. M. Schatz, A. Lincoln, A. O. Ballantyne, and D. A. Trauner. 2001. "Motor" impairment in Asperger syndrome: Evidence for a deficit in proprioception. *J Dev Behav Pediatr* 22 (2):92–101.

Weisberg, D. S., K. Hirsh-Pasek, and R. M. Golinkoff. 2013. Embracing complexity: Rethinking the relation between play and learning: Comment on Lillard et al. (2013). *Psychol Bull* 139 (1):35–9. doi: 10.1037/a0030077.

Weisberg, D. S., K. Hirsh-Pasek, R. M. Golinkoff, and B. D. McCandliss. 2014. Mise en place: Setting the stage for thought and action. *Trends Cogn Sci* 18 (6):276–8. doi: 10.1016/j.tics.2014.02.012.

Werner, E., G. Dawson, J. Munson, and J. Osterling. 2005. Variation in early developmental course in autism and its relation with behavioral outcome at 3–4 years of age. *J Autism Dev Disord* 35 (3):337–50.

Whyatt, C., and C. Craig. 2013. Sensory-motor problems in autism. *Front Integr Neurosci* 7:51. doi: 10.3389/fnint.2013.00051.

Whyatt, C. P., and C. M. Craig. 2012. Motor skills in children aged 7–10 years, diagnosed with autism spectrum disorder. *J Autism Dev Disord* 42 (9):1799–809. doi: 10.1007/s10803-011-1421-8.

Williams, J. H., A. Whiten, and T. Singh. 2004. A systematic review of action imitation in autistic spectrum disorder. *J Autism Dev Disord* 34 (3):285–99.

Yirmiya, N., I. Gamliel, T. Pilowsky, R. Feldman, S. Baron-Cohen, and M. Sigman. 2006. The development of siblings of children with autism at 4 and 14 months: Social engagement, communication, and cognition. *J Child Psychol Psychiatry* 47 (5):511–23. doi: 10.1111/j.1469-7610.2005.01528.x.

Yoder, P., W. L. Stone, T. Walden, and E. Malesa. 2009. Predicting social impairment and ASD diagnosis in younger siblings of children with autism spectrum disorder. *J Autism Dev Disord* 39 (10):1381–91. doi: 10.1007/s10803-009-0753-0.

18 Autism Sports and Educational Model for Inclusion (ASEMI)*

Marcelo Biasatti and Maximiliano Lombardo†

CONTENTS

Our Beginnings ... 271
Birth of AMYDI ... 273
Introduction to the Model ... 273
Structured Nature of Motoric Situations and Contexts ... 275
Combination of AMYDI with Other Existing Models ... 275
Interdisciplinary Team and Family Role ... 276
Stages of AMYDI ... 277
Stage 1: Development of Structured Sensory-Perceptive-Motor Abilities ... 277
Stage 2: Development of Semistructured Motor Activities ... 278
Stage 3: Development of Real Motor Activities ... 278
Stage 4: Playful Motor Inclusion ... 278
Main Objectives of AMYDI ... 279
Where to Apply AMYDI ... 279
Who Can Use the AMYDI Model? ... 279
References ... 280

This chapter provides a description of a physical education program implemented in Buenos Aires, Argentina. This program, specifically tailored for individuals with a diagnosis of autism spectrum disorders, builds bodily skills to first learn to sense the body through movements at the individual level, and then prepare the body for dyadic interactions at the clinic and the home. Through practice and evaluation of experts from an interdisciplinary team, we take the person through a step-by-step journey to find his or her way to social exchange outside the confines of the clinic or the home. We suggest that this step-by-step program, which is so successful in Argentina, could be of use to the schools and homes of the United States, where through team sports and socially oriented games the families, teachers, and children could learn to communicate with and be welcomed by their social medium.

OUR BEGINNINGS

In the years 2006–2007, several medical institutions in Buenos Aires, Argentina, launched interdisciplinary programs to begin the path toward providing a more holistic approach to autism spectrum disorder (ASD) interventions. Most notably, the Hospital Italiano formed a team led by Dr. Pallia and Dr. Baetti with a program that included physical exercise as part of a larger model for intervention in ASD. The goal was to strengthen different areas of mind–body integration (see Chapter 17) for a more inclusive approach that benefited the child, but also helped those caring for the child to

* In Spanish ASEMI would become AMYDI - and as such this will be referred to throughout.
† Translated from Spanish by E. B. Torres.

become the bridge between the child and society at large. This supportive network included the parents, caregivers, and schoolteachers, all of whom received guidance on how to deal with the needs of a child with ASD. One question posed by this team was how could society be made aware of complex issues facing children with ASD—issues such as motor difficulties?

Sports are something that anyone can relate to. The Argentinean society is very sports oriented, and as such, Buenos Aires has equipment that encourages people to exercise located throughout the city (Figure 18.1). Indeed, there is a culture of physical education in place that could help us advance these ideas in ASD. After all, ASD is defined in terms of social interaction deficits. Why not redefine it in terms of social inclusion? And then work toward that goal using interactive sports?

Since we are known to the hospital personnel as experts in the area of physical education, the newly formed medical team requested our intervention and asked if we were interested in this challenging project. Without hesitation, our answer was yes, and so we began a new path of learning about ASD, motility issues, and remediation strategies.

We reasoned that physical education provided a framework amenable to developing a step-by-step method to ultimately achieve inclusion of individuals with ASD within society. Our plan was to start with individualized sports practice for each individual, then gradually build skills toward interactions in dyads, and finally, include interactions in social groups. The playful aspects of the framework made it fun for the children, embedding the treatment within the context of a game rather than a therapy. Importantly, the structure of the exercises provided a controlled context to help the child become acquainted with his or her own bodily sensations and, as such, help the child begin the process of learning how to regularize them and better control them, eventually preparing the child for social exchange.

To our dismay, we found nothing related to this the matter in the literature of ASD. Interventions in ASD were primarily designed with specific goals in mind that did not include movements, their sensations, or any other motor aspects related to matters of coordination and control—so necessary to scaffold social behaviors. Indeed, although social behaviors are the core issue defining ASD, there had been no consideration as to how to connect physical exercise to social exchange. In that sense, we had to start from scratch and begin filling this void by developing a brand new program specifically tailored to the physical and sensorial needs of a child with ASD.

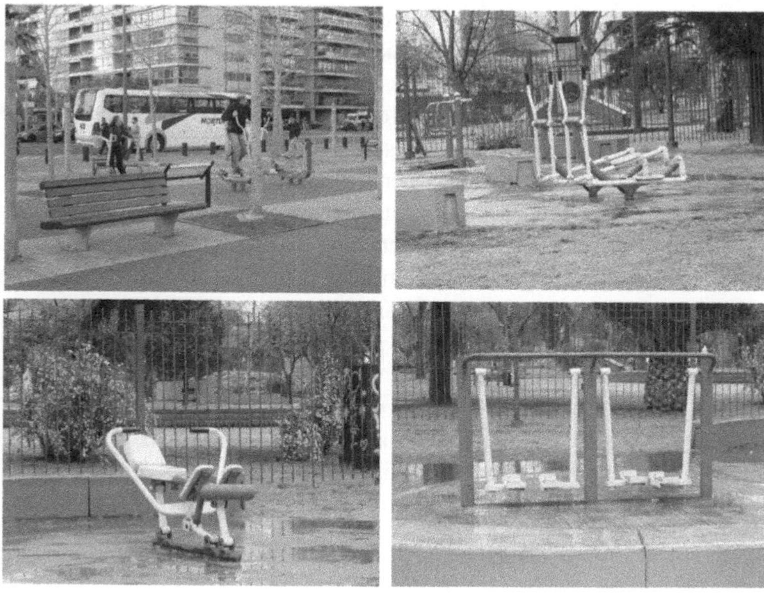

FIGURE 18.1 Buenos Aires is a sports-oriented city. Throughout the city, there are various places where people exercise in the open, perhaps while waiting for the bus, or in transit from work.

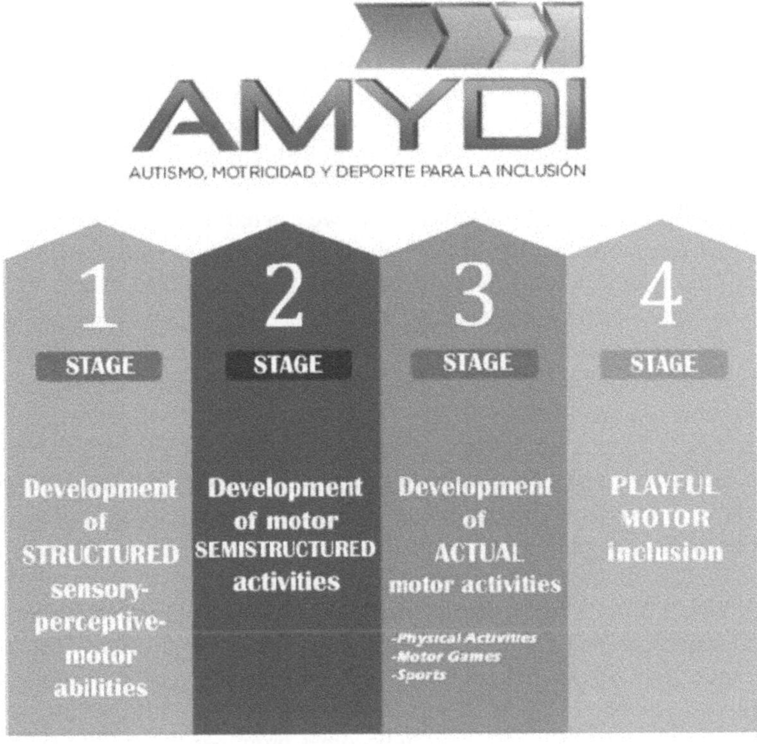

FIGURE 18.2 The AMYDI model has four well-defined stages, with the ultimate goal of social inclusion.

BIRTH OF AMYDI

We designed and launched our initial program, Autismo, Motricidad Y Deporte para la Inclusion (AMYDI) (Figure 18.2) at the Center for Pediatrics Mental Health of the Hospital Italiano de Buenos Aires, Argentina. Our program was part of a holistic approach to ASD that included music therapy, psychotherapy, psychopedagogy working with parents and teachers, and speech therapists, among other aspects of the overall child's development.

Tailoring our program in physical education to ASD has been very challenging, but by now, we understand well the needs of the children in the spectrum, the needs of their parents and teachers, and the general need for an individualized approach ultimately conducive of fruitful social exchange. The support we have received from the child psychiatric wards of the Hospital Italiano de Buenos Aires has been outstanding, and we owe a great deal of our success to the cohesive, cooperative environment that we encountered in the team of doctors and therapists that contacted us and trusted our judgment in the first place. Today the program is fully functioning beyond the confines of the clinical settings. It is functioning in the homes and schools of many Argentinian children with ASD.

INTRODUCTION TO THE MODEL

The main premise of the model is to use sports as the means to create and promote an environment of mutual cooperation between the child and others surrounding him or her. We start by admitting that the body sensation and motoric features of the child with ASD are fundamentally different than those from other children. Yet, as any human infant or child, the need for social contact and playful exchange can be evoked and used to the benefit of the child. One simply has to go about it along a different path and understand that this path is unique to each child. In this sense, there is an exploratory phase of mutual discovery in our model that involves not only a search for the child's preferences and predispositions to learn a given sport-physical routine, but also the possible ways in which this path is less arduous for the person teaching the child.

The main feature of sports-based teachings is that we can define specific goals and develop strategies to accomplish them together. As we teach the child a certain routine, the child also teaches us about the needs of his or her body and mind. Physical education is in this sense an excellent medium to experiment, test, and confirm hypotheses on many aspects of social exchange. We can use this context to build reciprocity, strengthen trust, and more generally, create important bonds that help us succeed as a dyad first and then later as a social group. Inclusion in society naturally falls out of this orderly schema (Figure 18.3).

Physical education is a practice of intervention to educate through movement. All proposals within this intervention must have a playful content that encourages the child to want to participate or to repeat motor actions. This playful, engaging component is based on the three areas of human behavior highlighted in Figure 18.3: cognitive area, socioaffective area, and psychomotor area. Together, they stimulate the well-balanced integral development of the child.

The cognitive area is stimulated through decision making, by helping the child develop the ability to anticipate consequences and solve motor problems. The socioaffective area helps the child recognize differences between teammates and opponents, increases self-esteem for the work done and the goals attained, and naturally leads the child to overcome his or her own limitations to accomplish such goals. The psychomotor area steadily becomes prominent, as movement is the means by which the individual is taught to solve situations more effectively.

In Torres's words and following the theme of the book, movements and their sensation are the "invisible glue" bringing these three areas together because of the omnipresence of motions in everything we do, even when the body is seemingly at rest.

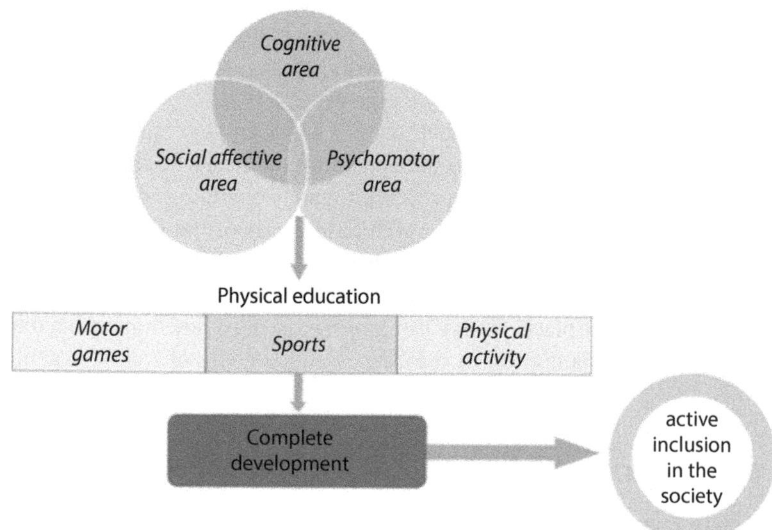

FIGURE 18.3 Three important areas the AMYDI model integrates using fundamental components of physical education seeking social inclusion as the main and ultimate goal of the program.

STRUCTURED NATURE OF MOTORIC SITUATIONS AND CONTEXTS

Parlebas's work is a source of inspiration here (Parlebas 1986, 2016), as he defined core features of motoric situations during games. In his work, he underscores the fact that every motoric situation or encounter raises the need for communication between two participants, or among two or more participants, such that one can naturally unveil the structure inherently present in any sports, game, or dyadic interaction. He used the term *psychomotor situations* to describe those situations in which the person alone interacts with the environment, perhaps using objects, but whereby other people are not included. The terms *comotoric interactions*, on the other hand, describe situations where the participants move in an environment where others may also move, but do not necessarily interact with the participant. In contrast, *sociomotor situations* are defined as those that require interactions with others in the social scene.

AMYDI uses these definitions and their structure to design the goals of the session in order to decide the most favorable outcomes for the individual child with ASD. These are considered a function of the child's predispositions and strengths, while being mindful of the child's needs.

COMBINATION OF AMYDI WITH OTHER EXISTING MODELS

AMYDI integrates elements from other models, such as Treatment and Education of Autistic and Communication related handicapped CHildren (TEACCH) and applied behavioral analysis. Each of these models places emphasis on different aspects of behavior that acquire maturity during the various stages of AMYDI. For example, to structure activities, we use basic principles of TEACCH (Cox and Schopler 1993) that facilitate the sensorial organization of the environment surrounding the child.

We use salient visual or auditory cues to help highlight the goals and evoke spontaneous responses without having to explicitly prompt the child all the time. This self-discovery process internally rewards the child and promotes self-esteem. The sensory-driven organization of the environment that TEACCH promotes is combined with the somewhat contrasting principles of ABA. There we use prompting and external reinforcers as needed, to reward the child in other ways that help promote chaining discrete action segments and organizing complex sequences, particularly at the early stages of the AMYDI model.

Two additional important aspects of complex social interactions that the model considers are executive function and social abilities. Executive function is important in deciding what the goal should be every step along the way, how to balance inhibition and facilitation of actions, how to plan ahead according to the consequences of self-generated actions versus the actions generated by others, and how to perform problem solving in the social context where others also move.

We teach the child with ASD how to plan acts, how to sequence various acts when executing each of them, how to weigh the consequences of each act on other impending acts, and how to explore more than one possible outcome to evaluate the consequences and implicitly build an error correction code (Figure 18.4). Social abilities refer to the capacity of the child with ASD to express feelings, wishes, and desires.

Through sports activities, we ensure that the child with ASD can express his or her thoughts and needs through bodily motions (whenever possible) without self-injurious behaviors or behaviors that may hurt others.

Another important aspect of the model is the combination and balancing of coordinating and conditioning capabilities. The former are related to the natural combination of synergies the body in motion produces when it is well coordinated. The learning of a sports routine is conducive of such coordination. The latter are related to conditional actions, actions that depend on others to be completed. These help the child become aware of the actions of others in relation to his or hers and of their potential consequences in the social context. In this sense, the balance of these aspects of playful sports contributes to the overall development of sensory-motor perception.* This is a fundamental premise of the AMYDI model.

* See also Juan Manuel Renda, "Fisiología de la Actividad Física," conceptos básicos y guía de estudio, Editorial UMET, Buenos Aires, 2015.

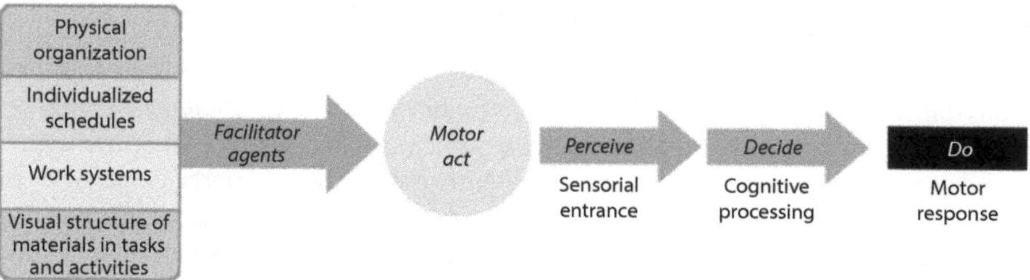

FIGURE 18.4 Schematics of AMYDI elements. Multidisiciplinary approach where all parties collaborate and interact to strengthen the child's sensorial and motoric capabilities for social exchange.

INTERDISCIPLINARY TEAM AND FAMILY ROLE

AMYDI is an interdisciplinary effort that combines the physical education required to build sports abilities and step-by-step social abilities with other forms of therapy by scaffolding them. As mentioned, these include music therapy, phonoaudiology, speech therapy, and elements of school education from educational psychology. Each expert in the team coordinates with the physical education teacher to plan the sessions in advance, to tailor the session to the individual child's needs. Figure 18.5 provides a schematic representation of these interactions aimed at increasing the chances of inclusion of the child with ASD into society at large.

Parents are also engaged in the AMYDI model, as they play a fundamental supporting role in the child's life and are often the only link between the child and the external world. The family is the main source of information to alert the AMYDI faculty of the child's initial predispositions and needs. Their input is critical to developing an appropriate plan of action that combines all areas of the therapy while taking advantage of the child's strengths. The child's strengths provide the entry point into the ASD restricted set of interests, and that entry point opens a window into the child's hidden and latent abilities. The parents are therefore a very important element to the success of the program.

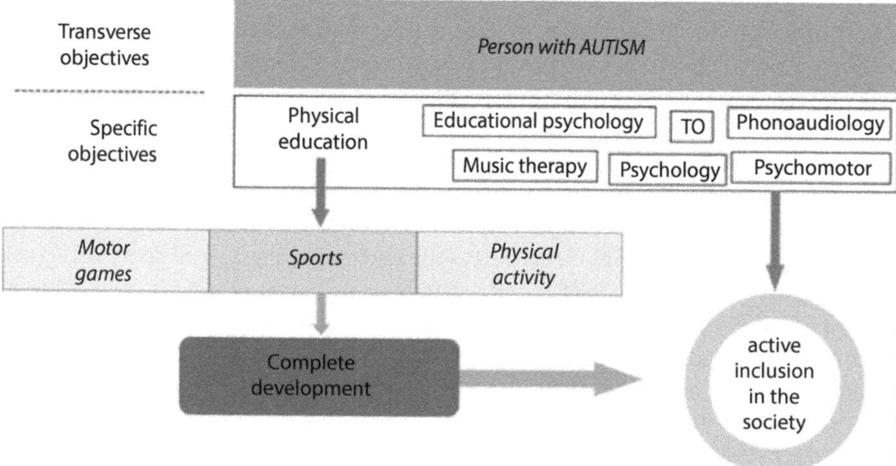

FIGURE 18.5 The common ultimate goal of active inclusion in society at large is preceded by step-by-step subgoals that gradually build the foundation for social exchange.

STAGES OF AMYDI

Stage 1: Development of Structured Sensory-Perceptive-Motor Abilities

In Stage 1 of AMYDI (Figure 18.2), the motoric tasks that AMYDI presents the child with are well defined with concrete goals that facilitate his or her achievement. They promote the organization of the child's body, the enhancement of motor sensing, and the ability to problem-solve. The situations that we evoke in this first stage elicit attention, evoke eye contact, and lead to self-regulation of the behavior. We use various exercises to stimulate the motor circuits across the body, help the child become acquainted with his or her body, and develop flexibility and physical strength during this process.* Figure 18.6 provides a schematic of the order we follow, along with examples of exercises that follow the TEACCH ideas of enhancing the salience of visual cues to evoke goals and facilitate their rapid identification during the play-alone time (Schopler et al. 1979). For example, in Figure 18.5 we visually enhance the salience of the hands contour so the child can better find the support he or she needs to guide the exercise. During this stage, there are times when the faculty assists the child and times when the dyadic exchange is promoted and enabled through goal-directed games. Figure 18.6 provides examples of interactions during this first stage.

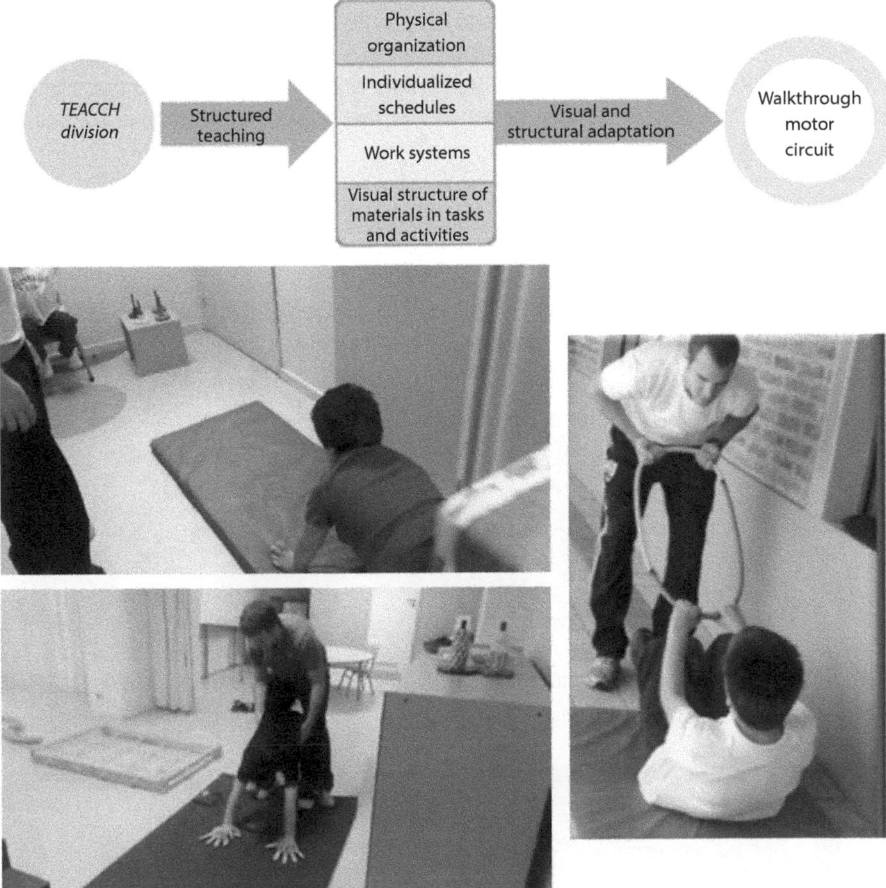

FIGURE 18.6 Stage 1: Well-structured games with sensory salience to help define goals in obvious ways. Exploring the motor circuitry step-by-step helps the child enhance bodily sensations from motions.

* See also Hans Dassel and Herbert Haag, "El circuit-training en la escuela," Editorial Kapeluz, Buenos Aires, 1975.

Stage 2: Development of Semistructured Motor Activities

Children who pass or do not require Stage 1 of the program initiate the path toward more open-ended situations in Stage 2. These involve playing in activities that have clear rules but are implemented within less structured environments when the children can begin to share their peripersonal space with others. The tasks during this stage promote self-esteem in the children. They habilitate and stimulate the child's abilities to self-discover rules of the game in a less structured way. He or she learns how to coordinate interactions with other children, and more generally self-discover the game's rules and organization. Here basic social abilities begin to develop, and the child gains confidence that he or she can indeed interact with others in the social scene. Figure 18.7 provides examples of such semistructured activities in different environments.

Stage 3: Development of Real Motor Activities

This stage is characterized by situations that closely resemble real motoric games and traditional games, including those that require cooperative exchange, turn taking, and more generally, sports tasks with more complex rules. The role of the faculty is to identify the strength of the child and his or her predisposition for a particular type of sport. Once this is determined, the activities conducive to a specific sport type are combined, and eventually a sport is used as a means to teach the child to identify, learn, and respect the rules of the game. The faculty works with the child to teach him or her how to interact with other children while following the rules. In this process, the child learns the spatiotemporal constraints of the game, and this helps him or her extend those to the highly dynamic social scene. Figure 18.8 provides examples of games that require learning and abiding by certain rules when interacting within a dyad or in a larger group.

Stage 4: Playful Motor Inclusion

The last stage of the program is the inclusion of the child with ASD into society at large through games and sports. Here the faculty searches for ways to generalize the sport rules the child learned step-by-step in stages 1–3 into wider societal situations. For instance, the child with ASD is

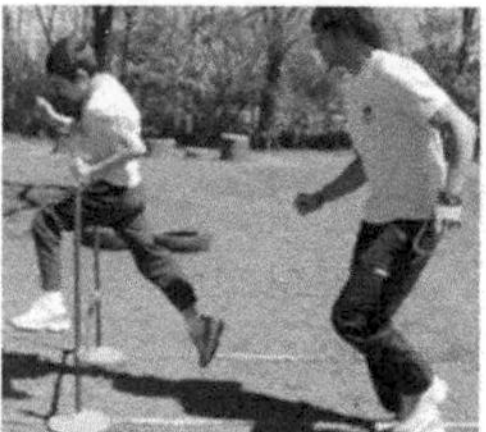
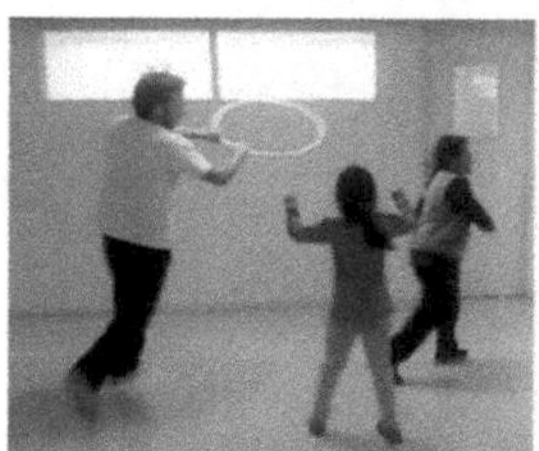
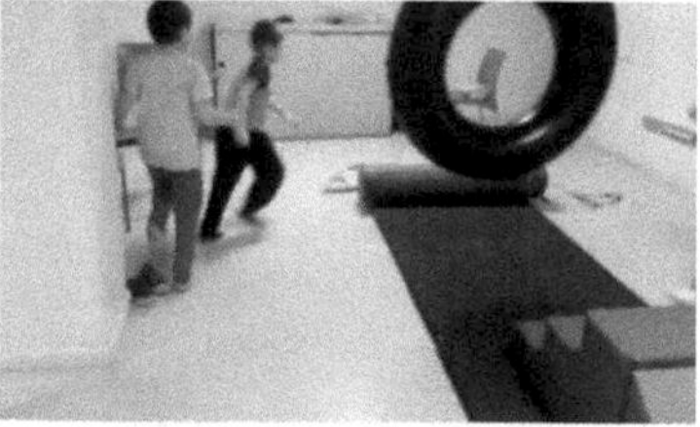

FIGURE 18.7 Stage 2: Semistructured games aiming at approaching real social situations.

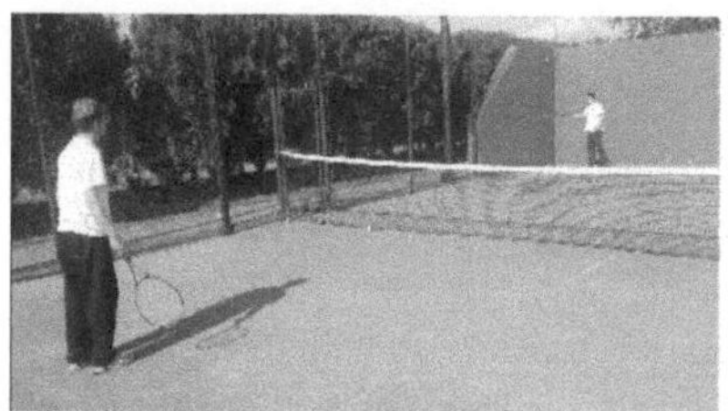
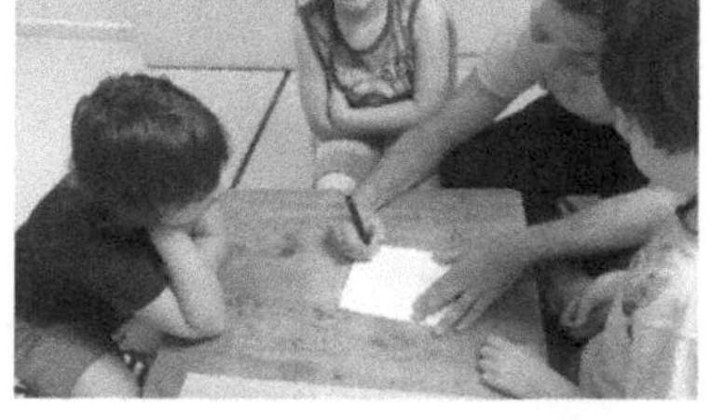

FIGURE 18.8 Stage 3: Real games with well-defined rules for a dyad or a group.

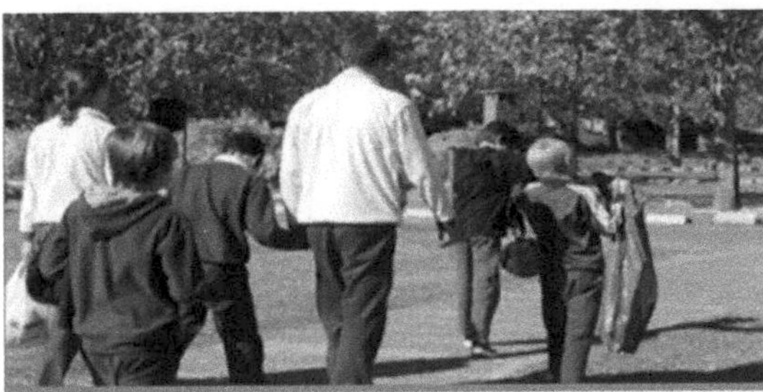
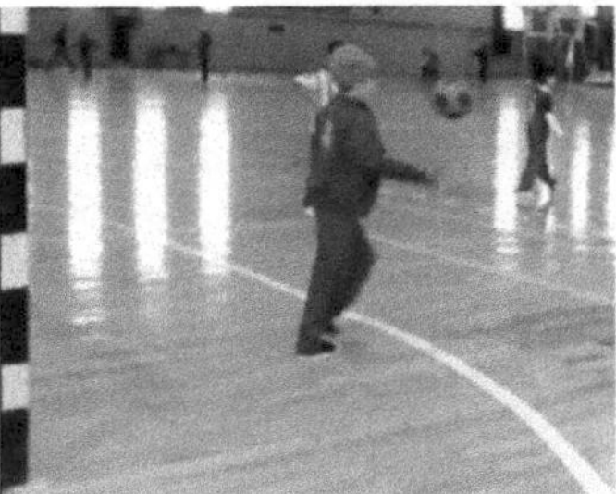

FIGURE 18.9 Stage 4: Real games in public places within novel social situations.

mainstreamed into sports facilities where other children play—these include public swimming facilities, track and field facilities, and basketball and volleyball courts. These facilities are public, and as such, the child with ASD may not necessarily know them at first. The idea is to prepare the child with ASD to face this type of uncertain social situation and facilitate the new exchange through the sports and game strategies that he or she has already learned (Figure 18.9).

Main Objectives of AMYDI

1. Provide a solid theoretical basis for the benefits of physical activity and motor and sport play in the development of various skills for people with ASD to facilitate opportunities for their active participation in society
2. Organize and collaborate toward each of the planning sessions
3. Identify each proposed activity as an achievable goal, and identify the activity that provides meaningful opportunities for inclusion
4. Identify each stage of the model to propose appropriate activities so that the teacher or therapist knows the level at which the child is and where the program should go from there

Where to Apply AMYDI

This AMYDI model can be used in all possible places where you can work through movement.

1. Clinics
2. Special needs schools
3. Hospitals
4. Foundations where children with ASD attend
5. Sports clubs
6. Schools
7. Public clubs, open areas, parks, and public places in society at large

Who Can Use the AMYDI Model?

While the AMYDI model was created by physical education teachers and expects the instructor to have basic knowledge of aspects of motor learning, maturation, and development, AMYDI is designed for interdisciplinary teamwork. Someone trained in AMYDI (even when lacking a degree in physical education) can carry out the four stages of the model, as its creators have drawn from other preexisting models and integrated into AMYDI what they consider essential to facilitate the path toward inclusion. Interdisciplinary work achieves the best results, as cooperation across different fields of expertise is at the core of the AMYDI principles and ensures the success of the program toward inclusion.

REFERENCES

Cox, R. D., and E. Schopler. 1993. Aggression and self-injurious behaviors in persons with autism—The TEACCH (Treatment and Education of Autistic and related Communications Handicapped Children) approach. *Acta Paedopsychiatr* 56 (2):85–90.

Parlebas, P. 1986. *Eléments de sociologie du sport: Sociologies.* 1st ed. Paris: Presses universitaires de France.

Parlebas, P. 2016. *Jeux traditionnels, sports et patrimoine culturel: cultures et éducation*. Paris: L'Harmattan.

Schopler, E., G. B. Mesibov, and University of North Carolina at Chapel Hill, Department of Psychiatry, Division TEACCH. 1979. *Individualized Assessment and Treatment for Autistic and Developmentally Disabled Children*. Baltimore: University Park Press.

19 Reframing Autism Spectrum Disorder for Teachers

An Interdisciplinary Task

Corinne G. Catalano

CONTENTS

Teacher Beliefs Matter 281
Empathy: Understanding the Child's Perspective 283
Teachers Want to Understand 284
Reframing Beliefs 284
References 285

In my roles of educational consultant and teacher educator, I am often asked if a student is doing something like rocking because he has autism. Others ask if a student's task avoidance is due to autism and share that they have been told by other professionals that children with autism are not intrinsically motivated. If we are going to change education for students with autism spectrum disorder, we must question teachers' beliefs and the meanings they place on differences they see in these students. Likewise, we must be concerned with how these interpretations impact how students are educated (Baglieri et al. 2011; Cochran-Smith and Dudley-Marling 2012).

TEACHER BELIEFS MATTER

The research in the field of teacher education reveals that teachers' beliefs serve as filters for the interpretation of information and experience, frames for defining problems or tasks, and guides for action and practice (Feiman-Nemser 1986; Fenstermacher 1978; Fives and Buehl 2012; Pajares 1992). Teachers often hold negative beliefs about students who differ from the mainstream norm by virtue of their race, ethnicity, social class, language, and ability (Ford et al. 2001; Langer et al. 2010; Milner 2005; Reeves 2006; Smith and Smith 2000). Therefore, the *beliefs* held by—or, at least, articulated by—special education teachers and general education teachers about students with autism spectrum disorder (ASD) and their education merit close examination. This focus is particularly compelling given that students with ASD are defined by the medical profession as those with persistent "deficits" in social communication and social interactions, as well as "abnormal" or unusual restricted, repetitive patterns of behaviors, interests, or activities (APA 2013). Because there is evidence that teachers' deficit views of students can jeopardize those students' learning opportunities (Irvine 1990; Milner 2005), the deficit-oriented definition used to identify students with ASD could have profoundly negative consequences for their learning.

As a mental health practitioner, educational consultant, inclusion advocate, researcher, teacher educator, parent of a child with a disability, and aunt of a child with ASD, I have had many different experiences that relate to autism. In this chapter, I share a few of these experiences and discuss the need for reframing teachers' beliefs about this wide spectrum of autism, as well as ideas for integrating research from a wide spectrum of disciplines.

When I first started in the field of special education, I had no idea that I would be involved in promoting change in our understanding of individuals with ASD. I received my master's degree in educational psychology and my certification as a school psychologist and was offered the opportunity to work part-time at a state university's lab school. This demonstration program, housed in a very small residence, was a very unique place. Twelve children with special needs between the ages of 3 and 8 were sent by their school districts to receive special education services in an out-of-district, self-contained setting. Many of these students had been diagnosed with autism. What made this place so special was that it was different from most out-of-district placements that were using behavioral interventions to "educate" children with pervasive developmental delays or autism. Teachers, therapists, and administrators regarded children's challenging behaviors as secondary to underlying, internal, developmental, biological, and relational processes, rather than as the primary focus of intervention (Costa and Witten 2009). This school was following an educational philosophy grounded in social constructivism. The children and the staff learned through their interactions with each other. Special educators, speech and language therapists, occupational therapists, and mental health professionals (myself included), worked side by side learning about the children from each other and co-constructing intervention plans based on each child's individual needs.

The woman who was the director of this program was very committed to social justice and access to high-quality education for all children. She challenged me in my role as a school psychologist to keep learning about child development and dyadic work with parents and children. She constantly made me defend what I thought I knew. Together, she and I began to explore the possibility of inclusive educational settings for several of the children in the program. It was through this exploration that I encountered my impetus for promoting change in the way teachers and school administrators viewed children diagnosed with ASD.

Jimmy, a 5½-year-old boy with autism, would soon be transitioning to kindergarten. This nonverbal child with a hyperreactive sensory system would be leaving our self-contained university-based preschool special education program and heading back to his home school district. For about a year, Jimmy had been spending part of his week in a private general education preschool classroom with the support of our staff. This opportunity to learn alongside his typically developing peers enhanced his engagement and play skills. Buoyed by the power of inclusion, Jimmy's parents were strong proponents of his inclusion in a general education kindergarten classroom. The staff in the district knew Jimmy's diagnosis and had observed him squeezing his arms and making loud "eee" sounds frequently throughout the day. They knew Jimmy as a child with autism, and they did not agree with the placement in a general education kindergarten classroom.

This pushback about including Jimmy is understandable when you examine the international research literature on teachers' beliefs about including students diagnosed with autism. Teachers believe that students with autism require the most significant accommodations and are substantially more difficult to include in general education classes than students with other disabilities (Cook 2001; Sansosti and Sansosti 2012; Stoiber et al. 1998). The literature also reveals that general education teachers—both preservice (Barned et al. 2011; Busby et al. 2012; Doody and Connor 2012) and in-service (Cook 2001; Humphrey and Symes 2013; Lindsay et al. 2013; Stoiber et al. 1998; Teffs and Whitbread 2009)—believe they lack adequate understanding of students with autism. Finally, the two diagnostic criteria for autism (repetitive, unusual behaviors and challenges with social communication) are the characteristics that general education teachers find most challenging (Al-Shammari 2006; Arif et al. 2013; Busby et al. 2012; Drysdale et al. 2007; Helps et al. 1999; Humphrey and Symes 2013; Robertson et al. 2003; Rodríguez et al. 2012; Segall and Campbell 2012; Teffs and Whitbread 2009; Gregor and Campbell 2001).

These types of beliefs impacted the district's decision to support Jimmy's transition to a general education classroom. Our interdisciplinary team, as well as Jimmy's parents, had worked collaboratively for 2 years so that we could understand Jimmy and attune to his internal state rather than his overt behaviors (Schore 2001). Using transdisciplinary practices, we had focused on developing Jimmy's capacity to experience, regulate (manage), and express emotions; form close and secure interpersonal relationships; and explore and master the environment and learn. So how were we going to share all this information? How could we turn this transition into a teachable moment for the staff in the school district?

EMPATHY: UNDERSTANDING THE CHILD'S PERSPECTIVE

At that time, I was enrolled in an infant mental health certificate program and was immersed in reading seminal pieces that used first-person narrative to help the reader gain an enhanced understanding of the child's internal life (Carter et al. 1991; Fraiberg et al. 1975; Stern 1990). With the support of my mentors, I decided to use this strategy to help the district's team attend to the numerous sensory, motor, and affective behaviors in a way that might allow them to think about why Jimmy was or was not doing something, or how he might be feeling when he was not engaged. Couser (2010) discusses the importance of the use of autobiography by individuals with disabilities and when we were preparing to support Jimmy's transition, I knew that Jimmy's voice would be the most powerful. However, at the time we needed Jimmy's voice, he did not have one. He could not speak and he could not write. He was only 5 years old, and he had such a complex developmental profile that most adults had a difficult time understanding it. Taking the liberty to speak for Jimmy was the only option we had to help him be heard and understood as an individual child rather than an autistic child. A few days before the transition planning meeting, I wrote a profile of Jimmy from his perspective, as I, my teammates, and Jimmy's parents understood it.

> Hello my name is Jimmy and I'm 5 and ½ years old. I can't make too many words to communicate with other people and this is very frustrating for me because I know a lot of things and have ideas about what I want to do. Sometimes I will look at someone, point to an object or nod my head to tell others that I need something or to answer a question. I'm getting better at using pictures and a few words to stand for ideas in my head.
>
> When people ask me questions and I can't respond it makes me feel uncomfortable. Many times I have to grab my arms, squeeze my body and make a loud "eee" sound when I feel like this. I usually need help answering the questions or at least I need a choice of pictures so I can show them my answer.
>
> I feel better when I get to do things with my body like jumping, climbing or crawling before I have to sit down to work or to be part of a group. It makes my body feel calmer and I feel like I am stronger and can do more things with my hands and fingers.
>
> I am most comfortable when things are familiar to me and I know what is going to happen next. For example, I know that after I play in the morning we will have circle time. Then I will wash my hands and sit at the table for snack. Sometimes things change. It really helps when people tell me and show me what will be different. They usually use the picture schedule. When things are really different and nobody tells me ahead of time I get scared and confused. I might cry or fall down or kick. I might even go to the window and look outside. I need to get away from everything that is confusing me. I really don't know what to do or how to tell people how confused I am.
>
> I really love writing my name on things I have made; it shows everyone it is mine. It helps when people remind me to write darker or when someone puts boxes on the paper for each letter. I like letters and I know them all and can even put them in alphabetical order. I can read some words like my classmates' names.
>
> I like being around other kids my age. It is fun to watch what they are doing. Sometimes I even try to copy them but lots of times I can't do that by myself. I want to tell them, "Please understand me and slow down. I am trying really hard and I want to learn."

Jimmy's school district listened. Jimmy was included in a general education kindergarten where his parents used this profile to explain Jimmy to his classmates and their parents. They helped all the new people in Jimmy's life look at his behaviors through a lens of understanding rather than through the lens of autism. Similar to our interdisciplinary team, his new teachers worked hard to understand Jimmy's hyperreactive sensory system and delayed motor planning as the sources of his "unusual" behaviors and limited verbal communication. Over the years, I have used this exercise of writing first-person profiles of young children as a transition tool for schools, as the foundation of a parent workshop series, and as part of my teaching in the field of teacher education (Catalano et al. 2002). I began to learn from teachers and parents that this type of narrative allowed them to deepen their understanding of the child, to gain empathy for the child, and to see beyond the label of ASD.

TEACHERS WANT TO UNDERSTAND

Because the diagnosis of ASD covers such a large spectrum, the diagnostic label cannot possibly provide sufficient information to a teacher about any individual child. According to research in the field of teacher education in the United States and abroad, general and special education teachers—both preservice and in-service—believe that understanding the needs of each student with ASD is essential to successfully teach these students (Able et al. 2015; Barned et al. 2011; Doody and Connor 2012; Lindsay et al. 2013; Lohrmann and Bambara 2006; Teffs and Whitbread 2009). For example, Lindsay et al. (2013) interviewed 13 general and special education teachers in Canada regarding their beliefs about including students with ASD in general education classrooms. Study participants repeatedly stressed the importance of knowing the needs of students with ASD to develop rapport with them and productively address situations in which students were upset or emotionally removed. One participant defined this task most clearly when stating, "If we don't really understand the core problems with the kids, you can't really teach them" (p. 356). Taking a different tack, Teffs and Whitbread (2009) used a web-based survey to investigate teachers' beliefs about teaching students with ASD in general education classrooms. Participants were 96 general education teachers teaching kindergarten through high school in the United States. These teachers reported that they needed to understand the social, behavior, and communication skills of students with ASD to appropriately meet their needs. In a study by Able et al. (2015) in which they conducted focus groups with 34 general and special education in-service elementary, middle, and high school teachers in the United States with experience teaching students with ASD in general education classrooms, the researchers found that the study participants believed they needed to understand the individual characteristics of students with ASD to support their inclusion. They further noted that during the focus groups, "teachers discussed how they were baffled by the range of ASD characteristics and were unclear about how to address individual students' personalities and needs" (p. 50).

Research involving those studying to become teachers revealed that teacher candidates believe that understanding the strengths and challenges of students with ASD is a necessary task to support their inclusion in general education classrooms. For instance, in a case study of a preservice general education teacher engaged in a practicum experience in Ireland, Doody and Connor (2012) reported that the candidate identified the need for knowledge of students with disabilities, including students with ASD, to feel confidence that she could teach these students. Similarly, Barned et al. (2011), who surveyed 15 preservice early childhood general education teachers in the United States about the inclusion of young children diagnosed with ASD, and then conducted interviews with 4 of them, also found that study participants believed general education teachers needed a deep understanding of students with ASD to teach them in inclusive classrooms. In brief, the research shows that both in-service and preservice teachers believe they need to gain a deeper understanding of the children they are being asked to teach. Receiving an individual education plan with a child's diagnosis and potential strategies to control challenging behaviors is not enough. Teachers are asking for more, and the field of teacher education needs to provide this by reframing the way we understand ASD through collaboration with those in the fields of occupational therapy, physical therapy, speech and language therapy, and mental health, as well as neuroscience.

REFRAMING BELIEFS

This need for reframing is theoretically grounded in the work of Stanley Greenspan and Serena Wieder (2009) and more recently part of the Self-Reg™ framework developed by Stuart Shanker (2016).

Shanker and his colleagues in Canada are explaining the neuroscience behind a child's reactive behaviors to teachers and school administrators across the country. Their first step is to engage these professionals in learning more about our body's responses to stress and all the possible causes of stress so that they can reframe what they observe in children. This means that instead of automatically looking at a behavior such as rocking as an "autistic behavior," they are able to wonder about what might be stressing a child. They are able to look at these behaviors through a different lens and identify what might be causing the child to self-sooth by rocking himself or herself. When we view a child's behavior as a "misbehavior," we view the child as being in control of their behavior. However, when we wonder about a child's individual differences rather than just their diagnosis, we begin to see these same behaviors as "stress behaviors." This shift in perspectives or beliefs changes the intervention. Instead of the primary focus being that of reducing the behavior, the focus is on reducing the stressor when possible, and also helping a child learn to find a sense of calm so that his or her brain is available to learn.

Adults with autism who are able to communicate are helping us think differently about young children who struggle with social communication and have repetitive patterns of behavior (Fleischmann 2012; Grandin and Panek 2013). The use of autobiography by individuals with disabilities in teacher preparation and professional development is critical in helping teachers have empathy for their students with a diagnosis of ASD. Empathy is the capacity to understand or feel what another being is experiencing from that being's frame of reference—it is the capacity to place oneself in another's position. Rather than viewing a child's behavior as criteria for a diagnosis or something to extinguish, teachers must be encouraged to wonder about what each behavior tells us about a child's inner life. Those who prepare teachers, as well as those who provide ongoing professional development for educational professionals, must engage teachers in examining research that adds to the complex conversation about autism. Many voices are asking us to inquire within each unique individual and reexamine how we understand autism (Donvan and Zucker 2016; Hamlin 2015; Prizant and Fields-Meyer 2015; Shanker 2016; Silberman 2015; Whitman 2004). It is time for us to listen.

REFERENCES

Able, H., M. A. Sreckovic, T. R. Schultz, J. D. Garwood, and J. Sherman. 2015. Views from the trenches: Teacher and student supports needed for full inclusion of students with ASD. *Teach Educ Spec Educ* 38 (1):44–57.

Al-Shammari, Z. 2006. Special education teachers' attitudes toward autistic students in the autism school in the state of Kuwait: A case study. *J Instruct Psychol* 33 (3):170.

APA (American Psychiatric Association). 2013. *Diagnostic and Statistical Manual of Mental Disorders*. 5th ed. Washington, DC: APA.

Arif, M. M., A. Niazy, B. Hassan, and F. Ahmed. 2013. Awareness of autism in primary school teachers. *Autism Res Treat* 2013:961595.

Baglieri, S., J. W. Valle, D. J. Connor, and D. J. Gallagher. 2011. Disability studies in education: The need for a plurality of perspectives on disability. *Remedial Spec Educ* 32 (4):267–78.

Barned, N. E., N. F. Knapp, and S. Neuharth-Pritchett. 2011. Knowledge and attitudes of early childhood preservice teachers regarding the inclusion of children with autism spectrum disorder. *J Early Child Teach Educ* 32 (4):302–21.

Busby, R., R. Ingram, R. Bowron, J. Oliver, and B. Lyons. 2012. Teaching elementary children with autism: Addressing teacher challenges and preparation needs. *Rural Educ* 33 (2):27–35.

Carter, S. L., J. D. Osofsky, and D. M. Hann. 1991. Speaking for the baby: A therapeutic intervention with adolescent mothers and their infants. *Infant Ment Health J* 12 (4):291–301.

Catalano, C. G., P. R. Hernandez, and P. Wolters. 2002. A child's self-statement: Who am I? *Exceptional Parent* 32 (4):60–5.

Cochran-Smith, M., and C. Dudley-Marling. 2012. Diversity in teacher education and special education: The issues that divide. *J Teach Educ* 63 (4):237–44.

Cook, B. G. 2001. A comparison of teachers' attitudes toward their included students with mild and severe disabilities. *J Spec Educ* 34 (4):203–13.

Costa, G., and M. R. Witten. 2009. Pervasive developmental disorders. In *Evidence Based Practice in Infant and Early Childhood Psychology*, ed. F. Robinson, A. Yasik, and B. Mowder. Hoboken, NJ: John Wiley & Son.

Couser, G. T. 2010. Disability, life narrative, and representation. In *The Disability Studies Reader*, ed. L. J. David. New York: Routledge.

Donvan, J., and C. Zucker. 2016. *In a Different Key: The Story of Autism*. New York: Crown.

Doody, O., and M. O'Connor. 2012. The influence of teacher practice placement on one's beliefs about intellectual disability: A student's reflection. *Support Learn* 27 (3):113–8.

Drysdale, M. T. B., A. Williams, and G. J. Meaney. 2007. Teachers' perceptions of integrating students with behaviour disorders: Challenges and strategies. *Exceptionality Educ Int* 17 (3):35–60.

Feiman-Nemser, S., and R. E. Floden. 1986. The cultures of teaching. In *Handbook of Research on Teaching*, ed. M. C. Wittrock, 505–26. New York: Macmillan.

Fenstermacher, G. D. 1978. 4: A philosophical consideration of recent research on teacher effectiveness. *Rev Res Educ* 6 (1):157–85.

Fives, H., and M. M. Buehl. 2012. Spring cleaning for the "messy" construct of teachers' beliefs: What are they? Which have been examined? What can they tell us. *APA Educ Psychol Handb* 2:471–99.

Fleischmann, A. 2012. *Carly's Voice: Breaking through Autism*. New York: Simon & Schuster.

Ford, D. Y., J. J. Harris III, C. A. Tyson, and M. F. Trotman. 2001. Beyond deficit thinking: Providing access for gifted African American students. *Roeper Rev* 24 (2):52–8.

Fraiberg, S., E. Adelson, and V. Shapiro. 1975. Ghosts in the nursery: A psychoanalytic approach to the problems of impaired infant-mother relationships. *J Am Acad Child Psychiatry* 14 (3):387–421.

Grandin, T., and R. Panek. 2013. *The Autistic Brain: Thinking across the Spectrum*. Boston: Houghton Mifflin Harcourt.

Greenspan, S. I., and S. Wieder. 2009. *Engaging Autism: Using the Floortime Approach to Help Children Relate, Communicate, and Think*. Boston: Da Capo Press.

Gregor, E. M. C., and E. Campbell. 2001. The attitudes of teachers in Scotland to the integration of children with autism into mainstream schools. *Autism* 5 (2):189–207.

Hamlin, T. 2015. *Autism and the Stress Effect: A 4-Step Lifestyle Approach to Transform Your Child's Health, Happiness and Vitality*. London: Jessica Kingsley Publishers.

Helps, S., I. C. Newsom-Davis, and M. Callias. 1999. Autism: The teacher's view. *Autism* 3 (3):287–98.

Humphrey, N., and W. Symes. 2013. Inclusive education for pupils with autistic spectrum disorders in secondary mainstream schools: Teacher attitudes, experience and knowledge. *Int J Inclusive Educ* 17 (1):32–46.

Irvine, J. J. 1990. *Black Students and School Failure: Policies, Practices, and Prescriptions*. New York: Praeger.

Langer, P., K. Escamilla, and L. Aragon. 2010. The University of Colorado Puebla experience: A study in changing attitudes and teaching strategies. *Biling Res J* 33 (1):82–94.

Lindsay, S., M. Proulx, N. Thomson, and H. Scott. 2013. Educators' challenges of including children with autism spectrum disorder in mainstream classrooms. *Int J Disabil Dev Educ* 60 (4):347–62.

Lohrmann, S., and L. M. Bambara. 2006. Elementary education teachers' beliefs about essential supports needed to successfully include students with developmental disabilities who engage in challenging behaviors. *Res Pract Persons Severe Disabil* 31 (2):157–73.

Milner, H. R. 2005. Stability and change in US prospective teachers' beliefs and decisions about diversity and learning to teach. *Teach Teach Educ* 21 (7):767–86.

Pajares, M. F. 1992. Teachers' beliefs and educational research: Cleaning up a messy construct. *Rev Educ Res* 62 (3):307–32.

Prizant, B. M., and T. Fields-Meyer. 2015. *Uniquely Human: A Different Way of Seeing Autism*. New York: Simon & Schuster.

Reeves, J. R. 2006. Secondary teacher attitudes toward including English-language learners in mainstream classrooms. *J Educ Res* 99 (3):131–43.

Robertson, K., B. Chamberlain, and C. Kasari. 2003. General education teachers' relationships with included students with autism. *J Autism Dev Disord* 33 (2):123–30.

Rodríguez, I. R., D. Saldana, and F. J. Moreno. 2012. Support, inclusion, and special education teachers' attitudes toward the education of students with autism spectrum disorders. *Autism Res Treat* 2012:259468.

Sansosti, J. M., and F. J. Sansosti. 2012. Inclusion for students with high-functioning autism spectrum disorders: Definitions and decision making. *Psychol Schools* 49 (10):917–31.

Schore, A. N. 2001. Effects of a secure attachment relationship on right brain development, affect regulation, and infant mental health. *Infant Ment Health J* 22 (1–2):7–66.

Segall, M. J., and J. M. Campbell. 2012. Factors relating to education professionals' classroom practices for the inclusion of students with autism spectrum disorders. *Res Autism Spectr Disord* 6 (3):1156–67.

Shanker, S. 2016. *Self-Reg: How to Help Your Child (and You) Break the Stress Cycle and Successfully Engage with Life*. London: Penguin.

Silberman, S. 2015. *Neurotribes: The Legacy of Autism and the Future of Neurodiversity*. London: Penguin.

Smith, M. K., and K. E. Smith. 2000. "I believe in inclusion, but …": Regular education early childhood teachers' perceptions of successful inclusion. *J Res Child Educ* 14 (2):161–80.

Stem, D. N. 1990. *Diary of a Baby*. New York: Basic Books.

Stoiber, K. C., M. Gettinger, and D. Goetz. 1998. Exploring factors influencing parents' and early childhood practitioners' beliefs about inclusion. *Early Child Res Q* 13 (1):107–24.

Teffs, E. E., and K. M. Whitbread. 2009. Level of preparation of general education teachers to include students with autism spectrum disorders. *Curr Issues Educ* 12:1–29.

Whitman, T. L. 2004. *The Development of Autism: A Self-Regulatory Perspective*. London: Jessica Kingsley Publishers.

Concluding Remarks to Section IV

Elizabeth B. Torres

As we approach a new era of precision medicine aiming at a personalized assessment and treatment of the patient, interventions to remediate autism spectrum disorder (ASD) will greatly benefit. The methods of practice in the United States are limited when used in isolation, but a comprehensive integrative approach to therapy, one that combines multiple interventions with diverse philosophies and tailors the treatment to the child's longitudinal progression, will be possible with the new methods developed by basic researchers. The new technological advances in wearable sensors and wellness and fitness devices for mobile-health concepts are beginning to be translated for use in neurodevelopmental disorders at large. Owing to the fast rate of growth and stunted development during the early years of life of infants with neurodevelopmental disorders, these new approaches will be critical for the cases that develop ASD. They will provide the types of longitudinally oriented outcome measures that insurance companies currently desire to provide coverage for diversification of therapies in ASD.

At the educational end, it will be necessary to educate teachers and school personnel on the intricacies of the autistic condition and the impact that societal rejection or apathy may have on the developing child. Beyond spotting the risk for ASD early enough to intervene, we must aim for an acceptance of the affected child and a new era that presumes competence and embraces the child and the family. If as a society we work together toward the main goal of supporting the person with ASD and better understanding the physiological underpinnings of this condition, we will be able to better our society at large. Perhaps learning from other cultures and opening our intervention programs to their ideas and diversity will help our endeavor.

Section V

Autism, the Untold Story from the Perspectives of Parents and Self-Advocates

Preface Section V

Caroline Whyatt

The preceding chapters have presented evidence for the role of sensory-motor difficulties in autism spectrum disorders (ASDs), specifically, why movement matters and how we, as an academic, clinical, or public community, can provide support. Through the presentation of novel research methods, theoretical exploration, and finally, a detailed statistical platform grounded on sound mathematical principles, the role of movement has been illustrated in the context of higher-level symptomatology across the ASD spectrum. Yet, this academic stance is arguably removed from the first- and secondhand accounts of sensory and motor difficulties that individuals with ASD face—accounts that are at the core of our scientific endeavor (Donnellan and Leary 1995, 2012; Donnellan et al. 2012; Robledo et al. 2012).

This section aims to give voice to parents, families, and indeed, individuals living with ASD on a daily basis. With moving accounts of the struggles and hurdles faced, these chapters aim to illustrate the pervasive and often debilitating effects of sensory and motor difficulties. First, a parent and advocate within the field provides a brief but welcome digression into the historical perspective of ASD, and contrasts her son's struggles with her own diagnosis of Parkinson's disease. The following five chapters provide the reader with intimate, and often raw, stories of struggle, pain, frustration, and love from five individual families. Juxtaposing individual stories of outstanding achievements with heartbreaking journeys of discovery and struggle, these parents provide a unique insight into daily life and the barriers artificially placed on these families, perhaps unintentionally, from society. Here we hear from families touched by ASD as a primary diagnosis, or children with Phelan-McDermid-Syndrome, a rare genetic disorder, that often also gives rise to the phenotype of ASD. These are the voices of those so often unheard by the academic and scientific communities—but the voices that need, and deserve, to be heard. Chapter 26 provides a researcher perspective of social difficulties faced by children and adults across the ASD spectrum, namely, bullying, while Chapter 27 questions our societal expectations and preconceptions of ASD. Combined, these chapters examine the daily impact of ASD, illustrating the impact of these "secondary" lower-level sensory and motor symptoms that are vehemently ignored by current clinical methods. The impact of societal and clinical pressures placed on the families is explored, and ultimately questioned—culminating in a chorus imploring understanding, love, and ultimately, acceptance.

REFERENCES

Donnellan, A. M., and M. R. Leary. 1995. *Movement Differences and Diversity in Autism/Mental Retardation: Appreciating and Accommodating People with Communication and Behavior Challenges*. Movin on Series. Madison, WI: DRI Press.

Donnellan, A. M., and M. R. Leary. 2012. *Autism: Sensory-Movement Differences and Diversity*. 1st ed. Cambridge, WI: Cambridge Book Review Press.

Donnellan, A. M., D. A. Hill, and M. R. Leary. 2012. Rethinking autism: Implications of sensory and movement differences for understanding and support. *Front Integr Neurosci* 6:124.

Robledo, J., A. M. Donnellan, and K. Strandt-Conroy. 2012. An exploration of sensory and movement differences from the perspective of individuals with autism. *Front Integr Neurosci* 6:107.

20 Seeing Movement
Implications of the Movement Sensing Perspective for Parents

Pat Amos

CONTENTS

Introduction 295
Why Movement Matters 296
Psychoanalysis to Behaviorism: The Paths Diverge 299
Impact of the DSM: A Carefully Curated Collection of Symptoms 302
Evolving Models: Brain-Based or Embodied? 306
The "Autism Quartet": Movement-Based Approaches 310
Variable Performance 311
Complex and Effortful Movement Strategies: Delayed Habituation 314
Marked Similarities to Other Neurological Conditions Involving Movement 317
A Strong Need for Relationship-Based Approaches 319
Conclusion 321
References 322

INTRODUCTION

On the occasion of his high school graduation, in the mid-1990s, I asked my oldest son to pose in his cap and gown for the obligatory out-of-focus parental photo. I knew better than to demand a smile—he staunchly maintains an unrevealing "poker face"—but felt the need for some reassurance that he appreciated the magnitude of his accomplishment. He was, after all, not an ordinary student but a person whose autism has frequently stacked the cards against him. So I gambled on a wide-open question: "On this special day, is there anything you would like to say about your life so far?" There was a long pause as he gazed off into the distance. Was the question too vague or confusing? But then he spoke softly, echoing the refrain from an old rock song, "What a long, strange trip it's been."

And so it was: strange for my son and others like him who describe an "inability to get consistent meaning through any of senses" (Williams 1996, 242) and recall childhoods in which "people were doing things for no reason I could make out" (Young 2011, 76); strange for parents trying to hear their child's voice amid a cacophony of theories, treatments, teaching methods, and marketing; strange for the advocates who chose a "puzzle head" logo for their cause; and strange for those researchers who started with the premise that a person with autism is fundamentally a bizarre collection of deficits awaiting redemption through remediation. This chapter briefly reviews the history of autism from the point of view of parents like myself, and attempts to place within it some of the observations we made as our children grew: observations for which the reigning behavioral, cognitive, and social narrative about autism, as well as the reigning diagnostic manual, could not find a convincing place. I suggest that by focusing on how people with autism interact with and make sense of their environments over time—by "seeing movement"—we can begin to explain those observations in dynamic ways and link them to a number of positive approaches that parents, teachers, and people with autism themselves are finding successful. When society as a whole begins to make more informed choices about how best to support the inclusion and self-determination of individuals with autism and other developmental differences, we will also be seeing movement in a historical sense. Then the lives of people with autism may no longer feel like a long, strange trip.

WHY MOVEMENT MATTERS

I have Parkinson's disease, which is understood to be a "movement disorder." When my son, who has an autism diagnosis, moves in similar ways, he is said to have "autistic behavior." Autistic behavior is considered "both volitional and meaningless; or as communicative acts signaling avoidance of interaction and evidence of diminished cognitive capacity; or as some combination of these, often to be targeted for reduction" (Donnellan et al. 2012, par. 2). My behavior, on the other hand, is said to be quite intelligent and adaptive, to offer evidence of my ability to carry on productively, and no one is expected to appear on my doorstep to enforce a protocol for its reduction. People cut me some slack when I am having difficulty organizing my body and hurrying up, because they "knew me when" and still recognize me as an competent person. My son has always had autism, so no one looks at him and sees a "before" picture; therefore, they often forget to cut him any slack. I also had what is considered a normal period of growing up, in which all the expected developmental milestones were met on time. For my son, development followed a different trajectory for which parents and siblings had no map. As our friend Barbara Moran says of her own autistic development, "My mind gets there in the end; but it takes the scenic route" (Donnellan and Leary 1995, 45).

The term *movement disorder* or, as I prefer, *movement difference* refers to an interference in the efficient, effective use of movement that is not caused by paralysis, weakness, or actual loss of some sensory apparatus (e.g., amputation or blindness) but by difficulties in the *regulation* of movement. The word *difference* is used as a reminder that these regulatory challenges are not necessarily considered problematic by the person who experiences them. They may have adapted effectively, by means that are harmless or even ingenious. They may not even recognize consciously that they have challenges to which their body has adapted, or that others are looking askance at their coping strategies. It is the process of social judgment itself, and the rejection and exclusion it encourages, that creates a feedback loop through which movement differences come to be perceived—by both observers and, in many cases, by the person observed—as disturbing, inexplicable, and even a source of shame.

Movement differences manifest in variable ways that can be hard to predict. Modern neuroscience includes sensory perception in the study of movement because the regulation of movement is inseparable from sensory perception; they are two sides of the same coin. While we tend to think of movement as the result of a one-way directive from the brain, it is also a sensory system in its own right—involving a dynamic, two-way relationship between the peripheral nervous system (PNS) and the brain and central nervous system (CNS). This is a radically different perspective from the long-standing assumption known in physiology as *classic reflex theory*, which held that CNS responses (called *efference*) are entirely explicable in terms of environmental stimuli (known as *afference*). Classic reflex theory took the relationship of afference and efference to be automatic and 1:1, with each perceptual stimulus calling forth its movement counterpart. Complex, higher-order activity was explained as *conditioning*, meaning that repetition through time would establish links that allow an entire sequence or chain of actions to be triggered, producing a reflex. This mechanism became known as "reflex chain theory." However, such simple mechanisms fail to account for our ability to reliably negotiate out surroundings—even at a basic level. For example, when we gaze at the scene before us, our eyes are rapidly moving from point to point. Yet we are spared the dizzying sensation that the scene itself is jumping about: some aspect of our perceptual system is holding it stable. By the middle of the last century, physiologists demonstrated that the existence of a more complicated perceptual process, dubbed *reafference*, could explain our ability to distinguish our own movements from those of the environment (Von Holst and Mittelstaedt 1950).

Reafference, the ongoing process of separating out our body's responses to external stimuli from the external stimuli themselves, allows us to perceive this difference that is crucial to behavior.

The principle of reafference illustrates that we can anticipate, and distinguish, sensory signals that are the result of our own movements. As such, we can perceive our own movement trajectories, our spatial orientation, and build an accurate representation of the external world, and our self-movement in relation it. Reafference creates feedback loops from which the CNS and PNS emerge not as simple input–output machines but as organized, dynamic systems. Indeed, using this feedback loop, we can adjust our behavior, modifying unproductive or dysfunctional links and chains. Without it, our behavior would be nothing but the sum of our reflex chains, totally and immediately under direct environmental control, rendering innovation, spontaneity, and the emergence of adjusted responses to novel goals impossible.

The attractive simplicity of reflex chain theory, however, continued to provide a very comfortable environment for researchers in certain fields. It is on this spot that classic behaviorism pitched its tent and staked its tenacious claim to an interpretation of learning and behavior based solely on external stimuli, and on this spot that modern cognitive psychology and neuroscience passed by as it slept (Thompson 1994). Konrad Lorenz, well-known for his studies of animal and human behavior and a colleague of reafference theorist Von Holst, found it ironic that many behavioral researchers had been lulled into insensate slumber by their own research designs:

> The preconceived opinion that the reflex and the conditioned reflex are the only elements of behavior determined a quite special, scarcely varied kind of experimental setup in which the central nervous system under investigation had no *opportunity* to show that it was capable of anything other than responding to the influence of external stimuli. In this way, it was quite unavoidable that the opinion *necessarily* developed and became consolidated, that the functioning of the central nervous system is restricted to receiving and responding to external stimuli.… The entire phenomenon of *spontaneity*, which is so crucial for the recognition of the *physiological* peculiarity of such a large fraction of all behavior, thus remained concealed from the very research workers who wished to learn about the physiology of behavior. (Lorenz 1996)

The modern movement approach proposes that the lists of behaviors used to define autism and related disabilities may originate not (as the received wisdom would have it) as inexplicable failures to respond appropriately to external stimuli, to be addressed by painstakingly breaking down, rehearsing, and chaining the "correct" actions, but in challenges to reafference. These challenges would cause differences in the neurological regulatory or tracking systems for predicting consequences of all types, and for relaying useful predictions to motor and other output systems. People with significant movement differences are often described as failing to understand cause and effect, but to explain their dilemma as if it represented a deficit in conscious thought processes is to miss the point.

It is crucial to note that these neurological tracking processes largely occur at a nonvolitional level, that is, "automatically" or without the formation of a conscious intention or a need to think through each step. While neural pathways corresponding to these regulatory challenges have been sought and identified in the brain and CNS over the last few decades, recent research has begun to focus productively on the presence of what is called *noise*—that is, random systemic interferences in information flow and transmission in the channels of the PNSs that relay the *signal*, or raw data of experience, to the brain and translate the brain's responses into further movement. This concept can be considered as analogous to your cell phone's signal bars indicating good (high signal and low noise) or bad (low signal and high noise) reception. Similarly, the nervous systems keep track of the signal-to-noise ratios arising from sensory processes, including possible interference from self-generated involuntary motions that are hard to keep under deliberate control.

Recent research has begun to focus productively on a range of movement classes with different degrees of deliberateness, ranging from spontaneous motions occurring largely beneath awareness to purposeful motions under successful control at will (Torres 2011). In the past, spontaneous random variations in motor performance were not considered relevant to the issue of intentional control.

However, contemporary research examines these variations and fluctuations in motor performance as a form of kinesthetic reafference (Torres et al. 2013a)—a way of sensing and mapping the environment through the bodily rhythms. Viewed from this perspective, the transition of spontaneous random fluctuations to well-structured and systematic patterns, the initial noise turns into signal within the system. Considered within the context of the cell phone analogy, this would be similar to going through a period of transient blackout, with high noise and no signal, to then gradually recovering good signal. The communication channels are open again and clear for exchange. Imagine what it would be like if those bars indicated corrupted signals most of the time (Brincker and Torres 2013).

When systems that track the balance between signal and noise are not working reliably, the person may be unable to correctly estimate the path and timing of a stimulus and regulate an efficient, effective response. Skewed estimates of a stimulus that are relayed to the systems regulating sensations may produce underreactions and overreactions in the form of hypo- or hypersensitive hearing, vision, smell, taste, touch, and sometimes extreme overreactions of "fight, flight, or freeze." The vestibular sense (which registers body balance and spatial movement) and proprioceptive sense (which registers body location and position) may operate differently under the stress of information that is distorted or corrupted by random noise. The confusing experiences that result may interfere with the ability to participate in everyday activities and to share them with others. Inaccurate estimates of a stimulus that are relayed to the body's motor system can produce challenges to self-synchrony (self-coordination), movements that undershoot or overshoot their target, as well as interruptions in the coordination of movement involved in typical social interactions (Maurer 1994, 1995, 1996).

Difficulties in establishing or maintaining self-synchrony inevitably play out as challenges to interactional synchrony (coordination with others). The emergence of relationship in human development is often described as a "dance" (Fogel 1993; Stern 1985) because its existence hinges on the crucial ability to establish and operate for predictable periods on a frequency that is in phase with that of prospective partners. The interactions of metaphorical (or real) dance partners must above all be timely; they must simultaneously be engaged in co-creating body maps that reflect a shared territory. The significance of our ability to coordinate our movement with others, from the moment of birth, is profound. In the words of child development and autism researcher Colwyn Trevarthen,

> Most impressively, an alert newborn can draw a sympathetic adult into synchronized negotiations of arbitrary action, which can develop in coming weeks and months into a mastery of the rituals and symbols of a germinal culture, long before any words are learned. (Trevarthen 2011, 121)

This complex synchrony of body language and timing underlying social communication, often referred to as the "dance of relationship" (Fogel 1993; Stern 1985), may become difficult to execute when movement differences obstruct the conversion of "arbitrary action" into shared and meaningful action. When the steps and routines of the dance are limited in this way, the resulting perception of social and communication deficits, and narrow or repetitive activities, can lead to an autism diagnosis.

It is not hard to imagine why individuals with movement differences would be judged as having deficits in communication and social interaction. These are finely tuned systems in which even a small difference in behavior can have an enormous impact. Grinning or frowning at the wrong time, talking out loud when you intended to whisper, jerking away from the hug you so desperately wanted, missing your split-second chance to jump into a conversation, shoving your homework at the teacher when you meant to hand it politely, or taking 10 seconds rather than the expected 2 seconds to respond to a question or comment can give an erroneous impression of a person's abilities and intentions that attracts unhelpful responses and pessimistic self-fulfilling prophecies. When these misperceptions begin early in life, the dance of relationships may be compromised in ways that further narrow the range of available emotional, communicative, and social learning experiences, with effects that become increasingly noticeable and confounding as a child grows up.

Focusing on symptoms of movement difference should not be considered a way of adding a new label or new traits to the lengthy list already attributed to autism (Donnellan et al. 2012). Too much "groundbreaking" autism research might be better described as the highly profitable strip mining of a continuous supply of new deficits for treatment. In contrast, the movement approach offers a way of moving beyond judgmental, categorical observations and remedial, proscriptive strategies, and toward an understanding of each person's unique experience and intact adaptive capabilities. It offers a framework for mutually exploring optimal accommodations and supports. Such exploration, which involves partnering with the individual as he or she seeks more reliable and coherent access to the world, is characteristic of a new generation of movement researchers (and their dedicated mentors, small in number but largely successful in handing down a nonconforming version of the autism narrative).

Many of these researchers, of both generations, are represented in this book. Of particular relevance to this chapter is the work of Elizabeth Torres and colleagues, who emphasize the neglected role of the PNS in human development and adaptation as a necessary complement to (and long overdue corrective for) prevailing brain-based models. Models of autism that are solely brain based tend to become static and closed, depicting autism as a fixed set of deficits specified in a person's genes and wired into his or her cerebral structure. Picturing autism symptoms as entrenched at a high neurological level, we "attack" them at a high level—appealing to abstract thinking and intentionality via flash cards and behavior charts and verbal prompts and reward schemes—only to run up against the distinct limitations of such interventions. By turning attention to the ongoing activities in the PNS, movement researchers are developing a dynamic model that views autism as the unfolding of self-regulatory challenges and the responses they call forth. Through neural systems that scaffold and support, but are different from, consciousness and volition, individuals with autism are understood to be negotiating solutions to those regulatory challenges based on their lived, embodied experiences. The body itself is seen as striving to harness random movement into reliable tools for exploration and communication. This model of PNS functioning in autism encourages us to intervene, as Torres et al. have done, not to backfill deficits but to help individuals self-discover more effective ways to experience and make sense of their body and their environment (Torres et al. 2013a, 2013c). The significance of seeing movement and of taking a nuanced, movement-informed approach to intervention becomes clear when viewed in light of the long, troubled history of the autism construct.

PSYCHOANALYSIS TO BEHAVIORISM: THE PATHS DIVERGE

The reason my son and I are observed with such different eyes has a lot to do with autism's history. The struggle to define what autism was, and was not, has involved an interplay of scientific, political, and social forces so diverse that, at times, the diagnosis has seemed like a blank slate on which almost any definition could be written and any etiology or treatment set forth. The term *autism* tentatively entered medicine in 1943, when the psychiatrist Leo Kanner of Johns Hopkins Hospital published a paper describing a rare group of patients whose condition "differs markedly and uniquely from anything reported so far" (Kanner 1943, 1995). Although Kanner declared this cohort to have an "innate" condition, he tended to depict the parents of the original 11 children he diagnosed in negative terms: "In the whole group, there are very few really warmhearted fathers and mothers" (1943, 250). His descriptions of parent–child interactions sounded sufficiently dysfunctional for autism to be claimed by the psychoanalytic establishment that exerted a strong force within psychiatry and psychology during that period. Autism came to be considered an acquired mental illness: a neurosis or psychosis brought on by poor parenting, especially poor mothering.

Prominent among advocates for a Freudian psychoanalytic approach was the child psychologist Bruno Bettelheim, whose highly influential book *The Empty Fortress: Infantile Autism and the Birth of the Self* (1967) blamed the development of autism on a lack of maternal affection. Mothers, portrayed as cold and rejecting, seemed to be the sinister cause lurking behind every aspect of autism, even those that were scarcely problematic. For example, in explaining the "motor behavior" of 10-year-old Julian, a child with autism described as climbing out of bed like "an infant" by slowly and tentatively touching his toes to the floor, Bettelheim asserted with confidence,

> It is not that these children lack some kind of body image or concept, (or) have no orientation in physical space.… Perhaps the clue lies in Julian's "feeling" for the ground though he has felt for it and reached it again and again in the past. He does it because he is not yet convinced the ground is there, because he doubts that anything is within his reach. Just as his mother was beyond his emotional reach so does everything else seem to be. (Bettelheim 1967, 451–452)

Bettelheim theorized that emotionally deficient mothers caused their sensitive children to withdraw psychologically into an inner "fortress" for self-preservation. Many children with autism were withdrawn physically from their homes and placed in residential treatment facilities in the hope that they would receive the nurturing needed to recover. Many parents, faced with the supposed evidence of their own inadequacy, were shamed, demoralized, and disempowered. Fortunately, by the mid-1960s some strong parent voices were raised in contradiction. A watershed moment was the publication of Bernard Rimland's *Infantile Autism: The Syndrome and Its Implications for a Neural Theory of Behavior* (1964), with a forward by Leo Kanner. Rimland, the parent of a son with autism, convincingly used scientific evidence to undermine existing theories of autism and propose that any viable explanation should be based on advances in neurology. Clara Claiborne Park's *The Siege* (1967), one of the earliest and most influential family accounts of autism, detailed her daughter's first 8 years in terms that made clear her autism was not induced by cold parenting. In 1965, the first national grassroots autism organization in the United States was formed by parents seeking greater respect, better understanding, and support.

Yet the view of autism as the product of dysfunctional families did not fade quickly or entirely; distinct traces still remain in the attitudes of many clinicians and the general public (Walden 2012). For example, although recent statistics alleging that parents of children with autism divorce at a uniquely high rate have now been shown to be inaccurate (Freedman et al. 2012), they continue to be cited widely as evidence of parental instability. Parents are very sensitive to these insinuations. It would be difficult to overemphasize the extent to which the experience of parent blaming has colored, and continues to color, the way parents perceive the politics of autism diagnosis and treatment. This may, at times, have led them to shy away too quickly from potentially respectful and constructive discussions of their children's inner or emotional lives and of the dance of relationship itself. My generation of parents, newly unburdened of the assumption that autism is a home-brewed mental illness, was soon encouraged to embrace its opposite. By the mid-1980s, the therapist assigned to my young son by our local disabilities support center cheerfully assured me that I would never have to worry about his acquiring a mental illness, because (and here the therapist held his thumb and index finger about half an inch apart) "the emotional life of a person with autism is this deep." A new cohort of professionals and parents had come to consider children with autism not as emotionally withdrawn, but as having a mere half inch of emotional capacity to draw on.

The roots of this profound change, like the first stirrings of organized parent advocacy, go back to the mid-1960s. As cracks formed in the initial consensus that autism equals bad parenting, the field opened up to new approaches. In 1965, *Life* magazine reported to the nation on a young assistant professor of psychology at the University of California, Los Angeles (UCLA) Neuropsychiatric Institute, O. Ivar Lovaas, and his behavioral approach to treating "a special form of schizophrenia called autism" (Grant 1965, par. 1). The claims were bold and very different. According to *Life*, Lovaas "argues that 'you have to put out the fire first before you worry how it started' … Lovaas feels that by 1) holding any mentally crippled child accountable for his behavior and 2) forcing him to act normal, he can push the child toward normality" (Grant 1965, par. 5). For these researchers, the problem was no longer assumed to be with the parents, who were now depicted in a positive light as potential teachers, but with the child. More specifically, it was located in the child's failure to act normal and could be overcome by enforcing normal behavior, a mandate that called on parents and therapists for "a willingness to use strong consequences, such as food and spankings, to be emotionally responsive, showing their anger as well as their love" (Lovaas et al. 1973, 159). Equally significant was the fact that an understanding of context and the individual's history of experience was considered unnecessary for effective intervention, largely because no significant context or history was thought to exist. As Lovaas would later recall,

> The fascinating part for me was to observe persons with eyes and ears, teeth and toenails, walking around yet presenting few of the behaviors one would call social or human. (Lovaas 1993, 620)

It was assumed that *nonhuman* behaviors occurred because the subject intended them, and that the subject intended them not because options and means of communication were scarce, but because a particular choice—even self-injury or aggression—was one he or she somehow found enjoyable. The task of behavioral intervention would therefore be to make each unwanted behavior as unrewarding as possible.

At that time, and continuing in certain venues today, behaviorism (aka "behavior modification" and, more recently, "applied behavior analysis") hewed closely to the 1913 definition of its founder, John B. Watson:

> Psychology as the behaviorist views it is a purely objective experimental branch of natural science. Its theoretical goal is the prediction and control of behavior. Introspection forms no essential part of its methods, nor is the scientific value of its data dependent upon the readiness with which they lend themselves to interpretation in terms of consciousness. The behaviorist, in his efforts to get a unitary scheme of animal response, recognizes no dividing line between man and brute. (Watson 1913, 158–167)

Watson's 1913 paper, often referred to as the Behaviorist Manifesto, limited psychology to the study of readily observable, external data at a time when sophisticated scientific tools for investigating the brain and nervous systems were unavailable. This is no longer the case today. It also ruled out introspection (self-observation) on the grounds that self-reporting was intrinsically unreliable and unscientific. When behavioral methods were initially applied to autism, this edict went unchallenged because the direct and consensual involvement of people with autism in research about themselves was unimaginable in most quarters. Whether lacking in supports to make communication possible, or defined as innately incapable of forming valid observations about themselves, people with autism must have seemed to early behaviorists to be the ideal research subjects for an approach that discounted self-observation as worthless. This situation too has changed. The expansion of both "hard" and "soft" assistive technology is making it possible for more people with autism to communicate important observations about their lives and treatment, and biases against accepting these self-reports are being confronted. The assertion that the field of psychology is destined to evolve in the direction of ever more efficient elimination of introspection has been discarded as "fictional history" and a "highly persuasive myth" by many psychologists today (Costall 2006, 635). A century after Watson, autism researchers are making respectable scientific use of many tools that incorporate self-observation, from verbal reports to questionnaires and surveys to functional magnetic resonance imaging (fMRI) (Deen and Pelphrey 2012; Eklund et al. 2016), and are increasingly willing and eager to accept those studied as participants in, not merely objects of, research. (It is one of the field's under-appreciated ironies that Watson himself departed academia for Madison Avenue, where he embraced the highly successful uses of introspective psychology that gave rise to modern advertising.)

Last but not least, Watson's sweeping scientific aspiration to "the prediction and control of behavior" has been replaced by a bow to more local, humbler gods. Developmental theories of learning no longer give pride of place to manipulating stimuli and reinforcers; Jerome Bruner, one of the leading psychological researchers of the late twentieth century, insisted that the proper business and "central concept of psychology" is "not stimuli and responses, not overtly observable behavior, not biological drives and their transformation, but meaning" (Bruner 1990, 2). The study of how children explore and relate to their bodies and environments—how they actively create embodied knowledge and a knowable, meaningful world—has become increasingly important (Thelen and Smith 1994).

At the midpoint between Watson's 1913 manifesto and the present, however, many members of the autism community found the assertions that we should concern ourselves only with surface behavior, and that all behavior is learned and maintained via rewards and consequences, to be appealingly simple after the convoluted explanations of unconscious and repressed motivations invoked by Bettelheim and his colleagues. Others found those same assertions to be unappealingly simplistic: methodologically open to ratifying the use of aversive control (Brown et al. 2008); unquestioning of the value, priority, and shifting cultural definitions of acting "normal"; overly confident in the objectivity and judgment of the scientific observer (based on a kind of "physics envy" that tries to model the human sciences on the "hard sciences" and their laboratory methods); willing to extract actions from the contexts that give them meaning and pigeonhole them as discrete, comparable "behaviors"; and unable to differentiate movements (such as tic-like or anxiety-driven responses or the spontaneously occurring transitional motions between goal-directed actions [Torres 2011]) that are not under direct volitional control, and are therefore poor candidates for reward and punishment.

Behaviorism demonstrated beyond a doubt that people with autism could learn and parents could teach; that was a crucial move. But behaviorism, which looked at first blush like the knight in shining armor that could restore parents' reputations and save us from wandering aimlessly in the labyrinths of psychoanalysis, may have functioned as an inhibiting factor in the consideration of a movement-based approach. In its agnosticism about the relevance or even the existence of inner lives, feelings, complex or intrinsic motivations, and a role for movement and perception in development, it can privilege those in power with the right to define and enforce normality. It may miss the golden opportunity to "see movement" and its sensation by moving beyond cosmetic, socially defined, culturally bounded norms toward an understanding of how people with autism actually self-discover and make sense of their worlds and how those worlds can expand beyond their immediate and perceived limits.

This complaint is not new and certainly not mine alone; we were warned almost a half century ago by Ludwig von Bertalanffy, the pioneering biologist who demonstrated that adaptations capable of opening new possibilities can emerge only within the dynamics of "open systems":

> It is well to realize the power and the limits of manipulating psychology and behavioral engineering.… If you manipulate a dog according to Pavlov, a cat according to Thorndike, or a rat according to Skinner, you will obtain the results described by these authors. That is, you select out of their behavioral repertoire such responses as may be controlled by punishment or reward, you *make* the animals into stimulus response machines or robots. The same, of course, is true of humans. (Bertalanffy 1967, 13)

Likewise, it may be useful to consider to what extent the perception of autism and its prognosis have been shaped by the methodologies and philosophies available to and adopted for its treatment, and the extent to which the outcomes of individuals with that label may represent self-fulfilling prophecies.

IMPACT OF THE DSM: A CAREFULLY CURATED COLLECTION OF SYMPTOMS

Just as the public's perceptions of autism were undergoing these massive shifts, the medical establishment began working to put in place a reliable, replicable way to diagnose it. The *Diagnostic and Statistical Manual of Mental Disorders*, Third Edition (DSM-III), the first iteration of that now ubiquitous manual to include autism as a distinct category (rather than a form of childhood schizophrenia, as in DSM-II), was hot off the presses when my son was diagnosed in 1980. It has since gone through two more editions and their revisions, taking us up to the release of DSM-5 in 2013.

From the DSM's introduction in 1952, questions have been raised about the meaning of "mental disorder" and the justification for including or excluding various conditions from its pages. To look up the diagnostic criteria for Parkinson's, for example, I have to turn instead to the World Health Organization's International Classification of Diseases (ICD), which is used worldwide for health care reporting and resource allocation and is now in its 10th edition. Parkinson's is considered a disease rather than a mental disorder because it involves a well-defined, clinically verifiable pathology: the nervous systems lose functioning in predictable ways via mechanisms studied by neurologists for more than 150 years. Signs of nonmotor issues in Parkinson's disease may emerge later, and therefore were not included in the earlier conceptualization of the diagnosis. Today, however, the Movement Disorders Society hosts entire halls of posters and talks on nonmotor issues, ranging from cognitive memory phenomena to mood-related disorders and even subtle sensory disturbances that frequently can foretell the onset of Parkinson's disease when motor issues are not as pronounced (Darweesh et al. 2016; Simuni et al. 2016). These new observations raise new and complex questions about the nature of disease, the nature of mental disorder, and the assumptions and prejudices that have automatically steered research and diagnosis for so long.

An autism diagnosis is currently a psychological construct—a description of a behavioral phenotype, based on observation and interpretation rather than on physical measurements—and remains far less defined at the physiological level; its pathways and mechanisms are not well understood and prognoses are not particularly helpful. Whether, or to what extent, the autism phenotype the DSM has constructed will match up with some future biobehavioral model remains to be seen. Much as a museum curator might display a group of puzzling artifacts reportedly found together, in the hope that their tentative association will encourage research and eventually lead to an interpretation of their function, the DSM's authors have continued to collect, curate, and rearrange groups of symptoms associated with the autism construct in the hope that they will one day prove meaningful at a deeper explanatory level. Not all collections of symptoms unveiled in the DSM are equally well received or productive; some are quickly disassembled and dispersed (as occurred with the Asperger's diagnosis from DSM-IV) because in practice they fail to capture systematic *endophenotypic* groups—that is, groups of behavioral symptoms with clear genetic connections. Other plausible, related collections of symptoms, such as "sensory processing disorder" (proposed in the run-up to DSM-5), have acquired professional lobbies but are still waiting in the wings for admission to a future edition.

This ongoing jostling to acquire display space among the DSM's diagnoses of mental disorders is, of course, partly related to funding: a condition listed in the DSM will need research. But it is also related to the history of American psychology. In contrast to the ICD, which has for more than 100 years been an international clinical tool with a global health mission, the DSM remains the more localized vehicle through which the American Psychiatric Association continues its epic struggle with a diverse and fragmented evidence base that, until 1980, "reflected the dominant psychoanalytic ideas of the time, emphasizing the role of experience, downplaying biology" (American Psychological Association 2009, 63). (The ICD has, of course, added a section for coding diagnoses of "mental disorders," on which it confers with editors of the DSM. Its autism language echoes each previous DSM; it is not seeking to break new diagnostic ground.) Autism's core collection of symptoms was first identified and studied in a pre-1980 psychoanalytic setting, so, not surprisingly, today diagnosticians bookmark "Neurodevelopmental Disorders" (subheading "Autism Spectrum Disorder") in the diagnostic manual of the American Psychiatric Association. For Parkinson's, convincingly claimed by neurology since the mid-1800s, the DSM defers to the ICD (but adds codes for "major or mild neurocognitive disorder due to Parkinson's disease"). Tourette syndrome, characterized by repetitive motor and vocal behaviors similar to those seen in autism (Hagerman et al. 2010; Niu et al. 2014), was, like autism, originally treated as a mental illness and is now more likely to be represented as a neurological condition and featured at meetings of the Movement Disorders Society. Due to its history, however, it too remains in the DSM as a neurodevelopmental disorder (subheading "Motor Disorders"). Autism and Tourette's, and Parkinson's have fallen and remain on different sides of what Joseph Martin of Harvard Medical School calls "an artificial wall" that has separated the "philosophical approaches and research and treatment methods" of neurology and psychiatry during the past century (Martin 2002, 695).

Researchers peering over this wall have created an approximately 40-year history of observations implicating neurologically based movement differences in the autism spectrum disorders (ASDs). In the article "Moving On: Autism and Movement Disturbance," Leary and Hill (1996) suggested the broad scope of potential inquiry through a thought-provoking comparison of known movement disorders with descriptions of behavior labeled autistic. More recently, a meta-analysis of 83 studies since 1981 concluded,

> The current overall findings portray motor coordination deficits as pervasive across diagnoses, thus, a cardinal feature of ASD. (Fournier et al. 2010, 1227)

And in 2013, a review of "motor research" found

> there is good evidence to suggest the presence of increased motor noise and timing deficits in autistic individuals and that these may lead to increased variability in temporal and spatial aspects of execution. (Gowen and Hamilton 2013)

Pioneering work in the 1970s and early 1980s (Damasio and Maurer 1978; Maurer and Damasio 1982; Vilensky et al. 1981) showed that children with autism walk in a manner similar to that of adults with Parkinson's, with slower movement and smaller steps, and experience similar postural differences. Yet it is probably not surprising that few references to movement have ever made the cut for inclusion in the DSM's definitions of autism—and then only as optional diagnostic criteria. These criteria refer to a few highly visible activities, such as hand flapping, rocking, or spinning, which have been termed, in the various DSM editions, "oddities of motor movement," "stereotyped body movements," "stereotyped and repetitive motor mannerisms," and in the DSM-5, "stereotyped or repetitive motor movements." Their detailed investigation has attracted little interest.

It can be conjectured that movement differences might not lend themselves well to prevailing diagnostic practices.

Despite this, the autism diagnosis today is overly reliant on the clinician's qualitative impressions of what a child *has*, and lacking in verifiable, replicable data about what a child physically *does*. Rather than being recorded as present or absent, gross motor or fine motor, movement differences need to be rigorously characterized and measured in relation to the environment, context, and task conditions under which they emerge, and as they evolve over time. Many movement differences—particularly in young children of diagnostic age—are not easily recognizable by the untrained eye; as long as major motor milestones are met, the *way* in which they are met goes unremarked (Teitelbaum et al. 1998, 2004). Many significant types of movements are also too small, and too fast, to be registered and recorded by an observer without special instrumentation (Torres 2011). The metrics and the technology exist to do this (Torres and Donnellan 2015)—movement is, at this point, far more measurable than the construct of autism itself—but without an understanding of why movement matters, this will not occur.

Indeed, basic science in autism remains unaware that the behavior that is observed, interpreted, debated, and scored to yield or not to yield a DSM diagnosis depends on sensory (kinesthetic) channels provided by the motor systems (Purves 2012). Without the dynamic movement information conveyed through these channels, behavior would not exist. This leaves users of the DSM unable to describe and interpret phenomena, since they are not physically measure it in an objective way. Indeed, the field continues to overlook the significance of movement because it does not appear within the spotlight surrounding current diagnostic preoccupations and priorities. The numerous movement differences that occur at transition points *between* activities, such as starting, stopping, or switching, may go unnoticed or be discounted as deliberate task avoidance because observers are focusing only on the activities—usually of a social nature—which they determined to be important a priori. Paying attention to movement would also entail a commitment to engage with insider perspectives and self-observation by exploring what a person intends and expects, and how they experience their body through movement, in recognition of the fact that "individuals with the autism label often describe experiences which are not immediately obvious to the rest of us (De Jaegher 2013) but which significantly affect our understanding of their behavior" (Donnellan et al. 2012, par. 8). In short, the process of seeing movement may have too many moving parts to fit neatly into the symptom or trait checklists of the DSM as currently envisioned. It remains to be seen whether future editions will seek to reduce the barrier between psychiatry and neurology by taking an interest in movement as a sensory channel. On a hopeful note, the DSM-5 does show an incipient preference for combining diagnostic traits and categories on the basis of probable "shared genetic variations and relationships between behaviour and neural circuitry" (Grinker 2010), rather than continuing to split categories like autism into highly speculative subtypes.

To date, all the DSM's autism definitions and examples can be characterized as rearrangements of the same triad of higher-order, socially defined impairments: deficits in social interaction (examples often cited are lack of eye contact and failure to take an interest in others), deficits in language and social communication (recurring examples include failure to sustain a conversation and the use of idiosyncratic words or phrases), and a restricted or repetitive repertoire of activities (examples repeatedly given are abnormal patterns of interest and an insistence on rituals or routines). The DSM-5 collapses the first two deficits into one, but the triad is still implicit. When my son received a label of infantile autism, as it was originally called, I looked up the DSM-III diagnostic criteria and found to my dismay that it meant he had demonstrated, among other symptoms, "bizarre responses to various aspects of the environment, e.g., resistance to change, peculiar interest in or attachments to animate or inanimate objects." What would it take, I wondered, to establish that someone's responses are bizarre, resistant, or peculiar, when we know so little about what they are responding to or what tools—cultural and physiological—they have at their disposal? It might turn out that their responses are adaptive or even creative, but at the very least, they would start to make sense.

Such descriptions presume to preinterpret behavior for us. In contrast, the ICD-9 is succinct and objectively descriptive in its neurological definition of Parkinson's, which reads (in part), [Parkinson's is] "a progressive motor disability manifested by tremors, shaking, muscular rigidity, and lack of postural reflexes." If we applied the same interpretive latitude and socially constructed language to the Parkinson's diagnostic criteria as we do to those of autism, we might get a statement like this: Parkinson's "is characterized by lack of attention to fine motor skills, bizarre and perseverative hand movements, persistent odd posture, refusal to keep pace with others, self-injurious behavior, and deficits in nonverbal communication (e.g. restricted use of gestures and facial expression)."

Parkinson's, of course, manifests in adult life and is progressive, while autism is developmental, playing out in complex interactions with the environment. Research over the past two decades has documented the presence of movement differences linked to autism in the earliest months of life. If I had lived, from birth, with challenges like those cited by the ICD-9, and if those challenges had been interpreted—and targeted for reduction—in terms of the imaginary DSM-style criteria just proposed, I wonder how my development and socialization would have progressed and what my worldview would be today. Would I have been a beneficiary of the supportive dance of relationships, meaningful inclusion in everyday experiences, and nurturing of intellect that developing humans need? It is surely a question worth asking.

Eventually, I came to realize that a DSM diagnosis was not intended as an exercise in cultural competence, and seeing things from my son's point of view was not the purpose of this system; the use of a term like *bizarre* was not questioned because the typical outside observer who would use the DSM knew "bizarre" when he or she saw it. The DSM's avowed mission was to create an orderly and replicable classification system for "mental disorders" out of a modest and scattered evidence base; the price to be paid was that the system would rely on readily visible surface traits or behaviors, as manifested with little reference to environment or context, which could be viewed synchronically (i.e., in a "slice of time") from a socially constructed perspective that privileges the observer. This is also a definition of what it means to pathologize behavior, that is, to extract it from its context (including the personal experiences and opinions of those diagnosed) and utilize it as a freestanding example of deviance, to which society's only imaginable response is attempted prevention or cure. In this regard, the DSM projected an image of autism that was in accord with the postpsychoanalytic *zeitgeist*, and highly influential among those who saw it as independent corroboration of the essential arbitrariness and meaninglessness—the bizarre nature—of autistic behavior. Perhaps not surprisingly, the marketing of a vast assortment of autism therapies and treatments—some of an equally bizarre nature—grew exponentially during this time, as did the tendency to approach intervention in a scattershot way, tossing a disparate mix of treatments at the target in the desperate hope that one might eventually score a hit. Parents' long-standing and unmet need was to find some central coherence in the autism narrative so that they could focus their time and effort on approaches that made sense—and that assumed their children made sense too.

EVOLVING MODELS: BRAIN-BASED OR EMBODIED?

During the 1990s, the "Decade of the Brain" (so named by President George H. W. Bush to promote awareness of research), vastly improved and noninvasive techniques for imaging the brain were developed. By the latter part of that decade, the fMRI procedure was being applied to many new populations, including individuals with autism. This rapid proliferation of autism research was encouraged by the DSM-IV's introduction, in 1994, of the diagnostic subcategory of Asperger's disorder. This diagnosis, which in practice often overlapped with the informal designation of "high-functioning autism," helped identify individuals whose speech and language use did not manifest the delays and difficulties often associated with autism. Since people with this diagnosis could better control their movements and take spoken instruction as required for brain imaging, as well as traditional pencil and paper tests, they were often used—without particular justification being offered—as a proxy for all those diagnosed on the autism spectrum. Having selected research subjects with less challenging (or at least less obvious) movement differences, and given them tasks that involved little to no movement, it was hard to resist jumping to the conclusion that their autism must be based in the brain and must represent the condition in its pure or essential form, uncluttered by secondary physical symptoms or intellectual disability. In this way, the constraints of the research techniques themselves were preemptively setting the parameters for, and thereby distorting, the conclusions that would eventually be reached. Looking for autism inside the brain also made sense to parents and to researchers because the diagnosis itself, through the DSM, had become so strongly associated with deficits in the higher-order processing needed for socialization, in particular social communication, empathy, and exploratory or play behavior.

Many people believed that the new imaging techniques would reveal a specific damaged or missing part of the brain to be the cause of autism. A major research focus from the mid-1980s to the early 2000s involved the search for a single deficit that was both innate and of sufficient magnitude to account for the triad of social, communicative, and perseverative symptoms appearing downstream. That deficit was generally portrayed as the lack of a key brain module (i.e., a collection of brain circuits dedicated, in advance, to a certain domain of knowledge) or special type of neuron required for the development of some key aspect of cognition, especially social cognition. The researcher who could name that deficit, and make it stick by proving it universal among, and in some way unique to, people with autism, would finally provide the core around which a theory-saturated field could crystallize. Among the many candidates for core deficit were the missing theory of mind (ToM) module (Baron-Cohen et al. 1985), resulting in the inability to recognize other people's point of view; the missing facial recognition module (Schultz et al. 2000), resulting in the inability to recognize other people's expressions of emotion; "weak central coherence" (Happe and Frith 2006) and its close cousin "poor executive function" (Ozonoff and McEvoy 1994), together suggesting the existence of a larger core deficit that causes poor contextualization of social *and* nonsocial information; and lately, missing or broken mirror neurons (Rizzolatti et al. 2009), presumably accounting for a failure to reflect the feelings of others.

In recent years, however, the utility of viewing autism in the static terms of missing modules or computer-like programs in the brain has been increasingly disputed. It has been noted that brain imaging studies have not found a consistent neural location for the ToM, and that many people with autism succeed in ToM tests and other tests of inference and empathy (Rogers et al. 2007).

Decreased brain activation during facial looking (compared with controls) is, some researchers argue, more parsimoniously explained by the shorter time typically spent looking at faces (Gernsbacher and Frymiare 2005, par. 18), which begs for an explanation of its own. Labels like "executive function" and "central coherence" are increasingly taken as umbrella terms for distributed neural systems rather than specific "things" or locales in the brain, and so fail to define a "single deficit." And the possibility that social life is all about mirror neurons has attracted greater enthusiasm in the social media than in socialization research (Fan et al. 2010; Southgate and Hamilton 2008). Many researchers now argue that the search to explain autism as the product of a single innate brain deficit has reached a dead end, particularly since there are profound methodological flaws in the fMRI paradigm (Eklund et al. 2016) that would render many of these studies and conclusions largely falsifiable.

Acknowledging this history, some current brain-based models of autism aim to address and characterize the more global processes being imaged through fMRI. In doing so, they hope to account for a range of observed phenomena broader and subtler than the autism triad. Neurologist Nancy Minshew and colleagues have honed such a model over decades of research (Minshew et al. 1997), disproving a long list of single causes before reaching the conclusion that

> autism is a selective impairment in the neural processing of complex information across domains and sensory modalities, with intact or enhanced simple abilities in the same domains as impairments. (Williams et al. 2006, par. 2)

This makes for a more complex story and fewer headlines than missing mirror neurons, but is worth tracking because it takes us to several interesting places. First, we are invited to consider how information is processed rather than to presume an innate blindness to certain areas of experience. This model takes seriously and brings to the fore the often ignored fact that, in autism, unusual challenges can exist side by side with perceptual advantages and exceptional skills. Rather than addressing a collection of deficits, it aims to address the wide variations and peaks of performance that seem to surprise many autism spectators, a phenomenon that Sue Rubin, whose autobiography became the Academy Award–nominated video *Autism Is a World*, wryly observes:

> It is funny how we are considered strange or different, even though our recollection of complex patterns, memory for precise detail, and overall capabilities many times exceed those of the people who are pointing or staring. (Young 2011, 107)

Another significant aspect of this information processing model is that the "complexity" that interferes with neural processing is not directly defined by content, intellectual or otherwise:

> The concept of complexity has more to do with the effect on the brain's mechanisms during processing of information than it does with the type of information (i.e., social or language) per se. (Williams et al. 2006, par. 2)

The model finds the key to autism in *how* and under what conditions information is processed, not necessarily in *what* information is processed. It is suggested that a highly sensitive processing system may become overwhelmed "when the information to be handled is inherently complex or becomes complex due to its amount or time constraints" (Williams et al. 2006, par. 2), and that "the dynamics of the task demands and situations imposed on the brain" (Williams et al. 2006, par. 3) are factors creating complexity. While social interaction *may* become complex in this sense, so might other types of experience. As Minshew states,

> Our paper strongly suggests that autism is not primarily a disorder of social interaction, but a global disorder affecting how the brain processes the information it receives—especially when the information becomes complicated. (NIH 2006)

This information processing model may come further than most current brain-based research from the presumption of highly specific, innate deficits—especially in the social realm—and therefore a few steps closer to a movement-informed approach. However, it implicates only high-level or late information processing in the brain, suggesting that information processed through the various supporting subsystems of the nervous systems is intact. This seems curious in light of the fact that the model specifies and requires the existence of constraints or glitches in the ways information becomes available to the brain. It might be useful to ask whether information could become "complex" in its dynamics and task demands if it becomes available through a noisy and dys-synchronized PNS, on which the cortically based mental processes must rely. It also might be useful to ask what a striving brain might do at the initial levels of cortical processing to compensate for signal distortions in the PNS. Perhaps it would come to rely on and strengthen attention and memory (because when many examples can be located, "held in mind" and compared, patterns may emerge despite noise), language (perhaps to label and track, and therefore support, the products of a highly developed memory), and visual-spatial domains (allowing a person to, as Temple Grandin [1995] put it, "think in pictures," using dynamic mental visualizations to fill in gaps in experiential information much as the eye fills in its blind spot). Interestingly, "attention, simple memory, simple language, and visual-spatial domains" are the four "domains of neuropsychologic functioning" that Minshew et al. (1997, abstract) have found to be at least as strong, and often enhanced, in subjects with autism compared with controls.

Despite the improbability of missing brain modules and the seeming incompleteness of the cortical processing model, research elaborating a brain basis for autism continues to capture an overwhelming share of the energy, attention, and vision within the field. Many of the most popular sources of autism information for the general public, from the advocacy group Autism Speaks to the online medical source WebMD, confidently refer to autism as a "brain disorder." This assurance that autism resides in the brain, linked with the widespread assumption that the brain of a person with autism must lack some basic capacity for social communication, seems a fair approximation of where most of the field stands today. Such a focus has been admirable in moving the discussion beyond "bad parents" or "badly behaved kids." Yet thinking of autism primarily in terms of deficits in the social brain may have unintended consequences. Parents and teachers may elect to shift their attention away from the child's presumably intractable lack of empathy and relationship, and redirect it toward exploiting the relative strength of rote memorization as applied to isolated facts, the application of rule-based systems of social etiquette as a stand-in for the give-and-take of actual friendships, and preestablished routines and protocols for all occasions. We have had several decades of educational activities of this kind, carried out in segregated settings, dependent on training students to cue off of artificial prompts, aspiring to social politeness in lieu of social understanding, and justified by the belief that children with autism are largely uninterested in imaginative play or socializing with peers, preferring to, for example, spend their days working alone at a screened-off computer station. The results, measured in quality of adult life, have been disappointing (Roux et al. 2015).

A strictly brain-based orientation to autism may likewise run the risk of encouraging overly abstract and insufficiently experiential approaches to intervention. Parents and teachers may come to perceive the delivery of knowledge to the child as a purely logical, cerebral task similar to data entry in a computer, at the expense of real, lived, and felt bodily experience and the emergence of autonomy. The belief that it is possible and even preferable to separate cognitive from affective information in teaching students with autism can yield strange results. One common and unfortunate example is the use of picture flash cards in an attempt to teach a deskbound student with autism to identify actions (i.e., running or jumping) as labels rather than as physical experiences involving affect, sensation, and appropriate contextual cues. The child may indeed learn to touch a certain card when he hears a certain sound. Yet, is the learning of "jumping" through the touching of the card, followed by a food reward, going to generalize to an actual physical context where a jumping action may be required? And what will it come to mean to a child who associates the word "jumping" not with play and interaction, but with sitting alone and moving an arm on demand?

It is this impasse that Stanley Greenspan and colleagues at the National Center for Clinical Infant Programs addressed in their influential 1992 overview "Reconsidering the Diagnosis and Treatment of Very Young Children with Autistic Spectrum or Pervasive Developmental Disorder":

> It is especially important to reconsider the notions that there is a fixed biological deficit in the capacity to form an interactive relationship.... With early diagnosis and a comprehensive integrated relationship-based treatment approach, children originally diagnosed as PDD [pervasive developmental disorder] are learning to relate to others with warmth, empathy and emotional flexibility—characteristics that run contrary to the very definition of PDD and that have been thought to be possible only for an exceptional few. (Greenspan 1992, 2–3)
>
> One needs to consider the hypothesis that the types of overly rigid and structured interventions that have been organized on behalf of these infants and children in part support rather than remediate their more mechanical behavior. (Greenspan 1992, 5)

Of course, it is not the fault of brain researchers that we often forget the brain has a body, or, as developmental neuroscientist Alan Fogel puts it, that we treat the mind "as a disembodied relationless computational machine, as an objective thing inside the head" (Fogel 1993, 4). Ours is a worldview that remains fractured by the Cartesian split between mind and body (much as psychiatry has been split from neurology) and in thrall to the spurious analogy of brain to computer and of learning to data input. Brains get respect. We tend to consider consciousness and volition as entirely brain based and as more significant, honorable aspects of the human experience than anything that occurs in the PNS (Gershon 1998), which is often pictured as merely a mechanical information conductor from the brain to the body parts being set in motion. Bodies are depicted as mere transport for the brain; a significant trope in science fiction is the brain that escapes its cumbersome body to merge with a computer and realize its true powers—fun to imagine but not worth a try, since even a nominally "living" brain without the wetware of constant physical sensing could not emerge into human consciousness or self-awareness as we know it. We forget that the PNS has its own vital and complex awareness, intelligence, and adaptive capability, based on the constant flow and sensing of movement and the ongoing mapping of the body as it moves through time and space. Knowledge emerges through this ongoing activity, on a scale and in a time frame that often leaves our conscious, volitional, abstracted "self" playing catch-up. It can be startling to consider the words of developmental neuroscientists Esther Thelen and Linda Smith, who insisted that

> Knowledge ... is not a thing, but a continuous process; not a structure, but an action, embedded in, and derived from, a history of actions. (Thelen and Smith 1994, 247)

Clearly, we need approaches to autism that are more active, dynamic, body based, experience driven, and responsive to the dance of relationship. Researchers will need to move beyond the widespread bias toward envisioning autism as fully rooted in the neural processing of key cortical regions of the brain that dominates current models of autism, and recognize that the brain-based model remains partial because it is disembodied. The missing piece may be a consideration of challenges in the PNS. Replicable, testable theories about what occurs there for children with autism have been scarce to nonexistent, resulting in a disinclination to attach much significance to sensory or motor phenomena, which tend to be reflected in diagnostic protocols as secondary or optional criteria. In contrast to studying people with autism as if only central cortical structures and connections contribute to development, researchers need to look at movement itself: as a sensory system in its own right, playing out at different levels in the PNS and interfacing with the CNS to create self-perception.

Responding to the current top-down brain- or CNS-based model of autism with a bottom-up PNS model opens up a significant new array of possible and positive approaches (Torres et al. 2013a). It suggests a new master narrative that parents can use as a guide to making sense of what their child is doing, and to helping their child make sense out of the raw stuff of experience. If autism involves challenges to the flow of reafferent (movement-based) kinesthetic information through the PNS, this would imply that movement and perception—the foundation of development—are not being integrated in typical ways, are evolving differently, and are presenting confusingly partial, selective, and intermittent information to the maturing brain and CNS, which in turn is responding with novel coping strategies—some of which may wind up on lists of "autistic behaviors" targeted for remediation. Potential patterns in these children's experiences—patterns they could use to scaffold development—may be buried in an abundance of random noise and slow to emerge, different from the schema being evolved by their nonautistic peers, and hard for their bodies to identify, predict, and act on—hence the frequently heard but misleading assertion that children with autism "do not understand cause and effect." As Torres et al. (2013c) have now demonstrated, they do indeed understand this concept when given the chance to explore and self-discover it, rather than presented with top-down adult direction.

People with autism themselves suggest that they are on high alert for patterns in their environments, but cannot necessarily be attuned to their presence or evaluate their significance by tapping directly into their socially defined meanings. Author Donna Williams explains,

> The inability to get consistent meaning through any of my senses in an environment that demanded that I did, meant that I developed another side; a side with an acute ability to respond, not to meaning but to patterns. (Williams 1996, 242)

It may be hard for developing children to tell which patterns arise through the unique properties of their own nervous systems, and which are shared by and meaningful to others. If children with autism truly are experiencing the world and forming concepts differently, then our task is to identify and work with the given state of each individual's movement as part of his or her perceptual system. Our aim must be to support reliable, coherent, self-directed experience that is both respected *and* connected with the experience of others—as Bruner might have said, to support the emergence of "meaning" (1990, 2). It also means that the autism triad of social, communicative, and perseverative deficits could be treated as secondary or downstream to these neurological challenges, rather than as innate and inevitable: we would not need to assume that deficits in sociability or a lack of empathy necessarily come with the territory. We could hypothesize that, for each child, the contents of that territory will be developed experientially through the mapping process itself.

THE "AUTISM QUARTET": MOVEMENT-BASED APPROACHES

While the DSM has proposed a disembodied, high-level "triad of impairments" to characterize autism, many parents with whom I have worked over the past 30 years have described elements of a different set of phenomena that seem to exist at a more fundamental and embodied level. Their observations have not been explained in any convincing way by the usual theories of autism as a cognitive and social deficit, nor has behavioral treatment tended to modify their persistence or impact it in a lasting or positive way, nor has the DSM given us adequate words to describe them. Yet these are phenomena that have an enormous impact on everyday life, and that parents struggle daily to understand better.

I have come to recognize these phenomena very well after many years of parenting children on the autism spectrum, helping to found and run advocacy organizations at the local, state, and national level, and working as a professional in the autism field. Recently, after creating a list of familiar parent observations, I realized that they could be grouped into a "quartet" of issues that may turn out to be related to the traditional autism triad; in fact, these issues may contribute significantly to the socially defined judgments on which the diagnostic triad was built. However, given parents' unique, in-depth longitudinal experience, the quartet tends to reflect a perspective that is more personalized and more questioning of the current master narrative about autism. Its components can be summarized as:

- Variable performance
- Complex and effortful movement strategies; delayed habituation
- Marked similarities to other neurological conditions
- A strong need for relationship-based approaches

All these observations involve us in the process of seeing movement. They are defined and some of their implications considered below.

Variable Performance

In Lewis Carroll's *Alice's Adventures in Wonderland*, there is a wonderful croquet game in which the lines between intentional and random activity become, like everything else in that topsy-turvy world, hopelessly muddled. Alice, a proper and rule-loving Victorian child, finds to her consternation that she has been enlisted into a game that is, quite literally, being played "live": a flamingo is the mallet, there is a hedgehog for the ball, and the Queen's guards serve as the hoops. Despite her knowledge of croquet and her motivation to succeed, all she can do is watch in dismay as these subsystems of the game disintegrate and merrily pursue their own ends. Alice can only persist, hoping for a fortunate moment when the trajectories of all these rogue actors can be reintegrated into a playable shot, however momentarily. The croquet game might offer an imaginative window onto the variable performance experienced by people with movement differences. The frustration of dependence on movement subsystems that are occasionally available and predictable, but generally respond only sporadically and chaotically, feels very familiar. Similarly, parents report occasional, unpredictable incidents when their child with autism surpasses his or her typical level of performance with a virtuoso display, such as the "nonspeaking" individual who suddenly makes a highly articulate statement, only to lapse back into silence, or the person who executes a perfectly coordinated gymnastic move once every few years. These may be occasions when a highly sensitive, easily disrupted nervous system beats the odds to achieve a win.

In fact, the existence of widely separated peaks and valleys in performance has contributed greatly to public perceptions of autism's "mystery," and to the misperception that autistic behavior is largely a willful refusal to cooperate and live up to one's potential. Parents report frustration at their own inability to reliably support the higher levels of performance occasionally glimpsed in their child, and this feeling may be exacerbated when others question their parenting skills or observations (e.g., "He didn't tantrum the last time we took him shopping, so why don't you just make him shape up?" or "How can you claim she reads at home when she doesn't read in school?"). Parents have to deal with the fact that what happens at one time, or in one setting, is not a good predictor of what will happen at another time or place; consolidation and generalization of skills is problematic, and we want to understand why.

The speech development of children with autism can prove particularly elusive to characterization and support. Many families report that their child's speech is not so much lost or gained once and for all, but rather emergent on certain occasions when all the necessary components seem to come together. The conditions required to attend, process, and respond to the environment through vocalized speech have to be calibrated just right, and today's "just right" might not be tomorrow's. A surprising number of parents whose children are described as nonspeaking report that their child *has* spoken in full sentences or paragraphs, but only a few times and never when asked directly. Some children, like my own son when he was small, can memorize and recite verbatim the entire text of a favorite story or dialogue of a favorite cartoon show, but seem unable to do the same with their home address. Some respond to speech better when it is sung than when it is spoken, and those with dysfluencies like my son's may be fluent when singing. On numerous occasions,

I have observed individuals vocalizing words in a seemingly meaningless fashion while, at the same time, holding a perfectly appropriate conversation via an assistive communication device. And while many professionals still insist that the window of opportunity for the emergence of speech closes around the age of 5, research supports the existence of individuals with autism who made significant breakthroughs into speech as late as age 12 (Pickett et al. 2009). A small cohort of people with autism even appear to have made impressive gains in their ability to speak during adulthood, but this possibility awaits further documentation and investigation.

Physical and social skills likewise puzzle parents with their tendency to come and go, or to remain highly compartmentalized. For example, the ability to manipulate and spin small objects with great dexterity may go hand in hand with illegible penmanship. During my son's early development, I was perplexed to discover that he was more alert and interactive when he was running a fever; other parents have since volunteered similar observations, but we have no idea why performance would appear to vary in this way. Sometimes the changes that emerge under certain conditions are dramatic: I was once the "therapeutic swimming" buddy of a little girl with autism who spontaneously made eye contact, laughed, and responded enthusiastically to my every suggestion while we were in the water, but despite my best efforts was unable to manage any of those things on dry land. And I seldom meet parents who do not critique the diagnostic process that identified their child with autism on the grounds that their child performs much better under conditions that could not be replicated in the diagnostician's office. Parents learn to build their routines and contingency plans around their children's variability, recognizing that good days and bad days emerge in ways that are complex and hard to predict. On good days, we are impressed by and grateful for the fragile balance that they seem to be working so hard to maintain; when things go wrong, it is generally because some part of the environment lacks or lost the ability to flex and accommodate their needs. Under the weight of novel and/or demand situations—like the diagnostician's office—that fragile balance disintegrates, and their nervous system either falls into a state of passive disengagement or is recruited into the anxiety-driven responses of "fight or flight."

Not surprisingly, a parent's enumeration of what a child can do—anywhere but here, anytime but now—can be frustrating for professionals too, and can give so-called "autism parents" a reputation for being difficult or unreasonable. On the other hand, professionals who observe a child with autism in a moment of high attunement with the environment and high achievement are often inclined to devalue and dismiss it as a useless "island of intelligence." In the language of the current DSM-5, some portion of a child's *negative* behavioral variability might be attributed to "extreme distress at small changes, difficulties with transitions, rigid thinking patterns," but there is no language characterizing those *positive* episodes when performance is suddenly and momentarily well beyond previous expectation. While parents are very interested in these phenomena, researchers have been wary because they lacked a framework through which to approach them. They generally are set aside as "exceptions that prove the rule" (a truly odd notion) or as further proof that autism is random and nonsensical.

In recent years, however, a cluster of research has suggested various types of neurological "short circuits" likely to produce the highly sensitive and context-dependent performance characteristic of autism (and similar conditions). Autism has been explored as an "intense world syndrome" (Markram et al. 2007) in which hyperreactivity and hyperplasticity of the nervous system result in excessively processed memories and overly intense responses to a surfeit of stimuli. It is as if the body tries to solve the problem of too much noise in the PNS by processing more stimuli, or processing stimuli more, in the hope of retrieving something it can recognize as signal. The intense world research suggests avoiding medication designed to increase neuronal and cognitive functioning, and (if medication is required) emphasizing those that slow and calm the nervous system. It also recommends that behavior be approached in a positive, rewarding, comforting manner, cautioning that direct punishment may "lock down" or deeply entrench highly intense and detrimental responses (Markram et al. 2007, par. 88).

Autism has also been dubbed a "temporo-spatial processing disorder (TSPD) of multisensory flows," meaning that it involves difficulty in "perceiving, imitating, understanding and producing emotional and verbal events on time, and therefore in interacting here and now with [the] human and social environment" (Gepner and Feron 2009, 1238). The split-second timing and acute sensitivity to environmental rhythms that allow neurologically typical individuals to go with the multisensory flow can falter in the TSPDs, which include—not surprisingly—Parkinson's disease, with its gradual disconnection of movement and perception from intention. As patterns in multisensory stimuli become increasingly difficult for people with Parkinson's to detect and respond to, neurologist Oliver Sacks noted that individuals often can be "activated and regulated, ordered and organised" by measures such as "stairs, steps painted on the ground, clocks, metronomes, and devices that count in a simple, regular, and orderly manner; or by co-action and co-ordination with a concrete, living activity or agent" (Sacks 1990, 347). I have known individuals with autism to experiment with and employ clickers, counters, and certain types of music as tools to successfully self-regulate and initiate movement; the effectiveness of moving in concert with a support person is just beginning to be appreciated. The possibility of adopting or adapting, for people with autism, accommodations already in use with people who have related movement differences would seem to be significant, yet this potential resource has scarcely begun to be tapped.

A related body of research is looking at the "binding window"—the window of time in which the input from different sensory modes occurs closely enough to be ascribed to the same event—which has been discovered to be twice as long for subjects with autism as for a typically developing control group (Foss-Feig et al. 2010). The admission of an overly generous array of sensory stimuli through this window may inhibit multisensory experiences from binding into a single well-integrated perception. Sights, sounds, and perhaps other sensory information would not match up smoothly to create reliable, shared meaning; at the same time, unrelated events might be perceived as connected, resulting in changes in information content that "endow social interaction with confusing and irrelevant associations" (Foss-Feig et al. 2010, 387–88). This would leave the person straining for coherence and, perhaps, adapting by trying to limit input to one perceptual stream at a time. This is a strategy frequently mentioned by people with autism, who report a strong preference for attending to visual and auditory information separately; sights and sounds experienced together are reported as overwhelming and difficult or impossible to process. In my son's words to a teacher, "If I look at you, I can't hear you. If you want me to hear you, I can't look at you." Applying a movement approach, we might decide that it is counterproductive to insist on eye contact while communicating verbally with a person with autism. We also might be less likely to take for granted the large amount of information that is embedded not in the content of our words to them but visually (i.e., in the context of our facial expressions and body language), and to remember that this visual information might not be processed simultaneously or accurately.

The existence of significant nonvolitional performance variability may also encourage us to rethink the ways classroom instruction and testing are set up, and to wonder about the ways in which typical education and treatment goals for people with autism are structured. Currently, success is defined and knowledge measured in predictable performances of a task (e.g., 8 times out of 10, with 90% accuracy and complete independence), with the person's precarious balance of internal state and task conditions destabilized by mounting pressure, time constraints, and increased demands for the instant replay of a successful act. We may find that we are inadvertently creating the very types of expectations and circumstances most likely to frustrate performance and lead to underestimations of capability and knowledge (Porges 2003).

A developing child with a TSPD or an enlarged binding window would presumably have a different set of developmental challenges to resolve than his or her neurotypical peers. For example, it seems possible that activities that appear to an observer to be pointlessly repetitious might not be perceived in that way by the child with autism, who may require many self-directed examples of a particular experience in order to integrate perceptually those aspects that belong together, and figure out which differences do not make a difference. More careful attention to movement and perception might open a window on how children with autism strive to explore and make sense of their worlds through play, and suggest more effective ways to enter into, support, and expand this core developmental activity, which has long been neglected in autism research and practice.

Exploring autism as an intense world, a TSPD, or the product of an enlarged binding window may throw light on one other aspect of variable performance in autism that is very familiar to parents and increasingly catching the attention of teachers and service providers: the emergence of intensely preferred interests. Many, if not most, people with autism seem to seek order and coherence through mastering at least one information system that structures and relates aspects of their experiential world, often with vast detail and precision. These information systems are often given the prosaic name of *preferred interests*, but some individuals with autism prefer the term *passions* (Stillman 2009). By including these interests as a form of variable performance, I hope to emphasize the way they seem to stand out in technicolor and three-dimensionally against a grey backdrop of topics in which the person may invest little or no emotion or even recognition, as well as the way he or she tends to mobilize or catalyze more self-regulated and organized performance. I have known youngsters who have enthusiastically accumulated an encyclopedic knowledge of everything from spiders to washing machines to traffic lights. My own son was mesmerized by the big metal storage tanks found around chemical manufacturing plants (a variant, perhaps, of the fascination most young children have with boxes, buckets, and bins, only more heroic in scale).

It may be significant that these passions frequently crystallize around preexisting systems of knowledge classification, such as road maps, train schedules, TV schedules, astronomical charts, calendars, the Linnaean classification system, the Dewey Decimal System, the top 40 songs on the hit parade, or sports statistics. When engaged with an intensely preferred interest, individuals frequently demonstrate an uncharacteristically high level of patience, motivation, attention, and time "on task," yet there is no body of research addressing how and why these very specialized topics emerge as such dynamic forces in many children's development. One hypothesis might be that such intense interests represent a coherent experience that the child has succeeded in rescuing from the noise and disorder of his or her nervous system. In a frighteningly intense and unpredictable world, that interest or passion may provide a hard-won platform that holds still, feels safe, and could be exploited as an anchor for stabilizing and exploring other aspects of perception. This would mean that, instead of discouraging such interests as perseverative or bizarre, or taking them away—as many programs do—to be controlled as rewards and withheld as punishment, we need to appreciate and engage with them as primary organizing systems.

The power of preferred or passionate interests has been independently discovered by many parents and professionals, given a variety of names, and mobilized successfully on behalf of different age groups, needs, and objectives. In developmental, individual difference, relationship-based (DIR) therapy, commonly known as "floor time," these interests become the key to coaxing the preschool child into increasingly sustained social interactions (Greenspan 1992; Greenspan and Benderly 1997; Greenspan and Wieder 2006; Greenspan et al. 1998; Wieder and Greenspan 2003). In pivotal response training (PRT), they supply the core motivation that triggers more intentional activity across other domains (Koegel et al. 1998; Koegel and Koegel 2006). Affinity therapy, widely popularized by the book *Life, Animated* (Suskind 2014), in which a young man on the autism spectrum develops an intense interest in Disney cartoon characters, clearly demonstrates the use of preferred interests to scaffold and explore complex emotions and social communication. Meanwhile, providers of adult vocational services have adopted a new job placement technique, called the discovery process, which draws on preferred interests to customize employment options (Callahan et al. 2005). It may be noteworthy that the frustrating performance variability experienced by people with autism appears to diminish in the presence of a preferred interest, however unusual or unlikely, as if that special area of expertise creates an optimal space in which the person can operate more effectively. A unified field theory of preferred interests has yet to be proposed, but the energy invested in them suggests that they matter.

Complex and Effortful Movement Strategies: Delayed Habituation

"My senses and body parts did not work as a unit" states self-advocate Tom Page, reflecting on his childhood (Young 2011, 166). Many parents express puzzlement and concern over the complex and often exhausting negotiations a child with autism seems to be having with his or her body. Instead of developing a predictable and (from a parent's point of view) efficient, labor-saving way to get things done, a child might approach everyday activities in ways that seem roundabout and indirect, adding extra steps, literally or figuratively. Parents may report a son or daughter's need to repeatedly pace outside a doorway before he or she can walk through, to touch or sniff a series of items each time he or she enters a room, to restart a task from the beginning if interrupted, or to engage in an elaborate repertoire of seemingly extraneous movements whenever it is time to transition from one activity to another. In addition, many routine activities do not seem to become habitual or easier over time. For example, while most adults can tie their shoes automatically while watching the TV news and talking to their partner, that everyday activity might require as much focus and effort for an adult with autism as it did when he or she was a child.

The recent work of Elizabeth Torres and colleagues (Torres et al. 2013a, 2013b, 2013c, 2016; Torres and Donnellan 2015; this volume) demonstrates that people with autism are receiving noisy, random feedback to and from their PNSs, barring them from creating a reliable internal map of the physical world and a feel for their bodies moving, through time and space, across that map. Without such a bodily sense, movement does not spontaneously adjust to task demands and our intricate body-based perception of time collapses into just two frames: the immediate present, surrounded by an uncharted and largely uninformative temporal expanse. While the movement systems of typically developing children adaptively self-organize in the direction of accumulating evidence toward predictive planning, these researchers find that children with autism are struggling with information that is processed in the "here and now," that is, with neurological systems that treat specific tasks as new whenever they are presented. Like the GPS in my car, they are constantly "recalculating." This does not mean that the children themselves have lost conscious awareness of their previous experiences; autism is not a form of amnesia (although such a possibility was once proposed). But despite past training with a given activity, the PNSs of these research subjects could utilize only the kinesthetic information available in the present moment (Brincker and Torres 2013, par. 6). Parents concur that repetition alone appears inadequate to acquire the automatic production of adaptive movement; the years of directed practice (and food rewards) that many children with autism receive are more likely to lead to prompt dependence than spontaneity.

At the brain level, researchers have used fMRI to document decreased overall connectivity and decreased activity in the cerebellum (a part of the brain focused on regulating movement) during simple motor task performance in children with autism compared with nonautistic peers, suggesting that these decreases may be associated with "difficulty shifting motor execution from cortical regions associated with effortful control to regions associated with habitual execution" and with "automating patterned motor behaviour" (Mostofsky et al. 2009). Others have called attention to motor patterns typical of earlier stages of development that are preserved in older children with autism, and have noted that in some children the level of motor development on the left and rights sides of the body may differ, manifesting as persistent asymmetry of movement or posture (Teitelbaum et al. 1998, 2004), as if development itself was occurring in a noisy, dys-synchronized way. All these findings would likely involve the person with autism in greater physical effort (due to repeatedly overshooting or undershooting the target) compared with the more fine-tuned and reliable efforts of nonautistic peers, as well as greater cognitive effort, since the person with autism must continue to attend to protocols and prompts to trigger and carry out activities that for others play out spontaneously.

A persistent theme in the autobiographical writings of people with autism is that of a body with a mind of its own. In its most extreme form, some people with autism recount frightening episodes in which their body "goes away," temporarily ceasing to provide the necessary feedback about where it is and what it is up to, and mention various "tricks" of movement they employ to regain that body awareness. (For ongoing examples, see the Proprioception Issues blog of the website Wrong Planet [wrongplanet.net].) It seems likely that at least some of the activity we have been calling aggressive or self-injurious may, in fact, represent panicked searches for missing sensory feedback, especially proprioception. Sue Rubin writes about her ongoing and strenuous efforts to "kill autism" in order to regain contact with her body, however temporarily (Rubin 1995). Nick Pentzell, a college student and frequent contributor to online publications, writes of his own sense of weary detachment from a body that defies him:

> I tell it to go to sleep, but it leaps on my bed. I tell it to want good and it goes for bad. I open the door to maturity and it slams it in my face. (Young 2011, 163)

Barbara Moran puts her own mind–body conflict memorably:

> If only people knew the reason why autistic people get upset so easily. Self-control is much harder because there is so much "self" to control. (Autism Support and Advocacy in Pennsylvania, n.d., available at http://www.aspergersyndrome.org/Article.aspx?j=50.)

Complex and effortful daily struggles with a recalcitrant, "memoryless" body may be a source of the frustration and fatigue that many parents observe in their children with autism. Fatigue is also one of the most common symptoms of Parkinson's, but adults with Parkinson's disease know how to ration their energy and how to make socially acceptable excuses when that energy flags; children do not. At a time in their lives when energy should be boundless, it is possible that fatigue itself is limiting opportunities to explore and causing children with autism to appear withdrawn and unsociable.

The movement perspective may help us take a fresh look at how these complex and effortful self-regulatory strategies—both conscious and unconscious, intentional and automatic—appear to the outside observer, and consider whether we have been misinterpreting them in ways that make the process of self-regulation harder. The common tendency to label as self-stimulatory, task avoidant, or attention seeking any behavior by people with autism that we find confusing may prevent us from seeing that a certain activity is internally triggered and nonvolitional (e.g., a complex motor tic, such as automatically reaching out to touch anyone who gets close), may be necessary to the individual's physiological self-regulation (as when my son corrects an imposed, overly rapid pace by rhythmically shaking an item in front of his eyes until his natural pace is restored), or may be a necessary adjunct to the performance of some other movement that the individual is trying to call forth. People with Parkinson's are well known for developing adjunct actions that only make sense as physiologically imposed detours on the way to the intended action. For example, when off my meds, I cannot simply reach out and hang up an item, such as a towel or coat. I can do a thorough task analysis, and raising four children has provided ample practice in hanging things up, yet the once habitual sequence of movements involved is, under those circumstances, inaccessible. The rather exhausting accommodation that works for me is to hold the item steady and jump so that it eventually lands on the bar or hook. I have seen children with autism enact what may represent similar self-taught accommodations—for example, clutching their jacket while jumping up and down in front of their coat hook at school—only to be admonished or punished for silliness and noncompliance.

People with Parkinson's and related conditions are also well known for devising ways to trigger movement patterns that have become inaccessible by means of allied and antagonistic reflexes, that is, distinct actions that share a common final pathway and can therefore work together to achieve an end, and distinct actions that inhibit the expression of another action (which also might be necessary to achieve an end). If you swing your arms wider while walking, for example, you will find that your legs respond by taking longer strides; this is a technique consciously employed by many people with Parkinson's. Some approaches to autism attempt to restart or reintegrate movement through similar techniques: Including modeling the action to be performed or "moving with" the person (i.e., supporting a nervous system that is challenged or "stuck" to ally with and cue off a smoothly functioning system), using indirection to trigger recalcitrant movements (as when a person must rock or pace for a period of time before plunging into a new activity pattern), and enhancing proprioception via touch, deep pressure, or rhythm (techniques used by many occupational therapists and neuromusicologists to help elicit and support the movement involved in speech and reciprocal social interactions).

Parents report that addressing the complex, effortful movement strategies of a child with autism requires intensive personalization that is itself complex and effortful. Many current programs and treatments generically marketed "for autism" do not feel this need to personalize interventions because their goal is to normalize: to stop seemingly extraneous behaviors or movement in their tracks. This "one-size-fits-all" approach to intervention does not ask what a person's movement might be supporting or regulating, and whether its suppression may impact other aspects of development. To think in terms of working *with* movement rather than working *against* behaviors, we may have to be prepared to travel with people with autism along what Barbara Moran calls "the scenic route," where the shortest distance between two points is not necessarily Euclid's straight line.

MARKED SIMILARITIES TO OTHER NEUROLOGICAL CONDITIONS INVOLVING MOVEMENT

As they cope with both childcare and the needs of aging family members, parents often observe that the behavior of a child with autism is uncannily similar to certain movement differences that emerge later in life. Research in the 1970s and 1980s demonstrated similarities between autism and many widely recognized features of Parkinson's disease (e.g., shorter and unusual gait, slower movement, unusual postures and hand motions and positions, and muted facial affect) (Damasio and Maurer 1978; Maurer and Damasio 1982; Vilensky et al. 1981). At the time, however, there was little context within the autism field for realizing the implications of these findings. In children with autism, slowness continued to be presumptively linked to cognitive deficiencies and task avoidance, unusual hand movements were framed as ritualistic or self-stimulatory behaviors, and the poker face was believed to signify lack of sociability. Rather than provoking further curiosity, these movement differences were routinely tagged for behavioral intervention with a goal of extinction. Ironically, by the time my son reached young adulthood, he was able to recognize clearly the similarity between his own movement patterns and his grandfather's decline into Alzheimer's, observing at one point, "Granddad is just like me now. He takes little steps, he talks very soft, and when you ask him something, he just says 'okay.'" Other useful comparisons can be made between autism and well-known movement disturbances, such as Tourette's and obsessive-compulsive disorder (OCD), as well as to traumatic brain injuries, with their intermittent good days and bad days.

Nowadays, most of us are familiar with the concept of creating accommodations for people with disabilities. The Americans with Disabilities Act greatly enhanced public awareness of accommodations, such as curb cuts and braille in elevators, by requiring that U.S. citizens with disabilities have access to public places. Accommodations have been defined as "adjustments or adaptations of an interaction, a task, situation, or the environment that assist a person to temporarily get around difficulties organizing and regulating sensory information or movement" (Donnellan et al. 2012, par. 18). Well-recognized movement differences such as Parkinson's are associated with a variety of successful accommodations, for example, the use of technology to alleviate struggles with handwriting, or the provision of an ergonomic workstation. It seems reasonable to consider whether the extensive literature concerning accommodations for Parkinson's and other familiar motor and sensory challenges (including visual and auditory impairments) could be mined productively in support of people with autism.

Historically, there have been two major barriers to such cross-disability activity. First, movement accommodations need to be adjusted on an ongoing basis; like movement itself, they are always in flux. What works for a person today may change tomorrow. The autism field, in contrast, has tended to overvalue replication over the types of exploration that lead to self-discovery under variable contexts. People are taught to carry out a task in the same prescribed and predictable way, based on the same predictable prompt, every time. There is little time or encouragement for individuals to test, add, discard, and remake coherent cause-and-effect interactions with the world through movement and perception. Successful accommodations for a person with autism, as with any other movement difference, will need to value exploration over replication, provide guidance rather than directives, seek the individual's optimal conditions for learning and performance, and emphasize self-exploration and real experience over artificial settings. Successful accommodations must be collaboratively designed with the person themselves; as the research of Torres et al. (2013c) very elegantly demonstrates, they must take account of the person's own self-explorations and self-designed solutions. In this body of research, it was only when the children spontaneously self-discovered cause and effect that the motor noise dampened and the randomness of motions turned into highly predictable actions. Four weeks later, they returned to the experiment and did even better than when they first started. Generalization and retention of their self-made movement accommodations had occurred. The message was clear: to impose or direct accommodations in a top-down manner is to seriously undermine their effectiveness. Prompting and external reward alone will not be conducive to autonomy, self-reliance, and independence.

A second barrier to the exploration of accommodations for people with autism lies in the presumptions we make based on the onset of a person's movement challenges. When we notice the emergence of movement differences in an adult, we continue to approach and respond to that person according to our years of shared experience. We feel confident that we know them, and are working within the context of that existing relationship. But when a child behaves in atypical ways from birth, we have no previous experience to work from. It becomes all too easy to presume the child's actions are randomly oppositional and pointless, leading to serious underestimations of their capabilities rather than to a search for movement accommodations.

The way out of this impasse is through a conscious decision, often referred to as a "presumption of competence." For parents, teachers, and support staff, this means approaching the child or adult with autism as a competent, social individual who is motivated to make sense of his or her experiences and has ways to communicate, even if we are still working out how to support those activities. It means that our attitudes matter deeply, that we cannot talk over people as if they do not understand, and that we must respond age appropriately rather than treat adults as children, or children as babies. For researchers, it means treating people with autism as stakeholders in, and not merely subjects of, their research. In the words of a slogan popularized by self-advocates, it demands "Nothing about us without us."

In a movement approach, accommodations are based on the presumption of competence. Rather than seeing the person as a collection of deficits to be remediated, we are invited to concentrate on the capabilities and motivations that are present and can be built on. The focus shifts from preemptively forcing change on the person with a disability, to changing the physical environment; the behavior, attitudes, and assumptions of other people; and the tools available for the person to use, so that change emerges in a dynamic, organic way. The movement approach aims to reduce noise and enhance reliability in the person's nervous systems so that, instead of more restrictions and extrinsic demands being placed on his or her activity, he or she can experience more degrees of freedom to explore, self-direct, and self-organize.

Accommodations come in many shapes and sizes, and are only limited by the imaginations of those designing them. Some involve technology, including many potentially useful communication devices, but others are low tech and involve changes in how we interact or what we do. It can be helpful to think of accommodations as falling into three main types. Environmental accommodations are the best known and often the easiest to identify. In essence, they change the environment so that it responds more effectively to the person's needs. Many parents and teachers of people with autism have learned, for example, that it may be helpful to dim bright lights, soundproof rooms, avoid sudden loud noises, replace visual clutter with visual systems of organization, use unscented cleaning products, and avoid unexpected rearrangements of everything from the living room furniture to today's class schedule. These accommodations may work because they simplify or clarify the signals, and reduce the noise, in an overburdened PNS. But there are, by my reckoning, two other, less familiar types of accommodations to which the movement differences of autism may respond. While environmental accommodations help the environment respond to the person, self-regulatory accommodations are strategies, systems, or devices that help the person himself of herself respond more effectively to his or her environment, both internal and external. Assistive technology, including augmentative and alternative communication (AAC), offers examples of systems and devices that enhance a person's ability to assert control or influence over his or her world. A self-regulatory accommodation might also take the form of an opportunity or means to more effectively control one's own body, for example, to squeeze a "fidget" ball or initiate deep-breathing exercises in response to stress. Each individual with autism is also likely to have created unrecognized self-regulatory accommodations of his or her own; to identify and understand them, we need to partner with and learn from that person.

Interactive accommodations, the third variety, involve changing the ways we and others relate to people with autism, based on an understanding of their sensory and movement differences. The so-called "soft" assistive technologies, which include changes in the behavior, attitudes, expectations, and interactive rhythm and timing of those who support a person with a disability, are examples of interactive accommodations. These are perhaps the least recognized and least understood of the accommodations, but parents report that their absence can be devastating. The willingness to cultivate accommodating *relationships*—to change and adapt oneself, rather than rush in to change someone else—can mark the difference between a successful teacher, aide, support person, physician, therapist, or caregiver, and a disaster of epic proportions. Sue Rubin writes about the profound effect of respectful relationships on her most basic abilities to learn and control her movements:

> When the teacher is well prepared and assumes all students are capable, I sit quietly and behave. When the teacher is disorganized and assumes we are stupid, I can't control my outbursts. Awful feelings come over me and I have to leave the classroom. (Rubin 1995)

Whether a family member is born with or acquires a movement difference, caregivers testify to the importance of keeping them included in a network of home and community relationships. Given its developmental significance and primary role in tapping into an individual's competence, relationship can perhaps be viewed as the *ur*-accommodation that creates the logic and the template for all the rest.

A Strong Need for Relationship-Based Approaches

The subject of relationships brings us to the last of our quartet of parent observations. Since a quartet is also a musical term, it may be fitting that these final notes concern the dance of relationship (Stern 1985). Through this universal parent–child dance beginning at birth, we are guided to explore the world and become aware of the possibilities of our lives. We learn to attach shared meanings to our emotions and experiences, to figure out what is and is not considered important, and to test our emerging ideas by seeing how others respond. Bit by bit, we develop motivation and direction as our daily experiments receive positive and gratifying responses. Relationships shape us—not in a coercive way, but as mutually engaged participants exploring the world together. We learn to trust, to give and take, and ultimately to empathize and "feel with" others (Amos 2013).

When my son was very young, it surprised me that sustaining this dance of relationship could take so much concentration. I had never met another baby who seemed so hard to woo, so difficult to comfort, so reactive to—rather than engaged by—touch and sound. As I got to know other parents of children with autism, I realized my experience was not unique. We traded advice on how to attract and hold our children's attention, learning by trial and error that it is vital to let them set the pace and to cue the interaction to their longer, slower rhythms. Then, as now, many parents also reported only fleeting success in one-way interactions demanding that the child "look at me," come here, toss the ball, say "juice," and so forth. These directives appear to have little meaning; if we instilled them via rewards and consequences, we felt a momentary sense of accomplishment, followed by a letdown when the child's responses tended to remain prompt dependent and inflexible over time. In other words, that sense of accomplishment may be ours alone, and not mutual. Parents' best successes seem to come not when we concentrate on the cultivation of certain skills, but when we work first and foremost on the cultivation of relationships, specifically, relationships in which the child is accommodated to explore and discover those aspects of experience for which he or she feels a natural affinity.

Of course, not all relationships are created equal or pursued with an appreciation of their true significance. In some interventions for children with autism, the opportunity for relationship is set aside as a reward to be earned by good behavior or considered an optional feature to be added to a child's academic or therapy program if time permits. The quality of a child's relationships may be considered a soft and fuzzy commodity unsuitable for observation, evaluation, or serious discussion in a tough-minded school or treatment program. And some parents, still haunted by the ghost of Bruno Bettelheim (1967) and psychoanalysis past, are relieved to remove that particular discussion from the table. However, an increasing number of educators and researchers in child development have come to recognize the dance of relationship as central to development for all children, and especially vital to pursue with those children who, due to movement differences, are most at risk of sitting out the dance.

If relationships are to become the foundation of how we approach, work with, and support a child who is developing differently, researchers and parents suggest that they must be *reciprocal.* Psychologist and psycholinguist Morton Ann Gernsbacher characterizes reciprocity as a "two-way street" and suggests that many parents and professionals "have neglected the reciprocal nature of reciprocity" (Gernsbacher 2006, 140). While one-way relationships based on controlling the actions of others can provide a type of structure around which to organize experience, their usefulness seems to be limited by their rigidity. Developmental psychologist Alan Fogel expresses this limitation with great insight:

> Information becomes available only through active engagement.... When relationships evolve into patterns in which participants perceive them as sequences of discrete exchanges of reward and cost it is quite likely that the creativity has gone out of them. They are no longer dynamic systems in which individuals grow, they have become prisons of the soul. (Fogel 1993, 89–90)

In considering the emergence of joint attention near the end of the first year of a typically developing child's life, Gernsbacher—herself the parent of a child with autism—argues that movement differences create a heightened need for reciprocity:

> But what about the child who is delayed in developing the ability to follow his parent's line of vision? What about the child who is delayed in developing the ability to make use of pointing gestures, that is, to follow a parent's manual point or to make his own pointing gesture? Or even to make his own reaching gesture? Experience suggests that this is when parents—and professionals—need to enact even more reciprocity, need to share even more of the child's world, need to follow even more of the child's lead, and need to become something of a detective to discern the ways that the child is expressing joint attention and social and emotional reciprocity. (Gernsbacher 2006, 145)

Relationship, to the degree that it is a mutual dance based on reciprocity, can be seen as the participatory process through which we co-create meaning. Since the final decades of the last century, developmental theories of learning have increasingly assigned a central role to meaning and its formation. Meaning—socially constructed, satisfying, and engaging—is unlikely to emerge from one-way relationships based on the manipulation of stimuli and reinforcement. Only those experiences that actively involve the child in making sense of his or her world may be considered to constitute actual, usable learning, because these are the experiences that become part of a person's self-organization and self-regulation, and can be interconnected in increasingly complex dynamics of development. Self-advocate Alberto Frugone puts it this way:

> It's necessary for me to gain real experience. While trying to perform an action, even if my gestures are difficult, I obtain valid practice. But it has to be a practical, contextual action not an artificial situation. (Biklen et al. 2005, 187)

This growing appreciation of the need to support self-regulation through real experience is evident in the increasing popularity of approaches such as DIR or floor time (Greenspan and Wieder 1997), which links relationship and the co-creation of meaning in an intentional practice that parents and other caregivers can self-monitor and, if needed, professionals can coach. Parents are encouraged to "follow the child's lead" by engaging actively and nondidactively around the child's strong interests, affirming what the child enjoys. To be successful, they must step out of the standard parenting role and into the role of the slightly older, slightly wiser friend, who can collaborate with the child to discover possibilities otherwise just beyond his or her reach, and provide the support needed to grow into new abilities. (The spirit of psychologist Lev Vygotsky [Vygotskiĭ and Cole 1978] seems to hover closely over this enterprise.) DIR emphasizes that relationship triggers and sustains development by helping the child with autism to organize and make sense of everyday experiences at the body level, and then building on that shared success to enlarge the child's frame of reference slowly, from within (Greenspan and Shanker 2007). It recognizes that experiences that do not make sense to the developing child because they are not integrated through movement, and which do not connect with anything beyond an artificial, extrinsic reward or punishment, generally remain unavailable for incorporation into other developmental processes. Their performance may be quickly dissipated. The frame of reference such unintegrated experiences create is still a dance of relationship, but as one movement expert memorably put it, it is "the box step" (Maurer, personal communication).

Torres and colleagues, coming from a neurological perspective on movement sensing, make essentially the same argument. In their recent research, they have devised task structures that serve to close an unreliable feedback loop in the PNS of young subjects with autism. With the link between certain (initially random) body movements and a desirable effect made highly salient, the children begin to evolve increasingly refined and targeted patterns of activity as they independently discover the link and systematically pursue increasing access to its compelling effect. When researchers "give spontaneity and self-discovery a chance in ASD" (Torres et al. 2013c) by setting the stage for self-directed exploration under mutually adaptive conditions, they find that random movement is gradually subsumed into goal-directed movement and, at an imperceptible level, random noise is transformed into well-structured, systematic noise: a signal controllable at will. Significantly, these advances in self-regulation are maintained over time, despite the absence of training based on external rewards.

Out of the lab, in everyday life, reciprocal relationships encourage spontaneity and self-discovery in strikingly similar ways: by assembling, on a flexible and moment-to-moment basis, the most adaptive conditions and accommodations for their emergence. More than a quarter century ago, a very influential occupational therapist named Jean Ayers observed about children with autism, "When the flow of sensation is disorganized, life can be like a rush-hour traffic jam" (Ayres and Robbins 1979, 5). People caught in the jam do not need a back-seat driver criticizing and shouting instructions as their panic grows; they need a calm companion to support them in discovering how to sort the signals from the noise.

CONCLUSION

My son was right: it *has* been a long, strange trip, one in which it was often hard to see the forest for the trees. Along the way, diagnosticians and researchers planted their flags of discovery at the locations of a multitude of behavioral deficits and cortical impairments, yet struggled to find some larger perspective within which to connect them. With our growing ability to envision how the dynamics of movement can affect a child's development and sense making, we finally may have reached a vantage point from which we can begin to redraw the autism map for modern travelers. Vast regions once in thrall to parent blaming or to blaming the person with autism—labeled, in the ancient mapmaking tradition, "Here be monsters"—may begin to open up for safe exploration. We may find ourselves talking more about how our children explore and make sense of the world, and about their emotional development, without the lingering fear that drawing attention to these challenges is either a self-indictment of our parenting skills or a wishful projection of our own aspirations, curiosity, and feelings onto beings who have none. We might chart those "islands of intelligence"—the unexpected but enticing phenomena that appear on the horizon when conditions are just right—and find that they are not illusory or free floating but connected, deep below the surface, to the mainland. We may learn to build sturdier bridges to reach them more reliably.

To build those bridges, we are going to have to look beyond brain-based and deficit-driven models of autism, understand sensing, and see movement: active, dynamic, and body based. The dance of relationship, through which we form a sense of self and understanding of others, emerges through coregulated movement. Perhaps autism research itself needs not only to study this dynamic, but also to incorporate more of the dance into its own practices. Movement researchers have observed that the congruence between their findings and the reports of self-advocates and parents "hinted at a latent, dispersed community already doing research on sensory motor disturbances in autism" (Torres and Donnellan 2015, par. 11). Bringing that diverse community together in an organized and effective way could lead to the emergence of dramatic, coregulated new developments; how appropriate and synergistic it would be to found a movement based on movement.

REFERENCES

American Psychological Association. 2009. ICD vs. DSM. *Monit Psychol* 40 (9):63.

Amos, P. 2013. Rhythm and timing in autism: Learning to dance. *Front Integr Neurosci* 7:27. doi: 10.3389/fnint.2013.00027.

Ayres, A. J., and J. Robbins. 1979. *Sensory Integration and the Child.* Los Angeles, CA: Western Psychological Services.

Baron-Cohen, S., A. M. Leslie, and U. Frith. 1985. Does the autistic child have a "theory of mind"? *Cognition* 21 (1):37–46. doi: 0010–0277(85)90022–8 [pii].

Bertalanffy, L. von. 1967. *Robots, Men, and Minds: Psychology in the Modern World.* New York: G. Braziller.

Bettelheim, B. 1967. The Empty Fortress: Infantile Autism and the Birth of the Self. New York: Free Press.

Biklen, D., R. Attfield, L. Bissonette, L. Blackman, J. Burke, A. Frugone, T. R. Mukhopadhyay, and S. Rubin. 2005. *Autism and the myth of the person alone.* New York: New York University.

Brincker, M., and E. B. Torres. 2013. Noise from the periphery in autism. *Front Integr Neurosci* 7:34. doi: 10.3389/fnint.2013.00034.

Brown, F., C. A. Michaels, C. M. Oliva, and S. B. Woolf. 2008. Personal paradigm shifts among ABA and PBS experts comparisons in treatment acceptability. *J Posit Behav Interv* 10 (4):212–27.

Bruner, J. S. 1990. *Acts of Meaning. The Jerusalem-Harvard Lectures.* Cambridge, MA: Harvard University Press.

Callahan, M., N. Shumpert, E. Condon, and M. Mast. 2005. *Discovery: Charting the Course to Employment.* Ocean Springs, MS: Marc Gold & Associates.

Costall, A. 2006. 'Introspectionism' and the mythical origins of scientific psychology. *Conscious Cogn* 15 (4): 634–54. doi: 10.1016/j.concog.2006.09.008.

Damasio, A. R., and R. G. Maurer. 1978. A neurological model for childhood autism. *Arch Neurol* 35 (12): 777–86.

Darweesh, S. K., P. J. Koudstaal, B. H. Stricker, A. Hofman, E. W. Steyerberg, and M. A. Ikram. 2016. Predicting Parkinson disease in the community using a nonmotor risk score. *Eur J Epidemiol* 31 (7): 679–84. doi: 10.1007/s10654–016–0130–1.

Deen, B., and K. Pelphrey. 2012. Perspective: Brain scans need a rethink. *Nature* 491 (7422):S20.

De Jaegher, H. 2013. Embodiment and sense-making in autism. *Front Integr Neurosci* 7:15.

Donnellan, A. M., D. A. Hill, and M. R. Leary. 2012. Rethinking autism: Implications of sensory and movement differences for understanding and support. *Front Integr Neurosci* 6:124. doi: 10.3389/fnint.2012.00124.

Donnellan, A. M., and M. R. Leary. 1995. *Movement Differences and Diversity in Autism/Mental Retardation: Appreciating and Accommodating People with Communication and Behavior Challenges.* Movin on Series. Madison, WI: DRI Press.

Eklund, A., T. E. Nichols, and H. Knutsson. 2016. Cluster failure: Why fMRI inferences for spatial extent have inflated false-positive rates. *Proc Natl Acad Sci USA* 113 (28):7900–5. doi: 10.1073/pnas.1602413113.

Fan, Y. T., J. Decety, C. Y. Yang, J. L. Liu, and Y. Cheng. 2010. Unbroken mirror neurons in autism spectrum disorders. *J Child Psychol Psychiatry* 51 (9):981–8. doi: 10.1111/j.1469–7610.2010.02269.x.

Fogel, A. 1993. *Developing through Relationships: Origins of Communication, Self, and Culture.* Chicago: University of Chicago Press.

Foss-Feig, J. H., L. D. Kwakye, C. J. Cascio, C. P. Burnette, H. Kadivar, W. L. Stone, and M. T. Wallace. 2010. An extended multisensory temporal binding window in autism spectrum disorders. *Exp Brain Res* 203 (2): 381–9. doi: 10.1007/s00221–010–2240–4.

Fournier, K. A., C. J. Hass, S. K. Naik, N. Lodha, and J. H. Cauraugh. 2010. Motor coordination in autism spectrum disorders: A synthesis and meta-analysis. *J Autism Dev Disord* 40 (10):1227–40. doi: 10.1007/s10803–010–0981–3.

Freedman, B. H., L. G. Kalb, B. Zablotsky, and E. A. Stuart. 2012. Relationship status among parents of children with autism spectrum disorders: A population-based study. *J Autism Dev Disord* 42 (4):539–48. doi: 10.1007/s10803–011–1269-y.

Gepner, B., and F. Feron. 2009. Autism: A world changing too fast for a mis-wired brain? *Neurosci Biobehav Rev* 33 (8):1227–42. doi: 10.1016/j.neubiorev.2009.06.006.

Gernsbacher, M. A. 2006. Toward a behavior of reciprocity. *J Dev Process* 1 (1):139–52.

Gernsbacher, M. A., and J. L. Frymiare. 2005. Does the autistic brain lack core modules? *J Dev Learn Disord* 9:3–16.

Gershon, M. D. 1998. *The Second Brain: The Scientific Basis of Gut Instinct and a Groundbreaking New Understanding of Nervous Disorders of the Stomach and Intestine.* 1st ed. New York: HarperCollins Publishers.

Gowen, E., and A. Hamilton. 2013. Motor abilities in autism: A review using a computational context. *J Autism Dev Disord* 43 (2):323–44. doi: 10.1007/s10803–012–1574–0.

Grandin, T. 1995. *Thinking in Pictures: And Other Reports from My Life with Autism.* 1st ed. New York: Doubleday.

Grant, A. 1965. Screams, slaps, and love. *Life*, 87–97.

Greenspan, S., and S. Shanker. 2007. The developmental pathways leading to pattern recognition, joint attention, language and cognition. *New Ideas Psychol* 25 (2):128–142.

Greenspan, S., and S. Wieder. 1997. Developmental patterns and outcomes in infants and children with disorders in relating and communicating: A chart review of 200 cases of children with autistic spectrum diagnoses. *J Dev Learn Disord* 1:1–38.

Greenspan, S. B. 1992. Reconsidering the diagnosis and treatment of very young children with autistic spectrum or pervasive developmental disorder. *Zero Three* 13 (2):1–9.

Greenspan, S. I., and B. L. Benderly. 1997. *The Growth of the Mind: And the Endangered Origins of Intelligence*. Reading, MA: Addison-Wesley.

Greenspan, S. I., and S. Wieder. 2006. *Infant and Early Childhood Mental Health: A Comprehensive, Developmental Approach to Assessment and Intervention. 1st ed.* Washington, DC: American Psychiatric Association.

Greenspan, S. I., S. Wieder, and R. Simons. 1998. *The Child with Special Needs: Encouraging Intellectual and Emotional Growth.* Reading, MA: Addison-Wesley.

Grinker, R. 2010. In retrospect: The five lives of the psychiatry manual. *Nature* 11:168–170. doi: doi:10.1038/468168a.

Hagerman, R., G. Hoem, and P. Hagerman. 2010. Fragile X and autism: Intertwined at the molecular level leading to targeted treatments. *Mol Autism* 1 (1):12. doi: 10.1186/2040–2392-1-12.

Happe, F., and U. Frith. 2006. The weak coherence account: Detail-focused cognitive style in autism spectrum disorders. *J Autism Dev Disord* 36 (1):5–25. doi: 10.1007/s10803–005–0039–0.

Kanner, L. 1943. Autistic disturbances of affective contact. *Acta Paedopsychiatr* 35 (4):100–36.

Kanner, L. 1995. Follow-up study of eleven autistic children originally reported in 1943. 1971 [in French]. *Psychiatr Enfant* 38 (2):421–61.

Koegel, L. K., R. L. Koegel, and C. M. Carter. 1998. Pivotal responses and the natural language teaching paradigm. *Semin Speech Lang* 19 (4):355–71; quiz 372; 424. doi: 10.1055/s-2008–1064054.

Koegel, R. L., and L. K. Koegel. 2006. *Pivotal Response Treatments for Autism: Communication, Social & Academic Development.* Baltimore: Paul H. Brookes.

Leary, M. R., and D. A. Hill. 1996. Moving on: Autism and movement disturbance. *Ment Retard* 34 (1):39–53.

Lorenz, K. 1996. *The natural science of the human species: An introduction to comparative behavioral research.* Cambridge, MA: MIT Press.

Lovaas, O. I. 1993. The development of a treatment-research project for developmentally disabled and autistic children. *J Appl Behav Anal* 26 (4):617–30. doi: 10.1901/jaba.1993.26-617.

Lovaas, O. I., R. Koegel, J. Q. Simmons, and J. S. Long. 1973. Some generalization and follow-up measures on autistic children in behavior therapy. *J Appl Behav Anal* 6 (1):131–65.

Markram, H., T. Rinaldi, and K. Markram. 2007. The intense world syndrome—An alternative hypothesis for autism. *Front Neurosci* 1 (1):77–96. doi: 10.3389/neuro.01.1.1.006.2007.

Martin, J. B. 2002. The integration of neurology, psychiatry, and neuroscience in the 21st century. *Am J Psychiatry* 159 (5):695–704. doi: 10.1176/appi.ajp.159.5.695.

Maurer, R. G. 1994. Autism, the brain, and the dance of relationships. Presented at the Autism National Committee 1994 Conference Rethinking Autism/PDD, King of Prussia, PA, April 22–23.

Maurer, R. G. 1995. Why study movement in autism? Presented at the NIH State-of-the-Science in Autism Conference, Bethesda, MD, April 11.

Maurer, R. G. 1996. Autism and the cerebellum: A neurophysiological basis for intervention. *The Communicator* (newsletter of the Autism National Committee), 1. http://www.autcom.org/articles/Cerebellum.html.

Maurer, R. G., and A. R. Damasio. 1982. Childhood autism from the point of view of behavioral neurology. *J Autism Dev Disord* 12 (2):195–205.

Minshew, N. J., G. Goldstein, and D. J. Siegel. 1997. Neuropsychologic functioning in autism: Profile of a complex information processing disorder. *J Int Neuropsychol Soc* 3 (4):303–16.

Mostofsky, S. H., S. K. Powell, D. J. Simmonds, M. C. Goldberg, B. Caffo, and J. J. Pekar. 2009. Decreased connectivity and cerebellar activity in autism during motor task performance. *Brain* 132 (Pt 9):2413–25. doi: 10.1093/brain/awp088.

NIH (National Institutes of Health). 2006. *Study provides evidence autism affects functioning entire brain.* https://www.nih.gov/news-events/news-releases/study-provides-evidence-autism-affects-functioning-entire-brain.

Niu, Y. Q., J. C. Yang, D. A. Hall, M. A. Leehey, F. Tassone, J. M. Olichney, R. J. Hagerman, and L. Zhang. 2014. Parkinsonism in fragile X-associated tremor/ataxia syndrome (FXTAS): Revisited. *Parkinsonism Relat Disord* 20 (4):456–9. doi: .10.1016/j.parkreldis.2014.01.006.

Ozonoff, S., and R. E. McEvoy. 1994. A longitudinal study of executive function and theory of mind development in autism. *Dev Psychopathol* 6 (3):415–31.

Park, C. C. 1967. *The Siege.* 1st ed. New York: Harcourt.

Pickett, E., O. Pullara, J. O'Grady, and B. Gordon. 2009. Speech acquisition in older nonverbal individuals with autism: A review of features, methods, and prognosis. *Cogn Behav Neurol* 22 (1):1–21 doi: 10.1097/WNN.0b013e318190d185.

Porges, S. W. 2003. The polyvagal theory: Phylogenetic contributions to social behavior. *Physiol Behav* 79 (3): 503–13.

Purves, D. 2012. *Neuroscience.* 5th ed. Sunderland, MA: Sinauer Associates.

Rimland, B. 1964. *Infantile Autism: The Syndrome and Its Implications for a Neural Theory of Behavior.* The Century Psychology Series. New York: Appleton-Century-Crofts.

Rizzolatti, G., M. Fabbri-Destro, and L. Cattaneo. 2009. Mirror neurons and their clinical relevance. *Nat Clin Pract Neurol* 5 (1):24–34. doi: 10.1038/ncpneuro0990.

Rogers, K., I. Dziobek, J. Hassenstab, O. T. Wolf, and A. Convit. 2007. Who cares? Revisiting empathy in Asperger syndrome. *J Autism Dev Disord* 37 (4):709–15. doi: 10.1007/s10803–006–0197–8.

Roux, A. M., P. T. Shattuck, J. E. Rast, J. A. Rava, A. D. Edwards, X. Wei, M. McCracken, and J. W. Yu. 2015. Characteristics of two-year college students on the autism spectrum and their support services experiences. *Autism Res Treat* 2015:391693. doi: 10.1155/2015/391693.

Rubin, S. 1995. Youth opinion: 'Killing autism is a constant battle.' *Los Angeles Times*, Issues Section, October 14. http://articles.latimes.com/1995-10-14/local/me-56785_1_constant-battle.

Sacks, O. 1990. *Awakenings*. 1st HarperPerennial ed. New York: HarperPerennial.

Schultz, R. T., I. Gauthier, A. Klin, R. K. Fulbright, A. W. Anderson, F. Volkmar, P. Skudlarski, C. Lacadie, D. J. Cohen, and J. C. Gore. 2000. Abnormal ventral temporal cortical activity during face discrimination among individuals with autism and Asperger syndrome. *Arch Gen Psychiatry* 57 (4):331–40.

Simuni, T., J. D. Long, C. Caspell-Garcia, C. S. Coffey, S. Lasch, C. M. Tanner, D. Jennings, K. D. Kieburtz, K. Marek, and PPMI Investigators. 2016. Predictors of time to initiation of symptomatic therapy in early Parkinson's disease. *Ann Clin Transl Neurol* 3 (7):482–94. doi: 10.1002/acn3.317.

Southgate, V., and A. F. Hamilton. 2008. Unbroken mirrors: Challenging a theory of autism. *Trends Cogn Sci* 12 (6):225–9. doi: 10.1016/j.tics.2008.03.005.

Stern, D. N. 1985. *The Interpersonal World of the Infant: A View from Psychoanalysis and Developmental Psychology*. New York: Basic Books.

Stillman, W. 2009. *Empowered Autism Parenting: Celebrating (and Defending) Your Child's Place in the World.* 1st ed. San Francisco: Jossey-Bass.

Suskind, R. 2014. *Life, Animated: A Story of Sidekicks, Heroes, and Autism. 1st ed.* New York: Kingswell.

Teitelbaum, O., T. Benton, P. K. Shah, A. Prince, J. L. Kelly, and P. Teitelbaum. 2004. Eshkol-Wachman movement notation in diagnosis: The early detection of Asperger's syndrome. *Proc Natl Acad Sci USA* 101 (32): 11909–14. doi: 10.1073/pnas.0403919101.

Teitelbaum, P., O. Teitelbaum, J. Nye, J. Fryman, and R. G. Maurer. 1998. Movement analysis in infancy may be useful for early diagnosis of autism. *Proc Natl Acad Sci USA* 95 (23):13982–7.

Thelen, E., and L. B. Smith. 1994. *A Dynamic Systems Approach to the Development of Cognition and Action.* MIT Press/Bradford Books Series in Cognitive Psychology. Cambridge, MA: MIT Press.

Thompson, R. A. 1994. Emotion regulation: A theme in search of definition. *Monogr Soc Res Child Dev* 59 (2–3): 25–52.

Torres, E. B. 2011. Two classes of movements in motor control. *Exp Brain Res* 215 (3–4):269–83. doi: 10.1007/s00221-011-2892-8.

Torres, E. B., and A. M. Donnellan. 2015. Editorial for research topic "Autism: The movement perspective." *Front Integr Neurosci* 9:12. doi: 10.3389/fnint.2015.00012.

Torres, E. B., J. Nguyen, C. Suresh, P. Yanovich, and A. Kolevzon. 2013b. Noise from the periphery in autism spectrum disorders of idiopathic origins and of known etiology. San Diego: Society for Neuroscience.

Torres, E. B., M. Brincker, R. W. Isenhower, P. Yanovich, K. A. Stigler, J. I. Nurnberger, D. N. Metaxas, and J. V. Jose. 2013a. Autism: The micro-movement perspective. *Front Integr Neurosci* 7:32. doi: 10.3389/fnint.2013.00032.

Torres, E. B., P. Yanovich, and D. N. Metaxas. 2013c. Give spontaneity and self-discovery a chance in ASD: Spontaneous peripheral limb variability as a proxy to evoke centrally driven intentional acts. *Front Integr Neurosci* 7:46. doi: 10.3389/fnint.2013.00046.

Torres, E. B., R. W. Isenhower, J. Nguyen, C. Whyatt, J. I. Nurnberger, J. V. Jose, S. M. Silverstein, T. V. Papathomas, J. Sage, and J. Cole. 2016. Toward precision psychiatry: Statistical platform for the personalized characterization of natural behaviors. *Front Neurol* 7:8 doi: 10.3389/fneur.2016.00008.

Trevarthen, C. 2011. What is it like to be a person who knows nothing? Defining the active intersubjective mind of a newborn human being. *Infant Child Dev* 20 (1):119–35. doi: doi: 10.1002/icd.689.

Vilensky, J. A., A. R. Damasio, and R. G. Maurer. 1981. Gait disturbances in patients with autistic behavior: A preliminary study. *Arch Neurol* 38 (10):646–9.

Von Holst, E., and H. Mittelstaedt. 1950. The principle of reafference: Interactions between the central nervous system and the peripheral organs. In *Perceptual Processing: Stimulus Equivalence and Pattern Recognition*, ed. P. C. Dodwell, 41–72. New York: Appleton-Century-Crofts.

Vygotskiĭ, L. S., and M. Cole. 1978. *Mind in Society: The Development of Higher Psychological Processes.* Cambridge, MA: Harvard University Press.

Walden, R. 2012. Autism: Origins unknown, but women still get the blame. *Women's Health Activist*, November–December.

Watson, J. B. 1913. Psychology as the behaviorist views it. *Psychol Rev* 20:158–67.

Wieder, S., and S. I. Greenspan. 2003. Climbing the symbolic ladder in the DIR model through floor time/interactive play. *Autism* 7 (4):425–35. doi: 10.1177/1362361303007004008.

Williams, D. 1996. *Autism, an Inside-Out Approach: An Innovative Look at the Mechanics of 'Autism' and Its Developmental 'Cousins'*. London: J. Kingsley.

Williams, D. L., G. Goldstein, and N. J. Minshew. 2006. Neuropsychologic functioning in children with autism: Further evidence for disordered complex information-processing. *Child Neuropsychol* 12 (4–5):279–98. doi: 10.1080/09297040600681190.

Young, S. R. 2011. *Real People, Regular Lives: Autism, Communication & Quality of Life*. Madison, WI: Lifeline Typing LLC.

21 Shiloh
The Outstanding Outlier

*Summer Pierce**

It was in March 2015 that we first met Shiloh and her family. As was the case with all other families, Shiloh's mother and grandparents formed a cohesive unit that became an extension of our own lab family. Full of joy, Shiloh and her family stole our hearts. Here is some of their journey in her mom's own words.

After 9 long months, we welcomed Shiloh into the world, a healthy baby girl weighing 7 pounds 14 ounces and measuring 21.5 inches. She was an instant source of pride and anxiety—a peculiar mix that I'm sure is familiar to most first-time parents. After years of working in the area of child development, I was thrilled to be a mom. Given my clinical experience, I couldn't help but watch as my daughter developed, noting when she gained new skills, from lifting her head and rolling over, to following my gaze. I remained unconsciously hypervigilant throughout her early months, drawing on my training and making mental notes from my experience with applied behavior analysis and occupational (OT), physical (PT), and speech therapies. Nevertheless, no amount of training could have prepared me for the emotional rollercoaster to come—I could not foresee that I would need to draw on my own career to help my own daughter toward fulfilling her potential.

It was when Shiloh was 7 months that I began to notice a plateau in her development. Trying my best to attribute this to first-time mother nerves, I silently noted that she was having difficulty sitting independently, and that her limited vocabulary seemed to have a singular underlying sound. I struggled to reconcile the fact that Shiloh was a sociable, smiling baby girl who was developing the beginnings of communication, with this plateau. Noting her floppy-like posture (hypotonia) and slightly large head (macrocephaly), (ABA), I knew it was time to seek the specialists. It was when Shiloh was around 1 year old that I made the difficult decision to take her for a consultation—our journey toward diagnosis had begun.

I began the long road with a team of specialists who mirrored my concerns and honed in on Shiloh's language and motor development. Shiloh began completing a range of short tests to examine areas of concern, but having weight behind my concern, I refused to wait for the results of this chain of events, and decided to take some matters into my own hands. I began Shiloh on a range of programs at my practice, including ABA strategies to help her learn animals, colors, shapes, numbers, and letters; speech therapy to enhance her language; and PT to help her progress through the remaining motor milestones. The change in Shiloh was gradual, but it was certainly noticeable. She learned to crawl, pull herself up to standing, and turn pages of books. Meanwhile, I bounced between consultations in search of an answer to my questions—with Shiloh not displaying any "typical signs" for a particular developmental issue, we moved between specialists, finding new complications at each turn. I was continually told that she was simply delayed, would grow out of it, or that the particular specialist I was seeing could do nothing to help. Finally, her pediatrician suggested a specific neurologist who he trusted and could see her quickly.

* Written by Caroline Whyatt on behalf of Summer Pierce.

It was during the initial consultation with this neurologist to address Shiloh's stalled development, that both an MRI scan and a microarray genetic consultation were suggested. The geneticists I consulted with could not point to any specific genetic complication to screen for and suggested a microarray screen. The MRI, which was initially completed more as a precautionary measure to screen for neurodevelopment difficulties, found evidence of a massive subdural hematoma—meaning that my 2-year-old had a buildup of blood, preventing the left-hand side of her brain from fully filling into her skull. Naturally, this became our primary concern, and so any thought of genetic testing became a distant memory. I listened in a fog as the specialist explained that they were "stunned" by how much progress Shiloh had made up to this point, with the subdural hematoma stunting her brain development—my Shiloh had somehow begun beating the odds. However, given the volume of liquid, which left one side of her brain resembling that of a 9-month-old child, surgery was recommended. Immediately.

The prospect of neurosurgery is terrifying for anyone, let alone a young child and her terrified mother, but when Shiloh was almost 2½ years old, she had surgery. A staggering 160 mL of blood was successfully drained from the cavity between her developing brain and skull. The buildup to the surgery was fraught with tension and anxiety, and was the most terrifying hour and half of my life. Shiloh's fighting spirit shone through the experience, and the surgery was a resounding success. The removal of the blood buildup quickly allowed her brain to begin the process of recovery, and it wasn't long until I saw an explosion in Shiloh's vocabulary, with her quickly acquiring more than 200 functional words. However, despite this radical change and progression in development, I noticed that Shiloh was still not making progress with independent walking. PT and OT had highlighted issues with hyperpronation of the bones of both of her feet—causing Shiloh to effectively stand on her ankles, severely hindering her progress. So at 3 years old, Shiloh went through a new round of surgery with a fantastic orthopedic team to correct the bone alignment in both feet. This was followed by a follow-up surgery 1 year later. Both surgeries were a success, and I gradually reduced the use of ankle supports and braces, allowing Shiloh to gain more functional independence. My initial concerns quelled, and I watched as my young fighter continued to overcome hurdles at every turn. Completing three surgeries by the age of 4, more than many in a lifetime, my daughter refused to comply with expectations—healing quickly, and free of the physical burden, forging ahead on the developmental path.

Despite all her progress, Shiloh was given a formal diagnosis of Phelan–McDermid syndrome at 4 years old. I decided to take Shiloh to the Cleveland Clinic for a consultation, as they were supposed to be one of the best pediatric neurology departments in the country. I vividly remember everything about the process. From the initial consultation with the pediatric neurologist at the Cleveland Clinic, to the brutal way the news was delivered over the phone months later. My life had been in turmoil with the range of surgeries since Shiloh's first developmental screening, and so I had foregone the genetic testing. Now, speaking with the consultant 3 years later, I was advised to progress with a microgenetic array screening. The appointment was a disaster. The doctor dismissed all the gains Shiloh had made since her neurosurgery, refused to acknowledge Shiloh's limited language, and acted as though my child wasn't even in the room. The one positive of the appointment was that we had a range of testing completed before we left. The results would take several weeks to process and the doctor would inform of me of the results. A month later, I got the phone call that would change my world entirely. I was not prepared—in any way—for the words to come: "rare genetic condition" and "Phelan–McDermid syndrome." The words rang through my head. Admitting to knowing nothing of this syndrome, the clinician then explained that he looked up the genetic disorder on Wikipedia and pronounced a sentence on my child (https://en.wikipedia.org/wiki/22q13_deletion_syndrome). He reinforced this devastating news by informing me that I could be assured that Shiloh would "never walk, talk, and will be retarded for the rest of her life"—a sentence that cut to the bone. Struggling to process and rationalize the extent of the repercussions on Shiloh's life, the severity of the prognosis, and the apparent lack of medical understanding, my mind began racing. As if Shiloh did not exist, this doctor effectively told me that my daughter was devoid of any prospects.

My daughter had become reduced to a piece of paper with genetic results that would restrict and limit her existence now and for years to come.

Still in a state of shock, at both the diagnosis and the cold, uninformed manner in which it had been delivered, I made an appointment with a geneticist in South Carolina. Accompanied by my father for moral support, we traveled to see yet another doctor. We sat patiently for the much awaited consultation to begin, not aware that this moment would change Shiloh's life, and our family, forever. Sitting in her grandfather's lap, Shiloh read a much loved Dr. Seuss book, oblivious to the gravity of the consultation. During the consultation, the doctor examined her genetic results and concluded that her deletion was more sizable than most, but his approach to us as a family was totally different. He watched Shiloh interact with both her grandfather and myself. He listened to her ask for Teddy Graham cookies, and even with her poorly articulated speech, he praised her. It was at this point we were told that Shiloh was the only child with her particular genetic deletion that he had come across that had any language at all. I was staggered by the revelation, and it helped me resolve to continue to push her as hard as I could to see what else we could accomplish.

It took a year of grieving for my life to make sense again—and long days researching the little known genetic condition. I instinctively attempted to draw on my own clinical experience to regain composure and rationalize the diagnosis, but failed miserably. Despite dedicating my life to working with children with a range of special needs, nothing prepared me for this moment. I reacted as I imagine any parent would. Despite the long and uneasy road I had up to this point, the diagnosis had ripped my world apart and left me mourning the loss of my "typically" developing child. With the support and love from my extended family and friends, I allowed myself the time to grieve, experiencing a range of emotions and dark days. I carried the words that were so brutally delivered by the clinician in my head—playing on repeat—constantly worrying about the stark prognosis that had been so confidently discussed. In hindsight, I am disappointed in the lack of support from the doctor at the Cleveland Clinic who first delivered the devastating news—after which I was left wondering, "What next?" Shiloh started kindergarten at age 5 in a self-contained classroom through the public school. We have been lucky enough to have access to all the resources she needs and have been blessed with amazing teachers. If it wasn't for the fact that Shiloh was in an established routine of OT, PT, speech therapy, and ABA through my clinical practice, I am not sure where we would be today. The initial year after her genetic diagnosis was full of emotional days and long nights, but we came through it as a stronger mother–daughter team. Gazing at the face of my young daughter, who loves to listen to fifties and sixties classics such as Frankie Vallie, the Four Seasons, and the Beach Boys; who loves to eat any and all food; and who can make me smile even on the most difficult of days, I realized we had simply needed time. Time to process, be angry, make sense of the information, and ask the hard questions. This time had allowed me to emerge fighting for the best chance at life I can give my daughter, but more importantly, accepting her for the amazing little person she is every day.

I later enrolled Shiloh in a clinical trial to examine the effectiveness of a novel drug in treating symptoms of Phelan–McDermid syndrome with the Seaver Center at Mount Sinai. As she had often before, Shiloh proved herself to be an outlier with her genetic disorder, surprising another set of doctors with her skills. We were informed, again, that she was the only child on the trial with language, functional or not. It was here that she was given several other diagnoses—autism spectrum disorder (ASD) included. At this point, Shiloh's progress had become so remarkable to the clinicians that her ASD diagnosis was "almost an afterthought." As a behavior analyst, I watched and shaped her behavior from the time she was a baby. "As such, she demonstrates no behavioral issues typical of ASD at all—no transition issues, no stereotypies, no self-injurious or aggressive behavior, etc. She was always compliant during testing," and tried hard to complete the work. Several clinicians who had worked with the team at the Seaver Center but had never come to the clinic came just to meet Shiloh. Each visit to Mount Sinai reinforced how amazing my little person is.

Today, we continue the diverse range of PT, OT, speech therapy, and ABA that we began when Shiloh was 1 year old, but complement these with a range of specialist interventions from across the country. For Shiloh, the diverse range, coupled with the consistency of these interventions, appears to be the key. Shiloh's perseverance and attitude have not faltered, and she has pushed through each session with a smile, and occasionally a dance. We have enrolled Shiloh in PT and OT programs that focus not only on functional outcomes for daily life, such as those provided through the schooling environment, but also on the development of the core fundamentals of motor control and proprioception, including establishing a frame of reference of her body, or a "body map." While Shiloh underwent regular PT and OT through her school, she appeared to lack an awareness of where her body was in space and time. These core fundamental principles are key to developing coherent motor control as they provide information for the coordination of your body in relation to itself, others, and objects within the environment. The establishment of this body map is therefore vital in the translation of motor learning into new contexts and the development of new skills. Through a reference from a client in my business, I found Euro-Peds, an intensive PT clinic in Michigan that has changed our lives. Use of Euro-Peds' high-pressure suit—inspired by NASA space suits that treat astronauts to remedy their proprioceptive readaptation to Earth's gravity field —is combined with the exercises to systematically provide Shiloh with pressure feedback to help her developing brain identify and map out her body through her senses of movement, pressure, and touch. This PT and OT program had a pronounced effect on Shiloh's motor coordination, leading to the development of new independent motor control and walking patterns that fall close to those of typical ranges, very different from her Phelan–McDermid syndrome fellows. Euro-Peds also targeted Shiloh's muscle strength, helping her build up the stamina to stand and walk independently for longer periods. Intensive weight-bearing exercises for 4 hours a day, 5 days a week, 3 weeks in a row is an impressive feat for anyone. Watching Shiloh pushing through with a smiling face, and her excitement to revisit year after year, is testament to the young fighter trapped in her soul.

A particular highlight in Shiloh's calendar is her weekly swimming lessons provided through the adapted aquatic program in Fairfax County (Virginia). These 30-minute sessions provide her with momentary freedom from the constraints placed upon her from numerous orthopedic complications. Seeing her dash around the pool, floating and splashing with so much joy, will always fill me with happiness and pride. Building on these weekly sessions, we work with WaterSafe Swim School in Seal Beach, California—a program started by Ginny Ferguson in 1988 who worked intensely with Shiloh, providing three lessons a day! This, along with her weekly lessons, has been an integral part of Shiloh's success and happiness—she loves being in the water, and this year was able to accomplish the amazing milestone of being completely water-safe! Through this, she has been given the ability to be independent in the water in a way that she isn't on land.

Throughout this journey of love and understanding, I have tried consistently to provide Shiloh every opportunity in which to explore her own potential. This consistency, coupled with a lot of fun times for Shiloh to just be Shiloh—to unwind and be frustrated—has seen my daughter blossom. I continue to witness her development, with new words entering her vocabulary, and bask in her personal triumphs. From the apparently small victories, such as when she independently climbed the stairs to her room while left alone for 2 minutes—which led to a proud but very panicked mom—to the large, with the completion of a 5k walk in under 60 minutes in the fall of 2015, Shiloh continues to challenge all expectations. Watching Shiloh cross the finish line of our 5k walk in Fairfax, Virginia, with no special arrangements made (other than having myself and her grandfather on either hand for support), was a huge accomplishment for all of us and marked a change in our trajectory. It was incredibly touching to have complete strangers run up to my child with tears in their eyes to congratulate her, without them being fully away of the breadth of that accomplishment. Shiloh's initial physical therapist that she had worked with prior to and shortly after her neurosurgery had told me to order a walker, as Shiloh was never going to walk by herself. Changing physical therapists at that point, I was lucky enough to find the first of many specialists for Shiloh who not only pushed her beyond the supposed "developmental ceilings" but also have surrounded her with enthusiasm, pride, and most importantly, unconditional love. Her exceptional progress has changed what the medical community thought possible for children with her genetic deletion, made us beam with pride, and importantly, raised a number of questions, namely, should we place these artificial ceilings on our child's expectations?

Shiloh has shown that despite a bleak prognosis from that horrible doctor 3 years ago, combined with numerous diagnoses, she has the ability not only to continually develop but also to thrive. Having acquired a functional vocabulary and independent walking despite the double diagnosis of hyperpronation and cerebral palsy, Shiloh has stunned us and overcome the medical expectations at every turn. Her progress has continually amazed specialists, and has led to questions of why and how.

As a mother and as a specialist in early intervention, I continue to believe that Shiloh's progress is due to the fact that I never gave up. I have never accepted no when it comes to her learning a new skill. It may take 3 days, it may take 8 months, or in the case of her walking, it may take 6 years, but we keep going. Shiloh began therapies from a very young age, and had been provided with a diverse and continuous range of options. I am always looking for new experiences for her, new ways to help her grow, and new ways for her to participate with the rest of the world. She is taking part in groundbreaking research projects—a true pioneer in our family. When I look back at the progress that Shiloh has made, I am immensely proud of her and will continue to support her—helping her to try her best. I mourned and grieved the loss of a typical child, but Shiloh was never going to be anything typical—she was born to break the mold, challenge expectations against all odds, and grow into our outstanding outlier. I know that other parents experience similar journeys because I work with them every day through my job. The integration of multiple therapies has had a profound positive effect on Shiloh's progress. Her life is work; between therapies and school, my child works harder in a day than I do in a week. Whenever possible, diversify and broaden the scope of what is offered—the main issue is where and how to get access to these therapies.

22 Ada Mae
Our Magical Fairy

*Jonathan Grashow and Kathryn Grashow**

This is the story of Ada Grashow—a loving, gentle soul touched by a rare genetic condition, Phelan–McDermid syndrome (PMS). This chapter gives voice to the Grashow family's journey to their happy ever after.

It was during January 2015 that we had the pleasure of first meeting Ada Mae and her family, including Ada's younger sister, Wilhelmina (Willa), and parents, Jon and Katie (See Figure 22.1). The family of four is a close-knit unit, sharing an infectious love with those around them. The lab instantly felt a strong attachment to the family, with time spent recalling stories from lands afar and playing "house." One of these heartfelt moments was particularly striking, hitting a cord with our team. During one session, a member of our team, Caroline, sat quietly coloring with Willa. Caroline, who had recently returned from spending a holiday break with her family in Ireland—including sitting through multiple repeats of Disney's latest hit, *Frozen*, with her 5-year-old niece—asked Willa if she had seen the film. After a brief pause, Willa stopped coloring. She responded that she had seen the film, and that her favorite princess was Elsa, before quickly returning her attention to the coloring task. Not providing the enthusiastic response to the mere mention of *Frozen* that many may be used to, Willa quietly went on to explain that it made her very sad. The story reminded her of Ada. To a young Willa, her sister Ada had been lost to her, paralleling the *Frozen* story line, but had never returned as Elsa had in the movie. The similarities were obvious to this young girl, and the film uniquely summarized the heartbreaking story of this family. Katie, overhearing the conversation from the lab room, confirmed that they had both watched the Disney hit together, struggling to hold back the tears and hugging each other close. Katie and Jon later explained that they have learned to avoid many mainstream TV shows and movies because the dramatic plots are too upsetting to be entertaining, given the family's real-life experiences. Ada was 4½ years old when she became "frozen," or regressed. This is their story.

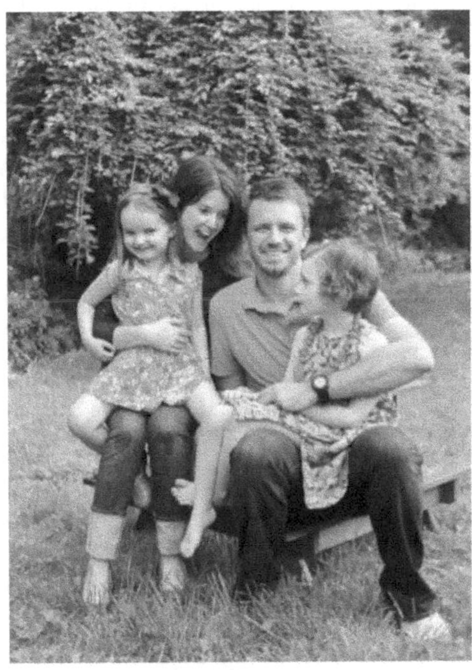

FIGURE 22.1 Right to left: Wilhelmina, Katie, Jon, and Ada Grashow.

Ada was born 3½ weeks premature after a relatively smooth pregnancy. We were concerned about the lack of movement Katie felt from the baby in her womb, finding it hard to identify with other expectant parents' reports of exuberant movement! After a very peaceful, typical delivery, Ada silently entered the world, without a loud cry that epitomizes most births. The medical professionals

* Written by Caroline Whyatt on behalf of Jonathan Grashow and Kathryn Grashow.

consistently reassured us throughout the quiet pregnancy and the peaceful labor that everything was progressing normally and Ada was healthy. In hindsight, this peaceful process foreshadowed Ada's quiet personality and later development.

For the first 3 weeks of Ada's life, nursing was a three-person collaboration. During each feeding session, Ada would fall asleep after a few successful sucks, apparently exhausted from the sheer effort. We quickly learned that Jon needed to actively work to keep Ada awake, removing her clothing, tickling her feet, and putting a wet cloth on her body as Katie fed her. Our work paid off, and after 3 weeks Ada began to display her healthy appetite without any extra support. Ada then progressed from one skill to the next, growing into a plump healthy baby girl and meeting all her developmental milestones as expected for her first 11 months.

As we approached Ada's first birthday, we noticed a plateau in her gross motor and language development. Despite mastering the ability to independently stand and bear weight, Ada displayed a persistent aversion to trying to walk—the next milestone toward independence. Similarly, she would happily babble nonstop, proving to be very talkative in her own language, yet there was a total lack of referential or meaningful verbalizations. When discussing our concerns with pediatricians, we were advised that Ada was likely just a "late bloomer" and that we should "wait it out" until she was 18 months old. Soon after Ada turned 1 year old, her health became progressively poor. She suffered from a series of ear infections and constant diarrhea. This time in Ada's childhood was painful and troublesome for the entire family. From the sleepless nights holding our crying daughter close, to the 5–10 daily diarrhea incidents, it was a trying time during which we felt a growing separation between our reality and that of other parents. Simply looking at our daughter, we could tell she was in pain. Over the course of the next 2 years, we worked with GI specialists to address her diarrhea to no avail, eventually implementing an elimination diet that resulted in the removal of gluten, dairy, and soy.

At 18 months old, the plateau of Ada's skills made her eligible for behavioral, physical, occupational, and speech therapy. This led to a mixture of emotions. The inappropriately harsh methods used, the brutally insensitive and judgmental language, and the unjustified expectations placed on Ada by some professionals broke our hearts. For example, at 18 months, Ada had finally developed the ability to walk while using a push toy for support. Working toward the end goal of independent walking, an evaluating physical therapist forced her to attempt to walk with reduced support from the push toy. This left Ada frustrated and crying with fear, looking directly at Katie with heartbroken eyes. Katie quickly interjected, stating that she didn't think Ada was ready, and was then told, "Ada might never walk because you are holding her back." Other therapists worked with Ada in supportive and empowering ways; we had to actively work to ensure that Ada's therapists were positive professionals. We learned through this initial foray into the world of therapy an important distinction between Ada being respectfully challenged and not being pushed too hard at the expense of her spirit.

During a consultation with a sleep specialist, we were told that rather than tending to Ada when she cried out in distress during the night, we should instead remove all additional furniture from the room and leave her, an especially troubling idea to us considering Ada's complete lack of safety awareness and tendency to self-harm. This idea that we were "not disciplining her enough", and feeding the problem by being attentive parents left us both in tears and with feelings of distrust toward the medical establishment. This interpretation of our parenting was at odds with all our instincts. It saddened us to realize that those professionals, in whom we placed our utmost trust and respect, seemed unaware of the reality of our daily challenges and, worse yet, treated us like it was our fault. It worried us that this was a common impression for parents in similar situations, and saddened us to think some may actually follow the counterintuitive advice of professionals, or believe that the issues faced by their children were truly their fault.

Despite the struggles facing Ada, she remained the happiest child we had ever met—a phrase echoed by a range of professionals. The stagnation of motor skills, coupled with a delay in language development, led to a referral for genetic testing to assess for Angleman syndrome and fragile X syndrome—two forms of a genetic neurodevelopmental disorder. Both returned negative results, and we continued to bounce between consultations in the hopes of finding an answer to the many questions we held. The system was ferocious. While therapists inferred that we were too soft and displayed an apparent disregard for Ada's autonomy and desires, clinicians captialized on our desire for the truth with aggressive promises of how they could help. Yet, after a few consultations it inevitably became clear that one of two outcomes would emerge. First, we would be told, "Everything looks normal"—a surprisingly common statement. Or second, we would be told, "This is just not my area of expertise." Exploring these dead ends was exhausting, demoralizing and made us feel as if we were unable to find our child the care she needed. Indeed, during a visit to a neurologist in Pittsburgh [Pennsylvania], we were solemnly informed that only a staggeringly low 35% of children who visit the neurology department ever receive a diagnosis. These statistics shocked us. We had begun this journey with the utmost faith and trust, believing that the medical profession was well placed to know why our child suffered and struggled so much. We were wrong, a fact that took time, money, and patience to learn. We resolved to continue to do all that we could for Ada, and that if a diagnosis—an answer to all our questions—never came, we would find a way to navigate these unchartered waters together.

It was after Ada had tubes inserted into her ears at 21 months to combat her near-constant ear infections that we witnessed a significant, positive change in our daughter. She became more playful and began acquiring words. She learned to walk independently a week before her second birthday, engaging with peers in a playgroup* and showing a significant improvement in her fine motor skills. It was at this stage that she began to take part in art activities, including making jewelry and painting. Meanwhile, the social environment of the playgroup led to the development of new strategies for interaction and play—she would observe activities from afar, and master them in secret alone, reducing the stress on group play sessions. Going into preschool at 3 years old, we had learned to manage Ada's dietary needs to minimize illness, and life had reached an even keel. We were entering Ada's "golden years," between 3 and 4½ years old. Achieving "best stacker and builder" in class—a badge of honor—she had integrated into preschool well, and continued her love for creating art, which seemed to be a meaningful mode of self-expression. We would spend hours making our own creations to display proudly around the home. She was now also using meaningful referential terminology with a vocabulary of more than 150 words.

Ada was affectionate and incredibly close to her baby sister, Willa, who arrived when Ada was 2 years old. Alternating between pushing Willa in a stroller and repeatedly running up and down the driveway or around our home, Ada's sense of independence was growing along with her warm personality. Life in our family started to settle, and we were in a new whirlwind of activity, from getting a pair of hamsters† for our girls, to road trips and days at the park. Willa had brought a new vibrancy to our family, while Ada made progress every day and her potential seemed unlimited. Little did we know this was to be short-lived. To this day, we feel guilt that we didn't appreciate that precious time with our Ada during those golden years.

Ada's regression was instant and alarming. Contracting a common, seemingly innocuous sinus infection, she suddenly migrated into herself and stopped all physical activity. Soon she became restless, emitting a high-pitched scream for hours on end, coupled with a rapid and complete deterioration of her vocabulary that left us at a loss as to how best to comfort our distressed daughter. She lost her ability to use her hands, which robbed her of all her favorite pastimes and the independence she had worked so hard to acquire. All the loving and calming strategies that had always soothed her were no longer effective. Her personality was gone, and it felt like our emotional bonds with her were disappearing. As sad as we were to lose our feelings of connectedness, we were saddened to an even greater

* Katie started a playgroup and preschool specifically for Ada to increase her socialization and interaction with peers. We would encourage other parents in a similar position to explore this option—there is often a lack of appropriate sources and outlets within the community for our kids.

† Ada pointed to the hamsters and verbally asked for them during a trip to the pet store—a major breakthrough for us—how could we possibly deny her request? It was a wonderful moment in our family journey.

degree imagining how alone Ada must have felt at that time. Ada was admitted to the hospital to undergo a range of immediate tests, including an EEG, MRI, spinal tap, skin biopsy, and another genetics test. Every test came back normal. Our mysterious nightmare continued, this time not knowing if our daughter was terminal. It was at this point that a new additional form of genetic testing was suggested—whole-exome sequencing—for which we were quoted a cost of $7000 out of pocket. Despite the cost, we felt we had no choice, and decided to opt for this more advanced assessment.

The following 6 months passed in a haze. Ada had fully regressed, and the daughter that had been running vibrantly around our family home, plastering artwork across our walls, and designing her own friendship bracelets had disappeared. She had in effect become frozen and wouldn't wake up. Watching videos of her younger self, Ada would smile and palm the screen, appearing to recognize the child that was trapped inside. We mourned the loss of our daughter, struggling to explain what had happened to friends, colleagues, and mostly to her baby sister, Willa. While cooking dinner one evening, Katie received the results from the genetic assessment—Ada was diagnosed with PMS. We finally had an answer, albeit an answer that raised so many more questions!

The next steps in our journey exposed us to the harsh reality of rare diseases, revealed our own personal limitations, and highlighted the lack of control we truly had to help our daughter. We attacked the Internet with a voracious appetite for any information we could find on PMS, from medical journal articles to parent support websites. After years of dreaming of finding a diagnosis so that we could help Ada more effectively, we instead found ourselves grieving over the lack of treatment possibilities and the limited expectations placed on the rest of our daughter's life. At our genetics appointment the following week to discuss Ada's genetic assessment further, we faced a lengthy discussion filled with scientific terminology. To Katie, who's background was in early childhood education, this frank scientific discussion caused her to panic due to the overwhelming foreign terminology and scary implications. Luckily, Jon, whose background was in bioengineering, was able to have the necessary conversations with the clinicians, while Katie actively listened, struggling to understand a single word of the clinician's explanation. We had thought that in receiving a diagnosis we would have something to work toward, a way to figure out the nature of Ada's difficulties, and thus a way to help. We relived the heartbreak later that evening, when we slowly came to realize that we had been struggling to find a truth, an answer, but were living in a mystery. Now, facing the everyday issues, such as knowing our 5-year-old daughter would likely never be potty trained, the responsibility of finding and providing the unique care she needed, and the realization that our daughter would require a lifetime of care, rocked us to our core.

It has been a long, drawn-out journey that is set to continue. We are conscious to not let Ada's diagnosis define her and instead focus on her amazingly unique perspective and undeniable friendly spirit. Each day presents new challenges, and we are learning to proactively create our own reality and sense of balance. Ada's regression has taught us that our main focus needs to be happiness rather than functional gains. In our eyes, Ada has shown wonderful improvement in the 3 years since her regression; she is once again able to feel and share happiness. She has shown improvement in "functional skills" as well, but is still a far cry from the abilities she possessed during her golden years. We feel it is important to cherish Ada for who she is today rather than focusing on hope that she will regain the skills she once had. We've learned to collaborate with Ada to develop effective "therapies" both at home and with professionals. For example, music has emerged as a consistent source of comfort for Ada, so Jon has learned to play the ukulele with pointers from Ada's music therapist. Another example is the integration of proprioceptive exercises, such as joint compressions and Anat Baniel Method (ABM) progressions with physical play. Through it all, we're careful to ensure that all of Ada's treatment is respectful of her developmental age, as opposed to her chronological age. We have found a fantastic team of therapists dedicated to helping Ada find her own voice and independence. This wonderful team allows Ada to take the alead in her future, by working with objects and activities that she enjoys. Rather than focusing on behavioral outcomes, we now focus more on what she may be trying to communicate to us. For instance, we recently noticed Ada did not want to sit at the table for dinner; she refused to eat and became increasingly upset. We interpreted this as a warning

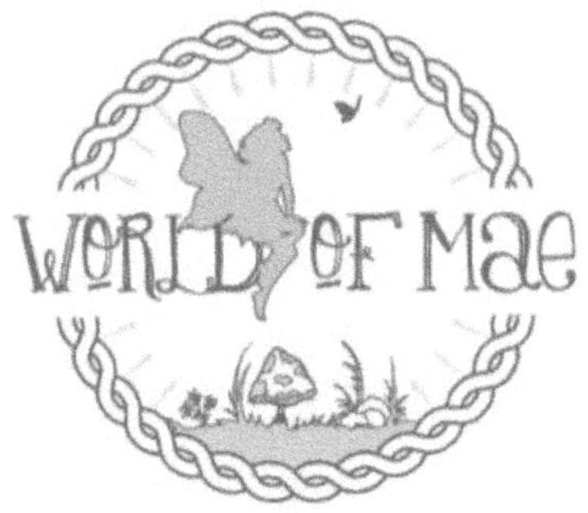

FIGURE 22.2 To find out more about our journey, please connect with our family via Facebook (https://www.facebook.com/worldofmae.home/) or Twitter (https://twitter.com/world_of_mae).

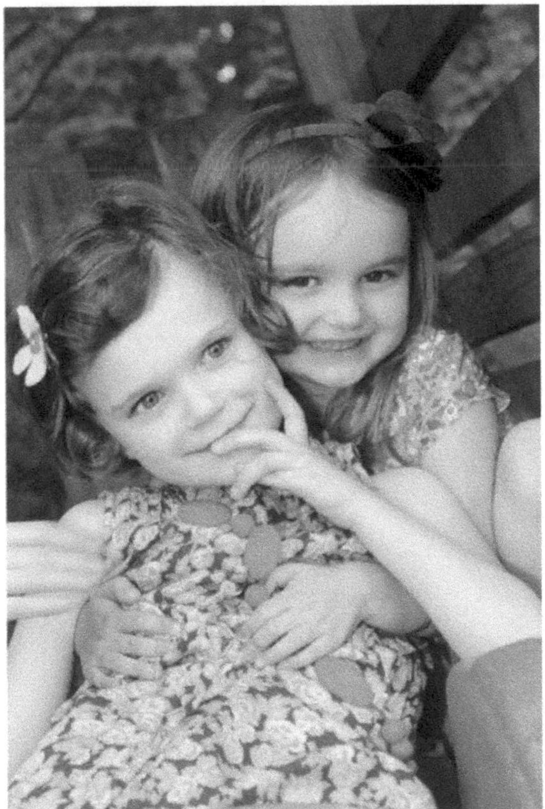

FIGURE 22.3 Sisters and best of friends: our fairy Ada and her elf Willa.

sign—and we later found out that she had strep throat. Previously, under the advice that we were not disciplining or being strict enough with Ada, we would have been told this was a disruptive, unacceptable behavior, and that we should ignore her protests and force her to eat. Under our new outlook, we viewed this behavior as a method of communication to achieve a new window into Ada's world. We feel empowered by therapists and physicians who look at the whole picture of our reality to effectively support us in creating the best life possible.

We continue to face daily challenges. Our overall goal remains the same—we just want our family to be happy. Rather than following previous advice to shape her behavior, we now spend our time finding ways to connect with each other. Ada's smile has started to melt away the frozen mask that she was trapped behind since her regression. We have a constant list of items or activities that have helped calm or break through to Ada at one time or another, and so we run through this list at all times—an activity that can be exhausting. We continue to live off a flash of her big smile and wide blue sparkling eyes, full of hope. Struggling to identify with families who often seem removed from the daily challenges of our life. We remain in a world that is largely not designed for us. Instead of focusing on our frustrations, we try to focus our energy on proactively forging a positive path forward, from inventing adaptations for our home, to finding opportunities for Ada to have consistent peer interactions, and starting a foundation, World of Mae (See Figure 22.2), to raise awareness and promote inclusion in our community. Annual World of Mae events are our way of spreading Ada's perseverance and bringing together people of all abilities and disabilities in celebration.

Willa has become Ada's ally and advocate, fiercely protective of her sister (See Figure 22.3). Having gone from the younger sister to effectively the older sister, we are comforted to see their compassionate and creatively unique bond is as strong as ever. We often refer to Ada as our "fairy" since she brings a magical and mysterious quality to our life, and Willa describes herself proudly as Ada's "elf" sister. The fairy tale of our life is sure to have many more chapters, and we're committed to living our version of "happily ever after."

23 It's a Girl's Life

Jadyn Waiser, Michelle Stern Waiser, and Anita Breslin*

Michelle Stern Wasier is an active advocate in the area of autism awareness and has become a close member of our team. Introduced in early 2015 through an ongoing research project, we have remained close to Michelle and Jadyn. This chapter gives voice to the emotional roller coaster and ongoing battle Jadyn and her family have experienced.

I am the proud mother of an exuberant 12-year-old girl, Jadyn. As with many families, we struggle to schedule a range of events, including running from gymnastic practice to dance or cheer on a nightly basis, all the while looking forward to a treat at the weekend of a girlie night in with a movie. Despite our hectic schedule, I am delighted that my young daughter engages in so many activities—at one time we weren't sure if Jadyn would ever speak, let alone have a better social life than her parents.

After a normal, peaceful pregnancy, Jadyn was born by a C-section in a flurry. My memories of the event are hazy, but I will never shake the moment I was told that she had been born blue, with her umbilical cord wrapped around her small neck twice. However, my maternal instincts and worry quickly subsided, with Jadyn soon declared a healthy, "chubby" baby weighing in at an impressive 8.5 pounds. The first months vanished from beneath us, and we slowly adjusted to being first-time parents. Jadyn went from strength to strength for the first 9 months, meeting all her early developmental milestones—although with some delay. It wasn't until we noticed that she had yet to crawl, and continued to feel very fragile—much like a rag doll [signs of hypotonia]—that we became slightly concerned. Voicing these concerns to our pediatricians, we were initially reassured that she was simply a late bloomer. This reassurance, however, was short-lived.

By 1 year old, her dad and I were dismayed that Jadyn was continuing to show no interest in any of the numerous toys that family and friends bestowed on her. More worryingly, we were still desperately waiting for her to utter "mumma" and "dadda," and noticed that we couldn't get Jadyn to make eye contact with us or respond to her name. Our pediatrician was less quick to reassure us this time round. Completing a range of tests, we were informed that in all likelihood, Jadyn could hear, and that her lack of spoken language or response to her name may be rooted in something deeper at 17 months, Jadyn began to crawl. We were quickly informed that this was a significantly delayed motor milestone, but what was more surprising as parents was the way that Jadyn choose to crawl. Up on all fours, her method of crawling looked exhausting to a spectator and was clearly an "atypical pattern," feeding our niggling concerns. Regardless, this was progress. At 19 months, her pediatrician referred Jadyn to the New Jersey Early Intervention (EI) program with a focus on physical therapy, occupational therapy, speech therapy, nutrition, and applied behavioral therapy. Unaware of what to expect, we started the home-based program and participated in all sessions enthusiastically. Coordinating our schedules, we had regular therapists at our home for up to 25 hours a week and became regular clients, actively soaking in all the advice, scouring baby books, and experimenting with a host of new techniques. We set aside our worries, and continued to ensure that Jadyn had a rich family life, following all recommendations from the therapists and medical profession—including the American Academy of Pediatrics vaccination schedule.

* Written by Caroline Whyatt on behalf of Jadyn Waiser, Michelle Stern Waiser, and Anita Breslin.

Twenty-one days—the exact number of days between Jadyn receiving the measles, mumps, and rubella (MMR) vaccination and her first seizure, on February 14, 2005. We are fully aware that there is no evidence for any connection between the MMR and autism,* but the controversy was fresh in 2005, fueling parental concern and distrust of the medical system. Was this a side effect? We never knew, and never will. Regardless, our life was never the same. The seizure instigated a range of assessments, with our medical team suddenly becoming growingly concerned with Jadyn's progress. It was a few months later, when Jadyn was 18 months old, that we were given the preliminary diagnosis of autism. Reluctant to give a confirmed diagnosis—as Jadyn was still so young—our clinical team increased the levels of EI, and worked closely with me as I had already left my job and career to be a stay-at-home mum and focus on her more. Working with a local team of experts, this initial diagnosis was confirmed through further behavioral diagnosis at a top children's hospital. All the while, we struggled to accept and understand.

Autism. It was a word that was unfamiliar to my entire family. Throughout my pregnancy, we had lengthy conversations with medical professionals about Down's syndrome and other genetic conditions, yet no one had ever broached the subject of autism. There were no support groups or credible sources of information—with families actively encouraged to stay away from the Internet for fear of reading something inaccurate. The MMR controversy had raised autism into the public spotlight, but we struggled to find any useful information. Every route informed us about boys with autism, but we had a daughter—were the rules different now?† We were confronted with out-of-date literature about refrigerator mothers and parenting styles, which only added to the confusion and led to self-doubt. We were on an emotional roller coaster with no option of getting off, and we had no idea what was to come. Our daughter wasn't even 2 years old, yet a train of questions about her future hit us square in the face. There was no prescription. No road map. No help. The charities couldn't provide one-on-one assistance, something we so desperately sought.‡ Nevertheless, throughout everything Jadyn was almost a toddler who needed nothing more than her family's love and support. We struggled to find our way into her world. With no sign of Jadyn acquiring verbal communication, I began an intense course of sign language night classes. Among others looking to learn a second language, I sat eager to learn nursery rhymes and how to teach our young daughter this method of communication. It was the day of Jadyn's third birthday that we enrolled her with a local public preschool disabled program, where she placed in an autism class using applied behavioral analysis (ABA) in an attempt to build her skill set.§

The first day was horrible. I imagine most mothers feel a void when they drop their child at nursery or preschool for the first time. Dropping off my daughter who had no skill set—couldn't say or respond to her name and had no form of communicating—to a group of people who were practical strangers was agonizing. The program had a strong focus on ABA, using the platform to help a range of children on the autism spectrum. Despite the tough beginnings, we patiently watched as Jadyn slowly acquired basic levels of sign language. The ability to communicate with our daughter for the first time was a truly thrilling experience. Using words such as *more* and *please*, we finally had a small window into Jadyn's world. These short phrases gave her more independence—a voice. Having relied heavily on our parental instincts, reading subtle cues to learn about Jadyn's

* Edit to Author's note: The MMR–autism link, initiated by discredited Dr. Wakefield, has been repeatedly refuted, with no substantial scientific evidence in support of such a claim. Indeed, an independent tribunal of the British General Medical Council found Dr. Wakefield guilty of scientific misconduct. The findings of this tribunal can be found here: General Medical Council, Fitness to Practice Panel Hearing, 24 May 2010, Andrew Wakefield, Determination of Serious Professional Misconduct: https://web.archive.org/web/20110809092833/http://www.gmc-uk.org/Wakefield_SPM_and_SANCTION.pdf_32595267.pdf.

† Current statistics indicate that the gender ratio of diagnosis is 4:1, with a disproportionately high number of males diagnosed with an ASD.

‡ Note: For those families within the New Jersey area, we would like to advocate the use of local support groups, such as www.POAC.net.

§ As part of New Jersey's state law, the public school district takes over when EI ends on a child's third birthday.

emotional state, we finally had a method to truly communicate. Smiling when watching her favorite shows, like Elmo, we knew Jadyn was a happy child, but having feedback to that affect lifted our hearts. As she began to use sign language appropriately, Jadyn met goals that we didn't even realize we had set. We then realized that we had no idea of what Jadyn could truly do—her potential was now, in our eyes, limitless.

After 3 years of acclimatizing Jadyn to independent life at a preschool ABA disabled program, she moved on in the public school system into a new elementary school—determined to expand her horizons with a self-contained classroom for children with learning and developmental disabilities rather than a strict ABA kindergarten platform. Moving away from the ABA platform, this lighter structure with less routine within the classroom environment challenged Jadyn at a new level. With a range of children of different ages and levels of ability, this environment also gave her an opportunity to explore her potential. Or so we hoped. Unfortunately, her behavioral challenges became gradually worse, culminating with Jadyn becoming increasingly disruptive, uncooperative, and finally, fiercely upset. These behavioral challenges bled out from the schooling environment into daily life; from screaming matches on the floor at Costco to temper tantrums around our home, we struggled to communicate and soothe our daughter. In hindsight, we appreciate the limitations of the public schooling system. In particular, the staff that meant well had very little training in dealing with disruptive behaviors. Moreover, we realized the school system was devoid of sign language. Our daughter had slowly developed a sign lexicon, yet the school staff was restricted to the most basic signs, such as thumbs up. We realized that Jadyn was once again trapped in her own world.

Our fears were only compounded by the lack of information sent home through the school system. With very little progress in key skills, we worried that Jadyn was lacking the appropriate support for her learning needs. Veering between believing that she was in the best place to begin her education and worrying relentlessly as new behavioral challenges amplified, we struggled to navigate the public school system. We would attend clinics and individualized education program (IEP) meetings at the school, where we would be asked to pick a few items from the Assessment of Basic Language and Learning Skills–Revised (ABLLS-R) for Jadyn to focus on. Using this system like a Chinese takeout menu, we were left dismayed by the lack of input and guidance from the education system in our daughter's development. Isolating skills to "master," we knew the team had their best intentions at heart, but we slowly realized this was no longer the avenue for Jadyn.

These thoughts, and our resolve to move Jadyn from the public school setting, were strengthened over the course of the next year, as we slowly explored a range of other options—though daunted by the potential cost of private education. Working closely with a psychologist and board-certified behavior analyst (BCBA) in the area of autism, Dr. Anita Breslin, we began exploring options.* This process culminated in a climatic manner, with Jadyn suffering a host of injuries as a result of a convulsive seizure in spring 2009—her last seizure to date, but one that had a lasting impact on our family.

Jadyn had been experiencing a range of nonconvulsive seizures (absence seizures), where she would appear to be mentally absent—as if in a world of her own. These could be difficult to detect, particularly within a schooling environment, difficulties that were further compounded by Jadyn's lack of verbal language—so the schooling team were often unaware of the underlying issue. However, in the spring of 2009, Jadyn suffered a convulsive seizure, along with a range of behavioral outbursts that left the staff simply not knowing what to do with the little girl with autism. Jadyn remained in the public school system until the end of second grade when—with the help of family—we privately enrolled her in a full-day clinic, SEARCH Consulting, led and founded by Carrie Khana, a BCBA and certified New Jersey special education teacher. Endorsing the use of ABA, and the use of set structures to facilitate routine, the SEARCH program was an emotional and financial stress

* Please see below for an insert by Dr. Breslin on Jadyn's experience.

on our family, but a true lifeline for Jadyn. At the time of enrollment, Jadyn was displaying signs of depression and growing levels of behavioral concerns. But soon, she was learning how to learn. Everything from how to follow instructions to how to sit quietly in a chair, we watched as our daughter gained a small range of new skills. Through the support and work of this team, our daughter acquired basic levels of verbal language at 7 years old—a moment that we will never forget. Hearing Jadyn's voice was a truly amazing experience—like putting a face to a name after 7 long years, did the voice match the person? It felt like we were meeting our daughter for the first time—this was Jadyn! It was through this program and the help of our wonderful specialists that we managed to secure Jadyn a place at Princeton Child Development Institute (PCDI). A moment that can only be described as a dream come true. Now, with an appropriate placement to aid her development, we watched Jadyn progress and develop into the young woman that she is today.

Today we have a very talkative daughter, who is known to burst into song. With a love for the theatre, Jadyn can recount the story and songs from many Broadway hit musicals. Sitting with her beloved pink iPad, Jadyn is like any other 12-year-old girl. Dressed in skinny jeans, her much loved UGGs, and pink sweater, she is every inch a "girly girl," color coordinating her medical alert bracelet* to match every outfit. This outside appearance can be half the battle. As a community, we struggle with perception of autism in society at large. First, the predominance of boys with autism leads to an inevitable conversation that yes, my daughter does have autism. And yes, girls get autism too. We fail to recognize that autism is not sexist, or racist or ageist—it is, after all, a lifelong disorder. Second, I then have to explain that although she may look great in her fashionable attire, her brain works a little differently and she may not respond or acknowledge you immediately. This often leads to confusion—when I have to point out that children with developmental challenges do not have neon signs or stripes and polka dots. It can be tiring, but on the whole, it is frustrating. News and mainstream media perpetuate the notion that autism is a male disorder and flash horror stories into the home of families worldwide. Just recently, we suffered the horrible loss of a young boy, Avonte Oqundo,† who ran from school and was later found dead in a river. This story is heartbreaking. Yet the media coverage can often be damning, casting autism in a light not too dissimilar to the notions of my parents' generation. We have come so far, yet in many ways so little, in our fight to educate and inform the mainstream public.

I watch as my daughter struggles to fit in—something I believe is familiar to many parents of children with autism. Girls can be cruel; more shockingly, so can their parents. As young children, it was the parents who didn't invite Jadyn to the class birthday party or sleepover. In the playground, it was the parents who didn't let her play with their children. These poor role models for their children need to realize that autism is not infectious. Now, almost a teenager, I watch as her peers mock and laugh at her expense. The phrase "mean girls" hasn't been popularized to the point of a hit Lindsey Lohan movie for no reason. I take comfort in the innocence of my daughter, naïve to the fact it is happening, but it will never quell my motherly anger. Seeing her try to join in activities with typical peers, only to watch as they move away from her laughing, breaks my heart. Seeing Jadyn follow, thinking it is an innocent game, only serves to worry me.

What does the future hold? It was a question that we have asked ourselves since Jadyn was first diagnosed. It seems all the more pertinent now. Nearly a teenager, often mocked by her peers, but with a sweet innocence, Jadyn remains relatively safe. Yet, we worry about what services will be in place for our daughter as she ages—presumably retaining this bittersweet innocence. Having a higher rate of autism than the rest of the country,‡ New Jersey offers considerable support for children through charities and specialist programs. However, a question remains over the future provision of care and

* People often fail to consider a health bracelet for autism. Clearly stating our contact details and that Jadyn has autism, with limited language, provides us with a peace of mind. We cannot recommend this enough.

† See http://www.nytimes.com/2014/01/22/nyregion/remains-found-in-queens-are-matched-to-missing-autistic-boy.html.

‡ The current rate of diagnosis of an autism spectrum disorder is 1 in 68 across the United States. In New Jersey, the rate is considerably higher at 1 in 45: http://www.autismnj.org/prevalence-rates.

support once our children reach 21 years old. I am grateful that through Jadyn's current academic placement she is eligible for an adult program. But, what happens after the fact? Where will she live? Her innocence, endearing yet heartbreaking as it can be, is a worry. We worry that without the correct support of people she can trust, our society can easily take advantage of adults on the spectrum. Considerable scientific evidence points toward growing diagnosis rates (Zablotsky et al. 2015)—how then do we plan for the future?

Jadyn's progress in a short time has been nothing short of phenomenal. We are active in a number of activities, including the Special Olympics and cheerleading with the New York Jets Junior Flight Crew. Being an athlete for New Jersey's Special Olympics gymnastic team, All-Stars, Jadyn is not shy of hard work and perseverance. Through these activities, we have become part of a diverse, close-knit community of wonderful families and volunteers, working around the clock to support our society. The experience, surrounded by this extended family, is a psychological boost—helping Jadyn explore her potential. This potential and courage [both Jadyn's and mine] were tested further when Jadyn tried out for the cheerleading squad of the New York Jets. During a random conversation with one of my close girlfriends, the potential of cheerleading for this groundbreaking team was mentioned. Inside I immediately thought, Jadyn can't do that … can she? Yes, she can. With the support of a wonderful mentor, Jenna,* Jadyn and I went to her first cheerleading session with the squad. The girls there were fantastic. They immediately accepted Jadyn as part of their sisterhood, and I watched with pride as Jadyn slowly learned the routine. Three years later, Jadyn holds a veteran position on the squad, with her teammates by her side—fiercely protective of my daughter. Game day crowds can be quite the struggle for Jadyn and myself, but with the help of our PCDI team, we have a strong routine and are a regular fixture during the season.

The home programming and on-site support from PCDI has taught our family how to deal with the new and unexpected events of our daily life. Using their strong ABA approach, we now use tokens to achieve goals across the week, "saving" these for the end-of-week treat. They also taught us how to help Jadyn learn. Viewing every new activity as a sequence of events, we break it down into a number of small steps, for instance, the simple act of brushing your teeth. We have sequentially broken this down into a list of 18 steps, starting at "Turn water on and wet toothbrush" through to "Clean sink." Independent showering has been broken down into 30 steps, beginning with "Get a clean towel, underwear, and a robe" through to "Put dirty clothes in hamper." These small steps, the use of routine, and charts have helped Jadyn grow in confidence and independence. We continue to change elements of our routine to help Jadyn become acquainted with variety. From changing the type of toothpaste to trying a new restaurant, these little changes (although difficult at first!) have helped Jadyn adapt. Now, we know that as long as the restaurant serves cheeseburgers, Jadyn will be content. Indeed, with the help of PCDI, we have even explored new environments. These include working with a local eye doctor and dentist to gradually simulate what will be expected, so she is now in a position to visit for a checkup with no fear or behavioral challenges. Beginning with an initial visit to simply sit in the room, through to meeting the doctor or dentist, to being shown some of the equipment, we have increased the demands throughout. We also plan ahead, from the little things to the big. For instance, through the support of PCDI we have slowly been teaching and mastered programs for Jadyn, including how to take a pill (using tic tacs), how to prepare for feminine hygiene issues, and importantly, how to use a cell phone.

These practical life skills are vital steps toward a level of self-independence that we had never considered for Jadyn. But throughout, we remember who she is—our daughter. We are simply providing her the tools to enable herself. We do not enforce any strict diets, or give any medication for behavioral challenges; rather, we work through them slowly. With the help of the PCDI team, we no longer need to avail ourselves of private speech, occupational or physical therapy, and certainly

* Jenna McBride is now working on her master's degree in an occupational therapy at Philadelphia University. She chose to pursue this career after working closely with our family and Jadyn.

do not believe in the 40 hours a week of therapy rule of thumb. All activities are built into Jadyn's program, freeing her evenings and weekends for her true love—theatrics. Having had no verbal language until age 7, we now struggle to keep Jadyn from bursting into flamboyant song. It is a pleasant problem and one I would never wish to change. Her love of the theatre and song has opened many doors. From our weekends at the local show to our evenings at dance class (jazz, ballet, and hip hop), we are keen to feed this enthusiasm.

My daughter has autism. It is now a phrase that I will say loud and proud. If you were to give me a magic pill to "cure" this side of my daughter, I wouldn't take it. I honestly do not know how I would fare with a "typically developing" kid. My daughter is her own person, there is no one like her, and autism is just one piece of her puzzle—not her defining quality. Her warm personality; her love of theatre, dance, and song; her excitement; and her innocence—perhaps influenced by her diagnosis—are the core pieces that make my daughter who she is. Moments like when she randomly and spontaneously thanked Caroline [coeditor] for joining us for a wonderful dinner on a gloomy March evening, before taking herself off to get ready for bed—those are the moments that lift my heart. I find so much happiness in the little joys of life—all thanks to my daughter. I may struggle to identify with my old girlfriends who spend evenings boasting about their son or daughter's grades—or sporting achievements—but I have a new world. A world where my daughter trying a new food or washing her plate herself is an achievement to be celebrated with a phone call to my parents or other families in our support network. A world where a trip to the theatre, which was once a yearly event, has become a nearly weekly occurrence earned through princess tokens scattered across my home. A world where I will stop to help the family that I meet in the Costco aisle—their son or daughter displaying strong behavioral challenges, often screaming on the floor—knowing all too well how difficult that can be. Our world is a world that I wish the public could see and understand. It was one of our clinicians, Dr. Audrey Mars, that struck a cord. When we first met Audrey after Jadyn's diagnosis, we were desperately using any means to get into her world. Audrey gently stated that we could try and try, but we would fail. Jadyn needed to come into our world, and we, as her parents, just needed the tools to enable and empower her. We have found these tools, and have connected with our daughter in a way that only 5 years ago we couldn't have imagined. We only hope that other families can find the right path for them, and that the next time you see a little girl who may seem awkward, you don't assume it can't be autism. After all, girls get autism too.

Insert by Dr. Anita Breslin, licensed psychologist and board-certified behavior analyst working in the New Jersey area

My journey into the world of autism began in 1979, the same year that the TV movie *Son-Rise: A Miracle of Love* was released. I was a full-time student at Douglass College, still contemplating various majors and trying to figure out what I was going to do with the rest of my life. Psychology and education were primary areas of interest for me, as were art and journalism. I didn't think I could find a job with a bachelor's degree in art, and after earning a D in a Media in America course, I relinquished my dreams of a career in journalism. It was a Field Work in Psychology class that gave me my first and very direct exposure to autism, and became the foundation of my chosen profession. I decided to complete my 1-day-per-week "practicum" for the course at the Douglass Developmental Disabilities Center (DDDC), a university-based school serving children and adolescents with autism. At that time, autism was a low-incidence disability, with one in several thousand children diagnosed with the condition.

While I am not a parent of a child with autism, I can honestly say that my first few days at the school were intriguing, mysterious, and devastating. I didn't know if I could handle the experience. I was assigned to work in the DDDC's preschool. The little boy to whom I had been assigned was absolutely beautiful. He appeared perfect in every way: curly brown hair, beautiful eyes, fair skin, and pudgy cheeks. I couldn't wait to learn as much about him as possible and do the best job I could as part of his educational team. It didn't take long for me to realize that this little boy was not ordinary. He hardly made eye contact, responded to his name, or showed an interest in toys. He did not respond to my initiations or seem aware of my presence. He seemed lost in his own world. Teaching him was an enormous challenge and very exhausting. The school incorporated ABA-based principles and teaching strategies to change his behavior. Gradually, I learned how to help him make and sustain eye contact, complete simple tasks most children seem to learn effortlessly, engage in leisure activities, and communicate his wants and needs.

Thirty-three years later, autism is no longer a low-incidence disability, and I have assessed more than 375 individuals with the condition. One in 68 children are now affected by autism. I learned about Jadyn Waiser when her mom, Michelle (Figure 23.1), contacted me with concerns about challenges Jadyn had been experiencing at school. I observed Jadyn engaging in frequent and persistent temper tantrums in the classroom. She engaged in screaming, crying, and shouting. Jadyn engaged in noncompliant behavior as well. Watching her was nothing short of exhausting. One thing was certainly very clear—Jadyn wasn't progressing. Her problem behaviors overwhelmed her days and were serious obstacles to learning anything. While school staff members had the best of intentions, they were not sufficiently trained to resolve Jadyn's behavioral challenges. It was clear that a change of placement was urgently warranted. Jadyn's parents were open to suggestions and highly responsive to my recommendations.

PCDI was determined to be an appropriate educational setting for Jadyn, and thankfully was located in close proximity to the Waisers' home. Jadyn was very fortunate to receive acceptance into this program shortly after my assessment was completed. Founded in the 1970s, PCDI provides full-time educational services to individuals with autism using the principles and proven strategies of ABA. Four years after her enrollment, Jadyn is an entirely different child. The gains she has made are nothing short of astounding. How do I know? I had the pleasure of observing her at PCDI a short time ago. Jadyn's progress, however, is not miraculous. In fact, Jadyn's skill acquisition and problem behavior reduction are entirely due to the skills and expertise of PCDI's instructional staff, trainers, and supervisors who painstakingly and systematically apply ABA techniques, gradually changing behavior, while also ensuring that these changes are displayed across all environments in which Jadyn is expected to function. Jadyn's current educational program includes more than 30 programs that have been individually designed and tailored for her. Data-driven teaching procedures are implemented at school, at home, and in the community. My observation of Jadyn at PCDI revealed that she completes a wide range of academic, leisure, self-help, and social activities. Jadyn has a full curriculum that includes instruction in reading, writing, language arts, mathematics, and science. She works quietly for lengthy periods of time, consistently follows her teachers' instructions, makes a wide range of choices, earns rewards throughout the day, and participates in small group activities. Jadyn's school days are filled with learning opportunities, and behavior problems have been eliminated. Jadyn continues to participate in a wide range of community-based experiences. She is a very active and productive young girl. Jadyn's autism is no longer an obstacle to learning.

Jadyn's story is not uncommon. Nearly every day, I am dealing with cases just like hers. There are so many children, adolescents, and adults with autism whose lives, unlike Jadyn's, are filled with struggle because they have not been fortunate to receive an appropriate education. We have the tools and knowledge to alleviate these difficulties. In the absence of effective evidence-based intervention, individuals with autism will continue to experience unnecessary challenges associated with this diagnosis, and families will continue to suffer the deleterious effects of this pervasive developmental disorder. I take comfort in knowing that Jadyn's life has been forever changed for the better thanks to PCDI's commitment to effective intervention. I should emphasize that had it not been for her proactive and informed parents, Jadyn would not

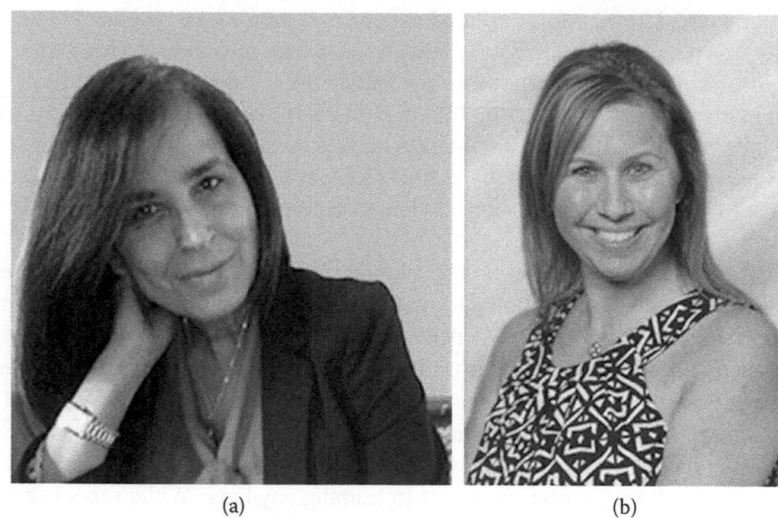

FIGURE 23.1 (a) Michelle Waiser and (b) Anita Breslin.

be where she is today. In fact, Michelle and Neal are the two main reasons for Jadyn's extremely positive outcome. There are no words to express the pride and satisfaction of knowing the Waiser family. I appreciate the opportunity Michelle and Neal gave me—the chance to meaningfully contribute to Jadyn's life by helping them access and secure the educational services Jadyn desperately required. For all the "Jadyns" out there, and for those yet to be born, I pray that they too are blessed with parents who never give up, who know when it's time to ask for help, and who will only rest when they have righted the wrongs and made a significant difference in the lives of their children.

REFERENCE

Zablotsky, B., Black, L. I., Maenner, M. J., Schieve, L. A., and Blumberg, S. J. 2015. Estimated prevalence of autism and other developmental disabilities following questionnaire changes in the 2014 National Health Interview Survey. *Natl Health Stat Rep* (87):1–21.

24 Treat the Whole, Not the Parts*

Our son Daniel is a healthy, smart, affectionate, fun-loving 6-year-old boy with a passion for the alphabet and trains. It isn't until you meet and spend time with Daniel that you also learn that he has autism—with difficulties in social situations, emotional regulation, and sensory processing. As a family, we face daily challenges, from the intense drama bundled up in our small boy that can be triggered from the most innocuous of daily events, to his delay processing sensory information, such as pain, through to struggles accessing and acquiring services. We have had many minor victories, and have watched as our son has settled into the school system, yet we bear the day-to-day stress of anticipating what could turn a good day bad and the anxiety of what the future holds for our son. Indeed, studies show that special needs parents suffer from PTSD, much like an embattled soldier. The need to be on high alert, to anticipate potential triggers of a meltdown and possible dangerous situations, means we continue to find our path.

After a long wait, we adopted Daniel a day after his birth in Maryland, bringing a new sense of family to our home in New Jersey. We beamed with pride as our son grew into a strong, healthy baby boy, who would smile readily, could be heard over the baby monitor happily babbling away in his crib, and would bounce for joy when we reached to lift him. As new parents, we diligently followed all advice as we watched our son go from strength to strength. Like most parents, one of our first parenting hurdles was dealing with teething pain. Daniel's response was typical; he struggled to sleep at night, crying with the pain. Hesitant to give him medication, we soon found that holding Daniel close in a warm hug seemed to quell his distress and soothe the pain. However, despite this typical response, our son would later display signs of poor pain perception and recognition—a more troublesome problem that would manifest in the years to come.

It was at his 9-month visit to our pediatrician for a routine wellness checkup that we were first alerted to the fact that Daniel may face challenges. During this visit, we completed the Modified Checklist for Autism in Toddlers (M-CHAT)—a particularly memorable and, in hindsight, pertinent moment in our journey. Focusing on the task at hand, we were perplexed to notice that Daniel did not fit neatly into the check boxes provided. When marking the presence or absence of behaviors in Daniel, we quickly realized that we needed to improvise by drawing a crude third column ("sometimes," "not always," "maybe"). Not knowing that this was screening for the key symptomatology of autism, we did know that Daniel did not fit our understanding of the "commercialized version" as seen in popular movies such as *Rain Man*. He displayed a clear attachment to both parents and grandparents, was highly affectionate and engaged in a social smile, and displayed no obvious repeated behaviors or rocking. We were unaware of what autism could look like in what people loosely call "high-functioning" individuals, and so we never considered that our son may go on to later receive a diagnosis. This ambiguity also posed a problem for the pediatrician and specialists that we would later work with. Daniel would "flirt" and smile with those evaluating him, engaging in social behaviors such as peekaboo—yet these overt skills masked a level of awkwardness that would not be overly apparent until his later years.

During this 9-month checkup, our pediatrician was concerned that Daniel had yet to master the art of independently rolling over. We were referred for an evaluation with early intervention (EI) services, which armed us with a range of tips to best teach Daniel this new skill, and it wasn't long before he had it mastered. This seemingly innocuous motor skill marked a turning point for Daniel—the beginning of a trend of being slightly behind on the trajectory of developmental

* Ghostwritten by Caroline Whyatt on behalf of the family. Note, names have been altered to retain anonymity.

milestones. This trend further manifested in delayed speech acquisition (not enough words for his age) at 18 months, leading to a second EI evaluation, where yet another motor delay was flagged —namely, that he couldn't climb the stairs. This time our parental confusion was palatable. Our son was 18 months old; we lived in a toddler-proof home, complete with stair gates! Did most parents know if their 18-month-old toddler could independently climb the stairs? This led to an experiment during our Florida vacation where I supervised stair sessions with Daniel, which confirmed that he could very much navigate the stairs alone—and that the stair gates at home would remain! This trend—of being just slightly behind a milestone—continued throughout Daniel's younger years, with a concern highlighted but quickly dismissed with the emergence of that particular skill or technique.

It was after this 18-month wellness checkup that we were provided with minimal services: one speech therapy session per week to address his speech delay—in an attempt to increase his lexicon to that expected of an 18-month old—and one occupational therapy session per month, for what we were unsure. This also began a trend of the EI team not clearly explaining or outlining their suspicions to us very concerned parents. We diligently began this course of EI, keen to support our son throughout. Very quickly, however, the speech and language therapist noted that Daniel had pronounced sensory-motor issues that were preventing her from effectively working with him—in particular, he had a strong need to pace around the room before he could settle. She immediately recommended we increase his levels of occupational therapy to help him learn how to sit and attend to the therapy session—a cue that concerned us both. It was during a later session that his speech therapist gently passed me a book called *The Out-of-Sync Child*, with suggestions that I may want to pay attention to references of sensory processing disorder (SPD) and consider visiting a specialist. Once the therapist left, I read through the book looking for signs of my son, scouring the pages for references to SPD and overlooking other disorders, such as autism. These subtle and convoluted hints throughout Daniel's early assessments left my husband and I confused, but suggested that warning signs were being observed, though not clearly communicated to us.

We began the arduous process of searching for a specialist, a process that hinted at the long journey to come. It wasn't until Daniel was 2½ years old that we finally managed to secure a visit with a neurodevelopmental pediatrician and received a diagnosis. Following a short play session, where the nurse practitioner asked Daniel to play with a doll and a truck, we were told that he was likely to have pervasive developmental disorder—not otherwise specified (PDD-NOS). This long title for a disorder that is no longer recognized in the *Diagnostic and Statistical Manual of Mental Disorders* was provided, along with details that Daniel's fine and gross motor skills were delayed, and he displayed a mixed profile of receptive and expressive language. Although appearing to tie in with areas of concern about our son, this title provided little information. It was through our own research that we realized that the nearly obsolete PDD-NOS label was potentially used as a "softer" label for autism—a pill that was presumably easier to swallow. We later heard a network joke that NOS loosely stood for "not all the symptoms." This striking example of miscommunication reflects a trend that we experienced throughout. Clinicians and professionals continually failed to tell us what they meant, opting instead to skirt around the issue. From the referring pediatrician saying let's just have EI check in on him, to the EI occupational therapists saying let's check on him once a month, through to the EI speech and language therapist passing me the *Out-of-Sync* book, not once did anyone mention concerns of autism spectrum disorder (ASD). Rather, we were left to assume that there were concerns about minor developmental delays and that he would simply "catch up." During our second consultation, armed with this new evidence, we stated, "It's autism," to which the neurodevelopmental pediatrician confirmed, "Yes, it's autism." There was no more talk of Asperger's or PDD-NOS.

Autism. This one word simultaneously provided a new perspective on the struggles our son had faced until this point and led to a new confusion. Our son had been, and continued to be, very social—something that was in direct contrast to the media's portrayal of autism. Our son, who would be bouncing for joy at the sight of you coming toward him in his crib, who ran excitedly to other children in the playground, who won over everyone with his cheeky smile, had autism. We had to relearn what autism was and meant. Looking back, we were provided with very little information on high-functioning autism, and so had no foundation to compare Daniel's behaviors to. His sociable demeanor and ability to talk led many to rule out this potential diagnosis, and created a sense of confusion over his developmental trajectory. It was the smart catch by our pediatrician of slightly delayed motor development at 9 months and the limited vocabulary at 18 months that began his journey, ultimately leading to the relatively early diagnosis. Nevertheless, to this day, we wonder why clinicians believe it is better to mask the issue, continuing to evade the problem at hand? The use of phrases such as "I don't know.... I don't have a crystal ball" when answering questions on your child's future development is simultaneously disheartening and angering to parents who want nothing more than a professional opinion. At a time when we as parents needed guidance, support, and yes, opinions, we were often left to wonder, what next? Alone.

Despite being armed with a confirmed diagnosis to open doors to specialist services, we faced a new set of challenges. Ranging from the mountains of overly complex, convoluted paperwork, to sourcing "local" in-network services, we found obstacles at every turn. With no manual for the administration of health insurance, I spent countless hours in an endless cycle of phone prompts, only to find dead ends—speaking to someone who more often than not did not hold any answers. We initially attempted to contact our case manager with the EI services, our first point of contact. Failing to get in touch with her, we called the main office in Trenton, or "the state," to get answers to our questions about the cost of services and what was available to our family. A struggle for answers and advice that continues today. Through this drawn-out process, we were eventually provided additional services, with developmental instruction two or three times a week and family training once a month. Unfortunately, subsequent dealings with our case manager were unpleasant—with a focus on the fact that we had went above her by calling Trenton, leading to a new tension and further difficulty securing services. Not once did she mention that she was sorry to learn our child had been diagnosed with ASD, nor did she ask how we were coping and processing this new information. Again, we felt alone in this journey.

At 36 months, Daniel began school. Up to this point, we had finally availed of home-based services through the EI program, which we complemented with hospital-based outpatient services through our health insurance. However, the EI program ceased when Daniel was 3 years old, leading us to depend on private avenues for all services. The lack of in-network service providers, coupled with long waiting lists, resulted in paying out of pocket on a sliding-scale fee. We also recognized that Daniel did not fit the commercialized version of autism, and so his needs were complex, and often overlooked by mainstream therapies. One such concern or need was Daniel's apparent delay in processing even the most critical sensory information—such as pain. Despite an appropriate pain response to teething, he had since displayed a slow reaction to this form of feedback—a worrying phenomenon that is a natural source of parental anxiety, and ranges in complexity and severity. Presumably present, even from the earliest years (thus references to SPD by the speech therapist), these difficulties in sensory processing have been largely overlooked by the medical profession, particularly once we had the official diagnosis of autism. This variation can be subtle, yet two of the more striking examples are solidly and vividly memorable. One such example occurred when he was approximately 4 years old, during a weekend trip to his grandparents' house. During the chaos of getting ready to leave, we took our eyes off Daniel for a millisecond. Once in the car, Daniel asked me to kiss his fingers—where a quick inspection revealed what looked like the small red line of a burn. His grandparents suspected that he touched the fireplace insert in their living room before leaving the house—much like Olaf the snowmen did in the movie *Frozen*, a favorite at the time. As he seemed content and settled, we started down the road to home. However, once well on our way he began crying out in pain—it was as if the pain had all hit him at once. Turning around, we made our way to his grandparents and tended to the burn with a cool washcloth. It was too late—it had blistered. I could not help but note the significant delay in his response, given the time between walking from the house, getting buckled in the car seat, and heading down the driveway. When he was later asked about the incident, if he was pretending to be Olaf, he got embarrassed and covered his eyes.

On later reflection, I realized I wasn't that surprised by the delay in processing the pain of the burn—we had a similar experience during heavy snowfall the previous year. Thinking nothing of my son playing aimlessly in the snow while I unloaded groceries from the car, I accompanied him into the house where he later began screaming. Worrying that he had accidentally touched something sharp buried in the snow, I took him to the sink and gently rinsed his hands to reveal no obvious cuts or injury. Noting the red cold color, I placed his hands firmly under my arms in an attempt to warm him, being instantly rewarded by him calming and moving closer. Again, this delayed response to pain was worrying, and led to an experiment. The next day, I decided to test my theory that he had a measurable pain delay. I took our son out to play in the snow, waiting for his natural response to freezing cold hands—warning him that his hands were going to get cold. The minutes passed, but no response or adverse reaction came. I brought him inside once I noticed his hands had become red, and quickly warmed him to avoid any pain—it was clear. I reached out to his teacher to work on wearing gloves—a skill that Daniel soon mastered. It should be noted, though, that when spring came Daniel had to be explicitly taught not to wear his gloves—as he was taught or "programmed" to do through applied behavioral analysis (ABA) teaching—a new, unforeseen difficulty. Speaking with his specialists, we were later informed that in these instances, when his brain received the delayed pain message, the feeling was magnified; therefore, his response was somewhat over the top. This processing delay resulted in his overwhelming surprise at the pain and intense response. It is like all the trains arriving at the station at one time instead of on schedule.

These sensory difficulties also manifest in a variety of ways that may be counterintuitive at first. This includes his apparent "lost in space" effect, where he loses sense of his body's position in space and time. We find he needs to be anchored to something through touch or pressure—this ranges from his need to sleep tightly pressed to someone (or the soft net of the bed rail that is there to keep him from falling out of bed), through to his need to have a long, tight squeeze or "snuggle" with one of us—almost to reset his sense of location. Akin to the stories of Temple Grandin's hug machine, we are now exploring alternative long-term solutions, including a weighted blanket, to help ground Daniel. Thus, despite the apparent overwhelming nature of sensory information in a number of contexts, he needs some everyday sensations to be enhanced to cope with his internal uncertainty.

This requirement to anticipate Daniel's needs and potential pain is something we have unconsciously developed. As a baby, we began predicting his need to eat, which we were later told to avoid by the speech therapist, who insisted that Daniel should learn to vocalize and request food and drink. Even now, as a healthy 6-year-old boy, we constantly remind and preempt his need for the bathroom. After several bathroom accidents, we now realize that it is not simply a case of pure laziness or "not wanting to go" that many children experience. Rather, on occasion, Daniel appears unable to tell or sense when he needs the bathroom—particularly if he is too distracted or engaged in something of high interest, like the iPad. Combined, we believe this anecdotal evidence suggests poor peripheral sensory feedback. Indeed, temperature, pain, sense of body in space, and control over bladder function (e.g., the micturition reflex) are all forms of sensory feedback. Delayed processing or sensory integration may be a core component of a number of Daniel's difficulties, as reflected in his delayed acquisition of developmental motor milestones. The vigorous bouncing and jumping in his crib that characterized his youth is now present in daily life. What was once considered a display of pure joy is now considered a display of happiness and a way to "kick-start" his nervous system. This literal and figurative jump starting of his system is part of his daily morning routine, and is present when he tires as a method to rev up his nervous system. These difficulties with sensory integration and its resulting intensity have an impact on his daily life and routine, including his social skills and engagement at this higher level. For example, I can vividly recall an instance when two of the neighborhood boys came over to our home for a visit. Daniel was so overwhelmed by the presence of his friends from the school bus—again, it was as if the sensory information was too intense, or over the top, leading to an overwhelming emotional response. I sat holding and comforting my young son, contemplating how, in this instant, the dichotomy of his excitement to be social and overwhelming inability to be so reflected the complexities of autism. Despite this complexity, we struggle to have such issues addressed. A year ago, we finally had our only consultation with a neurologist, in the hope of having Daniel's sensory processing professionally examined. This session proved to be an expensive 1 hour, 30 minutes—with an additional souvenir parking ticket—that was arguably fruitless. Spending the majority of the session simply talking to me, the neurologist paid very little attention to our son. The clinical observations consisted of what appeared to be relatively basic tests that overlooked the issues. At the end I was simply told, "It is autism," news that I had been given more than 2 years before.

The social anxiety that Daniel displayed, which seems to be in part a result of processing delay, continues to have a significant impact on Daniel's social skills. This manifests in a number of "classical" symptoms of autism, including the need to have a plan—in order to predict the sensory situation. In hindsight, subtle social difficulties were our first real "hint" of autism, with Daniel ignoring his toys and rarely engaging in pretend play, not always responding to his name, showing a lack of joint attention, and showing an inability to self-soothe as an infant. Nevertheless, his overt levels of engagement in social smile, clear attachment to others, and a strong desire to play and engage with friends added a level of ambiguity and confusion. It was this confusion of Daniel failing to fit the commercialized version of autism that led to early frustrations with the provision of interventions. With classes focused on expanding Daniel's food tastes—something that is difficult with a typical 2½-year-old—and applied behavior classes (ABA), we struggled with the singular focus on limited skills deemed necessary for school entry. While Daniel acquired new foundational skills, such as asking for help, we worried that his superb rote memory meant these ABA programs simply masked the problem. Indeed, we recognized that once Daniel learns something, he owns it; however, it is easy for a teacher or therapist to pass over novel contexts when you have an autistic child who is very bright and has an incredible ability to memorize. This is what is tricky about splinter skills. While Daniel could read or, more accurately put, "decode" in preschool at the second grade level and count to 100, in kindergarten it was discovered that he was never taught the difference between adults or grown-ups and children or kids. He also struggled with the differences between boy and girl. This is why I now insist that Daniel is asked questions in numerous ways to make sure he gets the concept; the English language is so tricky. Right now, it is important for him to get the foundations of our language because his splinter skills and rote memory could take him very far without anyone noticing what very basic and necessary foundational skills he is missing in his skill set. It is now a constant concern that Daniel is memorizing rather than understanding and comprehending.

Given this concern, and in light of Daniel's love of learning, we decided that public school would provide the best environment to allow our son a chance to fulfill his potential. Progressing from a contained classroom to a 50-50 split between the contained and general classroom, Daniel is now in his third year at school and has settled into the environment. We have witnessed his impressive academic advancements. Frustratingly, however, more than 3 years since Daniel's diagnosis, his delayed sensory processing continues to have a debilitating effect on his schooling and daily quality of life. He continues to struggle with the subtleties and unpredictability of social exchange, and has marked social anxiety. This underlying complexity has a direct impact on his relationships with peers at a social level and prevents him from learning in a group setting. Indeed, it is during the group teaching time with his peers that his academic achievements fall apart—a difficulty that prevents him from entering a mainstream classroom for the entire school day. We continue to struggle to have the underlying root of these issues addressed. Recommended providers of sensory-motor integration therapies, or specialist behaviorists, either are at such a distance that it is an unrealistic option or are a "boutique" center that is not covered by, or will not accept, even the most comprehensive of insurance coverage.

As a family, we continue to focus our efforts to help Daniel achieve his goals and further his progress at school. Nevertheless, the battle we face, as parents, to be heard, and also be told exactly what we need to do, continues. We are constantly negotiating between various interventions, struggling to move past the ABA platform—which is no longer prescribed for Daniel—to help him become an independent, future thinker. Indeed, we believe ABA for a child like Daniel can lead to behaviors that become too scripted, rote, and therefore robotic, with no understanding of concepts or reading comprehension. We have often voiced concern about Daniel's rote memory and the lack of generalization and/or transferability of these learned ABA skills to other contexts. However, sourcing and scheduling a range of boutique alternative therapies has become a full-time job, while I continue to be amazed by the sheer volume of paperwork facing parents seeking help and support. My wish, as a parent, is for a system that could enable, rather than disable, us in our mission to help our children. The hurdle of knowing your benefits, what your insurance will cover, and what options are available is mammoth. We believe there should be an insurance advocate at every employer's personnel department and at every hospital or large physician group that knows the individual's coverage for the ASD diagnosis. As ASD is a lifelong disability that requires coordinated care, health insurance companies should also assign families a case manager so that you can speak with the same person or, at the very least, the same department each time you call—someone familiar with your situation and, importantly, your needs.

It is through more novel research projects and work in the scientific community that we are finding acknowledgment of our concerns. The need to revolutionize and redefine our conceptualization of autism, not only as a heterogeneous disorder, but also as one with myriad additional features, including sensory-motor difficulties, is striking. Our hope is that research and clinical practice will begin an open dialogue. Our children need the support and assistance of others who can appreciate not only what they can do, but also what specific needs they have. These do not necessarily need to conform to the expectations of ABA therapy, and generic skills to aid in educational performance, but are often more subtle, including sensory processing, social skills training, and emotional regulation. Moreover, we need to view autism and all the idiosyncrasies of individuals living on the spectrum as an entire person—not simply a cognitive disorder or "floating head" that can be compartmentalized. Each person is unique. Each person is a full person. Treat the whole, not the parts.

25 Anthony's Story
Finding Normal

Cynthia Baeza

From the moment they first hear the news of conception, most parents are inclined to obsess over the health of their child. Many women may change their health habits for the better during their pregnancy. Newly endowed parents may check to see that there are 10 little fingers and 10 little toes as soon as they meet their newborn, wanting nothing more than to hear that everything is "normal." As a first-time parent, I was no different. Being the perfectionist and health fanatic that I was, I took careful measures to ensure my child was at optimal health. During my pregnancy, I devotedly refrained from caffeine, alcohol, unprotected sun exposure, mercury-tainted fish, carbonated drinks, and the majority of over-the-counter medications. During his first few weeks of life, I obsessively tried to keep my newborn away from germs by covering any surface his little face would make contact with using clean, sterile blankets and cloths—including furniture, myself, and other people. As he continued to grow through infancy, I made sure he was getting proper nutrition by breast-feeding as long as possible and buying organic baby food whenever I could afford it.

My caution and overprotectiveness had been working well to keep my little guy healthy and developing normally. Anthony was a very happy and social baby. He frequently made eye contact, even with strangers, and always had a smile on his face. Whenever we were out in public, it was not uncommon for someone to succeed at getting a giggle out of him or to comment on how well behaved he was. Tantrums were pretty rare occurrences, and when they did occur, they were usually due to hunger and easily subdued. Anthony was physically strong, healthy, and his psychoneurological development seemed to be unfolding smoothly. He was hitting all of his milestones on time: babbling by 3–4 months, saying "mama" by 7 months, walking by 10 months, and beginning to say words with meaning before 12 months. He passed all of his screenings and checkups. Thus, I had no concerns that anything was other than normal.

Then, at the age of 14–15 months, my sweet, beautiful boy went through an abrupt, inexplicable change. We had been living with my parents and my younger sister in Connecticut for a few months then, and Anthony had dealt wonderfully with the move. I could tell he enjoyed all the adult attention, aka "playtime," he was getting on a daily basis. One day, when my father came home from work, something strange and peculiar happened. Instead of running to him giggling with open arms, as was his usual greeting to grandpa, Anthony remained quiet, looking down, and did not respond to my father's cheerful greeting. He even repeatedly turned his face away when my father tried to look at him, asking, "What's wrong?"

This was the first sign of a stream of typical symptoms that would swiftly arise. In the days to follow, Anthony's behavior changed drastically: he stopped making eye contact, stopped responding to his name, stopped saying words that he had been saying, and stopped interacting with those around him. He became aloof and completely disconnected from the world, spending minutes to hours just staring blankly into space. He lost his keen, inherent interest in interacting with his family and other people, and became fixated on objects instead. It was as if his mind had been hijacked and trapped behind a glass box, having sight of the world around him but losing the ability to reach out and touch it.

As you can imagine, it took me a long time to accept that this was a lifelong disorder that had suddenly plagued my little boy. I was very familiar with the signs and symptoms of autism, as I had done a project and presentation on it during my last semester as an undergraduate bio major. Deep down, I knew what the signs were pointing to, but my mind stubbornly refused to see them. I convinced myself that it was just a stage he was going through, that maybe he just wasn't feeling well that week, and that he would revert back to his regular self once he was feeling better. Obviously, I was in denial. It's amazing how the mind will avert logic to prevent feelings of loss and hopelessness.

It wasn't until about a month went by and he did not pass a screening questionnaire during his doctor visit that I started to believe it could be autism. Although my parents and I had a difficult time with the news of his autism, we were lucky that it was detected early and that he began receiving early intervention services right away. With intense at-home services from an occupational therapist, speech therapist, and special teacher, Anthony slowly began to make progress. His giggly and cheerful personality began to shine through once again. He continued to have difficulty with social interaction, communication, and sensory issues, but some skills slowly began to reemerge. Seeing Anthony make progress and talking to his therapists about treatment options slowly gave me back some hope and eventually helped me come to terms with his diagnosis.

I believe acceptance is an essential step to making progress when faced with an autism diagnosis, or any diagnosis for that matter. However, acceptance should not elicit complacency. Ever since Anthony's diagnosis, I have set out on a journey to learn as much as possible about autism spectrum disorders, help my son cope with the difficulties and challenges he faces in any way I can, and hopefully contribute to the body of knowledge in the field and discover novel and effective treatments through a career in autism research.

Closely following his diagnosis, my family and I did everything we could to enrich Anthony's experience of the world, expose him to different sensory stimuli, help him conjure up new skills, and present him with opportunities for social interaction. We enrolled him in a playgroup, where we encouraged him to engage in reciprocal play with other children and adults. We started bringing him to open gym time at a gymnastics facility, which he highly enjoyed. We took him to the local library regularly. I even enrolled him in swimming lessons to foster his fascination with water. I believe all of these early, novel experiences gave Anthony a diverse framework for sensing and understanding his environment and helped him cope with his symptoms, including giving him a better sense of his body. Nonetheless, there would be many challenges to overcome on our journey with autism.

One area of difficulty, which carries over into many of the symptoms of autism, is a problem with sensory processing. Many children with autism have issues with altered sensitivity to certain stimuli, including hypersensitivity, hyposensitivity, or both. Anthony has had problems with both, and often within the same perceptual system. For example, his hearing was overly sensitive to loud mechanical sounds, such as blenders, but he could listen to loud music or singing without a problem. The sensitivity could also be present in certain body parts but not others. In his toddler years, Anthony was averse to touching certain textures with his hands, such as sand or Play-Doh, yet he would be willing to touch them with his bare feet. Sensory issues are often the culprit or catalyst for behavioral issues observed in autism. Although it is pretty rare for my son to cry or tantrum, when there is a tantrum or some kind of panic, it is usually linked to a sensory issue.

His sensitivity to certain sounds seems to often be the source of anxieties or phobias that pose a hindrance to daily living commonalities that most people take for granted. These anxieties tend to happen in stages, going through periods of high to low intensity, or vice versa. Although it is often more difficult to reduce a fearful reaction the first time, it will sometimes spring back up after it has been dormant for a while. For a long time, Anthony was deathly afraid of blow-dryers. He still leaves the room most of the time when I'm blow-drying my hair. When those newer, super powerful, and loud blow-dryers came out in public restrooms, he would cry and try to escape whenever someone activated one. It took us a long time to get him fully potty trained and using the bathroom in public. Then, recently, he went through a period where he was absolutely petrified of even entering a public restroom. He became terrified of any bathroom, except the one at home. This fear would cause him to hold his urine the entire school day and go scurrying to the bathroom as soon as he got home. Outings in public became very difficult, as he was often so afraid of entering a restroom that he would have accidents. These sensitivities to sounds continue to present challenges as Anthony grows, but they can be assuaged and overcome with gentle exposure, patience, and understanding.

Repetitive behaviors, aka "stimming," are a hallmark of autism and appear to be linked to sensory processing. Repetitive behaviors seem to occur as a coping mechanism and can be observed in times of boredom and understimulation, happiness and excitement, or in the presence of novelty and stress. Anthony has gone through a series of repetitive behaviors, which also tend to occur in stages, sometimes lasting months or years. The only one of these which really had me concerned was when he would repetitively tap hard objects against his teeth. This occurred for nearly a year and, after a lot of interference, was thankfully replaced by banging his hand—this was usually with softer objects. Currently, his obsession is swinging long objects around, such as cords or tubes, and manipulating them with his hands. He could enjoy this activity for hours and is often a lot more comfortable in novel environments when allowed an object to "stim" with. I personally, see nothing wrong with allowing stimming to occur as long as it is bringing the individual joy, is not harmful to themselves or others, and is not interfering with their learning. I think people should be more understanding of individuals on the spectrum, letting them cope in their own way, instead of trying to make them fit the mold of societal expectations.

Anthony's biggest challenge has always been his difficulty with communication and verbal language. Although he has no problem with perceptual language—he can understand pretty much everything that's being said to him or around him—Anthony has great difficulty forming spoken words. He has a few words that he can use functionally for requesting or labeling, but he is mostly nonverbal. This is probably the greatest challenge out of all his symptoms because he does not yet have a means to express what he is thinking, what he wants, or what he knows. It can be very frustrating, for both parties, if he is upset about something or is in some kind of pain and cannot tell us what's bothering him. His lack of language also makes forming social relationships with other children a challenge, as he is not able to interact with them verbally. If a child comes over to play with him, I sometimes have to explain, "Anthony doesn't know how to talk so he can't answer you, but he probably wants to play and he likes to run around if you want to play tag."

His inability to speak is the symptom that has taken the greatest emotional toll on me. I always thought he would learn to speak fluently. He showed a lot of potential from an early age, with frequent babbling and changing the intonation of his voice as if he were speaking his own language. I've had dreams where he would look at me and just start spewing out words fluently, telling me what's on his mind. Although my dream of him speaking verbally will never cease to exist, I have to face the reality that considering his current speaking ability at the age of 7, it is unlikely that he'll be able to communicate verbally in a fluent, comprehensible manner. His issue with speech seems to be a lack of motor control of his oral muscles. There also seems to be a problem in the processing of outgoing signals, since he frequently gets confused with which sounds he's trying to produce. For example, when requesting water, he will make the sound "ma" most of the time, but will sometimes say "wa" or "ta." His speech mainly consists of one-syllable words or word approximations, although he can put up to three syllables together when saying them one at a time, such as in "ba-na-na." Still, it is difficult for those who don't know him to understand him, and it is often challenging for my family and me as well.

He has been using a communication system on his iPad at school known as Proloquo2Go and doing well with it. It uses tags of pictures, symbols, and words that he can choose to convey his message. He has been using it successfully at school to answer questions and make requests, and we are planning to begin adding pictures and symbols for home use as well. One of the best features of this is that the app can read the words or sentences he forms aloud, which allows him to communicate with practically anyone who understands English. His use of this program greatly facilitates his ability to communicate and can reduce a lot of the frustrations of being misunderstood when he's trying to tell us something. We have also been working on teaching Anthony to type. He already recognizes many words by sight and seems to recognize the keyboard as a tool to get words on the screen and express his wants and needs; thus, I am very hopeful that he will learn to type. These tools would provide an unveiling window into his mind, a means of expressing his thoughts and ideas, and an outlet for him to reach out of his glass box and touch the world. They could give him a voice. I will never give up on improving his verbal speech abilities, but the thought of him being able to reveal what's on his mind in whatever method he can overwhelms me with joy. It would be a dream come true.

Anthony has really come a long way since the time of his diagnosis. He is a little boy with amazing ability to push through and surmount the challenges he faces every day, and do it with a smile on his face. I've done my best with my limited resources to give him the best possible odds of success. I believe some of the best ways to treat his autism are with exposure to novel, sensory-rich experiences, exposure to the community and community activities and events, and lots of love, praise, and positive attention. Anthony has been in everything from swimming lessons, to gymnastics, to horseback riding camp. He has visited three countries via airplane and loves to fly. I frequently take him out to museums, zoos, restaurants, birthday parties, beaches, pools, trampoline parks, playgrounds, and even theme parks. He'll sometimes have issues with noises or crowds at these places, but I help him deal with them and he slowly overcomes them. He'll sometimes eye someone else's food when out at a restaurant or cross the boundaries of personal space with strangers in public, but I slowly teach him what's acceptable and what's not. I think it's very sad that some families are so embarrassed or so fearful that they limit their special needs child's experience of the world and of society. How would my son ever learn the logistics of human social interactions if I don't bring him out into society? How would his brain develop better body awareness if he is always in the same environment and not exposed to new sensations? I believe enriching experiences such as these have helped him gain a better understanding of himself and the world around him and have likewise helped with his autism.

His therapies, such as occupational therapy (OT), speech, and applied behavioral analysis (ABA), have helped a great deal as well. I am very optimistic about the development of future therapies and am determined to dedicate my career to cultivating them and enhancing our understanding of the autistic brain. The work being done at the Sensory-Motor Integration Lab by Dr. Torres and her team is very innovative and makes me hopeful for a scientifically solid method of treating and diagnosing autism. Therapies that help fix the disconnect between sensory input to the brain and the motor output could prove wonders for my son and children like him. I have recently begun volunteering with the lab and cannot wait to contribute more to their research and their cause. I'm hopeful that in the future, the discoveries made with this work will allow us to help special needs children gain control of their bodies and greatly enhance their ability to interact with their environment and other people.

My journey as a mother of a child with autism has taught me a lot about life. I no longer seek to do everything to perfection or try to control the uncontrollable. I've learned that life almost never goes according to plan, but you have to face each unexpected challenge with ambition and resolve. It is the unplanned adversity you come across in life that builds inner strength and character. I'm a stronger person now than I ever thought I could be. Anthony is truly an inspiration to take things as they come. Despite the difficulties he faces, he doesn't let them faze him. He always has such a cheerful and positive demeanor that it is contagious to those around him. It is beyond words how much joy he brings to my life. The struggles we face only make every milestone and success more special. I've learned to cherish the small things. I've learned to share his joys by entering into his world and accepting his quirks along with his strengths. I've learned that normal is overrated. Whether he's wailing his arms above his head for joy or I'm walking around a fancy wedding reception with him riding piggyback, we have made our own normal.

26 Autism
A Bullying Perspective

Sejal Mistry and Caroline Whyatt

CONTENTS

Introduction 357
A Worrying Trend: Bullying toward the ASD Community 359
Our Hope for the Future 363
References 364

The previous chapters gave voice to families and individuals living with autism spectrum disorder (ASD) on a daily basis. These intimate accounts illustrate the complexities associated with a diagnosis of ASD, from the myriad symptoms often overlooked by the clinical field to the struggle to avail of treatment options available. Despite these tangible difficulties, a common thread is evident throughout: the struggle to adapt, and to find love, support, and acceptance from society—both for the family unit and at an individual level. From the account of Daniel, so eager to play with his classmates that it becomes overwhelming, to Jayden, innocently following her peers desperate to connect, these two highly emotional accounts appear to lie in direct contrast to our academic, clinical, and often public perception of ASD. This chapter explores the subtleties of socialization that are largely discounted by our traditional conceptualization of ASD, namely, bullying.

INTRODUCTION

Academically, bullying has been defined as inflicting repeated negative actions on an individual in either a direct (e.g., physical or verbal) or indirect (e.g., social exclusion) manner (Olweus 1994; Reid et al. 2004; Scarpaci 2006). Associated with a range of physiological and psychological side effects (Turner et al. 2013; Ilola et al. 2016), bullying is a growing worldwide concern among school-aged children (Raskauskas and Modell 2011), with approximately 20%–22% of school-aged children reported as victims of bullying (Raskauskas and Modell 2011; Lessne and Harmalkar 2013). Perhaps unsurprisingly, the estimated rate of victimization and bullying within the ASD community is notably higher than that in the broader population. Official statistics from the U.S. Department of Education indicate that approximately half (46.3%) of adolescents with ASD are a victim of bullying (Sterzing et al. 2012). Furthermore, estimates vary significantly across research sites—perhaps a by-product of the sample size or methodology employed—figures consistently indicate a higher prevalence of bullying reported toward the ASD community (Table 26.1).

This form of social interaction has a profound and wide-ranging impact on the ASD community. Indeed, during our recent research study we witnessed the impact and reach of this bullying epidemic firsthand via the reporting of social dynamics and struggles recorded through the Autism Diagnostic Observation Schedule (ADOS) (Lord et al. 2000). This semistructured interview provides a controlled environment for a clinician to probe specific traits of ASD, including social interactions and friendships under detailed categories, such as "social difficulties & annoyance," "friends, relationships, and marriage," and "responsibility." The ADOS is comprised of several modules, each probing a different aspect of social behavior. Each module is dependent on the

TABLE 26.1
Sample of Recent Estimates of Bullying Prevalence within the ASD Community

Study	Rate of Bullying Reported	Methodology	Experiment Format	Sample Size	Age of Children
Little 2002	94%	Parent reports	Questionnaire	411 (75% ASD), 15% nonverbal learning disability	4–17
Reid and Batten 2006	40%–59%	Parent reports and self-reports	Questionnaire and interview	1400 family responses; 28 children interviewed	N/A
Wainscot et al. 2008	87%	Self-reports	Interview	30	11–18
Carter 2009	65%	Self-reports	Questionnaire	34	5–21
Cappadocia et al. 2012	77%	Parent reports	Questionnaire	192	5–21
Zeedyk et al. 2014	75%	Self-reports	Interview	44	6–15
Zablotsky et al. 2014	63%	Parent reports	Questionnaire	1215	13

N/A, Not Available

child and may differ depending on the child's specific abilities. For example, module 3 incorporates a participant's ability to understand other's emotions and empathize. Lower scores indicate a clear understanding and an appropriate response to questions concerning emotional expression and empathy, while higher scores indicate minimal identification and communication regarding others' emotions. In particular, modules 3 and 4 explore facets of social interaction and can provide insight into friendships, relationships, and responsibility. It is in these sections that we notice an overwhelming prevalence of bullying emerging. A summary of the metrics recorded for such questions or categories throughout the ADOS administration is provided in Table 26.2. This small sample ($N = 18$) provides unanimous evidence of pronounced social difficulties in this group of individuals with ASD.

TABLE 26.2
Summary Metrics Recorded for Categories Probing Social Dynamics and Relationships Using the ADOS-2 (Lord et al. 2012)

SA Statistical Summary			
Category	**Average Score**	**Standard Deviation**	**Median**
Overall SA	10.00	3.56	10.5
Communication SA subscore	2.17	0.86	2.00
Reciprocal social interaction SA subscore	7.83	4.07	8.00
Restricted and repetitive behaviors	5.72	2.19	6.00
Overall scores	15.72	5.28	16.00

Note: Scored on a numerical scale, 0 is indicative of a "typical" response, while higher scores are indicative of pronounced difficulties. $N = 18$.

The algorithm behind ADOS score calculation aims to capture difficulties in communication, such as difficulties reporting events, holding conversations, and interpreting social gestures. High scores in this section indicate significant difficulties in understanding social dynamics, that is, a corrupted input of social information. Another feature of the ADOS algorithm incorporates reciprocal social interactions, along with eye contact, facial expressions, social responses, and quality of rapport. High scores in these sections indicate knowledge of social communication, but difficulty in reciprocating inner feelings, that is, a corrupted output of social information. Combined, difficulties in communication and reciprocal social interactions make overall social affect (SA) difficult. Overall, we see a high prevalence of difficulties with SA (see Table 26.2). The ability to both comprehend the social dynamics of a situation and respond appropriately seem to be difficult for children with ASD. Given these findings, it is no surprise that children with ASD are increasingly vulnerable to social abuse through bullying. This trend has garnered a growing research focus in ASD bullying, with questions raised over antibullying strategies, the type of victimization or bullying that individuals with ASD face, and why.

A WORRYING TREND: BULLYING TOWARD THE ASD COMMUNITY

Traditionally conceived as a strategy born out of an imbalance in power (Wolke and Lereya 2015), the causes and psychological underpinnings of bullying have been well documented. Literature indicates that victims of bullying are often targeted because they show signs of anxiety or insecurity (Glew et al. 2000), and generally demonstrate poor social skills, difficulty maintaining relationships with classmates, and increased loneliness (Nansel et al. 2001). Troublingly, a number of studies detail a clear and tangible intersection between such characteristics that make an individual prone to victimization and symptomatology of ASD. In particular, children diagnosed with ASD display behavioral difficulties with communication and socialization, and often engage in repetitive behavior (APA 2013)—characteristics that increase the likelihood of victimization (Schroeder et al. 2014). Furthermore, internalizing or hidden problems—behaviors that generate distress in an individual and are not visible to others—were found to be more significant predictors of victimization than ASD status (Zeedyk et al. 2014). This would suggest that children are bullied because of the symptoms of ASD, rather than the fact that they have ASD alone. In addition to egocentric factors, the peer environment or schooling system also appears to play a vital role in victimization. Zablotsky and colleagues recently (2014) reported that 89% of individuals with ASD who attend a general education school are victims of bullying, as opposed to 11% who attend special education. These figures may reflect two factors: (1) the overarching trend of increased bullying as correlated with external symptoms of ASD, and (2) the schooling environment may be a direct reflection of difficulties faced by individuals with ASD—namely, the struggle to be accepted.

Autism is a hidden condition that manifests in core behavioral symptomatology that, as mentioned, is known to include factors that may predict the prevalence or likelihood of being victimized (Schroeder et al. 2014). By defining ASD through such external and behavioral facets, society—public, academic, and clinical—retains a psychological perspective and dialogue for ASD. As noted throughout this book, this perspective is reinforced at all levels, from the diagnostic measures used to intervention programs provided and, importantly, our preconception of ASD. In particular, by retaining a psychological stance we paradoxically remove levels of autonomy, while placing "blame" or "intent" onto the individual with ASD—viewing behaviors as problematic, to be banished or reduced. Yet, if viewed within the context of sensory and movement models, we can begin to open a dialogue of physiological underpinnings, and consider behavioral difficulties through a new lens. For instance, individuals with ASD that have pronounced difficulty isolating and integrating sensory information to guide and control behaviors—from the presence of noisy and random input signals—will have behavioral repercussions. Core symptomatology, such as difficulty with social interactions or repetitive behaviors, may therefore be considered attempts to "dampen" the impact of sensory stimuli, or to "make sense" of the world. As noted in the example of Daniel in Chapter 24, the simultaneous overwhelming excitement of social encounters, mixed with the fact sensory information can seem overwhelming to the point of parental intervention, may point to some of the difficulties individuals with ASD face. These underlying physiological difficulties rooted in aspects such as sensory processing are a fundamental piece of the larger puzzle, and elements that are beyond the control of the individual. Rather, the individual is finding coping mechanisms or strategies to best accommodate these latent needs. By imposing restrictions and attempting to remove or modify behaviors, or placing intent and blame on the individual, society is perpetuating this stereotyping and victimization of the ASD community. Indeed, the role of sensory issues as a source of anxiety leading to the modification of behavioral patterns (Hebron et al. 2015; Humphrey and Hebron 2015) has been isolated as a potential predictor of victimization. As mentioned by Pat Amos in Chapter 20, no one would chastise her for having irregular movement patterns—her diagnosis of Parkinson's disease, a physiological condition affecting motor control, is accepted as the root of these difficulties, leading to acceptance, love, and support. In contrast, her son's similar movement irregularities are viewed and considered behavioral oddities that must be reduced or removed through programs that strip him of his autonomy.

We suggest it is now time for a new model of ASD, one that considers the physiological underpinnings, changing the public, academic, and clinical dialogue from one of behavioral intentions to one of acceptance and understanding. This extends to the schooling environment, where children and adolescents with ASD, during their formative years, are initially told to "conform" to societal expectations—with little negotiation. The first step may be education of the schooling system. Initially, rather than viewing an individual with ASD as a manifestation of his or her symptomologies of reduced social interaction or aversion to social settings, we may encourage questioning if the isolation is a by-product of victimization—a fact that may currently go unnoticed. Indeed, the methodology to examine levels of bullying within the ASD community (e.g., firsthand observation or direct reports vs. secondhand parent or teacher reports) produces radically varying results, indicative of the complexities associated with this social dynamic within a subgroup of individuals characterized as having difficulties with social interaction. Exemplified in the account of both Jadyn and Daniel, a struggle for acceptance mixed with pronounced social difficulties illustrates a complex dynamic that is artificially simplified with current models. With evidence of reduced social networks, and limited friend circles (Wainscot et al. 2008), individuals with ASD are known to have difficulty with isolation. Yet, due to the public, academic, and clinical interpretation of ASD, this isolation may be attributed to a social aversion—a foundation of ASD symptomatology. Indeed, while their interactions are not physical in nature, these children still do feel a sense of loneliness, reflected in scores presented in the categories "emotions" and "loneliness" that are explicitly scored during the ADOS administration (Table 26.1).

Further, antibullying strategies for the ASD population are in their infancy, with little research on the short- and long-term side effects of prolonged bullying in the ASD community (Humphrey and Hebron 2015). Only recently has ASD bullying research began to empirically establish risk and protective factors (Hebron et al. 2015). Within the wider population, schools typically apply a three-pronged approach, including engaging parents and other youth, creating policies and rules, and educating staff and peers. However, this education must be refined to aid the antibullying dialogue for ASD. In particular, we must educate children, teachers, and parents that the ASD community cannot help these internal factors, such as sensory, repetitive, or adaptive behaviors that may increase their likelihood of victimization.

To illustrate this point further, we draw on an excerpt from a recent ADOS report gathered as part of a research study to demonstrate this social complexity. In this example, we find evidence of a conscious victim of bullying, who is struggling to find a way in the world, seeking acceptance from his peers. As documented in Box 26.1, this participant demonstrates insight into his behaviors and the potential source of his isolation.

BOX 26.1 CONSCIOUS VICTIM: EXCERPT OF RESEARCH DIALOGUE FROM ADMINISTRATION OF THE ADOS

Examiner: So I have a question for you. Do you ever have issues with other kids from school?
Participant A: Sometimes.
Examiner: Are there ever things that other kids do that bother you?
Participant A: Yes.

Immediately, you can sense a change in the participant's mood. Before, he was confidently sitting up and making active eye contact with the examiner, but now you see him slouch and begin constantly moving around. This is reflected in the ADOS "Compulsions of Ritual" section, which identifies compulsions within the context of the participant's determination to carry out an action. This participant received a score of 1 on this sub-scale for "Compulsions of Ritual", indicative of unusual routinized speech or activities. The shift in both his posture and attitude triggers the examiner to approach the topic cautiously.

Examiner: Like what?
Participant A: Well ... a lot of times kids call me names. I don't really know what to do sometimes, but I usually tell the teacher.
Examiner: Are there things that you do that might irritate other kids?
Participant A: ... Yeah.
Examiner: Like what?
Participant A: Umm ... when I'm bored, sometimes I make noises. But eventually I remember and then I come back. I try really hard not to irritate others.
Examiner: So Participant A, tell me, what do you do so that you won't bother the other kids?
Participant A: Well ... I don't think I've really figured it out yet. But I'm working on it.

This insight, impressive for most, is eloquently illustrated with the participant alluding to an internal battle to resolve the behaviors he deems problematic in an attempt to "fit in." Yet, this raises an important question regarding the social expectations and pressures placed on the ASD community. Furthermore, a recent qualitative examination of victimization in ASD indicated that individuals across the spectrum had a pronounced difficulty articulating *why* someone may be bullied (Hebron et al. 2015). This inability to identify why or if someone is being bullied may play a vital role in the identification and characterization of bullying in ASD, and raises a *second* question regarding an individual's insight into the fact that he or she is indeed a victim of social isolation or bullying.

Inclusion in the mainstream, general education system may arguably result in higher levels of victimization as a by-product of egocentric factors, such as those outlined above, *and* reduced awareness of ASD by the wider population at large. Specifically, the overarching trend for higher levels of victimization or bullying associated with the general education system may be a by-product of higher inclusion within the mainstream classroom setting, and a pool of "higher-functioning" individuals. Arguably, higher levels of cognitive ability may translate into higher levels of awareness regarding bullying, leading to higher levels of parental knowledge, and thus reported cases. As such, along with reported cases, there may also be a problem with unreported or unconscious victimization—as illustrated in the example of Jadyn. In this heartbreaking example, we heard of a young girl struggling to be accepted by her peers —failing to read the social cues of the larger social group, and innocently vying for approval. This personal account again provides a unique insight into the paradoxical nature of ASD—one often overlooked by our traditional conceptualization of ASD: the simultaneous apparent aversion to and difficulty with social stimuli—a concept firmly ensconced within the academic literature, forming a core axis of the diagnostic process and criteria (Wing and Gould 1979; APA 2013)—with the overwhelming desire to socialize and fit in. By limiting our definition, and indeed understanding, of ASD, we may be providing a severe injustice to the ASD community. In failing to understand that individuals across the spectrum, irrespective of social difficulties, have an innate desire to be accepted socially, we may be supporting this dialogue and environment of unconscious victimization.

Again, we illustrate this point with an extract from the ADOS report, where a young girl diagnosed with ASD is visiting our research lab for the fourth time. Over the course of the year preceding this visit, the participant became close to our research team, enjoying the interactions—again, in contrast to the clinical and academic preconception of ASD—and recounts with brutal insight her limited social circle (Box 26.2).

BOX 26.2 UNCONSCIOUS VICTIM: EXCERPT OF RESEARCH DIALOGUE FROM ADMINISTRATION OF THE ADOS

Examiner: So Participant B, do you have some friends at school? Can you tell me about them?

Participant B: [*Clearly uncomfortable*] Well ... my friends are Mommy and Daddy. And Caroline [research team member].

Examiner: Wow, Participant B, that's so sweet! So I have another question for you. Do you have any friends from school?

Participant B: No ...

Examiner: Have you ever had problems getting along with people at school?

Participant B: Hmmm ... no trouble at school.

Examiner: That's great! Are there things you do that annoy others?

Participant B: I don't think so.

Examiner: Have you ever been bullied or teased?

Participant B: No.

This restricted social dynamic, yet insight, is reflected in a score of 1 (indicative of some attempt at getting and maintaining attention) under the heading "Amount of Social Overtures/ Maintenance of Attention."

Such questions regarding the impact of cognitive functioning, and thus mainstream schooling leading to higher levels of reported bullying, have been further illustrated through recent in-depth interviews that indicate that individuals across the ASD spectrum have a tenuous grasp on the concept of bullying (Hebron et al. 2015). Self-reported, firsthand accounts of bullying result in vastly different prevalence estimates (Van Roekel et al. 2010; Maïano et al. 2016), implying that individuals with ASD may have difficulty perceiving victimization. Combined, these points demonstrate the growing need for an education program to facilitate antibullying interventions in ASD. Unfortunately, examination of current antibullying interventions in place to protect the ASD community highlights a number of limitations, from the content and methods employed, to the statistical procedures used to examine effectiveness. For instance, a number of studies designing and examining such programs are limited in scope in terms of participant numbers (Rose et al. 2010; Blake et al. 2012), age range, ASD subdiagnosis, and geographical areas (Zeedyk et al. 2014), preventing generalizability. Furthermore, studies are often limited by dichotomous classifications, in which children are binomially divided into groups of "bullied" and "not bullied" (Hebron et al. 2015). While this reduces a complex social problem into a binary problem (Hebron et al. 2015), it fails to account for the different extents of bullying and discrepancies in knowledge. It is important to stress that while children with ASD may not be able to actively control their symptoms, these very symptoms may also impair their ability to detect or report bullying—as a typical child may do. This contributes to a negative feedback loop, where ASD may cause corrupted or noisy sensory input, which in turn results in external behavioral symptoms, which may further exacerbate victimization or bullying.

Finally, in line with difficulty perceiving victimization, a number of individuals with ASD may fall into a third category: the unconscious bully. Perceived as a lack of self-identification as examined through the ADOS subcategory "responsibility," this subset of individuals may fail to reflect on their behaviors and resulting impact on peers. Drawing on transcripts from an ADOS research session (Box 26.3) provides a window into this difficulty.

BOX 26.3 UNCONSCIOUS VICTIM: EXCERPT OF RESEARCH DIALOGUE FROM ADMINISTRATION OF THE ADOS

Examiner: So tell me, what type of things are you afraid of? Like, what might make you feel frightened or anxious?
Participant C: I would say people in my school.
Examiner: Who in your school makes you feel that way?
Participant C: I think the popular kids. So our school is basically divided into two groups … and it's the popular kids because I think they're rough.
Examiner: So you mean they're rough with you?
Participant C: I mean they like to fight each other. Like there's a lot of drama. There's … physical fighting and drama.
Examiner: So I know we started to talk about kids at school. Do they bully you at all?
Participant C: Well, sometimes they tell me to shut up.
Examiner: Is there anything you can do to help when they're on your nerves?
Participant C: Well, I usually go to the guidance counselor or the teacher.

At this point, the participant C becomes increasingly emotional. While talking about her school relationships, the examiner strikes a nerve, which results in a short comfort break during the session. The examiner reflects this in the "Anxiety" section of the ADOS. Anxiety includes initial wariness or self-consciousness, as well as signs of worry, upset, or concern. In this section, the participant scores a 1, indicating mild signs of anxiety of self-consciousness. However, the score for "responsibility," inferring an ability to self-reflect and identify the impact of one's own actions, was 2. This reflects a limited sense of responsibility for one's actions or may show a clear lack of responsibility relative to the child's age.

Examiner: That's good! So do you ever do anything that bugs the other kids?
Participant C: Well, not really. But there's this group of friends that sit near me during lunch. For some reason, when I seem to have fun, it seems to tick them off a lot. I don't really know why.
Examiner: So can you tell me about some of your friends? What are they like?
Participant C: Well some of them are very supportive. They're all from school. My one friend is really close to me.

OUR HOPE FOR THE FUTURE

Bullying and victimization are a concern for all members of society. Yet for those parents of individuals with ASD, that concern is tangible. From the external and internal factors that may make their children more prone to bullying, to the heartbreaking innocence as their children fail to identify with their own victimization, the dialogue surround bullying in the ASD community must change. We argue it is now time for a reconceptualization of ASD in general—moving from a psychological to a physiological construct—helping the public, academic, and clinical arenas have a new insight into this complex social world. With this, we suggest that it is time to begin viewing behavioral outputs or symptomatology not as something that is challenging and intended that must be reduced in individuals on the ASD spectrum, but rather as a coping mechanism to overcome latent physiological challenges. Working with education providers, parents, and importantly, peers, we call for antibullying programs that aim to enhance inclusivity not merely by reducing the autistic behaviors, but by educating others to the meaning of these—akin to our ability to understand movement and sensory problems in Parkinson's disease, or behaviors and language that may seem unacceptable at first in someone with Tourette's. As researchers, we also aim to give autonomy and identity back to those individuals that we have the pleasure to work with closely. By taking small steps toward education, we aim to provide each individual with a bespoke, tailored feedback protocol to help raise awareness and inclusivity. Working with the perceived power differential within the schooling environment, we produce custom-made pieces, including posters and short movies, where the participant is truly the star of the show. We build around a theme or an interest that may be deemed a repetitive behavior or restricted preoccupation, showcasing the impact the participant is having on not only our research, but also science. Displayed throughout the school setting, these pieces help educate the peers, while elevating the participant to a new status—one that encourages understanding, support, and ultimately, acceptance.

We believe it is small steps by society that will have a long-lasting impact for the ASD community. Cumulatively, these small steps may have a lasting and profound effect—one that we hope may change the lives of families and individuals living with ASD on a daily basis. We can only hope now is the time for this collective effort.

REFERENCES

APA (American Psychiatric Association). 2013. *Diagnostic and Statistical Manual of Mental Disorders*. 5th ed. Washington, DC: APA.

Blake, J. J., E. M. Lund, Q. Zhou, O.-M. Kwok, and M. R. Benz. 2012. National prevalence rates of bully victimization among students with disabilities in the United States. *School Psychol Q* 27 (4): 210.

Cappadocia, M. C., J. A. Weiss, and D. Pepler. 2012. Bullying experiences among children and youth with autism spectrum disorders. *J Autism Dev Disord* 42 (2):266–77.

Carter, S. 2009. Bullying of students with Asperger syndrome. *Issues Compr Pediatr Nurs* 32 (3):145–54.

Glew, G., F. Rivara, and C. Feudtner. 2000. Bullying: Children hurting children. *Pediatr Rev* 21 (6):183–9; quiz 190.

Hebron, J., N. Humphrey, and J. Oldfield. 2015. Vulnerability to bullying of children with autism spectrum conditions in mainstream education: A multi-informant qualitative exploration. *J Res Spec Educ Needs* 15 (3): 185–93.

Humphrey, N., and J. Hebron. 2015. Bullying of children and adolescents with autism spectrum conditions: A 'state of the field' review. *Int J Inclusive Educ* 19 (8):845–62.

Ilola, A.-M., L. Lempinen, J. Huttunen, T. Ristkari, and A. Sourander. 2016. Bullying and victimisation are common in four-year-old children and are associated with somatic symptoms and conduct and peer problems. *Acta Paediatr* 105 (5):522–8.

Lessne, D., and S. Harmalkar. 2013. Student reports of bullying and cyber-bullying: Results from the 2011 School Crime Supplement to the National Crime Victimization Survey. Web tables. NCES 2013-329. Washington, DC: National Center for Education Statistics.

Little, L. 2002. Middle-class mothers' perceptions of peer and sibling victimization among children with Asperger's syndrome and nonverbal learning disorders. *Issues Compr Pediatr Nurs* 25 (1):43–57.

Lord, C., P. C. DiLavore, and K. Gotham. 2012. Autism diagnostic observation schedule. Torrance, CA: Western Psychological Services.

Lord, C., S. Risi, L. Lambrecht, E. H. Cook Jr., B. L. Leventhal, P. C. DiLavore, A. Pickles, and M. Rutter. 2000. The Autism Diagnostic Observation Schedule-Generic: A standard measure of social and communication deficits associated with the spectrum of autism. *J Autism Dev Disord* 30 (3):205–23.

Maïano, C., A. Aimé, M.-C. Salvas, A. J. S. Morin, and C. L. Normand. 2016. Prevalence and correlates of bullying perpetration and victimization among school-aged youth with intellectual disabilities: A systematic review. *Res Dev Disabil* 49:181–95.

Nansel, T. R., M. Overpeck, R. S. Pilla, W. J. Ruan, B. Simons-Morton, and P. Scheidt. 2001. Bullying behaviors among US youth: Prevalence and association with psychosocial adjustment. *JAMA* 285 (16):2094–100.

Olweus, D. 1994. Bullying at school: Basic facts and effects of a school based intervention program. *J Child Psychol Psychiatry* 35 (7):1171–90.

Raskauskas, J., and S. Modell. 2011. Modifying anti-bullying programs to include students with disabilities. *Teach Exceptional Child* 44 (1):60.

Reid, B., and A. Batten. 2006. B is for bullied: The experiences of children with autism and their families. London: National Autistic Society.

Reid, P., J. Monsen, and I. Rivers. 2004. Psychology's contribution to understanding and managing bullying within schools. *Educ Psychol Pract* 20 (3):241–58.

Rose, C. A., L. E. Monda-Amaya, and D. L. Espelage. 2010. Bullying perpetration and victimization in special education: A review of the literature. *Remedial Spec Educ* 32 (2):114–30.

Scarpaci, R. T. 2006. Bullying effective strategies for its prevention: Put a halt to the name-calling, teasing, poking, and shoving, and make way for learning. *Kappa Delta Pi Rec* 42 (4):170–4.

Schroeder, J. H., M. C. Cappadocia, J. M. Bebko, D. J. Pepler, and J. A. Weiss. 2014. Shedding light on a pervasive problem: A review of research on bullying experiences among children with autism spectrum disorders. *J Autism Dev Disord* 44 (7):1520–34.

Sterzing, P. R., P. T. Shattuck, S. C. Narendorf, M. Wagner, and B. P. Cooper. 2012. Bullying involvement and autism spectrum disorders: Prevalence and correlates of bullying involvement among adolescents with an autism spectrum disorder. *Arch Pediatr Adolesc Med* 166 (11):1058–64.

Turner, M. G., M. L. Exum, R. Brame, and T. J. Holt. 2013. Bullying victimization and adolescent mental health: General and typological effects across sex. *J Crim Justice* 41 (1):53–9.

Van Roekel, E., R. H. J. Scholte, and R. Didden. 2010. Bullying among adolescents with autism spectrum disorders: Prevalence and perception. *J Autism Dev Disord* 40 (1):63–73.

Wainscot, J. J., P. Naylor, P. Sutcliffe, D. Tantam, and J. V. Williams. 2008. Relationships with peers and use of the school environment of mainstream secondary school pupils with Asperger syndrome (high-functioning autism): A case-control study. *Int J Psychol Psychol Ther* 8 (1):25–38.

Wing, L., and J. Gould. 1979. Severe impairments of social interaction and associated abnormalities in children: Epidemiology and classification. *J Autism Dev Disord* 9 (1):11–29.

Wolke, D., and S. T. Lereya. 2015. Long-term effects of bullying. *Arch Dis Child* 100 (9):879–85.

Zablotsky, B., C. P. Bradshaw, C. M. Anderson, and P. Law. 2014. Risk factors for bullying among children with autism spectrum disorders. *Autism* 18 (4):419–27.

Zeedyk, S. M., G. Rodriguez, L. A. Tipton, B. L. Baker, and J. Blacher. 2014. Bullying of youth with autism spectrum disorder, intellectual disability, or typical development: Victim and parent perspectives. *Res Autism Spectr Disord* 8 (9):1173–83.

27 Turning the Tables
Autism Shows the Social Deficit of Our Society

Elizabeth B. Torres

CONTENTS

Autism: The Current Definition....367
Two Different Goals: Very Different Outcomes....368
Follow the Money....370
Some Unforeseen Consequences of the Financial Conflicts of Interest Plaguing Autism Diagnoses and Treatments....370
Discrete Subjective Scales Cannot Capture Adaptive Change....371
Uncertain Outcomes of Psychotropic Medications and Behavioral Modifications....372
Politics and Economics....373
The Parents' Impossible Road to Diversified Treatments....373
Social Deficit of Our Society....375
References....376

The autistic condition, as currently defined by observation and dependent on a priori defined notions of social appropriateness, has gained prevalence of epidemic proportions worldwide. In the United States, the systems that diagnose and treat the condition follow a clinical model primarily based on a psychological or psychiatric construct. Such an approach leaves out bodily physiology and its sensory consequences in favor of descriptions and interpretations of observational data gathered by hand without proper scientific rigor. The clinical model thus constructed serves a fast-pace system to provide recommendations for treatment that directly impact the lives of the affected individuals and their core caregiver family unit, but fails to embrace them as active members of society at large. While limiting the potential contributions of the autistic person to our society, the current clinical model is also interfering with the scientific model and its progress, which has considerably stalled. This chapter exposes some of the contemporary issues surrounding the complex relationships between society at large and the autistic population in the context of a psychological or psychiatric model that is not working.

It's not science … it's politics and economics; that's what psychiatry is: politics and economics.

Dr. Thomas Szasz, Professor of Psychiatry

AUTISM: THE CURRENT DEFINITION

Defined as a deficit of social interactions, characterized by lack of communication and the presence of repetitive, restrictive behaviors (American Psychiatric Association 2013), autism spectrum disorders (ASDs) is now one of the neurodevelopmental disorders with higher prevalence in the United States. Soon enough, the so-called epidemic proportion of affected children will turn into affected young adults.

Indeed, the latest report on estimated prevalence of ASD based on 2014 data was 2.24%, "a significant increase from the estimated annualized prevalence of 1.25% based on 2011–2013 data" (Zablotsky et al. 2015a). How can we as scientists help address this societal problem?

The social definition of this neurodevelopmental problem affords more than one level of description and interaction. At present, the burden is placed on the affected person. One gets the feeling that "*they* are the ones with a problem: We ought to change *them* to conform to us" (Odom 2016). In this process, the majority of society may fall into one of several self-evident categories: mere spectators of a problem that has been portrayed in science as one of the biggest contemporary puzzles of the human brain with no foreseen solution in the near future, actuators on the problem to "cure" it or "reshape" it at all cost, people who care about the individual with autism and want to desperately help, and self-advocates who have somehow found a voice. However, there is an additional stand-alone category: those who profit or want to profit from this problem. These individuals inevitably drive the focus of other groups and society at large.

First, let us examine this problem using the lens of a researcher who tends to think outside of the box: An expectation comes from the systematic or frequent occurrence of events that surface so often and with such regularities that they reach statistical power of the kind that one can predict an outcome probabilistically and confirm it most of the time with high certainty. An oddity or unexpected outcome that does not conform to the preset expectation (e.g., a social norm) is indeed worrisome—particularly if the occurrence is so randomly heterogeneous that there is no pattern to classify it into something previously known. We do not know how to cope with it, so in a way, we lose our control over the situation. Let us then consider the implausible scenario that one morning we wake up only to find out that we lack total control over social situations and that, in the presence of such lack of control, we have acquired a social deficit ourselves: we have been labeled "autistic." As such, I wonder how we, as a society, should be treated. Should we all be reshaped through conditioning-based treatments? Should we all be medicated to eliminate this autistic condition? Should we all be deprived of our free will? And if so, who may be given the credentials to do this to us? Who will be authorized to treat us and reshape our behaviors to conform to expectations? What laws would protect us? And who will be dictating those laws? Scary, isn't it? The mere thought of it should make you wonder how a child with ASD, subject to all the above, feels about the rest of us.

Indeed, to have a true appreciation, we must flip roles and rethink this problem from the perspective of the affected child, that is, the human being that we (perhaps unknowingly) have robbed of any chance to be part of our "expected" social world. Let us have a look at the side of autism that very few of us in science come to think about.

TWO DIFFERENT GOALS: VERY DIFFERENT OUTCOMES

The main focus of psychiatry and clinical psychology is patient care. As such, these fields operate at a faster pace than basic scientific research. They must address real mental issues at a large scale and provide fast solutions to imminent crises. In these fields, time is of the essence. The basic scientific pursuit stands in stark contrast to this fast pace, as it requires careful testing and retesting of hypotheses through empirical verification and validation. The tenets, goals, and time frames of the scientific community are different from those of these two clinical fields. *Why is it then that these clinical fields drive our scientific quest today in areas concerning disorders of the nervous systems, such as ASDs?*

The nature of the clinical endeavor, its necessary accelerated pace, and the immediate need for treatment require a fast system of data gathering. As a result of these constraints, clinical practice gathers data through very subjective means. These include observation and interpretation of behavior accompanied by hand coding based on discrete numerical scales. These scales reflect a range of possible interpretations of what the clinician observes the patient doing in response to a given questionnaire or task. Additional metrics are often based on self-assessment, assessments by caregivers, or combinations of those and the clinician's assessment. This form of data gathering fits the clinical needs, but leaves out, by necessity, the vital detailed-level information required by scientists investigating the disorders of the nervous systems.

The naked eye has limited capacity for the conscious processing of visual information. While behaviors occur along a continuum, the information that is coded through such clinical reports (that which reaches consciousness) is intermittent, subjective, and lacking the precision to capture aspects of behaviors that occur largely beneath awareness. These include involuntary micromotions of the face and body that are much too fast or too subtle to be detected by the eye, as well as other physiological signals underlying behavior that are reachable only through instrumentation. Thus, although the scientists working within these clinical fields are forced to use the clinical data to validate their instrumentation-based data, the two are utterly dissimilar in more than one fundamental way.

First, owing to its subjective nature, the clinical data are difficult to reproduce with high reliability. For instance, while completing Autism Diagnostic Observation Schedule 2 (ADOS-2) training, I noted with dismay that it took nearly 30 minutes to reach a general consensus across 20 people (clinicians and researchers) on whether a child displayed behaviors indicative of anxiety. During this discussion, individuals drew on their own clinical perspective, leading to a variety of other possible outcomes being raised, illustrating the subjectivity of such metrics. Moreover, these assertions were based on discrete behavioral interpretation, not a continuous real-number-based scale reflecting physiological states in a standardized way.

Second, the fact that clinicians are trained to look for certain traits and expect certain outcomes may inherently skew data interpretation and thus scores. If the instrumentation-based data that the scientist gathers along a continuum uncover aspects of the phenomena that the clinical data failed to capture, there will be poor correspondence between the observed description of the behavior and the actual physical measurement of it. Therefore, we are left with an incomplete picture of the phenomena if we rely only on one side of the coin. However, if we use both approaches, it is vital that we maintain a level of independence between these two forms of data gathering and interpretation. Failure to do so will result in one form of data collection confounding the other, and vice versa, and thus continue to skew our inquiry, leading to the circular arguments we often have today.

Third, the above issues with clinical, observational data prevent blind reproduction of results across different labs—an important step of the scientific method to provide a natural system of checks and balances. Science relies on the openness of the data sharing and reproducibility of their results. Without that, there is no progress in science. Given the subjective nature of clinically derived data, it is difficult to ensure blind reproduction of data.

Lastly, external supervision by experts in different fields is commonplace within the scientific arenas that investigate the brain and body interrelations. This interdisciplinary endeavor contributes to the progress of the scientific inquiry, and the rigor of the scientific method. Yet, within the clinical arena a neutral observer from another field would be considered an intruder, and due to patient–practitioner confidentiality and privacy issues, the scientific model of external supervision is not possible.

The data gathering of the clinical practice is also subject to the flow of interpersonal relations, which also has the potential to bias the data-gathering process. The scientific counterpart of gathering data with instrumentation and anonymity is impervious to other social nuances. To the instrument registering the data, the subject's data are just streams of numbers. To the scientist analyzing it, the data are just that. There are no strings attached. *Why is it then that the scientist is forced to use the clinical data necessarily gathered under such confounding terms?*

There is no immediate correspondence between the goals of the clinical and scientific endeavors. Both branches of the medical field ultimately aim to cure disease in the long run, but in the short run, the goals of patient care and those of the scientific inquiry are much too different to accommodate each other. If science were to impose its standards on clinical practices, clinicians simply could not run their operation. Patients would not receive the care that they need when they need it, and clinical practices would be stalled. However, this is exactly what is happening today in the scientific pursue of neurodevelopmental disorders, such as ASDs. We scientists, forced to use the data gathered under the clinical model, are stalled. Our progress is stalled because our model is fundamentally different from the clinical model. The clinical data that we are forced to use are incomplete, skewed, plagued with confirmation bias, and gathered in ways that are difficult to reproduce. Using these data is not only interfering with scientific progress in our inquiry but also extremely costly. Science lacks the budget to run this operation.

FOLLOW THE MONEY

In psychiatry, there are well-known financial ties between the pharmaceutical companies and the makers of the *Diagnostic and Statistical Manual of Mental Disorders* (American Psychiatric Association 2013), dictating the diagnoses (Cosgrove et al. 2006, 2009a, 2009b, 2014a, 2014b; Cosgrove and Krimsky 2012). There are also conflicts of interests between the companies that make psychological testing tools and their creators in clinical psychology. Specifically, their creators receive royalties from tests conducted in such studies (Hus et al. 2014). Disclosing financial ties between psychiatry and Big Pharma or donating royalties to charity does not change the fact that the system is ill-conceived and deeply corrupted (Cosgrove and Wheeler 2013). Practitioners and researchers in these fields may have the best intentions to help the affected person, yet they have no control over the consequences of their actions or decisions. The ways in which the system is inherently structured give rise to hidden variables researchers and practitioners are not even aware of, so they cannot factor these into their decision-making process. As an example, in the cases of neurodevelopmental disorders, those administering the tests are a vital component of the interactions with the child under evaluation, yet there is no built-in supervision or proper assessment in the tests to determine the types of biases the examiners may introduce. For instance, during the administration of the ADOS-2—used to diagnose ASD—the examiner creates a controlled social environment for dyadic interaction with an examinee. However, despite the fact that the clinician administering the test is paid to do so, there is no control for any biases or inherent variability of the examiner's performance (see Chapter 7; Whyatt et al. 2015; Whyatt and Torres 2017). Moreover, in addition to being used for diagnostic and clinical purposes, these tools are often an integral piece of research. In particular, given the complex and stringent research standards imposed in the scientific community, research teams must first confirm diagnosis—for instance, of ASD—using clinical assessment tools. In this regard, the clinical method, designed with different goals and under different standards than the scientific method, is leading the basic scientific inquiry in ASD.

The financial burden on the scientific community is also felt. A number of such clinical tests have dual formats, that is, clinical versus research grade. This duality leads to inflation of the profits for the administration of the test, but also results in higher costs to do the science. Interestingly, the training procedures and rules for these tools are often more complex and demanding for the research-grade test—rather than the clinical test—which in and of itself questions the clinical world's approach to psychiatry.

SOME UNFORESEEN CONSEQUENCES OF THE FINANCIAL CONFLICTS OF INTEREST PLAGUING AUTISM DIAGNOSES AND TREATMENTS

Despite the known financial conflicts of interest, despite the lack of objective measures in their testing platforms, and despite the lack of external supervision and the condition of near impunity on the outcome of treatments, the fields of both psychiatry and clinical psychology exert an enormous power over the scientific community. For example, in the case of ASD, no research can get published unless the clinical scores are reported and correlated with the objective measures from instrumentation that scientists perform. Due to the aforementioned clinical model, the cost of a basic science research project with high statistical power is generally prohibitive. The scientific progress concerning neurodevelopmental research has stalled because of this circularity, where the errors and pitfalls of test scores and their limited or inconsistent statistics are unavoidably inserted into any empirical study of autism.

Mathematically, it is also incorrect to conduct correlations between these two disparate scales (discrete-linear clinical and continuous-nonlinear-dynamic physical). The discrete makeup of clinical scales generated by subjective methods assumes a normal distribution. This assumption tends to smooth out as noise the inherent fluctuations in data that come from a coping biological system, which is daily and rapidly changing during development. In the face of dynamic physical changes, the clinical scales are inherently static as they rely on absolute rather than incremental values (i.e., in the few cases where they are systematically and longitudinally used, they do not consider derivatives from visit to visit, reflecting change as the person ages).

The nervous systems of a child are changing at accelerated rates, following a rather nonlinear dynamic process with multiplicative stochastic signatures of variability (Torres et al. 2013a, 2016)—these cannot be empirically evaluated using clinical scales. It is thus inappropriate to correlate discrete, static, linearly conceived clinical scales—conceptualized under assumptions of additive statistics—with the continuous biological signals that are objectively captured from the physical body and/or brain of the person. We scientists are simply being forced to compare "apples and broccoli" at an extremely high cost.

DISCRETE SUBJECTIVE SCALES CANNOT CAPTURE ADAPTIVE CHANGE

Besides their pervasive influence on basic scientific research, psychiatry and clinical psychology hold an enormous power over the population at large. Society at large is impacted by their practices in nonobvious ways. One of these ways concerns the affected person and the supportive family unit. The disorder type that these fields dictate determines not only the kind of treatment the affected person may receive, but also the type of coverage the child's family may ultimately afford for such treatments. Since discrete scales are static, they cannot capture the types of nonlinear dynamic and stochastic changes of the nervous systems of the child under therapy. Such scales are unable to provide objective outcome measures reflecting underlying change in the nervous systems to assess the intervention's effectiveness, or to help insurance companies longitudinally assess the balance between benefits and risks of a given therapy.

For example, a child with ASD may need occupational therapy (OT) with a focus on sensory-motor issues, but this is not covered by insurance companies (Thomas et al. 2007, 2012; Benevides et al. 2015). Despite evidence of their disruption (Mostofsky et al. 2000; Minshew et al. 2004; Takarae et al. 2004; Gidley Larson et al. 2008; Haswell et al. 2009; Fournier et al. 2010; Torres 2012; Torres and Donnellan 2012; Brincker and Torres 2013; Mosconi et al. 2013; Torres et al. 2013a, 2016), sensory-motor issues are not considered part of the disorder by these two disciplines. In particular, any reference to sensory-motor issues is indirect—it occurs at a descriptive level in connection with motor use, for example, gestures, sensory aversions or interests, and repetitive or restricted behaviors. These difficulties are never examined in relation to the underlying physiological signatures from neurological interactions between the central (CNS) and the peripheral (PNS) nervous systems. Yet, the emergence of sensory-motor difficulties is a repercussion of physiological functioning. It is as though sensory and motor nerves transporting the signals along the nervous systems and enabling communication across the various structures for autonomic, automatic, and voluntary control did not exist within the framework of clinical metrics. Indeed, the fifth edition of the *Diagnostic and Statistical Manual of Mental Disorders* (DSM-5) criteria ignore the neuroanatomical and neurophysiological underpinnings of human behavior, which is reflected as well in their exclusion in diagnostic tools and tests, such as the ADOS (Lord et al. 2000). This conceptualization of ASD as a high-level description of subjective quantification of observed behaviors further drives the recommendations of coverage for therapies. As such, clinical scales and interpretations restrict the types of treatments a given family will have access to.

Without access to insurance coverage for treatments of sensory-motor disorders in neurodevelopment, the large majority of affected children grow up without sensory-motor-driven interventions. The child with autism will receive what is available through state programs after school age (Liptak et al. 2008; Lubetsky et al. 2014). A common intervention in this regard is applied behavioral analysis (ABA). Yet, that intervention was not designed to address issues concerning sensory-motor disturbances of the nervous system of the child. In fact, the very therapy renders some "behaviors" inappropriate or nonconforming with their protocols of what is appropriate. As such, they may "extinguish" those behaviors through punishment schedules. This is the case even when such seemingly odd behaviors may serve a purpose, for example, to comfort the child in the presence of sensory-motor issues unseen by the naked eye of the clinician. Under such uncertain conditions and lack of objective, physical measurements, it is possible that despite meaning well, the clinician's approach may in fact be harmful to the child.

Consider for a moment the excess of uncertainty that motor noise and randomness (Brincker and Torres 2013; Torres et al. 2013a) bring to the child's nervous system, and then amplify this with the type of uncertainty that prompting alone must bring to that child. Indeed, seasoned ABA therapists that have a tremendous interest in helping the children with ASD have privately communicated that anxiety, stress, and tantrums are commonplace during ABA sessions. We do not know the underlying physiological signatures of these manifestations, or how they impact the nervous systems of the developing child subject to such behavioral modifying therapies. When questioning some practitioners about this, the response invariably has been, "It's autism." Circular, isn't it? It is as circular as is the clinical criteria leading the scientific quest.

UNCERTAIN OUTCOMES OF PSYCHOTROPIC MEDICATIONS AND BEHAVIORAL MODIFICATIONS

An important aspect of neurodevelopmental disorders treated by psychiatrists and clinical psychologists is the profound impact that these treatments are bound to have in a developing human. As explained above, the manifestations of neurodevelopmental disorders coupled with the reliance on a discrete description or interpretation of symptomatic behaviors fails to provide enough information to make truly informed decisions on the course of treatment. Specifically, these discrete metrics fail to capture adaptive change—particularly at a time when physical growth and the development of the neural control of movement are changing at accelerated (nonlinear) rates (Kuczmarski et al. 2000, 2002). These pitfalls lead to an absence of proper methods to track the effectiveness of behavioral interventions, including as well the assessment of the risks of psychotropic drugs on the immature nervous system of an infant or a young child.

Pharmaceutical companies and the American Psychiatric Association are now by law forced to disclose their financial ties (by the health care overhaul legislation [Greenberg 2003]). Yet, disclosure is not enough to show the public the profound side effects of these drugs, which were not designed for children in the first place. Indeed, these drugs have measurable deleterious effects on the child's nervous systems (Torres and Denisova 2016). These effects are not considered or noticed by clinicians due to the inherent limitations of clinical tools, potentially compounded by profound financial ties that the clinical fields are known to have with pharmaceutical companies (Cosgrove et al. 2014b).

As in the case of psychotropic drugs, the behavioral modifying interventions imposed on the child are thought to have an impact on the child's development. As with psychotropic drugs, there is a paucity of objective methods to inform clinicians of the changes that the treatments exert on the child's nervous systems. As such, practitioners in those fields provide, rather blindly, a "one-size-fits-all" approach to disorders that are, by the very nature of the ways in which the disorders are defined, very heterogeneous. They are called "disorders on a spectrum," and yet, by default, early intervention programs given to each child with a diagnosis of a neurodevelopmental disorder provide similar treatment or behavioral intervention as any other child on that spectrum.

POLITICS AND ECONOMICS

These financial ties have implications on the lines of available therapies. In the United States, the type of coverage therapies received depends on the politics that affect the decision making of the judiciary branch of the government. As such, if a strong financial force backs a certain intervention, it is likely that taxpayers will end up covering those expenses. Yet, taxpayers are not well informed of the science behind such interventions. In a democratic system, being well informed is vital to decide and vote on lawmaking. That process is critical, as it has direct implications on the lives of those affected (i.e., the child and the family). Furthermore, because of the lack of information, ordinary citizens may not immediately foresee possible implications the legislation might have on other aspects of the problem that may affect their own lives, for example, have an impact on the educational systems or the resources needed for other areas of patient care.

THE PARENTS' IMPOSSIBLE ROAD TO DIVERSIFIED TREATMENTS

The processes involving treatment recommendation and the corresponding legislation of treatment coverage by insurance companies are very complex. Their rulings inevitably constrain the options available to the affected families. As a consequence, the family is left with no path to diversify treatments and increase the likelihood of improving the child's quality of life. A case in point is the intensive use of ABA nationwide. As explained before, this type of intervention was not designed to address the types of sensory-motor issues underlying the behaviors that this method attempts to modify. Indeed, a range of neurophysiological issues that have been scientifically established in children with ASD (Torres 2013; Torres et al. 2013a, 2013b, 2013c, 2016) are not factored into this intervention.

For instance, ABA is thought to improve structuring the child's actions. The therapy is based on animal conditioning models with stimulus–response associations made through schedules of reward and punishment (Hergenhahn 1973; Matson 2009; Raber 2011). Unfortunately, such methods, which rely on explicit instructions and external prompting, often rob the child of the opportunity to spontaneously self-discover cause and effect on their own (Torres et al. 2013d). This process is fundamental to engage more primitive structures of the autonomic nervous systems and promote a natural bridge between high-level CNS structures and low-level PNS structures that appear earlier in evolution than those in the neocortex.

Neurodevelopment occurs according to a phylogenetic order in the structures of the nervous systems. Within hours of life, the bodily rhythms of the newborn entrain with those of adult speech (Condon and Sander 1974). Likewise, rhythmic patterns of respiration, feeding (sucking), and cooing develop rapidly, contributing to the baby's survival (Barlow and Estep 2006). These motoric rhythms are controlled from the onset of life by primitive structures of the brainstem and central pattern generators developing in the spinal cord. They mature and allow survival before the baby can think in the abstract and make decisions. This level of bottom-up control (from autonomic to voluntary) scaffolds the gradual emergence of volitional control. Indeed, top-down operations, such as those driven by prompting, require the neocortical control and coordination of voluntary, automatic, and autonomic layers of the nervous systems, yet these functions develop from the bottom up, and these lower levels of control should not be assumed a priori before any type of intervention begins.

If the scaffolding of peripheral and subcortical structures of the nervous systems has a glitch during early neurodevelopment, it may be necessary to step back and "awaken," from the bottom up, those structures that evolutionarily mature earlier to enable reflexes, central pattern generators, and spontaneous motions to facilitate self-exploration and self-discovery. Yet, ABA is unable to accomplish such objective profiling and targeted intervention due to the very nature of the therapy. This therapy is based on extrinsic prompting, instructed from the top down using external reward-based associations under the assumption that the child's mental intentions already match the volitional control of the physical body. That matching between mental intention and physical action is the very end product of a maturation process that followed a typical path, but ASD is the by-product of a process that followed an atypical neurodevelopmental path. In this sense, therapeutic interventions such as ABA seem backward, failing to build on core principles of neurodevelopment.

Furthermore, in our own experience many of the ABA programs that are claimed to be successful in improving the child's performance (verbal or otherwise) filter out of admission children that are not likely to succeed. This practice was evident even in the very early work by Lovaas (1987) reported in the ABA literature (see the "Methods" section: "high agreement was not reached for subjects who scored *within the profoundly retarded range on intellectual functioning (PMA < 11 months); these subjects were excluded from the study*"). Such a screening method underscores the need for a broader and more diversified approach to interventions, so as to help those nonverbal children in the spectrum that are now underserved by the public school system. Their parents may gain access to special education and other resources through a rather expensive and tenuous litigation path that only a few can afford. That path is, however, not obvious to most. In fact, we discovered this through a long interview process sponsored by funds from the Innovative-Corps Program of the National Science Foundation, whereby 117 individuals in the ecosystem of autism were interviewed (including lawyers, parents, counseling services across the nation, board-certified behavior analysts (BCBAs), ABA schools, therapists from diverse areas such as physical and occupational, and insurance companies).

The ABA schools that I have personally visited in the New Jersey area (e.g., the Rutgers Douglass Developmental Disability Center and the Princeton Child Development Institute—quite successful at what they do, I must point out) already include some elements of OT and physical therapy (PT) in their practices. Yet, officially this is not recognized by any BCBA curricula. The curricula do not call either for experts from those fields or from the fields of sensory-motor neuroscience. Including sensory-motor physiology as part of the BCBA curricular training would help enrich their knowledge on the neurophysiology and neuroanatomy of the developing child's nervous systems.

Large bodies of scientific evidence from the fields of developmental neuroscience are not being actively utilized in the ABA model, a model that is based on the psychological construct that behavior—to be socially acceptable—must look a certain way. Without physically measuring the consequences of intervening in a coping nervous system with complex evolving physiology, this type of practice—necessarily skewed by one's interpretation and opinion of the observed responses of the child and blind to the nervous systems' physiological responses—can have very uncertain outcomes and unknown consequences in the long run. What is rather certain is that such practices are bound to target a very narrow aspect of the individual's existence and, as such, be severely incomplete.

Classical ABA seems to enhance a different skill set than that necessary to achieve functional goals and bodily awareness. As necessary as the skills that ABA teaches in the classroom may be, they do not necessarily transfer to other domains (Baer and Wolf 1987). This is particularly the case in activities of daily living, as well as those involving navigation and basic social exchange outside the school settings. Even simple daily tasks, such as taking a shower, tying one's shoes, or buttoning down a shirt, require other skills within the realm of visuomotor control, eye–hand coordination, sensory-motor integration, and bodily sensing (proper feedback from self-generated motions), all of which require an intrinsic element of autonomic control, self-initiation and stopping, and autonomous sensory-motor sequencing. Specific forms of neurological music therapy (NMT) (Thaut et al. 2014), OT, and PT interventions focusing on sensory-motor integration can enhance these important components that are so necessary to scaffold all naturalistic behaviors. However, unlike ABA, these therapies are not covered by insurance, or offered at the public schools (Zablotsky et al. 2015b). At present, they are very costly and only affordable by a very small segment of the very large number of individuals affected in the United States (Autism et al. 2012; Perou et al. 2013). It would be very interesting to know how the rest of the world is doing this.

SOCIAL DEFICIT OF OUR SOCIETY

One of the most poignant aspects of our research involving children on the spectrum of neurodevelopmental disorders like ASD is their enormous efforts to "fit in"; upon their exhausting and costly therapies (for the few that can afford them), the child might make it to mainstream classrooms in regular schools. Although a triumph for the child, the family, and all those involved (including devoted ABA therapists, occupational therapists, physical therapists, and a speech therapist), the large majority of these children are bullied, sometimes beaten up so badly that they regress considerably (see Chapter 26). They are generally evaded and dismissed by their peers (Zablotsky et al. 2014). The lack of awareness and education on the true physiological difficulties that underlie the observational diagnosis and treatments of autism prevents society from truly recognizing the nature of the struggles of the affected individuals and from assuming full responsibility to support this population. The perception created by the DSM and the ADOS criteria—portraying autism as a mental condition or a social deficit, often interpreted and perceived as a deliberate social withdrawal—does not help. The treatments geared to reshaping "socially unacceptable behaviors" without supporting the sensory-motor needs of the person are not helping the situation either. Rather, all of it exacerbates the stigmatization of the affected individual and leads to such a state of loneliness that only those who suffer it and those who listen to their testimony can truly come to understand it (Donnellan et al. 2012; Robledo et al. 2012; Amos 2013; Savarese 2013).

The influences that psychiatry and clinical psychology have on the legislation and finances behind neurodevelopmental disorders bring high uncertainties to the future life of any affected child and his or her family. First, due to the high costs associated with diagnosis and treatment during the early years of life, there is a paucity of programs implemented to address the disorders as the person evolves with aging. As such, there is no system in place to support the life of the person as an independent adult. Second, the development of the sensory-motor systems required for the acquisition of autonomy, self-control, and agency is not being promoted by any of the diagnoses and treatments currently available. In fact, the sensory-motor systems are negatively impacted by the deleterious side effects of psychotropic medications (Torres and Denisova 2016). Without this basic physiological foundation to scaffold self-autonomy and ultimately free will, there is little chance to welcome and foster the affected individual as an active, contributing member of our society. Thus, the forces at work to diagnose, treat, legislate, and finance all aspects related to neurodevelopmental disorders on a spectrum have yet to consider those disorders along the continuum of the human life span. The consequences of errors in their handling of the situation are merely starting to show. To this day, we do not know what the present treatments do to the brain or body of a developing child. Consequently, we do not know the resulting outcomes in the adult system. Somehow, by not properly supervising* what these fields have been doing with impunity for so long, we have failed the affected children and their families, but societally, we have actually failed ourselves. The consequences are soon to become self-evident in the nascent new generations of young and older adults on the spectrum that we, as a society, have neglected to embrace.

* Proper supervision would require multidisciplinary third-party neutral observers with no financial conflicts of interest and the integration of knowledge bases from different fields.

REFERENCES

American Psychiatric Association. 2013. *Diagnostic and Statistical Manual of Mental Disorders*. 5th ed. Washington, DC: American Psychiatric Association.

Amos, P. 2013. Rhythm and timing in autism: Learning to dance. *Front Integr Neurosci* 7:27.

Autism and Developmental Disabilities Monitoring Network Surveillance Year Principal Investigators and Centers for Disease Control and Prevention. 2012. Prevalence of autism spectrum disorders—Autism and developmental disabilities monitoring network, 14 sites, United States, 2008. *MMWR Surveill Summ* 61 (3):1–19.

Baer, D. M., and M. M. Wolf. 1987. Some still-current dimensions of applied behavior analysis. *J Appl Behav Anal* 20 (4):313–27.

Barlow, S. M., and M. Estep. 2006. Central pattern generation and the motor infrastructure for suck, respiration, and speech. *J Commun Disord* 39 (5):366–80.

Benevides, T. W., H. J. Carretta, and S. J. Lane. 2015. Unmet need for therapy among children with autism spectrum disorder: Results from the 2005–2006 and 2009–2010 National Survey of Children with Special Health Care Needs. *Matern Child Health J* 20:878.

Brincker, M., and E. B. Torres. 2013. Noise from the periphery in autism. *Front Integr Neurosci* 7:34.

Condon, W. S., and L. S. Sander. 1974. Neonate movement is synchronized with adult speech: Interactional participation and language acquisition. *Science* 183 (4120):99–101.

Cosgrove, L., A. F. Shaughnessy, E. E. Wheeler, S. Krimsky, S. M. Peters, D. J. Freeman-Coppadge, and J. R. Lexchin. 2014b. From caveat emptor to caveat venditor: Time to stop the influence of money on practice guideline development. *J Eval Clin Pract* 20 (6):809–12.

Cosgrove, L., and E. E. Wheeler. 2013. Industry's colonization of psychiatry: Ethical and practical implications of financial conflicts of interest in the DSM-5. *Fem Psychol* 23 (1):93–106.

Cosgrove, L., and S. Krimsky. 2012. A comparison of DSM-IV and DSM-5 panel members' financial associations with industry: A pernicious problem persists. *PLoS Med* 9 (3):e1001190.

Cosgrove, L., H. J. Bursztajn, and S. Krimsky. 2009a. Developing unbiased diagnostic and treatment guidelines in psychiatry. *N Engl J Med* 360 (19):2035–6.

Cosgrove, L., H. J. Bursztajn, S. Krimsky, M. Anaya, and J. Walker. 2009b. Conflicts of interest and disclosure in the American Psychiatric Association's Clinical Practice Guidelines. *Psychother Psychosom* 78 (4): 228–32.

Cosgrove, L., S. Krimsky, E. E. Wheeler, J. Kaitz, S. B. Greenspan, and N. L. DiPentima. 2014a. Tripartite conflicts of interest and high stakes patent extensions in the DSM-5. *Psychother Psychosom* 83 (2):106–13.

Cosgrove, L., S. Krimsky, M. Vijayaraghavan, and L. Schneider. 2006. Financial ties between DSM-IV panel members and the pharmaceutical industry. *Psychother Psychosom* 75 (3):154–60.

Donnellan, A. M., D. A. Hill, and M. R. Leary. 2012. Rethinking autism: Implications of sensory and movement differences for understanding and support. *Front Integr Neurosci* 6:124.

Fournier, K. A., C. J. Hass, S. K. Naik, N. Lodha, and J. H. Cauraugh. 2010. Motor coordination in autism spectrum disorders: A synthesis and meta-analysis. *J Autism Dev Disord* 40 (10):1227–40.

Gidley Larson, J. C., A. J. Bastian, O. Donchin, R. Shadmehr, and S. H. Mostofsky. 2008. Acquisition of internal models of motor tasks in children with autism. *Brain* 131 (Pt 11):2894–903.

Greenberg, D. S. 2003. Medicare overhaul wins congressional support. *Lancet* 362 (9398):1816.

Haswell, C. C., J. Izawa, L. R. Dowell, S. H. Mostofsky, and R. Shadmehr. 2009. Representation of internal models of action in the autistic brain. *Nat Neurosci* 12 (8):970–2.

Hergenhahn, B. R. 1973. *The Work of B. F. Skinner* [sound recording]. San Jose, CA: Lansford Publishing Co.

Hus, V., K. Gotham, and C. Lord. 2014. Standardizing ADOS domain scores: Separating severity of social affect and restricted and repetitive behaviors. *J Autism Dev Disord* 44 (10):2400–12.

Kuczmarski, R. J., C. L. Ogden, L. M. Grummer-Strawn, K. M. Flegal, S. S. Guo, R. Wei, Z. Mei, L. R. Curtin, A. F. Roche, and C. L. Johnson. 2000. CDC growth charts: United States. *Adv Data* (314):1–27.

Kuczmarski, R. J., C. L. Ogden, S. S. Guo, L. M. Grummer-Strawn, K. M. Flegal, Z. Mei, R. Wei, L. R. Curtin, A. F. Roche, and C. L. Johnson. 2002. 2000 CDC growth charts for the United States: Methods and development. *Vital Health Stat 11* (246):1–190.

Liptak, G. S., L. B. Benzoni, D. W. Mruzek, K. W. Nolan, M. A. Thingvoll, C. M. Wade, and G. E. Fryer. 2008. Disparities in diagnosis and access to health services for children with autism: Data from the National Survey of Children's Health. *J Dev Behav Pediatr* 29 (3):152–60.

Lord, C., S. Risi, L. Lambrecht, E. H. Cook Jr., B. L. Leventhal, P. C. DiLavore, A. Pickles, and M. Rutter. 2000. The Autism Diagnostic Observation Schedule-Generic: A standard measure of social and communication deficits associated with the spectrum of autism. *J Autism Dev Disord* 30 (3):205–23.

Lovaas, O. I. 1987. Behavioral treatment and normal educational and intellectual functioning in young autistic children. *J Consult Clin Psychol* 55 (1):3–9.

Lubetsky, M. J., B. L. Handen, M. Lubetsky, and J. J. McGonigle. 2014. Systems of care for individuals with autism spectrum disorder and serious behavioral disturbance through the lifespan. *Child Adolesc Psychiatr Clin N Am* 23 (1):97–110.

Matson, J. L. 2009. *Applied Behavior Analysis for Children with Autism Spectrum Disorders*. New York: Springer.

Minshew, N. J., K. Sung, B. L. Jones, and J. M. Furman. 2004. Underdevelopment of the postural control system in autism. *Neurology* 63 (11):2056–61.

Mosconi, M. W., B. Luna, M. Kay-Stacey, C. V. Nowinski, L. H. Rubin, C. Scudder, N. Minshew, and J. A. Sweeney. 2013. Saccade adaptation abnormalities implicate dysfunction of cerebellar-dependent learning mechanisms in autism spectrum disorders (ASD). *PLoS One* 8 (5):e63709.

Mostofsky, S. H., M. C. Goldberg, R. J. Landa, and M. B. Denckla. 2000. Evidence for a deficit in procedural learning in children and adolescents with autism: Implications for cerebellar contribution. *J Int Neuropsychol Soc* 6 (7):752–9.

Odom, S. L. 2016. Steve Silberman: *NeuroTribes: The Legacy of Autism and the Future of Neurodiversity*. *J Autism Dev Disord* 43 (1):1–534.

Perou, R., R. H. Bitsko, S. J. Blumberg, et al. 2013. Mental health surveillance among children—United States, 2005–2011. *MMWR Suppl* 62 (2):1–35.

Raber, J. 2011. *Animal Models of Behavioral Analysis*. Springer Protocols. New York: Humana Press.

Robledo, J., A. M. Donnellan, and K. Strandt-Conroy. 2012. An exploration of sensory and movement differences from the perspective of individuals with autism. *Front Integr Neurosci* 6:107.

Savarese, R. J. 2013. Moving the field: The sensorimotor perspective on autism (commentary on "Rethinking autism: Implications of sensory and motor differences," an article by Anne Donnellan, David Hill, and Martha Leary). *Front Integr Neurosci* 7:6.

Takarae, Y., N. J. Minshew, B. Luna, C. M. Krisky, and J. A. Sweeney. 2004. Pursuit eye movement deficits in autism. *Brain* 127 (Pt 12):2584–94.

Thaut, M. H., G. C. McIntosh, and V. Hoemberg. 2014. Neurobiological foundations of neurologic music therapy: Rhythmic entrainment and the motor system. *Front Psychol* 5:1185.

Thomas, K. C., A. R. Ellis, C. McLaurin, J. Daniels, and J. P. Morrissey. 2007. Access to care for autism-related services. *J Autism Dev Disord* 37 (10):1902–12.

Thomas, K. C., S. L. Parish, R. A. Rose, and M. Kilany. 2012. Access to care for children with autism in the context of state Medicaid reimbursement. *Matern Child Health J* 16 (8):1636–44.

Torres, E. B. 2012. Atypical signatures of motor variability found in an individual with ASD. *Neurocase* 1: 1–16.

Torres, E. B. 2013. Atypical signatures of motor variability found in an individual with ASD. *Neurocase* 19 (2): 150–65.

Torres, E. B., and A. M. Donnellan. 2012. Autism: The movement perspective. *Front Integr Neurosci.* 7 (32):1–374.

Torres, E. B., and K. Denisova. 2016. Motor noise is rich signal in autism research and pharmacological treatments. *Sci Rep* 6:37422.

Torres, E. B., J. Nguyen, C. Suresh, P. Yanovich, and A. Kolevzon. 2013c. Noise from the periphery in autism spectrum disorders of idiopathic origins and of known etiology. Presented at the Annual Meeting of the Society for Neuroscience, San Diego, November 9–13.

Torres, E. B., M. Brincker, R. W. Isenhower, P. Yanovich, K. A. Stigler, J. I. Nurnberger, D. N. Metaxas, and J. V. Jose. 2013a. Autism: The micro-movement perspective. *Front Integr Neurosci* 7:32.

Torres, E. B., P. Yanovich, and D. N. Metaxas. 2013d. Give spontaneity and self-discovery a chance in ASD: Spontaneous peripheral limb variability as a proxy to evoke centrally driven intentional acts. *Front Integr Neurosci* 7:46.

Torres, E. B., R. W. Isenhower, J. Nguyen, C. Whyatt, J. I. Nurnberger, J. V. Jose, S. M. Silverstein, T. V. Papathomas, J. Sage, and J. Cole. 2016. Toward precision psychiatry: Statistical platform for the personalized characterization of natural behaviors. *Front Neurol* 7:8.

Torres, E. B., R. W. Isenhower, P. Yanovich, G. Rehrig, K. Stigler, J. Nurnberger, and J. V. Jose. 2013b. Strategies to develop putative biomarkers to characterize the female phenotype with autism spectrum disorders. *J Neurophysiol* 110 (7):1646–62.

Whyatt, C., A. Mars, E. DiCicco-Bloom, and E. B. Torres. 2015. Objective characterization of sensory-motor physiology underlying dyadic interactions during the Autism Diagnostic Observation Schedule-2: Implications for research and clinical diagnosis. Presented at the Annual Meeting of the Society for Neuroscience, Chicago, October 17–21.

Whyatt, C. and E.B. Torres. 2017. *The social-dance: decomposing naturalistic dyadic interaction dynamics to the 'micro-level'*. Fourth International Symposium on Movement and Computing, MOCO'17, 28–30 June. London, UK: ACM.

Zablotsky, B., B. A. Pringle, L. J. Colpe, M. D. Kogan, C. Rice, and S. J. Blumberg. 2015b. Service and treatment use among children diagnosed with autism spectrum disorders. *J Dev Behav Pediatr* 36 (2):98–105.

Zablotsky, B., C. P. Bradshaw, C. M. Anderson, and P. Law. 2014. Risk factors for bullying among children with autism spectrum disorders. *Autism* 18 (4):419–27.

Zablotsky, B., L. I. Black, M. J. Maenner, L. A. Schieve, and S. J. Blumberg. 2015a. Estimated prevalence of autism and other developmental disabilities following questionnaire changes in the 2014 National Health Interview Survey. *Natl Health Stat Rep* (87):1–21.

Conclusions

Elizabeth B. Torres and Caroline Whyatt

As we continue our journey through the first 20 years of the twenty-first century, the field of Neuroscience is undergoing rapid changes at all fronts. New technologies ranging from optogenetics to a plethora of wireless sensors are bound to revolutionize the ways in which we gather data from the brain and from the body the brain senses to enable its voluntary control. New analytics entering this landscape of big data will help profile the development and growth of the nervous systems, particularly during neurodevelopment. As such, autism spectrum disorders (ASD) at large are poised for radical change along a positive and optimistic pathway ahead.

While seminal literature and works have guided the field to new discoveries and enabled a new era of ASD understanding in the academic and public domain, this book has begun to highlight the imminent revolution in ASD. It is the byproduct of a superb collaborative effort among parents, therapists, clinicians, and researchers from all areas of science, physics, engineering, and applied mathematics, inviting us to learn about the coping nervous systems of the developing child and the new technological advances, enabling new designs for data-driven accommodations and support.

The book invites the reader and user to go far beyond subjective descriptions and interpretations of ordinal data gathered by hand into the realm of objective data harnessed, in tandem, from the brain and body. This new avenue of exploration will help researchers better understand the functioning of the nervous systems as the person behaves, naturally moves, and senses back the responses from natural interactions with the surrounding environment. Specifically, this book has introduced how movement, specifically movement sensing, may have a profound and reverberating impact on the various axes of development; axes characteristic of ASD. Viewed from this perspective, the authors unite in a singular message—that it is time to re-shift our focus and conceptualization to one that considers the needs and development of the individual from a more holistic approach. This departure from traditional isolated domains of constrained symptomatology opens new possibilities—for therapies, diagnosis, and data-driven research. For instance, by introducing the movement-sensing dyad of the child and clinician, or the child and parent, this book creates a new basic unit of social exchange—a core feature of ASD symptomatology and research. This unit is now quantifiable and longitudinally tractable in data-driven ways. Moving beyond mere descriptions of social exchange, and subjective attribution of preconceived 'social appropriateness', this dyadic exchange can now be objective profiled and steered in real time using sensory feedback derived from the person's self-generated movements, with noninvasive technology. This new platform paves the way for a reconceptualization of both diagnostics and intervention strategies within a mobile health framework.

Informed from data that are harnessed directly from the nervous systems of the person, these new dynamic analyses of development, combined with probabilistic conceptualizations and characterizations of 'traditional' axes of symptomatology such as social exchange in ASD will inevitably bring positive outcomes for the affected individual and may improve the attitude of society at large. Indeed, through a personalized dynamic and probabilistic approach to diagnose and track treatment outcomes in ASD, we enter a new era of potential development of true target therapies aimed at minimizing off-target side effects. Together, we close this editorial with a constructive message as we begin the process of societal education with the immediate goal of better understanding and embracing ASD as one of the many human conditions.

Index

A

ABA, *see* Applied behavioral analysis
ABIDE I database, 14
ABLLS-R, *see* Assessment of Basic Language and Learning Skills–Revised
Action evaluation and discrimination, *see* Imitation fidelity, action evaluation and discrimination as indexes of
ADHD, *see* Attention deficit hyperactivity disorder
ADI, *see* Autism Diagnostic Interview
ADI-R, *see* Autism Diagnostic Interview–Revised
ADOS, *see* Autism Diagnostic Observation Schedule
ADOS-G, *see* Autism Diagnostic Observation Schedule–Generic
Alternative and augmentative communication (AAC) methods, 141
Ambulatory integral model, *see* Argentinian ambulatory integral model to treat autism spectrum disorders
Americans with Disabilities Act, 317
AMYDI, *see* Autismo, Motricidad Y Deporte para la Inclusion
Analysis of variance (ANOVA), 157, 169
ANS, *see* Autonomic nervous system
Applied behavioral analysis (ABA), 253, 372
Argentinian ambulatory integral model to treat autism spectrum disorders, 253–269
  applied behavioral analysis, 253
  cognitive and academic program, 256–257
  communication skills program, 258–259
  developmental, individual difference, relationship-based model, 253
  motor skills program, 262–264
  musical therapy for sensory modulation, program of, 260–261
  parent support program, 265
  self-reliance and sensory regulation, program for, 264
  social skills program, 259–260
Artificial intelligence, 82
ASC, *see* Autism spectrum condition
ASD, *see* Autism spectrum disorder
ASEMI, *see* Autism Sports and Educational Model for Inclusion
Asperger's syndrome (AS), 23, 140
Assessment of Basic Language and Learning Skills–Revised (ABLLS-R), 341
Attention deficit hyperactivity disorder (ADHD), 9, 13, 179, 201
Augmentative and alternative communication (AAC), 319
Autism Diagnostic Interview (ADI), 90
Autism Diagnostic Interview–Revised (ADI-R), 90
Autism Diagnostic Observation Schedule (ADOS), 103–118
  affect versus motor control, 113–115
  bullying perspective and, 357
  combining of psychological and physiological perspectives, 107–110
  definition and working conceptualization of social skills, 104–106
  emotional task, 115
  inertial measurement units, 107
  microlevels of exchange, importance of considering, 115
  multilayered, bidirectional approach to social dynamics, 106–110
  psychological perspective, 104
  severity scores, 9
  SPIBA and the micromovement data type, 110–113
  tell-a-story task, 115
Autism Diagnostic Observation Schedule–Generic (ADOS-G), 90
Autismo, Motricidad Y Deporte para la Inclusion (AMYDI), 273; *see also* Autism Sports and Educational Model for Inclusion
Autism phenotype, 23–41
  associated motor symptoms, 29–32
  associated secondary symptoms, role of, 24–25
  associated sensory symptoms, 28–29
  behavior (physiological stance), 26–28
  development of behavior, 26–28
  fragile X disorders, 34
  missing link, 34
  Parkinson's disease as model for ASD, 32–33
  psychological versus physiological, 25–26
  secondary by-products, 33
  time for a new model, evidence suggesting, 34–35
  underdeveloped nervous systems, by-product of, 28–32
Autism spectrum condition (ASC), 141
Autism spectrum disorder (ASD)
  biophysical rhythms, 69
  characterization of, 23, 103, 230
  cognitive theories in, 44–45
  complexities associated with, 357
  core motor sensing traits in, 197
  diagnosis, 329
  DSM-5 definition of, 140
  handwriting in, 49
  holistic approach to, 271
  life functions in individuals with, 120–121
  micromovements, 221
  motor functioning in, 43–44
  motoric development and social cognition, 89
  music therapy for, 232–233
  prescription of drugs to treat, 179
  range of impairments, 43
  research, 153
  rhythm and movement for, 229
  social skills in, 75
  statistical distributions, 157
  teacher beliefs and, 281
  time for a new model, evidence suggesting, 34–35
  top-down approach, 57
  video technology and, 244

Autism Sports and Educational Model for Inclusion (ASEMI), 271–280
beginnings, 271–272
birth of AMYDI, 273
combination of AMYDI with other existing models, 275
interdisciplinary team and family role, 276
introduction to the model, 273–274
main objectives of AMYDI, 279
stage 1 (development of structured sensory-perceptive-motor abilities, 277
stage 2 (development of semistructured motor activities, 278
stage 3 (development of real motor activities, 278
stage 4 (playful motor inclusion, 278–279
structured nature of motoric situations and contexts, 275
users of AMYDI model, 279
where to apply AMYDI, 279
Autonomic nervous system (ANS), 3
Autopoesis, 120

B

BCBA, *see* Board-certified behavior analyst
Behavior, development of, 26–28
Behaviorist Manifesto, 301
Board-certified behavior analyst (BCBA), 341, 374
Brainstem origin of autism, 119–137
affective neuroscience, 119
arousal and social engagement (locus coeruleus and related systems), 128–129
autopoesis of conscious experience, 120–124
brain for purposeful movement, questions on development of, 131
case history, 131–132
consensuality, 120
coordination of multiple action units, 125
disrupted movements in autism, 121–122
exteroception from the distance receptors, 125
higher-order abstractions, 123
human communication and social understanding, 122–124
identifying and supporting problems arising from disruption of motives, 130–131
inferior olive, 126–127
intelligent moving, timing and serial ordering in, 124–125
intrinsic and environmental factors affecting ASD, 129–130
locating motor-affective intelligence, 124–129
methods of therapy and education that support hopes for movement, 130
microkinesic descriptive methods, research using, 120
miscoordination of movements, 120
motor control, brainstem neurophysiological system for, 125–126
nucleus ambiguus and related systems, 127–128
primary process conscious acts, 123
proprioception of the body in motion, 125
prospective control of movement, characteristics of, 120–124
visceroception of information, 125
weakened central coherence, 129
Bullying perspective, 357–365
ADOS, 357
antibullying strategies, 360
conscious victim, 361
hope for the future, 363–364
recent estimates of bullying prevalence, 358
trend, 359–363
unconscious victim, 362, 363

C

CDC, *see* U.S. Centers for Disease Control and Prevention
Central limit theorem (CLT), 157, 162–163
Central nervous system (CNS), 3, 64, 178
Classic reflex theory, 296
Cognitive theories, 43–55
assessment of handwriting proficiency, 49–51
cognitive theories in ASD, 44–45
difference in cognitive style, 45
handwriting in ASD, 49
how children with ASD sequence their movements, 45–46
interpretation of motor sequencing patterns, 46–47
motor functioning in ASD, 43–44
movement organization and sequencing, 45
theory of mind, 45
visuomotor integration, 47–49
Competence, presuming, 146–147
Computational psychiatry, 156
Conditional random fields (CRFs), 82
Conditioning, 296
Consensuality, 120
Core motor sensing traits in ASD, new strategies for detection and treatments of, *see* Nervous systems' rhythms, inherent noise hidden in (core motor sensing traits in ASD and)
Cortical plasticity, music and, 231–232
CRFs, *see* Conditional random fields

D

Data analysis, motivation to change methods of, *see* Visual search and autism, excess success for study on
Developmental, individual difference, relationship-based (DIR) model, 253
Diagnostic and Statistical Manual of Mental Disorders (DSM), 13
Diagnostic and Statistical Manual of Mental Disorders, Third Edition (DSM-III), 302
Diagnostic and Statistical Manual of Mental Disorders (DSM-5), 23, 156, 230
Difference, relationship-based (DIR) therapy, 314
Dynamical systems (DS), 27

E

Efference, 296
Electrodermal activity (EDA), 66
Emotional (EMO) task, 115
Empathy, 283–284
Ex-afference, 6

Excess success, *see* Visual search and autism, excess success for study on
Exteroception from the distance receptors, 125

F

Facial imitation, 95–98
Facial recognition models, 67
Finding normal (Anthony's story), 353–356
"Floor time," 314
Fragile X disorders (FXDs), 34
Functional magnetic resonance imaging (fMRI), 68, 157, 301
Functional speech communication, use of music therapy to help with (example), 235–236

G

GABA-mediated synchrony, *see* Intention and action, gap between
Girl's life, 339–346

H

Handwriting proficiency, assessment of, 49–51
  characterizing handwriting difficulties in ASD, 50
  features of poor handwriting, 49–50
  handwriting impairment explained within cognitive theoretical frameworks, 50–51
  predictors of handwriting impairment in ASD, 50
HARKing, *see* Hypothesizing after the results are known
Hidden Markov models (HMMs), 82
Hodgkin–Huxley (HK) model, 156
Hypermobility syndrome, 264
Hypothesizing after the results are known (HARKing), 168, 175

I

IEP meetings, *see* Individualized education program meetings
Imitation fidelity, action evaluation and discrimination as indexes of, 89–102
  facial imitation, 95–98
  investigation in autism, 93
  kinematics, 92–93
  measuring imitation, 92
  object movement reenactment, 93
  outcome variables, 93–94
  relationship between imitation and autism, 91–92
  relationship between imitation and autism (copying values), 98–99
  "universals," 90
Impulse control, use of music therapy to help with (example), 237
Individualized education program (IEP) meetings, 341
Inertial measurement units (IMUs), 107
Infant Regulatory Scoring Systems (IRSS), 80
Intention and action, gap between, 139–150
  altered connectivity in autism, 142–143
  altered GABA-mediated synchrony in autism, 143–145
  alternative and augmentative communication methods, 141
  connectivity and GABA-mediated synchrony, 142–145
  diagnostic considerations, 140–141
  external behavior versus internal states of mind, 141–142
  instructional strategies (playing to strengths), 145–146
  network synchronization, disruptions of, 145
  pervasive developmental disorders, 140
  presuming competence, 146–147
Interspike interval (ISI) analyses, 224
IQ scores, 13, 14
IRSS, *see* Infant Regulatory Scoring Systems
ISI analyses, *see* Interspike interval analyses

K

Kinematic measures (imitation fidelity), 92
Kolmogorov–Smirnov (K-S) distance, 157
Kolmogorov–Smirnov test, 161–162

L

Law of large numbers, 162–163
Lognormal multiplicative distribution function, 161

M

Magical fairy (Ada Mae), 333–338
Maternal Regulatory Scoring Systems (MRSS), 80
M-CHAT, *see* Modified Checklist for Autism in Toddlers
Mean squared error (MSE), 174
Mentalizing theory, 45
Micromovements, 64, 221–227
  continuous signals to "spiking" information, 223–224
  data type, 110–113
  interspike interval analyses, 224
  random versus periodic behavior of motor output fluctuations, 224–226
  simulating patterns and empirically verifying them, 224–226
Mirror neuron system (MNS), 76, 77–78
Modified Checklist for Autism in Toddlers (M-CHAT), 347
Motor reductionism, 17–18
Movement variability, reason for studying, 3–21
  autism research, 12
  continuous reentrant historicity, integration, and (voluntary) control, 7–8
  ex-afference, 6
  input, movements as, 7
  institutional barriers, 13–16
  methodological and conceptual barriers, 12–16
  movements as richly layered reafference, 4–10
  new data and new analyses, need for, 10–12
  output, movements as, 6–7
  physiological perspective, 15
  reafference principle, 5–6
  voluntary control and stability, 8–10
  warning against motor reductionism and neat cognitive modularity, warning against, 17–18
MRSS, *see* Maternal Regulatory Scoring Systems
MSE, *see* Mean squared error
Music therapy, *see* Rhythm and movement for autism spectrum disorder

N

Necrotizing enterocolitis (NEC), 190
Neonatal intensive care unit (NICU), 190
Nervous systems' rhythms, inherent noise hidden in (core motor sensing traits in ASD and), 197–215
  bridging of mind–body dichotomy, 209–210
  choice of pointing and gait in examples, 200–203
  deafferented subject (Ian Waterman), 205–206
  discrete segments to continuous, naturalistic behaviors, 202–203
  motor dysfunction assessment, background on, 198–199
  noise in the periphery, 203–205
  phenotypic feature of, 200
  shift from random and noisy motor patterns to predictable motor signals, 206–209
Nervous systems' rhythms, non-Gaussian statistical distributions arising from, 155–164
  central limit theorem, 162–163
  computational psychiatry, 156
  gamma additive distribution function, 159–160
  Gaussian distribution, 158
  general additive probability distribution function, 161
  geometric mean, 162
  Kolmogorov–Smirnov test, 161–162
  law of large numbers, 162–163
  lognormal multiplicative distribution function, 161
  personalized medicine, 155
  Poisson random process, 158–162
  precision psychiatry, 156
  scale parameter, 160
  symmetric distribution, 158
  Weibull additive distribution function, 160
Neurological music therapy (NMT), 374
NICU, *see* Neonatal intensive care
Non-Gaussian statistical distributions, *see* Nervous systems' rhythms, non-Gaussian statistical distributions arising from
Normalcy, *see* Finding normal (Anthony's story)

O

Object movement reenactment (OMR), 93
Obsessive-compulsive disorder (OCD), 317
Occupational therapist (OT), 264, 371
Outstanding outlier (Shiloh), 327–331

P

Parents, implications of the movement sensing perspective for, 295–326
  augmentative and alternative communication, 319
  "autism parents," 312
  "autism quartet," 310–317
  Behaviorist Manifesto, 301
  classic reflex theory, 296
  conditioning, 296
  delayed habituation, 314–317
  efference, 296
  emotionally deficient mothers, 300
  evolving models, 306–310
  extreme overreactions, 298
  "floor time," 314
  impact of the DSM, 302–306
  labels, 307
  marked similarities to other neurological conditions involving movement, 317–321
  movement difference (term), 296
  nonhuman behaviors, 301
  "open systems," 302
  "physics envy," 302
  pivotal response training, 314
  profound change, 300
  psychoanalysis to behaviorism (diverging paths), 299–302
  reafference, 296
  reflex chain theory, 296
  relationship-based approaches, need for, 319–321
  theory of mind module, 306
  variable performance, 311
  why movement matters, 296–299
Parkinson's disease (PD), 31, 32–33
Parvalbumin (PV), 144
PCDI, *see* Princeton Child Development Institute institute
PDD-NOS, *see* Pervasive developmental disorder—not otherwise specified
PDDs, *see* Pervasive developmental disorders
PDFs, *see* Probability density functions
PECS, *see* Picture Exchange Communication System
Peripheral nervous system (PNS), 3, 64
Personalized medicine, 155
Pervasive developmental disorder—not otherwise specified (PDD-NOS), 140, 348
Pervasive developmental disorders (PDDs), 140
Phelan–McDermid syndrome, 328, 329
Phenotype, 23–41
  associated motor symptoms, 29–32
  associated secondary symptoms, role of, 24–25
  associated sensory symptoms, 28–29
  behavior (physiological stance), 26–28
  development of behavior, 26–28
  fragile X disorders, 34
  missing link, 34
  Parkinson's disease as model for ASD, 32–33
  psychological versus physiological, 25–26
  secondary by-products, 33
  time for a new model, evidence suggesting, 34–35
  underdeveloped nervous systems, by-product of, 28–32
Phoneme production, use of music therapy to help with (example), 236
"Physics envy," 302
Picture Exchange Communication System (PECS), 249, 253
Pivotal response training (PRT), 314
PNS, *see* Peripheral nervous system
Poisson random process (PRP), 158–162
  gamma additive distribution function, 159–160
  general additive probability distribution function, 161
  Kolmogorov–Smirnov test, 161–162
  lognormal multiplicative distribution function, 161
  Weibull additive distribution function, 160
Precision psychiatry, 156
Princeton Child Development Institute (PCDI), 342

Probability density functions (PDFs), 157
Problems with basic brain science methods (contemporary), progress in ASD research and treatments impeded by, 177–195
  neurodevelopmental disorders, 179
  neuromotor control to predictive social behavior, 189–190
  orderly development of control levels in infant's nervous systems, 190–191
  problem 1 (linear, static models imposed on neurodevelopmental data), 179–181
  problem 2 (imposition of normality in data that are not normally distributed), 182–186
  problem 3 (activity required for spontaneously self-supervised and self-corrective internal models), 186–191
  problem 4 (lack of a proper taxonomy of control levels in motor research), 191–192
  problem 5 (lack of models to assess and track social interactions), 192–193
  psychotropic drugs, prescribing of, 179
Proprioception of the body in motion, 125
PRP, *see* Poisson random process
PRT, *see* Pivotal response training
Psychotropic drugs, prescribing of, 179
Psychotropic medications and behavioral modifications, uncertain outcomes of, 372–373
Purposeful self, disorder of the intrinsic motive processes of, *see* Brainstem origin of autism
PV, *see* Parvalbumin

R

Reafference, 296
Reflex chain theory, 296
Rhythm and movement for autism spectrum disorder, 229–241
  clinical case vignettes, 234
  cognition/attention, 237
  functional speech communication, use of music therapy to help with (example), 235–236
  improving initiation of motor output (example), 234–235
  impulse control, use of music therapy to help with (example), 237
  music and cortical plasticity, 231–232
  music therapy for autism spectrum disorder, 232–233
  naturally evoking sustained motor output through music (example), 234
  phoneme production, use of music therapy to help with (example), 236
  rhythm for motor movement, 230–231
  speech, 235–236
  switching attention, use of music therapy to help with (example), 237
  treating issues with motor inhibition (example), 235
  working memory, use of music therapy to help with (example), 237

S

SEARCH Consulting, 341
Secondary by-products, 33
Seeing movement, *see* Parents, implications of the movement sensing perspective for
Self-making, 120
Sensory processing disorder (SPD), 348
SHANK3 deletion syndrome, 264
Social encounter, perspectives of, 63–71
  behaviorist account (psychological perspective), 65–66
  computational neuroscientist account, 67–68
  electrodermal activity, 66
  facial recognition models, 67
  guessing mental states of the other party, 68–70
  integrating of accounts to explore deeper layers of detail, 70
  physiologist account, 66–67
  research areas, 64–68
Social skills, definition and working conceptualization of, 104–106
Social skills, redefining the role of sensory-motor control on, 73–88
  artificial intelligence, 82
  conditional random fields, 82
  correlational methods, 81
  description of social skills, 73–74
  hidden Markov models, 82
  measurement of social interaction, 80–82
  microlevel evolving social dyadic interactions, specialized techniques to examine, 81–82
  mirror neuron system, 77–78
  motor perspective, 82–83
  origins of social skills, 75–80
  role of active movement in development, 78–80
  social dance (temporal interdependence), 78
  social dialogue (content interdependence), 75–77
  social signal processing, 82
  social skills in autism spectrum disorders, 75
Society, social deficit of, 367–378
  applied behavioral analysis, 372
  board-certified behavior analysts, 374
  current definition of autism, 367–368
  different goals, different outcomes, 368–370
  failure of discrete subjective scales to capture adaptive change, 371–372
  financial conflicts of interest, unforeseen consequences of, 370–371
  following the money, 370
  neurological music therapy, 374
  parents' impossible road to diversified treatments, 373–375
  politics and economics, 373
  psychotropic medications and behavioral modifications, uncertain outcomes of, 372–373
  social deficit of our society, 375
SPD, *see* Sensory processing disorder
Special Olympics, 343
Speech pacing, use of music therapy to help with (example), 236
Spike trains, 223
Statistical platform for individualized behavioral analysis (SPIBA), 13, 110
"Stuck thoughts," 245

Superior temporal sulcus (STS), 145
Switching attention, use of music therapy to help with (example), 237
Synchronicity, 81, 112, 224

T

Teachers, reframing of autism spectrum disorder for, 281–287
  beliefs impacting decision making, 282
  empathy, 283–284
  pushback, 282
  reframing beliefs, 284–285
  teacher beliefs matter, 281–283
  teachers want to understand, 284
Tell-a-story (TS) task, 115
Temporo-spatial processing disorder (TSPD), 312
Theory of mind (ToM), 68, 75, 210, 306
Tourette syndrome, 303
Treating the whole (not the parts), 347–352
Treatment and Education of Autistic and Communication related handicapped Children (TEACCH), 253

U

U.S. Centers for Disease Control and Prevention (CDC), 140

V

Video technology, 243–251
  autistic neurology, compatibility with, 244–245
  Dakota, 249–250
  David, 247–248
  generalization, 245
  Max, 248–249
  Monty, 245–247
  Picture Exchange Communication System, 249
  PowerPoint presentation, 246
  Sam, 247
  "stuck thoughts," 245
  "tornado video," 245–246
Visceroception of information, 125
Visual search and autism, excess success for study on, 165–176
  alternative approach, 171–175
  excess success, 165–168
  hypothesizing after the results are known, 168, 175
  noise fitting, 171
  "questionable research practices," 168
  trusting your data, 168–171

W

Weakened central coherence, 129
Working memory, use of music therapy to help with (example), 237
World Health Organization (WHO), 179